Pocket Guide to Home Care Standards

Complete Guidelines
for Clinical Practice,
Documentation,
and Reimbursement

Pocket Guide to Home Care Standards

Complete Guidelines
for Clinical Practice,
Documentation,
and Reimbursement

Springhouse Corporation
Springhouse, Pennsylvania

STAFF

Publisher
Judith A. Schilling McCann, RN, MSN

Design Director
John Hubbard

Editorial Director
David Moreau

Clinical Manager
Joan M. Robinson, RN, MSN, CCRN

Clinical Editors
Gwynn Sinkinson, RNC, MSN, CRNP (project manager); Shari Cammon, RN, MSN, CCRN; Jill Curry, RN, BSN, CCRN; Maryann Foley, RN, BSN

Editors
Rachel Anderson, Cynthia C. Breuninger, Catherine Harold, Laura Poole

Copy Editors
Jaime Stockslager (supervisor), Jeri Albert, Virginia Baskerville, Heather Ditch, Amy Furman, Barbara Hodgson, Kimberly A.J. Johnson, Malinda LaPrade, Maria Neithercott, Judith Orioli, Pamela Wingrod, Helen Winton

Designers
Arlene Putterman (associate design director), Lynn Foulk (designer and project manager), Joseph John Clark, Donna Morris

Projects Coordinator
Liz Schaeffer

Electronic Production Services
Diane Paluba (manager), Joyce Rossi Biletz

Manufacturing
Deborah Meiris (director), Patricia K. Dorshaw (manager), Otto Mezei (book production manager)

Editorial and Design Assistants
Tom Hasenmayer, Beverly Lane, Beth Janae Orr, Elfriede Young

Indexer
Manjit Sahai

The clinical procedures described and recommended in this publication are based on research and consultation with medical and nursing authorities. To the best of our knowledge, these procedures reflect currently accepted clinical practice; nevertheless, they can't be considered absolute and universal recommendations. For individual application, treatment recommendations must be considered in light of the patient's clinical condition and, before administration of new or infrequently used drugs, in light of latest package-insert information. The authors and the publisher disclaim responsibility for any adverse effects resulting directly or indirectly from the suggested procedures, from any undetected errors, or from the reader's misunderstanding of the text.

Printed in the United States of America.

PGHCS - D N O S

03 02 01 00   10 9 8 7 6 5 4 3 2 1

Library of Congress Cataloging-in-Publication Data
Pocket guide to home care standards: complete guidelines for clinical practice, documentation, and reimbursement.
        p. ; cm.
    Includes bibliographical references and index.
    1. Home care services — Standards — United States — Handbooks, manuals, etc. 2. Home nursing — Standards — United States — Handbook, manuals, etc.
    I. Springhouse Corporation.
    [DNLM: 1. Home Care Services — organization & administration — Handbooks. 2. Home Care Services — Standards — Handbooks.   WY 49 P7393 2001]
RA645.35 P63 2001
362.1'4 — dc21   00-041967
ISBN 1-58255-039-5 (alk. paper)   CIP

Contents

■ Contributors

Cathy Bellehumeur, JD
Senior Vice President and General
    Counsel and Corporate
    Compliance Officer
Option Care, Inc.
Bannockburn, Ill.

Marie Bluebond, RN, BS
Administrator
Center for Women's Health
Langhorne, Pa.

Jeri L. Brandt, RN, PhD
Associate Professor of Nursing
Nebraska Wesleyan University
Lincoln

Marie O. Brewer, RN
Homecare Manager
WellStar Home Health
Marietta, Ga.

Kathleen Cummings, BSN, CRNH
Director of Hospice Programs
Fairview Home Care and Hospice
Minneapolis

**Denise Del Serra Detato, RN, MBA,
    MSN, CNA**
Director of Clinical Operations
Staffbuilders
Bala Cynwyd, Pa.

Carole R. Eldridge, RN
President
E-Quipping: Education for the
    Workplace
Granbury, Tex.

Debra Lynn Hagan, RN
Admission Team Leader
Coram Healthcare
Malvern, Pa.

Jane Haggerty, RNC, MSN
Public Health Nurse/Project
    Coordinator
La Salle Neighborhood Nursing
    Center
Philadelphia

Linda A. Hines-Roberts, RN
Case Manager
Legend Healthcare-Equipnet
Sharon Hill, Pa.

Edward J. Hoey, RN, BSN, CRNI
Care Team Leader
Thomas Jefferson University Hospital
Philadelphia

Carol June Hooker, RN, MS
Staff Nurse, Home Health
Absolute Nursing Care
Silver Spring, Md.

Kathleen J. Hudson, RN, MSN
Nursing Instructor
Illinois Eastern Community Colleges
Mt. Carmel, Ill.

Bette L. Hughes, RN, BSN
Nursing Instructor (Clinical) and
    Home Care Nurse
Northwest State Community College
    and Community Hospitals of
    Williams County
Archbold, Ohio

Cynthia Lange Ingham, RN, BSN
Public Health Nursing Supervisor
Children with Special Health Needs,
  Vermont Department of Health
Burlington

Lori Jordan, RN
Nurse Manager
Coram Healthcare
Malvern, Pa.

Bonnie Kosman, RN, MSN, CS, CDE
Administrator
Lehigh Valley Home Care and Lehigh
  Valley Hospice
Allentown, Pa.

Ruth Lagonegro, RN, BSN
Home Care Staff Nurse
Community Nurse-Home Care
  Department
Grand View Hospital
Sellersville, Pa.

Carole Leone, RN, MS
Staff Nurse
Barnes-Jewish Hospital
St. Louis

Jeanne Lewis, RN,C
Coordinator of Maternal Home Care
  Program
Grand View Hospital
Sellersville, Pa.

Dawna Martich, RN, BSN, MSN
Clinical Trainer
Diabetes Treatment Centers of
  America
Pittsburgh

Sue Masoorli, RN
President
Perivascular Nurse Consultants, Inc.
Philadelphia

**Melinda Granger Oberleitner, RN,
  DNS, OCN**
Associate Professor and Acting
  Department Head of Nursing
College of Nursing and Allied Health
  Professions
University of Louisiana at Lafayette

Donna S. Olson, RN, BSN, PHN
Consultant and Educator
San Diego Hospice Palliative Home
  Health

Gail P. Poirrier, RN, DNS
Acting Dean and Professor
College of Nursing and Allied Health
  Professions
University of Louisiana at Lafayette

Susan Poole, BSN, MS, CRNI, CNSN
Senior Director of Professional
  Services
Option Care, Inc.
Bannockburn, Ill.

**Theresa A. Posani, RN, MS, CS, CNA,
  CCRN**
Critical Care Clinical Nurse
  Specialist
Presbyterian Hospital of Dallas

Marisue Rayno, RN, MSN
Nursing Instructor
St. Luke's Hospital School of Nursing
Bethlehem, Pa.

Mary Jean Ricci, RN,C, MSN
Assistant Professor of Nursing
Holy Family College
Philadelphia

Rosemarie Rorvik, RN, BSN
Quality Improvement Coordinator
and Educator and Independent
Nurse Consultant
Warminster, Pa.

Susan Semb, RN, MSN, CS, NP
Diabetes Program Coordinator
SunPlus Home Health Services
San Diego

Marilyn Smith-Stoner, RN, MSN, ABD
Vice President of Clinical Operations
Ramona Visiting Nurses Association
and Hospice
Hemet, Ca.

Amy L. Swett, RN, AD
Community Health Educator and
Independent Nurse Consultant
Mechanicsburg, Pa.

Allison Jones Terry, RN, MSN
Nursing Coordinator
MidSouth Home Health Agency
Montgomery, Ala.

Elizabeth Hazen Willburn, RN, BSN,
MSN
Home Care Consultant
Lincoln, Nebr.

Kenny Mallow Williamson, RNC,
MSN
Nurse Consultant
CIF, Inc.
Clay, Ala.

■ Foreword

Sweeping changes brought on by the Prospective Payment System continue to have a significant and sustained impact on the way home care nurses deliver care. No longer can we afford the luxury of extra visits for our patients. Care must be focused and targeted to the patient's health needs so that he can assume self-care in the shortest time possible.

Pocket Guide to Home Care Standards can help you in your daily practice because it provides a reliable template for obtaining full reimbursement for your services under a wide range of health conditions.

Part I offers an overview of the home health system, presenting essential information for any novice or experienced home care nurse. The home care system is complex and always changing. Understanding its structure and function will help you understand the origins of regulations and requirements that affect your clinical practice. Recognizing the importance of interdisciplinary collaboration in home care, part I also describes the responsibilities and duties of the many providers that form the interdisciplinary team. In addition, it reviews legal and ethical issues of home care practice, methods you can use to maintain quality in home care delivery, documentation guidelines, and practical tips on how to conduct a home care visit.

Part II focuses on the clinical management of patients in their homes. Organized by clinical specialty (adult, maternal-neonatal, pediatric, and psychiatric disorders and treatments), these sections describe what the nurse must consider before making the home visit, common interventions that may be part of the home visit, and follow-up activities that must be considered after the home visit has ended.

Part III presents clinical pathways for 26 of the most common disorders seen by home care nurses, ranging from asthma, chronic renal failure, and hypertension to myocardial infarction, pneumonia, and sepsis.

Part IV provides several appendices, including the ICD-9-CM 5th-digit subclassifications, hospice care, resources for patients and caregivers, and DME coverage, among others.

As home care nurses, we are being challenged to do more with less, while remaining committed to providing the highest quality of care for patients and their families. Our goal is to help them regain their independence in self-care and promote the quality of life. We can make this happen by using tools designed to help us provide comprehensive, focused care for our patients. *Pocket Guide to Home Care Standards* is one such tool. I urge you to use it every day in your clinical practice.

Joan D. Mason, RN, MSN
Coordinator, Advanced Practice
Nursing—Home Health Nursing
New York University
New York

■ How to use this book

Pocket Guide to Home Care Standards: Complete Guidelines for Clinical Practice, Documentation, and Reimbursement is a portable, quick-reference resource designed primarily for health care professionals who have skill in performing home care but would like to document more effectively for business purposes. Nurses in the field can use the book to prepare for a visit or to review which details need to be documented to ensure meeting continuous quality improvement (CQI) and reimbursement criteria. Its easy-to-scan format makes *Pocket Guide to Home Care Standards* an ideal resource for case management, staff education, and supervisory personnel who need to access specific, pertinent information quickly.

Part I reviews home care essentials relevant to every home care visit you make. Chapter 1 provides an in-depth discussion of home care and the current health care environment. Chapter 2 identifies the members of the home care team and details each discipline's responsibilities in the home care environment. Chapter 3 discusses specific methods for maintaining and demonstrating quality in home care. Chapter 4 identifies common legal pitfalls that home care personnel encounter as well as effective strategies to prevent and minimize problems. Chapter 5 takes you step by step through preparing for and conducting home care visits. Chapter 6 discusses current methods of documenting home care, exploring the advantages and disadvantages of each.

Part II contains guidelines for adult, maternal-neonatal, pediatric, and psychiatric disorders and treatments, presented alphabetically within their respective sections. Each entry provides:
● a description of the health problem or treatment
● a previsit checklist of potential physician orders and needed equipment and supplies
● safety requirements to consider
● major diagnostic codes that may apply (when appropriate, the reader is also referred to Appendix A for fifth-digit subclassifications of these codes)
● a defense of the patient's homebound status
● selected nursing diagnoses and patient outcomes
● skilled nursing services that focus on such topics as physical assessment, evaluation of findings, patient teaching, and coordination of care
● interdisciplinary actions taken by other members of the health care team, including areas of overlap (for example, a physical therapist may evaluate a patient's wound or vital signs, and a nurse may teach crutch-walking skills)
● a discharge plan that outlines expected endpoints of care for the disorder or treatment (these may range from a return to a previous level of health to death with dignity)
● documentation requirements that list what third-party payers and CQI reviewers are looking for
● reimbursement reminders, including tips on what to include on billing and requisition forms, validations for delayed progress, and cost-saving mea-

sures) and insurance hints (what information to have on hand when speaking with case managers for third-party payers).

Part III explains how clinical pathways are developed and refined, how they impact home care, how the information they gather is used, and how nurses can document effectively on them. It then presents 26 clinical pathways especially designed for use by home care nurses.

Part IV contains several helpful appendices (fifth-digit subclassifications for ICD-9-CM billing codes; hospice care; resources for professionals, patients, and caregivers; durable medical equipment coverage; NANDA diagnoses listed according to Gordon's functional health patterns; and an English-Spanish medical translation guide).

Finally, it offers a generous list of selected references for further reading and a well-organized index to help you locate important information quickly.

Note: Throughout the sections devoted to nursing diagnoses and patient outcomes, abbreviations in parentheses are used to identify which health care team members can help the patient and family achieve the outcome. Health care team members are abbreviated as follows:

Dietitian (D)
Enterostomal therapist (ET)
Home care aide (HCA)
Lactation consultant (LC)
Nurse (N)
Occupational therapist (OT)
Pharmacist (PH)
Physical therapist (PT)
Physician (MD)
Podiatrist (PO)
Respiratory therapist (RT)
Social worker (SW)
Speech pathologist (SP)
Spiritual counselor (SC).

Home care essentials

1 Understanding home care

From its origins as a religious charity in the 19th century, home health care has evolved into a highly technical, highly regulated field that requires nurses and other health care professionals to function with considerable autonomy, fiscal responsibility, and clinical skill.

Most recently, the evolution of home care has been driven by a national push to cut health care costs. For a growing population of ever sicker patients, home care has become a viable — even a preferable — alternative to care delivered in a hospital or other costly institution.

In addition to being less costly, home care offers a level of comfort, personal attention, and individual control not available in a hospital. Many highly technical services can be delivered at home. Most services are supported by a range of public and private funding sources. For these reasons, the demand for home care agencies and trained home care workers has boomed in recent years and continues to do so.

Today, home care in the United States encompasses a wide variety of services that supplement or circumvent institutional care. Services are delivered by nurses, physicians, physical and occupational therapists, respiratory therapists, pharmacists, home care aides, social workers, durable medical equipment suppliers, and more. These health care professionals work together in multidisciplinary teams with patients and families to promote, maintain, or restore health; to maximize independence; to minimize the effects of illness; and to care for patients who are dying. Currently, almost 2.5 million people are receiving health care at home.

If you've chosen to practice nursing in the home setting, you know that you need not only clinical expertise but also financial and administrative acumen. This chapter helps to supplement your knowledge by reviewing the types of agencies that administer home care, the types of funding available to pay for home care, and the credentials by which home care agencies maintain their status.

Types of home care agencies

As the home care sector of the medical industry expands, the types of agencies that administer home care services are expanding as well. (See *Types of home care agencies,* pages 4 and 5.) Today, home care agencies may be official, voluntary, or private. They may be for-profit or not-for-profit, independent or affiliated with another health care facility. Some even specialize in certain types of home care, such as hospice, nutritional therapy, infusion therapy, and companion services.

Official agencies

Official agencies are established by law and function as a part of state, county, municipal, or local government. Typically, official agencies are public, not-for-profit, freestanding organizations. State and local health departments are examples of official agencies.

Typically, official agencies primarily serve poor and indigent people. Home care services may be included in the agency's overall public health caseload, or they may be handled through a distinct division of the organization. Because the services are funded by municipal, county, or state governments, their availability may be influenced by changes in public funding or political control.

Voluntary agencies

Most voluntary agencies are public, not-for-profit organizations that exist to serve a defined geographic or service area. The Visiting Nurses Association is an example of a voluntary agency. Like official agencies, voluntary agencies provide community and public health services and home health care.

Most voluntary agencies are governed by a board of directors made up of respected community leaders. No tax revenue is used to support the agency. Instead, funding comes from nontaxable sources, such as donations, endowments, grants, and some third-party insurers (possibly including Medicare and Medicaid).

In the past, voluntary agencies made and received virtually all of their referrals from their own geographic — or catchment — areas. Today, however, the boundaries of each agency's geographic area have become blurred by the influence of a growing number of for-profit and institutional agencies competing for referrals in the same area.

Private agencies

These days, almost half of all home care agencies are freestanding, for-profit businesses. Although some are independent corporations, many others are affiliated with a complex network of proprietary agency chains and hospital organizations.

Proprietary agencies

A proprietary home care agency is a for-profit corporation managed by a paid board of directors and a chief executive who may or may not have a background in health care. Proprietary agencies commonly provide many multidisciplinary services, including skilled nursing care, physical therapy, occupational therapy, respiratory therapy, and home care aide services. Some specialize in such services as renal dialysis, hospice, wound management, and home infusion therapies.

Proprietary agencies typically receive funding from third-party payers, such as Medicare, Blue Cross, and other insurers. Some also rely heavily on pri-

(Text continues on page 6.)

Types of home care agencies

Although the structure and organization of home care agencies is complex and subject to change, the chart below highlights the characteristics of the major types of home care agencies. If Medicare certifies the agency, it must comply with Medicare regulations.

DESCRIPTION	GOVERNING SOURCE
Official agency • Governmental agency • Public • Not-for-profit • Usually freestanding • Public health department or separate division	State, county, municipal, or local community legal statutes
Voluntary agency • Usually public • Not-for-profit • Serves a specified geographic area	Board of directors from local community
Private for-profit agency • Individual, corporate, or other organizational ownership • For-profit • Freestanding, institution-based, or part of local, state, or national chain	Chief executive and paid board of directors appointed by owner
Private not-for-profit agency • Individual, corporate, or other organizational ownership • Not-for-profit • Freestanding, institution-based, or part of local, state, or national chain	Paid board of directors appointed by owner
Private institution-based agency • Department or division of sponsoring institution • For-profit, not-for-profit, or a combination, depending on institution • Separate provider of services	Sponsoring institution's board of directors or trustees
Hospice agency • Institution-based, separate department, or freestanding • For-profit or not-for-profit	Advisory panel or board of directors from the community or the sponsoring institution

FUNDING	SERVICES
• State tax revenues • County tax revenues • Municipal tax revenues • Local tax revenues	• Disease prevention, including vaccinations • Health promotion • Communicable disease investigation, control, and quarantine • Environmental health surveillance and health code enforcement • Skilled care • Maternal-child health • Family planning
• Donations • Endowments • Grants • Third-party reimbursement	• Skilled care • Screening activities • Community health activities • Specialty services, such as maternal-child health
• Third-party reimbursement • Private pay	• Skilled care • Home care aide and homemaker services • Private duty • Specialty services, such as wound management, dialysis, and infusion therapies
• Third-party reimbursement • Private pay	• Skilled care • Home care aide and homemaker services • Private duty • Specialty services, such as wound management, dialysis, and infusion therapies
• Third-party reimbursement • Private pay • Endowments • Fund-raising (via sponsoring institution)	• Skilled care • Home care aide and homemaker services • Private duty • Specialty services, such as wound management, dialysis, and infusion therapies
• Third-party reimbursement • Private pay • Donations • Grants	• Skilled care for terminally ill patients and their families • Medical and social services • Counseling • Home care aide and homemaker services • Volunteer support • Respite care • Bereavement services

vate payment from patients or their families. In the latter case, payment is usually for prolonged private duty nursing services rather than for intermittent visits.

Not-for-profit agencies

Not-for-profit agencies provide services similar to those offered by proprietary agencies. The difference is that the agency's not-for-profit status means that any excess income isn't taxed but rather is funneled back into the organization. Not-for-profit agencies may be governed and owned by an individual, a corporation, or an organization. A board of directors manages the agency.

Institutional agencies

A home care agency may function as a department or an affiliate of a hospital or other institution. The agency is considered a separate service provider, with its own certification and provider numbers. However, it's still governed and regulated by the sponsoring institution's board of directors or its trustees, and it must adhere to the sponsoring institution's philosophy and mission.

An institutional agency may be for-profit or not-for-profit, often based on the status of the sponsoring institution. Either way, most referrals come from the inpatient population of the institution itself. Payment comes from various sources but commonly relies heavily on Medicare.

Institutional agencies have proliferated in recent years and continue to do so. About two-thirds of the nation's hospitals offer standard home care services, such as postpartum checkups, postoperative teaching, and follow-up for newly diagnosed chronic illnesses

such as diabetes. Almost a quarter of hospitals also offer specialized home care services, such as infusion therapy, wound management, ostomy care, home dialysis, and psychiatric home care.

Hospice agencies

Hospice agencies may be affiliated with a sponsoring institution or they may be independent. Their structure and organization vary widely. For example, a hospice agency might be:

• an inpatient unit in a hospital, subacute care facility, or nursing home
• a community-based agency, such as a not-for-profit volunteer organization
• a freestanding inpatient facility
• a home care agency that employs specially trained health care providers
• a corporation that provides hospice care
• an alliance or network of hospice care providers that contracts with a managed health care program.

Regardless of the organization's structure, hospice services focus on palliative and supportive care for terminally ill patients and their families. Compared to other home care services, hospice services typically receive more liberal funding definitions (homebound status, for instance), wider coverage of equipment (such as wheelchairs), and the availability of services even after the patient dies (grief and bereavement counseling for family members). Payment for hospice care typically comes from Medicare, Medicaid, or private health insurance.

Reimbursement for home care

Naturally, patients and their families can pay for home care services directly if they choose to do so. Usually, however, the funds come from public or private third-party payers. (See *Who pays for home care?*)

Public third-party payers

Public third-party payers include Medicare, Medicaid, the Older Americans Act, the Veterans Health Administration, social services block grant programs, and community agencies.

Medicare

Most Americans who are over age 65 or disabled are eligible for the federal Medicare program. This program will pay for a range of home care services if the patient and the services meet certain requirements. Specifically, the patient must be homebound, be under a physician's care, and have a medical need for covered services.

Depending on the patient's condition, Medicare may pay for intermittent skilled nursing; physical, occupational, or speech therapy; medical social work; psychiatric nursing; and medical equipment and supplies. The referring physician must authorize and periodically review the patient's care plan. Except for hospice care, the services delivered must be intermittent or part-time. They also must be provided by a Medicare-certified home care agency to qualify for reimbursement.

Who pays for home care?

Reimbursement for home care typically comes from public or private third-party payers such as those listed here.

Public payers
- Medicare
- Medicaid
- Older Americans Act
- Veterans Health Administration
- Block grants to states for social services programs
- Community agencies

Private payers
- Commercial health insurance
- Managed care organizations
- Civilian Health and Medical Program of the Uniformed Services
- Workers' compensation

Medicaid

Medicaid is a federal and state medical assistance program for people with low incomes. Each state administers its own program and forms its own set of eligibility requirements. States are only mandated to provide home care services to residents who are "categorically needy" or who receive federally assisted income maintenance payments, such as Social Security Income and Aid to Families with Dependent Children (AFDC).

A categorically needy person is one who has reached a certain age, is blind or otherwise disabled, and has an income below the federal poverty level but above the level that qualifies for mandatory coverage. Persons under age 21 who meet income and resource requirements for AFDC, yet for other reasons aren't eligible for AFDC, also qualify as categorically needy.

Under federal Medicaid rules, covered home care services include part-time nursing, home care aide services, and medical supplies and equipment. At the state's option, Medicaid may also cover audiology; physical, occupational, or speech therapy; and medical social services.

Older Americans Act

The Older Americans Act of 1965 provides federal funds for state and local social service programs that enable frail or disabled older adults to maintain their independence. Funding is available for home care aide services, personal care, meal delivery, and chore, escort, and shopping services for residents age 60 and over who have the greatest social and financial need.

Typically, patients or their families request services through a local Area Agency on Aging, which may provide the services directly or may provide a referral to another local organization. Increasingly, patients are being asked to share the cost of these services in proportion to their income.

Veterans Health Administration

Veterans who are at least 50% disabled by a service-related condition are eligible for home health care from the Veterans Health Administration (VHA). A physician must authorize the services, and the services must be delivered through the VHA's network of hospital-based home care agencies.

Block grants to states for social services programs

Each year, states receive federal social services block grants for state-identified service needs. The federal government allocates these funds, within a federal limit, based on each state's population. Some funds typically are directed into programs that provide home care aide and homemaker services. Information about current block funds is available from state health departments and the local Area Agency on Aging.

Community agencies

Community agencies, along with state and local governments, also provide funds for home health and supportive care. Depending on the patient's eligibility and financial status, these organizations may pay for all or a portion of the needed services. Hospital discharge planners, social workers, and the local Area Agency on Aging can provide information about community agencies that fund home care. Certain community-based agencies, such as churches and shelters for the homeless or women and children fleeing domestic abuse, may also provide home care services. Funding for these programs may come from grants, religious organizations, or charitable trusts such as the Robert Woods Johnson Foundation.

Private third-party payers

Private third-party payers include commercial health insurance companies, managed care organizations (MCOs), the Civilian Health and Medical Program of the Uniformed Services (CHAMPUS), and workers' compensation.

Commercial health insurance

Commercial health insurance policies typically cover some home care services for acute needs. Benefits for long-term services vary and may provide only partial payment. In other words, the patient or another payer must supply the portion not covered by insurance.

Commercial health insurance policies occasionally cover personal care services. Most commercial and private insurance plans cover comprehensive hospice services, including nursing, social work, therapies, personal care, drugs, and medical supplies. Most plans don't require cost-sharing for hospice care.

MEDIGAP PLANS

Because Medicare doesn't cover all of the services a patient may need, many patients purchase insurance — called a Medigap plan — to pay for some of the services not covered by Medicare. Various Medigap plans are available; the more services covered by the plan, the higher the plan premium.

In general, Medigap plans are most helpful for patients who are recovering from acute illness, injury, or surgery. Some Medigap policies offer at-home recovery benefits, which cover some physician-ordered personal care services when the policyholder receives Medicare-covered home health care. In a general sense, however, these plans aren't designed to cover extended long-term care.

LONG-TERM CARE INSURANCE

A better shield against the catastrophic expense of lengthy home care is long-term care insurance. Although long-term care policies originally covered only nursing home care, they're increasingly covering in-home services as well, including personal care, companionship, and other services. Covered services vary with each plan.

MCOs

MCOs and other prepaid group health plans increasingly include benefits for home care services. Indeed, the managed care plan's policy may encourage an earlier hospital discharge and an increasing emphasis on less costly home care services. Most MCOs contract with home care agencies to provide preapproved services.

CHAMPUS

On a cost-shared basis, CHAMPUS covers skilled nursing care and other professional home care services for dependents of active military personnel and for military retirees and their dependents and survivors. CHAMPUS also offers a comprehensive hospice benefit that covers nursing, social work, counseling services, therapies, personal care, drugs, and medical supplies and equipment.

Workers' compensation

If a patient's need for home care results directly from a work-related injury, the state-run workers' compensation program will most likely cover at least some of the required services. All workers' compensation policies cover medical benefits and rehabilitation.

Regulation of home care

To compete in today's health care market, home care agencies must submit to multiple regulatory authorities. For example, to receive Medicare funding, an agency must gain Medicare certification. It may also need a state license and a certificate of need. To win sig-

Tighter purse strings, tougher scrutiny

Rampant fraud in the health care system has prompted the U.S. Congress, in the Balanced Budget Act of 1997, to launch an era of increased scrutiny and heightened control over home care agencies. Although specific guidelines remain incomplete, their effects promise to be far-reaching.

For example, home care agencies must reenroll in the Medicare program every 3 years so they can be held to newer, more stringent standards. In addition, audits of home care agencies are expected to double, and claim reviews will rise by 25%. Providers who overcharge Medicare or Medicaid must repay the overcharged amount.

The Health Care Financing Administration (HCFA) also hopes to control costs with a prospective payment system for home care visits that eliminates open-ended billing. HCFA also hopes to separate Medicare payments into two divi-

sions, one for care following a hospital stay and one for care needed for a chronic condition. This separation is intended to better highlight necessary — and unnecessary — services. The combined effect of these provisions will likely require many agencies to significantly reduce their average per-visit and per-patient cost.

Other measures proposed to ensure appropriate payment include:
- clearly defined limits on hours and days on which home care is provided
- standardized guidelines for frequency and duration of home care
- clarification of part-time and intermittent nursing care
- reimbursement based on the location of service rather than the agency's location to prevent higher urban reimbursement rates for services provided in lower-cost rural settings.

nificant referrals and major contracts, it also needs approval from independent accrediting bodies.

Home care agencies are regulated by other federal entities as well. They include the Centers for Disease Control and Prevention, the Clinical Laboratory Improvement Act (1988), the Food and Drug Administration, the Occupational Safety and Health Administration, and the Department of Labor. Together, federal, state, and private organizations function to certify, accredit, license, and regulate the delivery of home care services. In the future, the regulation of home care delivery promises to become even more

stringent. (See *Tighter purse strings, tougher scrutiny*.)

Certification

Any agency that wishes to receive Medicare reimbursement must first receive certification from the Health Care Financing Administration (HCFA), the federal agency that administers all Medicare and Medicaid programs. To receive certification, the agency must submit to an on-site evaluation and demonstrate competence in each of these 12 areas:
- informing patients of their rights

- complying with federal, state, and local laws and professional standards
- creating an organizational structure and administrative procedures that are clear and effective
- completing an annual review of the agency's policies and relationships with other health care providers
- forming an acceptance policy for patients based on a written plan of care that adheres to a physician's orders and is reviewed by both the agency and the physician at least every 62 days
- defining the scope and supervision of services from registered nurses and licensed practical nurses
- defining the scope and supervision of services from physical and occupational therapists and speech pathologists
- defining the scope and supervision of medical social services
- defining the scope and supervision of home care aide services and ensuring aides' training and competency
- demonstrating qualifications to furnish outpatient physical therapy or speech pathology
- maintaining appropriate clinical records for appropriate lengths of time
- evaluating the agency's total program at least yearly, including a review of policies, administrative practices, and clinical records.

Hospice agencies must receive a specific type of certification before they can receive reimbursement from Medicare. Hospice certification requires:
- centralized authority
- medical direction
- patient-focused plans of care
- provisions for staff development and performance improvement
- use of an interdisciplinary approach
- emphasis on home care.

In addition, to stay certified, the hospice patient population must maintain a ratio of 80 home-care days to 20 inpatient-care days. Inpatient care must still be available for pain control, symptom management, and provision of respite — but for short-term care only.

Licensure

Most states require home care agencies to obtain a state license; some also require a certificate of need. (See *Certificate of need,* page 12.) Usually, state licensure laws and regulations closely parallel those governing Medicare certification. In states that require a license, it must be obtained before the agency requests Medicare certification. If agency officials don't want Medicare certification, the agency may not need a state license even if state licensing laws exist.

To obtain a state license, an agency typically submits an application that includes information about its owners and directors. A state licensing team then visits the facility and evaluates:
- skill level of key staff
- scope of services to be provided directly and indirectly
- compliance with applicable state and federal laws
- appropriate level of liability insurance
- necessary record-keeping ability.

If the agency passes the evaluation, a license will be issued, usually for a 1-year period. If the agency has deficits but an acceptable plan to remedy them, the licensing team may issue a provisional license. If the agency receives but later loses its state license, it forfeits any Medicare reimbursement for

Certificate of need

Some states require home care agencies to obtain a certificate of need in addition to a state license. A certificate of need states that a certain geographic area needs the agency's services and that no other agency is available to provide them. The agency must file an application outlining this need with the state licensing department. Typically, licensing departments use certificates of need to control the number of licenses issued and thus prevent duplication of services. In general, state health-planning officials review certificate-of-need applications using these parameters:
• identification of a need for service in the state health plan
• needs of the intended population
• availability of less costly or more effective alternatives
• immediate and long-term viability of the project
• adequacy of support available, including staff, community, and professionals.

Based on the results of the evaluation, the planning agency may grant the application, deny it, or accept it with certain conditions. If the home care agency disagrees, the decision can be appealed by hearing or in court.

services rendered during the time spent without a state license.

Accreditation

Accreditation provides concrete evidence of an agency's commitment to high quality care. To become accredited, a home care agency must request and pay for evaluation by an accrediting authority. Several independent authorities accredit home care agencies, including the Joint Commission on the Accreditation of Healthcare Organizations (JCAHO), the Community Health Accreditation Program (CHAP), the Accreditation Commission for Home Care (ACHC), and the National Home-Caring Council.

JCAHO

JCAHO is the best known of the accrediting authorities. More than 5,000 home care agencies (both Medicare-certified and non-Medicare-certified) are involved in the JCAHO accreditation system. To earn and maintain accreditation, an agency must undergo an on-site survey by a JCAHO team at least every 3 years. The survey team also spends significant time on home visits, observing care as it's delivered. A surveyor may track a patient throughout the entire course of care, both in person and through the patient care record.

The standards by which a home care agency is judged are basically twofold: patient-focused and organization-focused functions. Using these two categories, surveyors evaluate 26 performance areas, scoring each on a 5-point scale on which a score of 1 is most favorable. (See *JCAHO performance areas.*) The sum of the agency's scores, along with other performance considerations, determines its accreditation status. In the near future, JCAHO plans to institute surprise inspections, giving less than 24 hours' notice before arriving to evaluate some agency functions.

JCAHO performance areas

The Joint Commission on the Accreditation of Healthcare Organizations (JCAHO) evaluates home care agencies on each performance area listed below. The rating scale ranges from 1 (substantial compliance) to 5 (no compliance).

PATIENT-FOCUSED FUNCTIONS	ORGANIZATIONAL FUNCTIONS
• **Rights and ethics** • **Assessment** – Patient assessment – Assessment of specific patient populations • **Care, treatment, and services** – Care planning – Preparing and dispensing drugs – Drug administration – Patient drug monitoring – Nutritional care – Diagnostic services • **Education** – Education program management – Patient education – Education about specific care issues • **Continuum of care and services**	• **Improving organizational performance** – Planning and designing – Measuring – Assessing – Improving • **Leadership** – Governance – Operations – Role in improving performance • **Environmental safety and equipment management** – Environmental safety – Equipment management • **Management of human resources** • **Management of information** – Information-management planning – Patient-specific data and information • **Surveillance, prevention, and control of infection**

CHAP

CHAP is the oldest accrediting organization for community and home care agencies. Established in 1965 as a division of the National League for Nursing, it became an independent agency in 1987. In 1992, it became the first private organization empowered by the Department of Health and Human Services to accredit home care agencies. Therefore, if an agency meets the criteria for CHAP accreditation, it also meets the certificate of participation qualifications for Medicare. In most cases, the standards for accreditation by CHAP exceed those of HCFA.

To obtain CHAP accreditation, an agency must uphold four CHAP standards of excellence:

• consistent consumer-oriented philosophy, with the agency's purpose and mission reflected in its structure and function
• high-quality services and products
• adequate and effectively organized human, financial, and physical resources
• long-term viability.

It also must meet CHAP's core standards, which address:

- education and credentialling of management
- policies and procedures for public disclosure and patient rights
- human resource management
- ongoing performance improvement
- contracts and agreements
- staffing patterns
- adequacy of financial controls and resources
- adequacy of financial information systems and strategic planning and evaluation
- risk assessment and management
- marketing strategies and initiatives
- data collection and effective incorporation of data
- management information systems
- corporate support of innovations.

Any home care agency, regardless of its type or specialization, can apply for and receive CHAP accreditation. The accreditation process requires four steps: submission of an application and fee, submission of a self-study that compares the agency to CHAP standards, submission to an unannounced 4- to 5-day site visit, and determination of accreditation status by the CHAP review board. Accreditation lasts for 3 years, and unannounced site visits occur annually during the first term.

ACHC

ACHC, an independent, private, not-for-profit organization, was established in 1986 by the North Carolina Association for Home Care in response to provider concerns about quality in-home aide services and because of a desire for an alternative to JCAHO review. Currently, ACHC accredits multiservice Medicare-certified and non-Medicare-certified agencies, home infusion companies, home care aide programs, home medical equipment suppliers, hospices, and companies that specialize in services and products for patients who have had breast surgery.

The goal of the program is to ensure that agencies who provide home care can replicate hospital standards in the home for noncritical patients and that they give primary caregivers and family members an opportunity to take part in care planning. The home care experience should increase patient independence, improve quality of life, and decrease overall health care costs while improving care.

National HomeCaring Council

The National HomeCaring Council sets standards and provides voluntary accreditation for paraprofessionals and private duty nurses who work in home care. As with other accreditation organizations, the process includes four steps: application, self-study, site visitation, and review by the accreditation committee. Accreditation lasts for 3 years.

Naturally, your agency's structure, funding sources, and adherence to regulations are largely the responsibility of agency officials. By fulfilling those responsibilities, your agency provides the foundation you need to deliver high-quality, multidisciplinary home care.

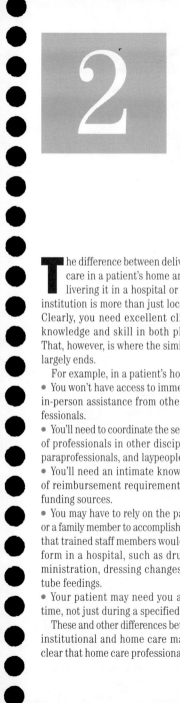

2 Identifying the home care team

The difference between delivering care in a patient's home and delivering it in a hospital or other institution is more than just location. Clearly, you need excellent clinical knowledge and skill in both places. That, however, is where the similarity largely ends.

For example, in a patient's home:
• You won't have access to immediate in-person assistance from other professionals.
• You'll need to coordinate the services of professionals in other disciplines, paraprofessionals, and laypeople.
• You'll need an intimate knowledge of reimbursement requirements and funding sources.
• You may have to rely on the patient or a family member to accomplish tasks that trained staff members would perform in a hospital, such as drug administration, dressing changes, and tube feedings.
• Your patient may need you at any time, not just during a specified shift.

These and other differences between institutional and home care make it clear that home care professionals are a distinctive group with particular attributes. (See *Characteristics of home care professionals,* page 16.) In short, to participate effectively in delivering home care, you need a broad range of valuable professional traits — traits that may differ from those needed in a hospital. One of the most valuable of those traits is the ability to function as part of a team.

Even more than in hospital care, home care depends on clear communication and planned coordination between teams of professionals and paraprofessionals working together to care for patients and their families who may have complex, multidimensional problems. Typically, each patient has both a core team and an extended team — what some people call a direct care team and a support team.

The core team includes a physician, a registered nurse, and professionals from other disciplines as defined by the patient's needs. They may include a physical therapist, an occupational therapist, a speech pathologist, a respiratory therapist, a medical social worker, licensed practical or vocational

Characteristics of home care professionals

Good home care professionals share certain characteristics, including:

• flexibility, openness, creativity, and willingness to apply skills and knowledge in a manner unique to each patient

• ability to function independently and yet recognize personal limitations and those of the scope of practice, seeking guidance when necessary

• ability to evaluate broad aspects of a situation and to communicate them clearly and concisely, both verbally and in writing, to other team members

• adaptability in applying skills and knowledge to each unique patient and home setting, focusing on the patient's specific areas of need and improvising in situations that may be atypical or challenging

• ability to independently plan time to meet patient goals despite varying locations, visit times, commuting times, and communication styles

• flexibility and openness to changes in schedules and priorities, prompted by either the agency or the patient

• respect for and comfort with the patient's home, regardless of its condition

• ability to assess the setting, establish limits, and feel secure in an environment in which you are a guest

• interest in the patient's full home environment — including location, safety, finances, relationships, and more — and

how its influence could affect his rate of recovery or adaptation

• ability to establish rapport and trust with patients and their families while working to develop and achieve mutual plans and goals

• creativity in motivating patients, fostering positive attitudes, and promoting independence and compliance with the plan of care

• continued professional interest in therapeutic discoveries and developments, and enthusiasm about incorporating them into the practice when appropriate

• ability to evaluate the limitations of and response to the current treatment plan, including unexpected results, adverse effects, or complications that need immediate care, additional home visits, or follow-up

• ability to converse with patients, family members, and significant others about the treatment plan, options for care, and changes that should prompt a call to you, the physician, or the agency

• knowledge and understanding of current and changing regulations regarding reimbursement criteria, length of service, visit frequency, covered equipment and services, out-of-pocket patient expenses, and discharge from service

• broad knowledge of community agencies and resources for referrals, transportation, equipment, meals, and more.

nurses, and home care aides. Typically, the registered nurse plays the leading role in coordinating the patient's core team.

The extended team includes members of the core team plus formal or informal caregivers or participants in the plan of care. They may include case managers, other registered nurses, clinical supervisors, nursing managers, directors of professional services, schedulers, and any other staff members who enable the core team to perform their duties.

Ongoing communication through case or team conferences, thorough documentation, adherence to each discipline's professional standards, and compliance with regulatory, accrediting, and governmental standards helps to ensure coordinated, effective delivery of home care. (See *Standards for home care professionals*.)

Perhaps the most important element in creating an effective team is a clear understanding of each team member's role. Therefore, this chapter reviews the basic roles and requirements of home care administrators, physicians, case managers, nurses, physical therapists, occupational therapists, speech pathologists, medical social workers, home care aides, and more.

Home care administrator

The administrator of your home care agency may be called an administrator, director, director of professional services, manager, chief executive, or one of numerous other titles. Regardless, the administrator should be a licensed physician, a registered nurse, or a person with training and experience in health service administration. The person should also have at least 1 year of administrative and supervisory experience in either home care or another health-related program. (See *Becoming a certified administrator,* page 18.)

Medicare and the Joint Commission on the Accreditation of Healthcare Organizations (JCAHO) define the ad-

Standards for home care professionals

If you're on a core home care team, make sure you uphold these standards at all times:

• Keep all patient information confidential.

• Document all interventions and responses.

• Ask for help if you aren't sure about a procedure or treatment.

• Report changes in a patient's condition to the appropriate team member, such as the care manager or physician.

• Participate in team meetings and case conferences.

• Perform your assigned role on the team.

• Cooperate and coordinate with all team members.

• Consider the patient an equal partner in decision making, planning, and meeting goals.

• Provide care that adheres to state and federal guidelines and to your discipline's scope of practice.

• Uphold the professional standards established by your discipline.

• Take part in quality assurance or performance improvement activities, as requested.

• Take part in continuing education, in-service programs, seminars, and other learning opportunities.

• Maintain your license or certification to practice in the home setting.

ministrator as someone who organizes and directs the agency's functions, acts as liaison between the agency's governing body and its contracted profes-

Becoming a certified administrator

One way to demonstrate your qualifications as a nurse administrator is to obtain voluntary certification from the American Nurses Credentialing Center. This organization offers two levels of certification for nurse administrators. Both are valid for 5 years, after which you can obtain recertification by providing evidence of continuing education or by achieving a passing score on an examination.

CNA

To become a certified nurse administrator (CNA), you must:
• have a baccalaureate or higher degree in nursing
• have held a full-time nurse manager or nurse executive position for the equivalent of 24 months during the past 5 years
• demonstrate 20 contact hours of continuing education applicable to nursing administration during the past 2 years, with a total of 30 hours in the past 5 years, or hold a master's degree in nursing administration
• achieve a passing score on a written examination.

CNAA

To become a certified nurse administrator, advanced (CNAA), you must:
• have a master's degree (if not in nursing, then the baccalaureate degree must be in nursing)
• have held an executive position for 24 months during the past 5 years, performing activities that are congruent with published tasks for this level
• demonstrate 30 contact hours of continuing education applicable to nursing administration during the past 2 years if you don't have a master's degree in nursing administration
• achieve a passing score on a written examination.

---

sionals and staff, maintains appropriate numbers of qualified staff, supervises staff evaluation, ensures the accuracy of public information materials and activities, and oversees the budgeting and accounting systems.

The Community Health Accreditation Program says that an agency's chief executive should match one of these two descriptions:
• Master's degree in a health-related or business field with at least 2 years of administrative experience
• Bachelor's degree in a health-related field with at least 5 years of administrative experience.

Some states have requirements for home care administrators as well.

An administrator's role varies somewhat with the needs of the agency. In all cases, however, the administrator is directly or indirectly responsible for all of the agency's clinical and business activities. This person is accountable for all internally delegated tasks.

Because of this detailed level of responsibility, the agency administrator should be available at all times. In other words, another person—usually a supervising physician or public health nurse—should be empowered in writing to act in the administrator's absence. This chain of command should be readily available, in writing, to all employees.

Physician

The physician plays a pivotal role in home care, both in directing the services provided and in justifying reimbursement for them. The Health Care Financing Administration (HCFA) defines a physician as someone who holds a Doctor of Medicine, Doctor of Osteopathy, or Doctor of Podiatry degree and who has the legal authority to practice medicine (and surgery, if needed) in the state.

Most insurers, including Medicare, require that home care be medically necessary. Thus, the physician's administrative role is to:

• certify that the patient needs care
• confirm that the patient is home-bound
• sign the plan of care form that details services to be provided (HCFA form 485).

Beyond these duties, the physician's role is much as it would be in any health care setting. Specifically, the physician diagnoses health problems that need care and then prescribes what care and drugs should be delivered. The physician must be informed of all care planned and provided and any changes in the patient's condition and the plan of care.

Case manager

Typically, two types of case managers are involved in the delivery of home care: the fiscal case manager and the clinical case manager. These two professionals collaborate to provide quality, cost-effective patient care.

Fiscal case manager

The fiscal case manager helps patients obtain services in the most cost-effective manner, usually by performing these functions:

• evaluating the patient's eligibility for home care
• validating the proposed plan of care
• defining the payment system
• contracting with the home care agency
• coordinating benefits among payers
• evaluating the program and auditing the providers.

Clinical case manager

The clinical case manager is responsible for providing quality patient care by performing these four roles, as defined by the Case Management Society of America:

• *assessor,* which involves collecting appropriate data and determining their affect on outcomes
• *planner,* which involves promoting patient, family, and caregiver participation; determining a viable treatment plan; developing quantifiable outcomes; and performing regular evaluation and revision of the care plan
• *facilitator,* which involves communicating with all team members and

maintaining cooperative relationships with all involved parties
• *advocate,* which involves supporting the patient's interests in all aspects of care (including resource allocation, financial issues, and care needs) and promoting independence within the patient's abilities.

In addition to providing continuous assessment and outcome-oriented care planning, the clinical case manager coordinates care inside and outside the agency, implements the care plan, allocates resources (including community referrals), and evaluates the quality and appropriateness of care. In short, the clinical case manager usually is directly involved with patient care. Typically, the clinical case manager is also responsible for reporting assessment data to the fiscal case manager. In fact, clinical and fiscal case managers usually need to communicate frequently to coordinate the patient's care with reimbursement.

Primary care provider

In the home setting, a primary care provider assesses patient needs, provides direct care according to a physician's order, communicates progress and changes to the physician, and acts as liaison between the patient and everyone involved in his care. Depending on the patient's specific needs, the primary care provider may be a registered nurse, a licensed practical (or vocational) nurse, a physical therapist, an occupational therapist, or a speech pathologist, all of whom are considered "skilled" by Medicare.

According to most third-party payers, including Medicare, services qualify as "skilled care" if they must be provided by a registered nurse, a licensed practical or vocational nurse being supervised by a registered nurse, or a physical, occupational, or speech pathologist in order to be safe and effective. If a service can be provided by a layperson without supervision, it isn't a skilled service. The complexity of the skill, the patient's condition, and the accepted standards of medical practice help to determine whether a service is skilled or not. In general, however, skilled services involve teaching, training, assessing, and observing as well as hands-on care.

Registered nurse

According to the HCFA's conditions of participation for home care nursing, a registered nurse is responsible for:
• performing the initial patient evaluation
• reevaluating the patient's needs regularly
• initiating the plan of care
• revising the plan of care, as needed
• providing appropriate skilled services
• employing preventive and rehabilitative nursing strategies
• performing clinical documentation
• coordinating services
• communicating changes in the patient's condition or needs to other team members
• providing patient and family counseling
• participating in in-service programs
• supervising and educating other nursing personnel.

The scope of practice for a registered nurse in the home care setting may be as a generalist or a specialist.

Generalist home care nurse

A generalist home care nurse approaches the patient in a holistic manner, assessing him within the influence of the immediate and extended environment. Activities involve teaching, managing resources directly or indirectly related to the patient's condition, monitoring technical and instrumental care, collaborating with other providers and disciplines to promote continuity of care, and supervising other support personnel.

A generalist nurse might have a caseload of patients ranging from infants to elderly adults with a variety of illnesses and conditions, such as heart failure, diabetes, wounds, or postoperative needs. The generalist home care nurse may seek voluntary certification from the American Nurses Credentialing Center. (See *Seeking certification in home care nursing,* page 22.)

Clinical specialist in home care nursing

The clinical specialist in home care nursing typically has a graduate degree and a different role from that of the generalist nurse. Indeed, the clinical specialist may need to perform all the tasks of a generalist home care nurse and more. That is because the clinical specialist has extensive clinical experience with individuals, families, and groups — plus expertise in case management, consultation, collaboration, and education of patients, staff, and other health professionals. The clinical specialist is also proficient in planning, implementing, and evaluating programs, resources, services, and research for health care delivery to patients with complex problems.

Commonly, a home care clinical specialist consults with the generalist nurse who is delivering care to a high-risk patient. For example, a patient with a complicated, nonhealing wound requires a weekly visit from an enterostomal therapist and daily wound care by a generalist home care nurse.

In addition to providing direct patient care and consultation, the home care clinical specialist monitors and evaluates performance improvement processes and risk management. Other activities may include research, education, identification of trends, consideration of ethical issues, and facilitation of multidisciplinary and interagency treatment plans stalled by barriers to care.

Licensed practical nurse

A licensed practical nurse (LPN), sometimes called a licensed vocational nurse (LVN), provides follow-up care for stable patients. An LPN or LVN is responsible for:
- providing services based on agency policy
- performing clinical documentation
- assisting with specialized procedures
- preparing equipment and materials for treatments using aseptic technique
- helping patients learn self-care activities.

Physical therapist

A physical therapist can provide a homebound patient with a profession-

Seeking certification in home care nursing

Through the American Nurses Credentialing Center, you can become certified as either a home care nurse generalist or as a clinical specialist in home care nursing. Use this table to compare the requirements for each one.

HOME CARE NURSE GENERALIST	CLINICAL SPECIALIST IN HOME CARE NURSING
CERTIFICATION CRITERIA	
• Active RN license	• Active RN license
• At least a baccalaureate degree in nursing	• At least a master's degree in nursing
• At least 2 years of practice as a licensed RN	• *Either* at least 1,000 hours of practice in home care nursing after gaining the master's degree and during the past 2 years *or* graduation from clinical specialist master's degree nursing program with up to 50% of clinical practice applied toward the 1,000-hour practice requirement
• At least 1,500 hours of practice in home care nursing during the past 3 years in direct patient care, clinical management, supervision, education, research, or direction of others to achieve or help achieve patient goals	• Average of 8 hours per week of direct patient care or clinical management in home care nursing
• At least 8 hours per week of current practice in home care nursing	
• At least 20 contact hours of continuing education applicable to the specialty area during the past 2 years	
TEST TOPICS	
• Program management	• Practice
• Concepts and models	• Education
• Clinical management	• Consultation
• Trends, issues, and research	• Research
	• Administration
	• Issues and trends

al evaluation, from which an intervention plan can be developed to promote strength, function, and mobility. In some cases, a physical therapist may be the only professional actively providing services, although those services are always under a physician's supervision. In other cases, the physical therapist works with team members to promote optimal mobility, range of motion, strength, and return of function. Physical therapists participate as active members in patient care conferences,

and a physical therapist may supervise physical therapy assistants in states that license them.

Responsibilities

A physical therapist's responsibilities in home care are based on state laws and practice standards. Specific responsibilities and duties include:
• performing an initial evaluation and assessment, with full documentation of the patient's baseline status

• developing an appropriate plan of care that includes needed skilled interventions

• reviewing the plan of care with the patient, caregivers, and the physician

• providing skilled services consistent with the plan of care (See *Physical therapy: Skilled services.*)

• evaluating, implementing, and documenting changes in the plan of care

• updating the plan of care at least every 30 days and as the patient's condition changes

• documenting the patient's ongoing status in the clinical record

• supervising and communicating with physical therapy assistants

• giving instructions to other care providers, such as home care aides

• communicating problems, progress, and outcomes to other team members

• recommending follow-up and coordinating services

• maintaining knowledge of community resources and making referrals as needed

• documenting the final evaluation and assessment

• assessing the competence of support personnel

• maintaining patient confidentiality

• participating in conferences, in-service programs, chart audits, performance improvement, and peer review activities

• participating in continuing education.

As with other providers of skilled services, physical therapists must provide complete documentation at each visit or patient encounter. This documentation may take the form of progress notes, visit records, care summaries, physicians' orders, plans of care, or out-

---

Physical therapy: Skilled services

Federal regulations consider these physical therapy procedures to be skilled services when the patient's condition and the underlying factors involved warrant them:

• assessment

• therapeutic exercise program

• gait evaluation and training, including repetitive exercises, exercises to maintain strength and endurance, and assistive walking when part of the initial maintenance plan

• range-of-motion exercises when part of an active treatment plan that addresses loss of motion or mobility because of a disease, illness, or injury

• maintenance therapy that involves complex and sophisticated procedures

• ultrasound, short-wave, and microwave diathermy treatments

• hot packs, infrared treatments, paraffin baths, and whirlpool baths to address a complicated condition.

---

come measurement tools. It should include treatment provided, patient and caregiver responses to treatment, progression toward goals, updated outcomes if needed, visit frequency, start and finish times, the total time spent with the patient, and the contents of patient conferences with other team members, family members, or other care providers or supervisors.

Occupational therapist

An occupational therapist evaluates patients who have lost the ability to in-

Documentation topics for occupational therapy

At the first evaluation, an occupational therapist assesses the patient's level of impairment in the areas listed here, documents the amount of help the patient needs in each area, and outlines a plan of services and goals.

Activities of daily living (ADLs)
• Bathing
• Bed mobility
• Dressing
• Feeding
• Functional transfers
• Grooming
• Toileting

Instrumental ADLs
• Homemaking
• Home safety awareness
• Money management

Performance components of ADLs
• Cognition
• Coordination
• Perception
• Range of motion
• Safety judgments
• Sensory processing
• Strength
• Upper limb sensation

Environmental issues
• Adaptive equipment
• Assistive devices
• Caregiver or community service presence
• Home accessibility

dependently perform activities of daily living — such as eating, toileting, dressing, and bathing — and develops a plan of intervention to help them regain those abilities. An occupational therapist may also help patients with instrumental activities of daily living, such as money management, homemaking, and transportation. Patients with many different problems can benefit from the services of an occupational therapist, including those with head trauma, cerebrovascular accident, chronic lung disease, joint replacement, amputation, and developmental disabilities.

Responsibilities

In practice, occupational therapists have responsibilities analogous to those of physical therapists:
• evaluating the patient's level of function
• recommending a plan of intervention to the physician
• obtaining orders to proceed with planned treatment
• providing appropriate skilled services
• supervising the activities of occupational therapy assistants
• evaluating the patient's progress
• documenting occupational therapy issues at the initial evaluation and throughout care (See *Documentation topics for occupational therapy*.)
• advising and consulting with the patient, family, and members of the home care team
• keeping all team members informed
• providing community referrals as needed
• maintaining patient confidentiality

- participating in conferences, in-service programs, chart audits, performance improvement, peer review activities, and continuing education.

Speech pathologist

A speech pathologist works with patients who have trouble communicating because of injury or disease. In some circumstances, such as after a cerebrovascular accident or head trauma, the speech pathologist may be the only home care professional working with the patient.

Responsibilities

A speech pathologist evaluates a patient's speech, language, and oral-pharyngeal status; conducts hearing screenings; develops treatment plans to address deficits; implements treatments (including selecting, dispensing, and adjusting assistive devices); recommends prosthetic and augmentative devices; and makes referrals to appropriate community resources.

Like other team members, a speech pathologist also attends team meetings, communicates with other team members, documents treatments and outcomes, evaluates the patient's progress, and participates in in-service programs and continuing education.

Medical social worker

A medical social worker typically has a master's degree from a school of social work accredited by the Council on Social Worker Education, plus at least 1 year of social work experience in a health care setting. The services offered by this professional help patients and their families to maintain practices or relationships that are culturally, spiritually, or ethnically meaningful to them. Thus, social workers seek to minimize or eliminate the social or emotional stresses that result from illness or its treatments.

Responsibilities

Some social workers provide individual or family counseling if needed. They help patients and families obtain needed community resources to improve their ability to function or progress in treatment. In addition to helping patients directly, social workers help physicians and other team members to understand the social and emotional factors that affect their patients.

To meet the HCFA's conditions of participation, a medical social worker or a supervised assistant must be made available for visits in the patient's home if the patient's plan of care specifies a need for social services. The social worker may contract with the home care agency or may be an employee of the agency.

Regulations also specify that a medical social worker should:

- assess the social and emotional aspects of the patient's illness and care
- assess the influence of the patient's home environment, finances, and available community resources
- help develop the plan of care
- prepare clinical and progress notes
- work with the patient's family
- provide or obtain counseling services as needed

When your patient needs a social worker

A medical social worker can help you address these types of patient problems:
• adverse reactions to illness
• problems adjusting to changes in functional status
• problems adjusting to illness
• relationship problems, including isolation
• mental illness
• barriers to medical care, such as lack of transportation or an inability to obtain prescribed drugs
• caregiver problems, such role strain and personal stress
• financial problems
• problems involving housing and living arrangements, including institutionalization
• neglect and physical, emotional, and sexual abuse
• substance abuse
• vocational and educational problems.

• make use of appropriate community resources
• remove obvious barriers to treatment or recovery
• participate in discharge planning and in-service programs
• act as a consultant to other agency personnel.

To perform these duties with excellence, the social worker should adopt the standards of the National Association of Social Workers. One standard recommends that social workers know about chronic, acute, and terminal illnesses; physical disabilities; and their age-specific effects on patients and families. Another standard recommends that home care social workers should support and advocate for appropriate home care for people with chronic, acute, or terminal illnesses.

The third standard recommends that social services provided independently in a patient's home should be delivered by a social worker with an appropriate license or certification.

Finally, the standards recommend that home care social workers integrate social work intervention with interventions from other members of the interdisciplinary team, that they work to achieve an appropriate continuum of care, and that they serve patients, the agency staff, and the community. Taken together, these standards exceed those of the federal government.

Clearly, medical social workers address a wide range of patient problems. (See *When your patient needs a social worker.*) The social workers' activities may include assessing social, economic, environmental, and emotional influences on the patient; developing a treatment plan and helping to obtain needed services; advocating for the patient and intervening in crises; providing counseling, education, and support; collaborating with other team members; and participating in discharge planning and case management.

Home care aide

Home care aides provide personal care — not skilled care — to patients who can't care for themselves. Aides perform such tasks as giving bed baths, assisting with tub baths and showers, shampooing hair, administering nail and skin care, performing oral hygiene, transferring patients, and toileting. Home care aides also provide basic monitoring of patient status, including weight, temperature, pulse, and respiration. They promptly report any adverse changes to a team supervisor such as a nurse.

Services provided by a home care aide also can support skilled care delivered by other members of the home care team: performing range-of-motion exercises based on the physical therapist's instruction, for example. Usually, home care aides spend more time with patients and their families than any other member of the home care team.

Preparation

The care provided by home care aides — and the preparation required to provide it — are strictly regulated by the government. To ensure the competency of home care aides, conditions of participation require that they complete an approved 75-hour training program (usually given by a registered nurse) that includes at least 16 hours of supervised clinical or practical training before providing any patient care. The government also requires that home care aides receive a competency or performance evaluation at least every 12 months. It must include all areas covered in the training program. (See *Competency areas for home care aides.*) If an aide fails any of the required skills, the aide can't administer home care unless directly supervised by a registered nurse.

Competency areas for home care aides

Medicare requires that home care aides master these core concepts:
- communication
- observing, reporting, and documenting patient status and care delivered
- methods for obtaining and documenting vital signs
- basic principles and procedures needed to control infection
- basic body functions and changes that should be reported immediately to a supervisor
- ways to preserve a clean, healthy environment
- ways to recognize emergencies and what to do about them
- patient's physical, emotional, and developmental needs; privacy; respect for person and property; and ways to meet all these needs
- safe and appropriate techniques for performing personal hygiene and grooming (bed, sponge, tub or shower bath; shampoo; nail and skin care; oral hygiene; toileting; elimination)
- safe techniques for transfer and ambulation
- normal range of motion and positioning
- adequate fluid and nutritional intake.

Any agency that doesn't offer the required training program must obtain proof that a newly hired home care aide has successfully completed the program before allowing the aide to provide home care. Also, the agency must require its education or in-service department to devise a method for annually ensuring and documenting the ongoing competence of its home care aides.

Responsibilities

Medicare defines the personal care provided by home care aides to include:
- bathing, dressing, grooming, hair care, nail care, and oral hygiene needed to facilitate treatment or prevent a decline in the patient's health
- changing bed linens if a patient is incontinent
- shaving
- applying deodorant
- applying lotions or powders to the skin
- giving foot and ear care
- feeding the patient
- helping with elimination, including giving enemas (unless the patient's condition warrants nursing care)
- giving routine catheter and ostomy care
- helping with ambulation, transfers, and positioning in bed.

A home care aide may also perform simple dressing changes, help with drugs that the patient takes, help with activities that support other skilled services (such as routine maintenance exercises and practice of functional communication skills), and provide routine care of prosthetic and orthotic devices.

Supervision

The HCFA's conditions of participation require that home care aides be supervised while providing home care. This supervision takes several forms. For one thing, a registered nurse as-

signs the home care aide to a specific patient. For another, the nurse prepares specific, written patient care instructions that the aide must follow exactly. Only with current physician's orders, a specific patient assignment, and written instructions can the home care aide provide care, and then only within the realm of services allowed by state law.

In addition, a nurse or other primary care provider must visit the home of a patient receiving home care aide services. If the patient receives only home care aide services and no skilled services, then a registered nurse must make a supervisory visit to the patient's home at least every 62 days. The home care aide must be present so the nurse can evaluate the care given.

If the patient receives skilled services along with home care aide services, then the registered nurse must make a supervisory visit to the home at least once every 14 days, more often if the patient's condition or the plan of care changes. The home care aide may be present during this supervisory visit but isn't *required* to be present. The agency administrator may assign one nurse to conduct all such visits or may require all nurses to conduct supervisory visits in their assigned areas. (If the patient receives only physical, speech, or occupational therapy, a skilled therapist may make the supervisory visit instead of a registered nurse.)

Specialized home care roles

With training, experience, or both, home care nurses can take on specialized roles.

Discharge planners

Discharge planners coordinate the referrals of patients who need additional care after being released from an inpatient facility. The desired outcome is to provide care in the setting that best promotes independence, safety, and cost-effectiveness — whenever possible, at home. Discharge planners make sure the patient has everything needed to safely return home and receive effective, cost-conscious care.

Home care aide trainers

Trainers or supervisors of home care aides provide education and training in keeping with strict Medicare regulations. The regulations affect the aides, the nurse, the training supplied by the nurse, and the assessment of competency. In general, home care aide trainers or supervisors must be registered nurses with at least 2 years of nursing experience, at least 1 of which must be in the provision of home care.

Home care coordinators

Sometimes called clinical liaison coordinators, home care coordinators help to educate physicians, staff, and the community about the role of home care in the broader health care arena. Medicare exerts fairly strict control over these external educators; most regulations involve meticulous record keeping about time, program contents, and audience approached.

Patient educators

Patient educators provide specialty education that directly helps patients and indirectly helps the staff. They can be specialists in diabetes education, asthma education, maternal-child education, or any other special niches an agency serves.

Psychiatric nurses

Psychiatric nurses provide evaluation, psychotherapy, and teaching activities for patients who have diagnosed psychiatric disorders and a need for active treatment. These nurses must meet certain criteria and be certified before the agency can receive Medicare reimbursement for their services.

Quality assurance managers

These managers may be responsible for auditing, compliance, ongoing monitoring of compliance, documentation review, and similar quality surveillance processes.

Staff development coordinators

These professionals typically are responsible for continuing education and staff competency. Specific roles vary according to each agency's needs.

Other team members

Other team members may be involved in delivering home care.

Dentists

Dentists can evaluate patients' ability to consume and chew food, especially patients who have mouth-altering diseases such as cancer of the tongue. A dentist may also evaluate the fit of a patient's dentures or other dental appliance to ensure optimal functioning—and optimal nutrition.

Dietitians

Dietitians and nutritionists are registered professionals who provide consultation and home visits to patients to promote optimal nutrition and diet modification, including supplementation and recommendations for enteral and parenteral nutrition therapies. In some agencies, a dietitian or nutritionist may be an integral member of the home care team.

Homemakers

In most states, homemakers provide no direct or hands-on patient care. Instead they perform such chores as cleaning, preparing meals, running errands, and buying groceries for patients.

Pharmacists

Licensed pharmacists can provide expert information about drugs to the health care team. They also evaluate the regimens of patients who take multiple drugs, assess for therapeutic effects, and screen for adverse drug reactions and interactions. Pharmacists also provide in-service education, consultation, and assistance with case conferences.

Podiatrists

These licensed health care providers specialize in foot care. They commonly trim the toenails of high-risk patients, such as those who are elderly or have diabetes. They also may treat foot injuries or perform minor surgery. In most states, they can prescribe drugs or treatments to be administered by licensed nursing staff.

Psychologists

Psychologists are licensed in most states and, in the home care arena, can help change behaviors in patients with diagnosed mental illness or mental retardation. A psychologist may also administer psychological tests to patients with suspected head trauma or dementia to assist with diagnosis and treatment.

Respiratory therapists

Licensed respiratory therapists evaluate a patient's respiratory status, provide teaching about respiratory equipment (such as home oxygen therapy and nebulizer therapy), and provide respiratory care measures such as chest physiotherapy.

Volunteers

Volunteers can provide unskilled care that the patient or family can't perform, such as running errands, doing laundry, and preparing meals. With training, volunteers can also provide respite care for several hours or even several days to allow family caregivers time to rest while caring for a loved one.

3

Maintaining quality in home care

Most people think of quality as a relatively simple concept. They know it when they see it. When it comes to home care, however, defining quality may not be so easy. Why? Because the various people involved in home care may have varying perspectives on what makes it successful.

For instance, patients and their families may judge quality based on whether they receive the services they want. Or, they may judge quality based on whether nurses, aides, and therapists arrive on time and maintain pleasant attitudes. A family who pays directly for services may assess quality differently than a family whose insurance is paying for services.

In contrast, third-party payers and government officials may define quality by the number of visits made within a specified period of time. From this perspective, quality care involves not only patient outcomes but also cost control. Sometimes this perspective differs from that of health care professionals, who tend to judge quality based on whether the patient returns to an independent or a pre-illness level of functioning—no matter how many services it takes to achieve that goal.

Accrediting and certifying organizations tend to have yet another perspective, based primarily on whether a home care agency and its staff adhere to required standards. From this perspective, quality home care may be directly linked to timely documentation and other largely administrative tasks.

As with most topics on which people have varying opinions, the truth about quality in-home care almost certainly incorporates elements of all perspectives. Thus, each home care agency must balance the requirements of governing bodies with the expectations of patients, the professional commitment of its staff, and the standards established by accrediting and certifying agencies. Naturally, the drive for quality home care affects and is affected by the agency's staffing needs and patterns, patient population and mix, financial and legal liability, length of stay issues, peer review, continuing education, policies and procedures, and documentation issues.

Measures of quality

No matter whose perspective you take, one fact is clear. To remain competitive, home care agencies must provide patient-centered, outcome-oriented services that can be measured and continuously improved. In a general sense, attaining this goal requires three initiatives: Meeting the standards of governing bodies; developing and implementing policies, protocols, and procedures; and soliciting input from selected groups of health care professionals. Many agencies group these initiatives and other quality-seeking steps in what is called a performance improvement (PI) program (also known as continuous quality improvement or total quality management).

Standards

The foundation on which all quality-seeking efforts must rest is adherence to the requirements of the home care agency's governing bodies. Usually, that means the Health Care Financing Administration (HCFA), which administers Medicare and Medicaid.

To receive funds from these programs, the agency must follow HCFA's conditions of participation. In short, conditions of participation require home care agencies to pursue outcomes-based PI so they can continuously upgrade processes, outcomes of care, and patient satisfaction.

Conditions of participation are patient-centered and supported by patient outcome data or performance measures. They're mirrored by the requirements of such accrediting bodies as the Joint Commission on the Accreditation of Healthcare Organizations (JCAHO) and the Community Health Accreditation Program (CHAP). In each case, the goal is to improve outcomes for patients.

Because the requirements of JCAHO and CHAP meet or exceed those of the conditions of participation, HCFA has given these independent accrediting organizations "deemed status." Any agency accredited by these organizations also receives deemed status, which means that they're no longer subject to routine inspection by state survey agencies.

Policies, protocols, and procedures

Sound policies, procedures, and protocols are crucial to achieve the agency's overall quality goals. (See *Understanding policies, protocols, and procedures.*) In fact, Medicare mandates that home care agencies establish policies, protocols, and procedures in the following areas:
- types of services provided
- geographic area served by the agency
- patient admission and discharge criteria
- medical supervision, including the physician's role in the plan of care
- plans of care, including criteria for the initial visit, recertification, and plan revision
- responsible personnel (including physicians) and the time frames of plans of care
- emergency management plans for patients
- documentation, including required forms, sequence of completion, security and confidentiality, approved abbreviations, and length of time that records are kept

- personnel criteria, such as licensure, experience, education, health requirements, insurance, and transportation needs
- program evaluation requirements.

Other regulatory bodies, including state agencies, may require policies, protocols, and procedures in these areas as well:

- infection control, including reporting and following up
- criteria for terminating service
- requirements of a quality management program
- emergency preparedness plan
- procedures required of each discipline involved
- resources for patient education
- case or team conferences
- billing and administrative practices
- specific safety management issues.

Committees

To ensure that its policies, protocols, and procedures are appropriate and congruent with standards imposed by regulatory bodies, a home care agency may assemble various committees to develop policies, review them, or both. (See *Home care committees,* pages 34 and 35.)

In some agencies, these committees may overlap, or additional committees may be established depending on the agency's organizational structure and needs. Small agencies don't have several committees but rather one committee that oversees all PI initiatives, with specific staff devoted to problem-solving or developing policies and procedures. Regardless, all of the agency's staff must work together to make sure the home care agency provides quality care.

Understanding policies, protocols, and procedures

Policies provide a clear picture of an agency's values and its commitment to patients, staff, and standards important to daily operation. They provide direction and define the conditions and mechanisms necessary for the agency to function. Typically, policies address role definitions and responsibilities in matters involving patient care and support services.

Care plans or clinical pathways consist of protocols and procedures. *Protocols* detail the steps required to manage a specific issue or problem. They provide standard guidelines for action and continuity, thus helping to ensure quality. *Procedures* include statements about how to perform specified tasks. They're typically based on clinical, scientific, and technical rationales.

Elements of quality

In today's competitive health care environment, home care agencies must be able to prove that they provide quality care — and that they continuously strive to improve it. Usually, that proof comes via data gathered as part of a PI plan designed by the agency. Obviously, however, an agency's level of quality stems largely from the performance of its staff. That is why quality also hinges on hiring the right staff, ensuring their competency, providing them with a full orientation, ensuring that they maintain quality performance lev-

Home care committees

Your agency may convene several committees to manage and evaluate the services it provides, or it may have a single performance improvement committee with designated action teams to accomplish goals.

COMMITTEE AND MEMBERS	TASKS
PROFESSIONAL ADVISORY COMMITTEE	
• Physician (Medical director) • Registered nurse • Representative from each of the agency's disciplines • Consumer representative • Performance improvement nurse	• Establish and review policies at least annually. • Evaluate specific policies related to each discipline. • Consult with management. • Assist with devising solutions. • Assist in evaluating agency programs. • Help maintain liaisons with other health care professionals.
PROGRAM EVALUATION COMMITTEE	
• Selected members of the professional advisory committee • Representative from each discipline involved with services being evaluated	• Review the agency's appropriateness, adequacy, and effectiveness. • Review active and closed clinical records. • Report findings and recommendations. • Develop action plans for short- and long-term correction of problem areas.
UTILIZATION REVIEW COMMITTEE	
• Representative professionals who supply care	• Review clinical records at least quarterly. • Report findings to program evaluation committee, professional advisory committee, or both.
PERFORMANCE IMPROVEMENT COMMITTEE	
• Administrative and clinical staff (possibly rotating) • Selected members of the professional advisory committee or another quality- or performance-oriented committee	• Meet monthly or bimonthly. • Review all processes related to direct or indirect patient care. • Gather monitoring data. • Identify data trends and provide information to appropriate discipline. • Report to professional advisory committee.
PROFESSIONAL STANDARDS AND ETHICS COMMITTEE	
• Representatives of expert health care professionals, including home care aides	• Research, review, and make recommendations for clinical standards of practice. • Review clinical standards, protocols, and plans of care or treatment. • Obtain professional competency standards for each discipline. • Act as a resource for identifying and standardizing patient education material. • Assist with development of an orientation program.

Home care committees *(continued)*	
COMMITTEE AND MEMBERS	**TASKS**
SAFETY COMMITTEE	
• Representative from each department in the agency • Representative from senior management	• Review safety issues, such as back injury, automobile safety, safety in the home, and high-risk neighborhoods. • Review effectiveness of safety management plan at least annually. • Identify safety indicators to be included in performance improvement program. • Report to the governing body.

els, retaining them, establishing protocols for them to follow, and administering peer reviews.

Following a PI plan

According to JCAHO, PI should take place in a continuous cycle that involves creating objectives and processes, collecting and analyzing data, setting priorities for improvement, making improvements, and evaluating their effect. All of these elements should be included in some form in a PI plan.

Ideally, the plan should also have clear leadership assignments, an effective design, and practical methods of data collection and analysis for specific, defined activities. (See *Practical methods of data collection and analysis,* page 36.) PIs can be made at any point in the process as problems become evident. Tools used to identify problems include incident reports, infection surveillance logs, chart audits, problem logs, on-call logs, reimbursement audits, patient satisfaction surveys, and employee satisfaction surveys.

Certain types of data collection may be mandated by a regulating authority. For instance, the Outcome and Assessment Information Set, commonly known as OASIS, must be collected for every patient on admission, every 2 months and, if he has a significant change in condition, at discharge. Typically, OASIS data is assembled from documentation.

Required or not, data should be collected for all processes important to your agency's scope of services. How often you collect data depends largely on the process or outcome involved. Analysis of the data offers information about how current staff performance compares with previous performance, how the agency compares in quality with other agencies providing the same services, and how the agency compares to data found in the literature.

Serious problems or trends that could be revealed by an agency's performance plan — and that deserve immediate corrective action — include:
• variance in clinical outcomes when compared to published databases
• significant and undesirable variation in performance from recognized standards
• confirmed blood transfusion reactions
• significant adverse drug reactions
• significant drug incidents

Practical methods of data collection and analysis

Here are two simple methods for collecting and analyzing data that will help your agency pinpoint problems and implement performance improvements.

FOCUS method

F — Find a process to improve.
O — Organize a team that knows the process.
C — Clarify current knowledge of the process.
U — Understand the sources of variation in the process.
S — Select a way to improve the process.

PDCA method

P — Plan change by studying the process, deciding what could improve it, and identifying data to assist in that process.
D — Design and implement the plan on a small scale.
C — Check the results of the change and modify it if needed.
A — Act on the change or repeat the data collection and analysis cycle.

- problems with medical equipment and products
- serious patient or employee injuries
- denial of claims.

Naturally, when problems relate to the performance of a particular person, agency officials must take individual action. When problems relate to policies, procedures, or other systematic issues, officials must address these wider issues. Either action must be documented as part of the performance evaluation process. In addition, HCFA's conditions of participation require each agency to summarize its PI activities in an annual agency evaluation.

Hiring the right staff

For any home care agency, high-quality services depend on a dedicated, skilled professional staff. Obtaining such a staff involves an arduous process of defining jobs and evaluating candidates.

First, the agency's staffing manager determines that a position needs to be filled. The manager defines the position in detail, including its key responsibilities and the minimum requirements needed to qualify for the job. After the requisition is approved by the agency's governing authority, the staffing manager recruits candidates for the job, inside the agency, outside the agency, or both.

As candidates respond to the recruitment effort, the manager may acknowledge receipt of their resumes while prescreening certain applicants. A good prescreening interview concentrates only on unclear or incomplete areas of the applicant's application. It usually takes only about 10 minutes, and it may conclude with an appointment for a more lengthy interview. All interesting candidates undergo this comprehensive interview. The staffing manager also may check the final candidates' references and validate their education and licensure.

Based on interviews and experience, the staffing manager chooses a candidate and offers the job. Naturally, the offer must include the starting salary and starting date. Some agencies send a written offer to the candidate that may require the new employee's signature.

Ensuring competency

Ensuring the competency of an agency's home care staff goes well beyond simply making sure they have the appropriate licenses. Indeed, many home care nurses must develop competency in particular service areas to be accepted by the agency's governing authority.

For instance, some agencies require that initial assessments be made only by registered nurses with specialized competency in assessment. A hospice nurse must have extensive knowledge about the dying process and about palliative therapies but doesn't need extensive knowledge about and experience in inserting vascular access devices and maintaining them.

To meet HCFA's conditions of participation, an agency's home care aides must receive at least 12 hours of continuing education each year. Plus, some states require continuing education for relicensure for professional nurses.

Typically, agencies help to ensure core competency levels by defining jobs clearly, observing the staff at work (or in simulated settings), performing periodic assessments, and issuing performance evaluations. If an individual competency issue arises, the agency should work with the individual staff member. If an agency-wide competency issue arises, an agency-wide response should follow.

For example, if 7 of the agency's 10 nurses score poorly in documentation, the agency should design a solution, apply it to all staff members, and evaluate it as part of the overall PI plan. Naturally, praising staff members for PIs helps to build motivation and morale.

Providing appropriate orientation

Even a competent professional may have trouble meeting an agency's competency standards without an appropriate orientation at the start of a new job. Such an orientation should include not only written and verbal information, but also time spent with a manager and coworkers. (See *Elements of an orientation,* page 38.) The new employee should understand the new job and the expectations of agency officials before being asked to perform independently.

In addition to arranging this hands-on introduction, agency officials should clearly document their expectations and goals for the new employee — on the first day of employment. Then, at designated periods (commonly 30, 60, and 90 days) the employee should receive written performance evaluations that reflect the original goals. This process should help the new employee start off successfully while ensuring staff competency for the agency.

Providing continuing education

Perhaps the most common method that home care agencies use to foster competency and continuous improvement is continuing education. Agency staff may offer the program internally, or the agency may contract with another organization to provide it. The program

Elements of an orientation

Each new employee should receive a full orientation that includes:

• an overview of the agency's services, mission, plans, and goals

• an explanation of services provided by the agency, including guidelines for referrals, visits, testing, and other disciplines involved

• patient confidentiality requirements

• job description and expectations, including dress code, availability, discipline measures, payment schedules, benefits, and continuing education requirements

• employee's role in the agency team

• outline of agency teamwork and methods of communicating about patient care

• education about specific services the employee will be providing

• review of all policies and procedures for technical procedures, productivity, therapy management, equipment management, and performance improvement

• education about infection control, including standard precautions and tuberculosis prevention standards

• education about safety management, including hazard communication standards and ergonomics

• review of community resources

• review of documentation and medical records procedures

• explanation of on-call procedures

• completion of skills checklists or tests that allow employee to demonstrate understanding and agency officials to document understanding

• provision of supervised home visits.

may include in-service programs, staff presentations, journal articles, video or audio tapes, teleconferences, product demonstrations from manufacturers, and self-study programs. New products, new treatments, revised standards, and evolving ethical issues provide excellent opportunities to improve staff knowledge and solicit feedback.

In general, each continuing education opportunity should include these elements:

• overview of the topic

• rationale for the topic

• pretest, if appropriate

• objectives to be achieved

• topic outline

• provisions for note-taking

• interactive teaching methods (such as audiovisual aids, role playing, group discussion, demonstration, and hands-on practice)

• summary

• posttest, as appropriate

• participant evaluation of the program.

Summaries of the program evaluations should be used in the PI process to obtain feedback from staff, to identify needed areas of training, and to develop more efficient use of training resources.

If you want to participate in a continuing education program outside your agency, you'll need to submit verification that you attended and completed the program. You'll most likely receive a certificate that shows you completed the course. Your agency will probably want to keep a copy of it in your employment file to verify competency.

Documenting performance

Although JCAHO requires only annual staff evaluations, the National Home-Caring Council requires that agency staff receive a written performance evaluation after 6 months (or less) on the job and annually thereafter. Usually, the evaluation is created by the employee's supervisor and signed by both supervisor and employee. An increasing number of agencies are experimenting with self-evaluation.

The purpose of performance evaluations is to give employees a periodic opportunity to clarify their responsibilities. It also helps agency managers learn about employees' personal goals, ambitions, and attitudes toward their jobs and the agency. Strong working relationships between supervisors and employees help make this process honest and valuable, both to employees and to the agency.

A performance evaluation should include:

• detailed job description
• rating (such as *exceeds expectations, competent,* or *needs improvement*) for each area of the job description
• comments to explain or support each rating
• employee's response to comments and ratings
• areas for improvement and long- and short-term goals to be achieved
• date and signature of supervisor and employee.

To keep performance reviews as objective as possible, they should be based largely on data collected from the following sources:

• supervisory visits
• chart audits

• client satisfaction surveys that apply to the employee
• incident reports involving employee activities
• problem log entries involving employee activities
• exceptional service comments.

Implementing standards

One of the best ways to ensure quality performance — and agency recognition of it — is to follow appropriate standards and guidelines for general practice and specialty procedures. For example, by following the American Nurses Association's Standards of Clinical Nursing Practice, you can demonstrate and prove a certain level of competency. If you specialize in infusion therapy, oncology nursing, or pediatric nursing, you can use standards issued by the related nursing societies as a performance benchmark.

In addition to following standards, you can use adherence to professional guidelines to demonstrate quality performance. Guidelines may be issued by a variety of organizations — the American Diabetes Association, for example — and typically provide flexible recommendations that can be adapted to meet specific patient needs. (See *Exploring the National Guideline Clearinghouse,* page 40.) Naturally, the standards and guidelines you follow must reflect current practice, be acceptable to your agency, and be incorporated into agency policies and procedures.

Retaining staff

Recruiting and maintaining a competent, motivated staff is a home care agency's most difficult and costly task.

Exploring the National Guideline Clearinghouse

If you want the latest evidence-based clinical practice guidelines from more than 100 professional organizations, try exploring the National Guideline Clearinghouse at either *www.ngc.org* or *www.guideline.gov*. There you'll find more than 380 guidelines and related materials for clinical practice. Plus, you can download them for free. The National Guideline Clearinghouse is a joint venture of the Agency for Healthcare Research and Quality (formerly the Agency for Health Care Policy and Research), the American Medical Association, and the American Association of Health Plans.

- compliance with governing regulations, such as HCFA
- adherence to agency policies and procedures
- identification of patient needs, both met and unmet
- identification of trends in care for individuals and groups.

From this information, the reviewer determines the agency's strengths and weaknesses and then communicates those findings to agency officials and staff. As with all the efforts reviewed in this chapter, this process provides yet another way to help ensure that patients and their families are receiving the best possible care.

That is why good home care agencies do everything they can to retain valuable staff members. Staff retention efforts commonly involve financial rewards, such as salary increases or bonuses for meeting agency objectives or improving performance.

Agencies may offer other enticements as well, such as tuition reimbursement, awards for research or publication, and employee recognition programs. They may also offer flexible benefits packages that include such innovative programs as job sharing and flexible shifts.

Performing peer reviews

JCAHO is a peer-review organization. In a peer review, a qualified person from outside the agency selects a random sample of clinical records and examines them for the following:

Recognizing legal pitfalls

Over the years, many lawsuits have been brought against nurses and their employers for alleged malpractice, which is a form of professional negligence or omission of duty that causes harm to a patient. Some of the most common lawsuits involving nurses stem from injuries sustained when a nurse fails to prevent a fall, doesn't follow a physician's order or an established protocol, makes an error in drug administration, uses equipment improperly, fails to monitor appropriately, or fails to communicate adequately. (See *Tips to prevent lawsuits,* pages 42 and 43.)

Legal issues that may be especially prominent in home care include agency compliance, patient rights, patient abuse, restraints, noncompliance, incompetent caregivers, and supervision of home care aides.

Agency compliance

Home care agencies in the United States must comply with applicable laws, rules, and regulations established by the Health Care Financing Administration (HCFA) and federal, state, and other regulatory bodies that have jurisdiction over the home care industry. In fact, HCFA recommends that home care agencies create corporate compliance plans that outline a set of rules and procedures to reduce fraud and illegal conduct. Compliance plans typically contain a code of conduct that clearly identifies appropriate, lawful behaviors and practices. For example, the code of conduct probably requires all employees, subcontractors, and vendors to:

- follow agency policies and procedures
- obey all applicable local, state, and federal rules and regulations
- adhere to the standards of the applicable professional practice act
- maintain the confidentiality of patient information
- notify a designated agency official about any known or suspected wrongdoing.

The agency's compliance plan may provide for the appointment of a corporate compliance officer to disseminate the plan and monitor employee behavior. The plan may also forbid delegation of authority to people likely to pursue illegal activities. It may stipulate that employees must learn about the plan in an in-service program and then receive ongoing updates as the plan evolves.

Tips to prevent lawsuits

Here is how to reduce or eliminate the threat of a malpractice judgment in the most common types of legal action taken against nurses. Make sure you clearly document all assessment findings and nursing actions.

REASON FOR LAWSUIT	PREVENTIVE ACTION
Patient falls	• Carefully assess all patients for a risk of falling. • Take necessary precautions when caring for any patient with an increased risk of falling.
Failure to follow physician's orders or established protocols	• If you don't understand a physician's order, ask questions until you do. • If you question the wisdom of an order or protocol, bring it to the attention of the physician or your supervisor.
Medication errors	• Obtain the patient's complete drug history, including allergies, at the start of care. Document other drugs the patient takes and other drugs you see in the home. • Routinely review all of the patient's drugs to identify possible ineffective drug therapy, adverse reactions, allergies, or contraindications. • Make sure you have a valid physician's order for each drug you administer. • Make sure all medication orders include the patient's name, drug name, dosage, and route of administration. • If you're unfamiliar with a drug or an administration route, consult a reputable text or pharmacist. • If you don't understand a physician's order, ask questions until you do. • If you make an error or the patient has a drug reaction, complete an incident report within 24 hours. Recount the facts of the incident in your clinical notes. • Preserve the drug, supplies, and I.V. bag as is for possible investigation. • If asked by your agency's risk managers, help them determine why the mistake occurred and what plan could correct or prevent it in the future.
Improper use of equipment	• Know how to operate a device before you use it. • If you have misgivings about using a device, refuse to do so unless the situation is extraordinary. • Remove questionable equipment from the patient's home, and have it examined and, if necessary, repaired. • Report all equipment-related adverse effects to your supervisor or risk manager. • Report and document all equipment-related injuries.

Tips to prevent lawsuits *(continued)*	
REASON FOR LAWSUIT	**PREVENTIVE ACTION**
Failure to monitor sufficiently	• Adhere to the frequency of monitoring specified in physician's orders, in agency policies and procedures, and by the patient's condition. • Document the frequency of monitoring and the patient's status.
Failure to communicate	• Promptly report changes in the patient's symptoms and signs of distress to the physician. • Document all assessments and telephone conversations with the physician.

Your agency will give you a copy of its compliance plan and ask you to sign a document acknowledging that you received it. The compliance officer or administrator should also clearly explain the avenues by which you should report criminal conduct.

Patient rights

Since the mid-1960s, many legislative, judicial, and medical events have advanced the rights of patients in the United States. If you breach these rights, you may be sued. Some of the patient rights most important in home care include privacy, informed consent, advance directives, and do-not-resuscitate (DNR) orders.

Privacy

Although the U.S. Constitution doesn't formally sanction a right to privacy, this right has been developing since the early 1890s and has been supported by a series of Supreme Court decisions. Today, the concept of privacy includes several issues, such as the right to information about one's health status,

freedom from unwanted intrusion by health care workers, and freedom from disclosure of private facts by health care personnel. Because patients are cared for in their homes, the risk for invasion of privacy is perhaps highest among home care providers.

The concept of privacy also gives home care patients the right to:
• choose a health care provider
• be admitted to care only if the agency has sufficient resources
• participate in planning and revising services
• request and receive information about the diagnosis and applicable services, including alternative treatments and associated risks
• be informed — verbally and in writing — before care begins about the extent to which the agency expects Medicare or another payer to pay for services and the amount that may be required from the patient
• receive quality service free from discrimination based on age, race, color, creed, national origin, religion, gender, sexual preference, or disability
• receive care from a health care team that is qualified and experienced

Tips for upholding a patient's rights

How can you uphold your patient's rights? Start by following these tips:

• Help the patient understand his illness, the goals of planned treatments, and his ultimate prognosis.

• Develop a plan of care that incorporates both the physician's orders and the patient's goals and wishes.

• Make sure your nursing diagnoses meet your patient's needs and the physician's orders.

• Involve the patient and family in making decisions about care, interventions, risks, and outcomes.

• Communicate in terms the patient and family can understand and from which they can make sound decisions.

• Act as the patient's advocate.

• Openly discuss the patient's ability to follow health care instructions, with the patient, family, and other health care personnel involved in the patient's care.

• Give repeated instructions and ask for multiple return demonstrations over a specified time to make sure the patient and family can meet the plan of care.

• Carefully document all aspects of teaching, including return demonstrations, to provide evidence of the patient's ability to follow the plan of care.

• If the patient or family members can't follow instructions or adequately perform tasks, inform the physician and suggest using additional ancillary personnel, providing additional services, or exploring the benefits of an alternative care setting.

• Reveal information about the patient's health status only with his consent or as permitted by state law.

• receive the names, titles, and functions of each member of the team

• be treated with respect, dignity, and consideration

• have his personal property treated with respect

• be informed about advance directives

• be able to formulate an advance directive

• expect the confidentiality of all records, communications, and personal information

• receive information about proposed changes in service that result from an altered health status or available resources

• be informed of the frequency of services being performed and any changes in the schedule

• refuse all or some services and treatments and be informed of the possible consequences

• be fully informed about policies regarding payment for services

• be informed — verbally and in writing — as soon as possible and no more than 30 days after the agency finds out, about changes in the cost of items and services for which the patient may have to pay

• have a family member or guardian exercise the patient's rights, if he's been judged incompetent

• have access to health records upon written request, unless contraindicated in the medical record

• be notified before being transferred to another home care provider or having home services terminated

• initiate grievances and make suggestions in policies and services without fear of reprisal or discrimination

• be informed of the state's home health agency hotline telephone number and hours of operation.

All members of the home care team must understand patient rights and know how to protect them. (See *Tips for upholding a patient's rights.*) At the start of home care, give the patient a written outline of his rights and review it with him. Keep the patient fully informed about his care, and do your best to clarify issues on which the patient is confused or ill informed. You have a legal and ethical responsibility to make sure that the patient, a caregiver, or both, have a clear understanding of the patient's condition and the services being provided.

Confidentiality

As the use of electronic patient records increases, worries over patient confidentiality are also increasing. While legislators and health care groups debate how to best ensure the security of electronic patient data, your most prudent course of action is to know and uphold your state's laws and your agency's policies about confidentiality. Most agencies have requirements like these:

• Records must be maintained and secured in a safe place and used only for intended purposes and only by those authorized to use them.

• Access to confidential information in a patient's record is given only to those involved in planning, providing, or evaluating the patient's care.

• Confidential patient or family information may be released to third-party payers, government agencies, and other agencies not involved in the patient's

care only with permission from the patient and family.

• Original patient records are kept in the agency's office. Staff members should only take copies of authorized information into the field.

• When travel folders are used, they must be stored in secure containers in locked vehicles during transport.

Failure to strictly comply with your agency's policies and state and federal laws could lead to criminal, civil, or disciplinary action; termination of employment; or all of the above.

Informed consent

One of the most important patient rights is the right to accept or refuse care. Except during an emergency, a patient or his legal representative must voluntarily authorize health care providers to render treatment by giving informed consent. If you render care without a patient's informed consent, you could be sued for battery (touching a person without legal permission to do so) even if the result turns out to be positive.

Consent isn't as simple as the patient merely saying "yes" or signing a hospital form. The law requires that the patient give *informed* consent. This makes you responsible to give the patient as many material facts as necessary for him to reasonably understand his situation and to make an informed choice among his treatment options. (See *Elements of informed consent*, page 46.) You must obtain informed consent for all procedures and treatments.

The patient may give either express or implied consent. Express consent is given through direct words, either ver-

Elements of informed consent

To give informed consent, your patient must sign a consent statement, and he must receive the following information in terms he can comprehend:

• a brief but complete explanation of the care, treatment, or procedure to be performed

• the name and qualifications of the person who will be performing the care, treatment, or procedure and any names and qualifications of others who may be assisting with care

• an explanation of any serious harm that may occur during the care, treatment, or procedure, including death if it's a realistic outcome, as well as pain and discomfort during and after the care, treatment, or procedure

• a description of alternatives to the recommended care, treatment, or procedure, including the risks of doing nothing at all

• an explanation of the risks incurred by refusing the recommended care, treatment, or procedure

• assurance that he may refuse the recommended care, treatment, or procedure without having other types of care or support discontinued

• the fact that he may refuse to continue care even after the care, treatment, or procedure begins.

it. Verbally expressed consent is unlikely to protect you if the patient or his family argues a lack of informed consent.

Implied consent is inferred by the patient's conduct or assumed in an emergency. For example, if you tell a patient that he needs an injection and he holds out his arm, his actions have given you implied consent. To protect yourself legally, you should never rely on implied consent except in an emergency or for a minor whose parent or guardian can't be reached. Remember, however, that the patient must be unable to make his wishes known and that a delay in treatment must threaten permanent harm. The treatment you give must be something a reasonable patient would allow, and you must have no reason to believe the patient would deny care if he could.

To make sure you maintain a patient's informed consent throughout home care, follow these guidelines:

• Continuously assess the patient's competence.

• Communicate openly with the patient.

• Clearly explain each procedure, its risks and alternatives, and the risks of not doing it.

• Respect the patient's right to refuse.

• Know your state's laws regarding patient refusals of life-sustaining treatments.

• Remember that informed consent is fluid and can be changed.

• If you think your patient has misunderstood something you explained, clarify it.

• Tell your supervisor or the physician if the patient withdraws consent or you have reason to believe that the stan-

bally or in writing. For example, when a patient says "okay" after you tell him that he needs an insulin injection, he has given you express consent. As a rule, express consent is the type usually sought by health care providers. In home care, you should obtain the patient's written consent on your first vis-

dards of informed consent haven't been met.

• Don't try to talk a reluctant patient through his reluctance. Instead, notify the physician.

• Thoroughly document all interactions, actions, responses, and communication with the patient and caregivers.

Even if a patient has given informed consent, he still has the right to refuse care at any time. He need only to notify you or your agency that he no longer wants your services. If he does so, carefully explain the ramifications of his choice. Document the details of the patient's decision fully and notify his physician. In rare cases, if the danger of stopping care poses too great a threat for the patient, the law may allow it to continue — but you may need a court order.

Advance directives

The Patient Self-Determination Act of 1991 requires Medicare- and Medicaid-funded health care providers to ask patients if they have an advance directive and to provide appropriate forms if the patient needs them. (See *Handling advance directives,* page 48.) An advance directive is a legal document that expresses a patient's wishes about his health care. In most states, it takes the form of a living will or a durable power of attorney for health care; usually, the patient should have both.

A living will specifies the types of treatments a patient wants — and doesn't want — if he becomes unable to make decisions for himself because of terminal illness or a persistent vegetative state. It recognizes the patient's wish not to prolong life artificially through life-support or food and water supplied artificially. A living will provides instructions directly to the medical team and caregivers.

In a durable power of attorney for health care, the patient appoints a particular person to make medical decisions for him if he becomes unable to do so. In most states, the patient's physician can't perform this role. The document becomes effective when the patient is temporarily or permanently unable to make decisions about his treatment. It's no longer in effect when the patient can resume making decisions.

Before or during admission and before you provide any care, you must take the following steps:

• Ask whether the patient has an advance directive.

• If he has one, place a copy in his chart. Or, place a prominent note in the chart that says whether or not he has an advance directive.

• If he doesn't have one, verbally review and provide written information about advance directives.

• Provide the patient with appropriate forms or tell him where to obtain them.

• Have the patient indicate his understanding of the information you provide by signing a document provided by your agency.

Many nurses and other health care providers find the regulatory aspect of advance directives much easier to handle than the emotional aspect. After all, the issues outlined in an advance directive are highly personal, especially the exact circumstances under which the document is to be invoked. It's crucially important, however, that you overcome your discomfort and talk with

Handling advance directives

To handle advance directives safely and correctly, follow these tips:
• Review your state's statutes concerning do-not-resuscitate orders, durable powers of attorney for health care, and living wills.
• Ask your agency's attorney to hold an in-service program so that all providers can become fully aware of the statutory requirements and the means by which advance directives are enforced.
• Review the agency's policy and procedure manual for any guidelines about advance directives.
• Follow all agency policies carefully.
• Immediately inform your supervisor and the patient's physician about the existence of an advance directive.
• Document the existence of the advance directive in the patient's record.
• Obtain a copy of the advance directive and place it in the patient's record.
• Make sure other home care providers know the document exists.
• Make sure the patient has signed and dated the advance directive and that the appropriate number of witnesses were present, as required by state law.

• Avoid acting as a witness to the document; your status as a care provider may invalidate the document.
• Ask the patient to review and sign the advance directive annually.
• If the patient revokes the document verbally, document it in writing and notify the agency and attending physician immediately, even if the patient's competence is unclear.
• Read the document to determine the scope of the provisions and clarify them, if necessary, while the patient is still capable of doing so.
• Document any clarification supplied by the patient about the document.
• If someone other than the patient prepared or signed the advance directive, document it in the patient's record; certify that the signatory is the patient's legal guardian.
• If the advance directive goes into effect, help family members in this time of crisis by being available and by answering as many of their questions as possible. Give them time to accept the consequences of the patient's directive.

your patients about their wishes. In most states, family members aren't permitted to override a patient's written requests unless they can prove that the document is invalid. So, completing an advance directive is the best way for a patient to be sure his wishes will be carried out.

DNR orders

One type of treatment a patient may choose to specifically refuse is cardiopulmonary resuscitation. A DNR order is a written physician's order instructing the home care team not to resuscitate a patient whose heart or breathing stops. Typically, a DNR order is considered appropriate when the patient has a terminal medical condition or is in a permanently unconscious

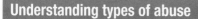

Understanding types of abuse

Abuse raises many difficult issues, including the emotions that stem from discovering it, the personal and professional uncertainty about when to report it, the struggle to understand it, and the broad definitions that may apply. To help understand the types of abuse and neglect you may see, review these definitions.

Abuse

Material or financial abuse: Stealing funds or property, such as eating meals given to the patient by a community meal service and using the patient's medical card to obtain drugs for use by someone other than the patient

Physical abuse: Intentional infliction of physical harm, such as bruising, burning, and sexual molestation

Psychological abuse: Emotional harm inflicted by verbal aggression, insult, instilling fear, or berating a person

Self-abuse: Self-inflicted harm such as refusing to eat

Neglect

Active neglect: Intentional infliction of harm by neglecting to provide something the patient needs, such as withholding food or a prescribed drug

Neglect: Paying too little attention or being remiss in care, such as leaving a patient to lie in wet bed linens for several hours and ignoring the patient's request for analgesia

Passive neglect: Unintentional infliction of harm caused by caregiver inability, lack of knowledge, or laziness — such as failing to give personal care at regular intervals

or vegetative state as well as when resuscitation would be considered medically futile.

The patient's physician is responsible for explaining his diagnosis and prognosis, for describing the purpose of a DNR order, and for outlining the circumstances during which such an order would be invoked. However, your agency will most likely impose these requirements when you work with DNR orders. A DNR order must be:
• obtained from the physician and placed in the patient's medical record
• reviewed and confirmed with the patient and caregiver
• reviewed upon recertification of home care services and with any sig-

nificant change in the patient's condition.

Remember that a patient, custodial parent, or legal guardian can revoke a DNR order at any time.

Patient abuse

Abuse refers to the mistreatment of a person that ultimately results in physical or emotional pain or injury. (See *Understanding types of abuse.*) You may be the first person to identify signs of neglect or abuse. If you do see signs, you're required by law to make a "good faith" report of your suspicions. In other words, if you report suspected neglect or abuse in good faith, the law will protect you from retribution if your suspicions are unfounded. You don't need inconclusive evidence before reporting neglect or abuse; you just need evidence that a reasonable person would consider suspicious.

Your agency almost certainly has policies and procedures for you to follow if you suspect that a patient is being neglected or abused. It should include these elements:

• interventions to minimize the risk of neglect or abuse
• signs of neglect and abuse, including self-neglect and self-abuse
• instructions to immediately report any knowledge or suspicion of abuse to your supervisor
• instructions to consult with the patient's physician when indicated
• an explanation of when referral to community services is appropriate and instruction to report all such referrals to the patient's physician.

As in all other areas, you must maintain patient confidentiality during the reporting and investigation of patient neglect or abuse. Also, appropriate disciplinary action must be taken against any employee involved in patient neglect or abuse.

Restraints

Home health care personnel must work to provide the most benefit and minimize possible harm to all patients — especially those who are elderly or suffering from dementia.

Physical restraints

A physical restraint is something — a device or piece of cloth, for example — used to restrict a patient's freedom of movement that can't be easily removed. If a patient may need to be restrained at home, explain the appropriate devices to the patient and caregiver. When a restraint is in place, make sure you or someone else assesses the patient at least once every 2 hours to ensure the patient's safety, comfort, body alignment, circulation, and skin integrity and assess the need for continued restraint. Also, make sure the patient has a call device within reach.

If you believe that restraints are being used in a neglectful or an abusive manner, document your concerns and reeducate the caregiver about how to use restraints properly. If your concerns continue, you'll need to report the problem to your supervisor.

Chemical restraints

A chemical restraint is a psychoactive drug used to minimize behavioral problems that make a patient dangerous to himself or others. State and federal laws bar you from using chemical restraints to treat depression, psychosis, Alzheimer's disease, and other dementias. Also, never use a chemical restraint as a substitute for delivering patient care or educating a caregiver to give care.

Chemical restraints have a number of potential drawbacks, including an increased risk of falling and being injured, urine retention, skin breakdown, visual disturbances, constipation, and hallucinations. Urge caregivers to use alternatives to chemical restraints whenever possible by developing a toileting schedule; providing smaller, more frequent meals; finding other methods for pain control; controlling external stimuli; and attending promptly to the patient's needs.

Before you resort to using any type of restraint, try to circumvent the need for it. For example, try occupying the patient with repetitive tasks. Ask family members or volunteers to spend time with the patient. Or, place alarms on doors to prevent the patient from slipping out. These actions help to preserve the patient's freedom and dignity while promoting kindness and compassion.

If you must restrain a patient, obtain a physician's order that specifies the type of restraint to be used, why it's needed, when it should be used, and for how long it should be used. Fully document your physical and psychosocial assessment of the patient, all measures you took to avoid using a restraint, and the behavior that warranted use of the restraint.

Noncompliance

Noncompliance by patients and caregivers is a significant concern in home care. In too many cases, a patient's outcome is hampered by his or his caregiver's inability or unwillingness to follow instructions, take or administer ordered drugs, and refrain from or perform activities as requested.

Many patients have trouble adapting to treatment, drug, and dosage changes as well as selecting food they aren't used to eating. Make every effort to ensure compliance through teaching and demonstration that is relevant to the patient's immediate needs. If appropriate, try teaching for brief periods and addressing specific concerns at each visit. Reeducate the patient or caregiver as specific problems arise.

If you find that a patient or caregiver is repeatedly noncompliant, listen carefully for clues that reveal the reason. Perhaps the patient doesn't understand something about the care he needs. Perhaps he has too little money to buy the drugs he needs. Document any statements the patient makes about noncompliance. Also document your response to noncompliance and the methods you employed to correct the problem. Inform the patient and family about the consequences of noncompliance; document this discussion. Have a second person validate issues pertinent to the patient's noncompliance, as appropriate.

If the patient's noncompliance causes his condition to deteriorate rapidly or causes him undue stress and suffering, explore other care settings as needed. Throughout, document thoroughly and adhere strictly to your agency's policies.

Incompetent caregivers

In acute care settings, you rarely encounter an incompetent caregiver. In the home care setting, however, this happens a lot. This is because home caregivers are commonly family members, friends, neighbors, and paid unprofessional help. To help minimize the effects of caregiver incompetence, you'll need to involve caregivers in

Supervising a home care aide

When supervising a home care aide, check to make sure that she's:
• developing a good rapport with the patient and family
• delivering service with which the patient is satisfied
• maintaining the patient's personal hygiene
• keeping the patient's environment clean and orderly
• responding to patient requests in a timely manner
• using equipment and supplies effectively and efficiently
• completing assignments in an organized and timely manner
• writing concise, legible documentation
• producing documentation that demonstrates knowledge of the assignment
• using proper body mechanics
• complying with the agency's policies and procedures
• reporting adverse reactions, problems, or changes in the patient's condition.

the patient's plan of care from the beginning.

Commonly, caregiver incompetence stems from a lack of knowledge. You can help remedy this problem by:
• providing instructions — including written information — at the caregiver's level of comprehension
• reviewing important procedures at each visit
• asking the caregiver to demonstrate procedures

• reminding the caregiver about the patient's goals
• praising the caregiver for what he does correctly and for his contribution to the care of the patient
• asking questions and being a good listener
• developing alternatives for care that the caregiver finds more comfortable or easier to understand
• clarifying what the caregiver is expected to do
• addressing the consequences of noncompliance
• using physical therapy, speech therapy, occupational therapy, social services, or home care aides, if possible, to ease the caregiver's burden.

A caregiver's incompetence may also stem from a physical or mental inability to perform the needed tasks. If so, investigate other caregivers, other care settings, and the possibility of expanding the services provided by your agency. Document your concerns, possible options, referrals, and your consultation with the patient's physician.

Home care aide supervision

According to Medicare's conditions of participation for home care agencies, home care aides require supervision. If an aide receives inadequate supervision and an injury results, you and your agency could be liable.

If the patient is receiving a skilled service, supervision of home care aides typically takes the form of a supervisory visit that occurs at least once every two weeks. (See *Supervising a home care aide.*) The aide need not be present at this visit. Take the opportunity to talk with the patient and family about the aide and the care she delivers. If the aide is present, observe her directly and provide teaching and discussion as needed.

If the patient receives no skilled service, you should make a supervisory visit at least once every 62 days while an aide is working in the patient's home. Assess patient and family relationships with the aide, assess the aide's delivery of care, and determine whether patient outcomes are being met. Make sure you always document supervision of a home care aide in the patient's chart.

Litigation

If you're served with a subpoena, summons, or other legal notice, alert your supervisor immediately. Don't give out any information—written or verbal—on the topic of the legal action unless directed to do so by the agency's attorney. Refer all inquiries to the agency's attorney.

If, despite your best efforts, you're named as a defendant in a patient's lawsuit, you may need your own attorney. If so, keep these tips in mind:
- Choose an attorney who specializes in the appropriate area of law.
- Make sure your attorney has no conflicts of interest in your case.
- Inquire up front about your attorney's fees.
- Choose an attorney who answers your questions and concerns promptly.
- If you don't understand something your attorney says, ask for a different explanation.

- Expect your attorney to respect your objectives, including whether or not to settle your case. If you choose not to settle, ask how much the ongoing litigation will cost.
- Provide your attorney with all the facts surrounding the case; don't try to judge what is important.
- Tell your attorney where and how to contact you.
- Tell your attorney what information you want to know and who you've authorized to discuss the case with him.
- Don't discuss your case with your friends.
- Discuss who will review the home care records.
- Ask whether there will be a jury and what evidence the jury will hear.
- Ask about mediation and other alternative dispute resolutions.

Although the threat of a lawsuit is real and, for many nurses, frightening, it need not monopolize your professional life. In all likelihood, you're already doing what you need to do to prevent a legal judgment against you:
- upholding accepted standards of nursing practice, adhering to your agency's policies and procedures, and following physicians' orders
- assessing thoroughly, intervening appropriately, and documenting carefully
- developing caring, trusting relationships with your patients and their families.

Preparing for and conducting home visits

When a patient meets his insurer's eligibility requirements and your agency agrees to provide home care, you and other members of the team assume a great responsibility: to provide safe, timely, cost-effective, appropriate care that adheres to your scope of practice, your agency's policies and procedures, and the insurer's requirements. To achieve this goal, you need to understand how patients qualify for home care, how to execute your role on the home care team, and how to conduct safe home visits.

Home care qualification

Home care services begin when the agency receives a patient referral. It may originate with the discharging facility, a physician, or the patient's family or friends. A typical patient referral

includes a physician's order (which is required for reimbursement), patient history and diagnosis, special treatment needs, drugs and supplies, goals and expected outcomes, insurance coverage, and demographic data. Nursing administration at your agency then decides whether the agency can meet the patient's medical, nursing, and social needs in the home, based on the referral information, agency policies, and insurance coverage.

Next, you or another nurse will confirm that the patient is eligible for services by visiting the home. Remember, however, that this first visit is considered administrative and, thus, isn't covered by insurance. That is why you should use all the information at your disposal to determine eligibility before you go to the patient's home. For instance, if you call to schedule the first home visit and the patient says she can't be there because she has to drive her car across town to be serviced, you know that the patient isn't homebound and, therefore, isn't eligible for Medicare reimbursement. You may also want to consult with the patient's physician about the patient's need for services. You may need to investigate other sources of funding.

Keep in mind that not every patient referred for home care is eligible or appropriate. You and other agency officials need to make sure the agency and the patient's needs meet Medicare's conditions of participation or the requirements of another third party payer.

Medicare requirements

To receive reimbursement from Medicare, your agency must be certified by Medicare, and the patient must meet the following criteria:

• The patient must be age 65 or older or permanently disabled.
• The patient must need part-time (up to 8 hours daily or 35 hours weekly) or intermittent (at least once every 60 to 90 days) skilled service. These services include nursing, physical therapy, and speech therapy. Occupational therapy is considered a skilled service when a nurse, physical therapist, or speech pathologist establishes the need for it.
• The patient must be homebound. (See *Is your patient homebound?*)
• The services must be covered by Medicare's home health benefit (no custodial or maintenance care, for instance) and be deemed reasonable and necessary.
• The patient must have a physician's certification and a plan of care (Health Care Financing Administration [HCFA] form 485). The plan of care must contain all data pertinent to the patient's condition and must specify the type, frequency, and duration of services and the type of professional who will pro-

Is your patient homebound?

For your agency to obtain Medicare reimbursement, your patient must fit Medicare's definition of homebound, which means being confined to one's home — although not necessarily bedridden — for medical reasons.

A patient is homebound if:
• He can't leave home.
• He leaves home only with great effort and difficulty.
• He leaves home infrequently, for a short time, or to receive medical care.

A patient isn't homebound if:
• He leaves home frequently for social activities.
• He drives a car.
• He goes to an adult day-care center for nonmedical reasons.
• He goes to a relative's home regularly.
• He goes grocery shopping or does other business regularly.
• He stays home because of feebleness or insecurity (unless he also meets one of the criteria that qualifies him as being homebound).

vide them. The physician who signs the plan of care should be the attending physician and should see the patient periodically. The plan must be updated, or recertified, every 60 to 62 days, typically by a nurse or physical therapist and approved by a physician. If visits occur 5 to 7 days per week, the plan must specify an end date. Medicare will consider the patient discharged from home care if a physician's order doesn't specify a need for visits at least once every 90 days.

Why patients aren't accepted for home care

Not all patients referred for home care will end up receiving it. Here are some common reasons why.
- The patient refuses care.
- The patient doesn't need skilled care.
- The patient lives outside the geographic area served.
- The patient isn't under a physician's care.
- The agency can't provide the needed services.
- The attitude of the patient, the caregiver, or both isn't conducive to therapeutic home care.
- The patient's needs can't be met at home.
- The requested services aren't reasonable or necessary to treat an illness or injury.

- Medicare must be the primary payer, and the patient must have no other primary insurance.
- The patient must not need a level of care that can only be provided in a hospital or an extended care facility.
- The patient, caregiver, or both must be physically and emotionally able and willing to take part in the plan of care and respond to medical emergencies.
- A primary caregiver must be available to the patient whenever professionals aren't present.
- The patient must have shelter, food, clothing, and protection, and the patient's home environment must be conducive to safe, proper, and effective care.
- The patient's environment must not risk the safety of the home care team.

- The patient must live inside the agency's service area.
- For Medicare to cover hospice care, the patient must be eligible for Medicare Part A, have a life expectancy of less than 6 months, live within range of a Medicare-certified hospice program, have a written plan of care that is reviewed regularly, and activate Medicare's hospice benefit.

Covered skills

If the patient is a Medicare beneficiary, Medicare is the correct payer, and the patient meets the criteria for homebound status, Medicare will pay for the following 15 skills:

- observation or assessment that requires the skills of a professional nurse
- management and evaluation of the patient's plan of care
- patient teaching, injections, disease processes, and preventive measures
- wound care
- ostomy care
- skilled nursing visits
- drug administration and instruction
- home care aide visits
- medical social worker visits
- catheter insertion and maintenance
- oxygen administration
- case management to eliminate multiple visits to the emergency department or hospital
- suctioning
- safety evaluation of the home
- physical, occupational, or speech therapy.

If the patient meets Medicare's criteria for home care coverage and needs one or more of the services listed here, your agency can refuse to provide home care only for certain reasons. (See *Why patients aren't accepted for home care.*) Those reasons don't include the person's age, race, sex, color, creed, religion, national origin, disability, sexual preference, or ability to pay. If a patient doesn't receive home care, referrals to other community resources may be helpful.

Managed care requirements

Most managed care organizations have requirements similar to those of Medicare. However, some may differ. For instance:
• The managed care plan typically authorizes a specific number of visits eligible for reimbursement.
• If the patient needs more visits or needs them more often, the plan must approve them.
• The plan typically must approve equipment, supplies, and support services (such as homemaker and nonmedical services) in advance.

Your role in home care

To fulfill your role as a home care nurse, you'll need to be able to accomplish a number of tasks beyond delivering whatever care the patient needs. For example, you'll need to be able to discern what other services the patient may need. You'll need to help determine the frequency and duration of home visits that are necessary to meet the patient's needs. You'll need to perform an initial assessment and ongoing evaluation of the patient's condition. And you'll need to prepare the patient for discharge.

Needed services

At your initial visit and throughout home care, you are responsible for determining the patient's need for service. Usually, you'll be the one making referrals for other disciplines, such as physical therapy and occupational therapy. (See *Common reasons for referrals,* page 58.) For each of these disciplines, specific instructions for visit frequency, duration of service, and care to be provided must be written in the patient's plan of care and signed by the physician.

Visit frequency and duration of service

You'll also need to make judgments about the frequency and duration of visits. Frequency refers to the number of visits per discipline in a specified number of days, weeks, or months. Duration refers to the number of days, weeks, or months that services will be rendered.

Frequency

The appropriate frequency of visits is determined by several factors:
• the patient's condition, including functional limitations, activity requirements, and restrictions
• acuity of the condition being treated
• ability of the patient and family to provide care and learn new concepts and skills
• physician's orders
• your judgment of the patient's needs and home environment
• requirements of the reimbursement source.

Typically, the frequency of visits declines as the patient's condition

Common reasons for referrals

When you evaluate a patient's need for home care services, part of your job involves assessing his need for other services, such as physical therapy, speech therapy, occupational therapy, and home care aide visits. Here are some common reasons for making referrals to these other disciplines.

DISCIPLINE	REASONS FOR REFERRAL
Physical therapy	• Unsafe ambulation or transfers • Home assessment for safety and necessary modifications • Assessment for use of or teaching about assistive devices • Significant change in patient's mobility status • Problems with balance and coordination • Loss of function in one or more limbs • Need for restorative therapy • Worsening of chronic condition that decreases physical function • Impaired pulmonary function that necessitates chest physiotherapy and instruction • Need for specialized tests such as ultrasound • Need for caregiver instruction in proper body mechanics • Need for instructions in easiest and most efficient methods to accomplish activities of daily living (ADLs)
Speech therapy	• Impaired or lost communication skills • Weakness of facial or throat muscles and difficulty swallowing • Loss of phonation • Changes in receptive or expressive abilities • Memory deficits • Difficulty reading, writing, or seeing • Apraxia • Neurologic impairment • Hearing loss
Occupational therapy	• Impaired ability to perform ADLs • Decreased strength and range of motion in arms • Impaired fine motor skills, sensation, or cognitive and perceptual motor abilities • Need for reality orientation planning • Impaired body image • Impaired ability to write, use the telephone, and make needs known • Need for teaching about joint protection techniques, pain management skills, or energy conservation • Need for home adaptations
Home care aide visits	• Need for help with personal care (primary indication) • Need for simple dressing changes • Need for help with medications and activities supported by skilled disciplines

improves and goals are achieved. If you believe, however, that the patient's condition warrants additional visits, you'll need to obtain a physician's order for the altered plan of care. Make sure your documentation reflects the need for increased visits.

If a managed care organization is paying for care, the patient's insurance plan will probably specify the visit frequency; you'll confirm it at your first visit to the patient's home. If you feel the patient needs more than the number of visits that have been approved, you'll need to contact the managed care organization and explain the medical need for additional visits.

Duration

The duration of home care is typically set by the payer as well. For Medicare, the duration is 62 days. During that time, the patient's plan of care is reviewed to determine whether more time is needed to meet the goals of care. If so, you and the patient's physician will need to complete a progress report that contains orders for 62 more days. This progress report is called a recertification.

For other insurers, duration may differ. A managed care plan may stipulate any duration of service based on the reason why the patient needs home care. Visits that extend beyond the approved duration must be approved beforehand by the managed care organization, or they may not be covered by the patient's insurance.

Assessment and evaluation

You'll probably be responsible for many important aspects of the patient's care, such as:

Assigning ICD-9 codes

The Health Care Financing Administration (HCFA), which administers Medicare, requires you to use a set of numbers called International Classification of Diseases (ICD-9) codes to translate the patient's diagnoses on HCFA form 485, the one you use to prepare a plan of treatment. These codes are recognized throughout the medical, insurance, and health finance community. Here is what you need to do to use them properly.

• Identify each service, procedure, or supply with an ICD-9 code.

• Code the primary diagnosis first, followed by the secondary diagnosis, tertiary diagnosis, and so on.

• List as supplementary information any coexisting conditions that affect the patient's treatment, procedure, or visit.

• Carry the code to the fourth or fifth digit if possible.

• Code a chronic disease when applicable to the patient's treatment. For example, code 402.01 (hypertension with congestive heart failure) adequately supports the need for skilled care.

• completing the initial nursing assessment, typically within 24 hours after the start of care

• developing the plan of care using HCFA form 485 after consulting the physician's treatment plan and the patient and caregivers (See *Assigning ICD-9 codes.*)

• assessing the patient at each visit

• evaluating the need for changes in the plan of care or visit frequency

Criteria for discharge from home care

Your patient may be discharged from home care if he meets any of the following criteria:

• Therapeutic goals have been achieved or are no longer attainable.

• The patient's medical condition requires services that can't be provided intermittently at home.

• The home environment has changed and is no longer consistent with safe or proper patient care.

• The patient or caregiver isn't able or willing to participate in the plan of care.

• The patient or caregiver repeatedly fails to comply with the physician's orders.

• Medical orders aren't recertified.

• The patient moves out of the service area and needs referrals to community resources in the new location.

• The patient, caregiver, or attending physician requests that services be terminated.

• Continuing to provide services creates a real or potential safety risk for the home care staff.

• The patient wasn't home for two or more scheduled visits and failed to notify the agency.

• The patient is referred to another facility or service because the home care agency can't meet the patient's needs.

• The patient dies.

• supervising the home care aide at the first visit and every 14 days thereafter

• reporting all changes in the patient's condition to the physician

• making referrals for medical equipment and supervising a timely, efficient response.

Remember that HCFA form 485, on which you generate the patient's plan of care, is a legal document that specifies physician's orders, goals for the patient, visit frequency and duration, needed drugs, and specific orders for evaluation by other services such as medical social services. The physician must sign this document and return it to the agency, typically within 14 days. If the patient's condition changes or he needs services for longer than planned, you'll need to fill out another HCFA form 485 and have the patient recertified.

Any time you send a new or revised order to the physician, keep a copy in the patient's chart. The same procedure applies for verbal orders; as soon as you receive one, write down the date; the patient's name, address, and medical number; the physician's full name and address; and the order. Sign and date the order, place a copy in the patient's chart, and send the original to the physician to be signed. Typically, the physician must return the signed order to the agency within 14 days. When it arrives, someone at the agency will stamp it with the date it was received, place it in the patient's chart, and discard the copy.

Discharge plan

Usually, a patient's discharge from home care is planned from the beginning. The payer, home care agency, patient, and family should all know the discharge date. However, keep in mind that a patient may be discharged from home health care for a variety of reasons. (See *Criteria for discharge from home care.*)

Under certain circumstances, the patient may not be discharged but instead placed on hold. This could happen if a managed care plan approves it, if the patient is rehospitalized and a diagnosis is confirmed, or if a therapist is waiting for the arrival of a device, such as a prosthesis, after which home care will continue.

Visit safety

When you work in a patient's home, you have less control over the environment and less control over your patient than you would in a hospital or other facility. What is more, you must consider yourself a guest in your patient's home, and treat him with respect even if his customs and lifestyle choices are foreign to you. Each person has differing thoughts about religion, diet, spending money, cleaning house, disciplining children, and performing health care practices. You may find a sense of humor and a nonjudgmental attitude to be some of your most useful tools when working in home care.

Other useful and necessary tools are those you use to ensure your safety and the safety of your patients and their families. In the home environment, safety is a more complex issue than it is in a controlled setting. There is more for you to think about and watch for and, occasionally, you may face danger. Even in safe homes, you need to maintain a level of watchfulness that is rarely necessary in health care facilities.

Agency safety measures

Especially if you work in a high-risk area, agency officials will do what they can to safeguard you. Before you visit a patient's home, agency personnel may:
- assess the level of risk in the neighborhood where you're going, possibly by hiring a safety consultant to assess risk levels in communities throughout the service area
- consult reports from workers who have visited that neighborhood
- work with the district's community relations officer to assess risk neighborhoods served by the agency
- establish close ties with law enforcement officers in high-risk areas
- communicate openly with local police to help guide the actions of visiting home care workers
- hire retired police officers or other trained people to act as escorts for home care workers
- adopt a policy of sending two people rather than one into high-risk areas
- require workers to call in at the end of their day or at designated times
- provide you with a cellular phone and immediate backup if you find yourself in a dangerous situation
- provide training in personal safety awareness, drug awareness, and proactive safety measures
- provide basic safety equipment. (See *Elements of a safety tool kit,* page 62.)

By taking these and other concrete steps, agency administrators show their concern for your safety. They also should be willing to stop sending you

Elements of a safety tool kit

Your agency may supply you with safety tools such as the ones listed here:
• handheld alarm that emits a loud noise when activated
• cellular phone
• large and powerful flashlight to help identify house numbers and street names in the dark
• smaller flashlight to help assess the patient's home and navigate dark halls or stairs
• capsicum (pepper) spray, if you're willing to use it and your agency and local authorities allow it.

If your agency doesn't supply you with these tools, consider obtaining them on your own to help ensure your safety.

into an area where you feel threatened or uneasy.

Personal safety measures

Although your agency can do much to promote your safety, on-the-spot decisions ultimately fall on you. In a potentially threatening situation, it's up to you to handle yourself and the situation appropriately. To help ensure your personal safety, take these steps:
• Never give patients or caregivers (active or discharged) your personal address or phone number. Instead, tell patients and caregivers to contact you through your agency and give them the 24-hour phone number.
• Tell your supervisor or director if you think a safety problem could develop with a patient or caregiver.

• If your schedule changes, notify your agency immediately, even if you're in an apparently safe neighborhood.

In addition to these objectives, you should also work to maintain the three cardinal rules that will help keep you safe when delivering home care: Be prepared, be alert, and be able to think and act without hesitation or panic. To prepare yourself, become familiar with the types of hazards you could encounter. Plan how to avoid or minimize them. Also, develop a plan for how to defend yourself or make a quick exit from a threatening situation.

The best way to stay alert is to be watchful for real problems and to avoid worrying about imagined or possible problems. Excessive worrying about what could happen may raise your risk of danger by taking your mind off what is actually happening around you.

In many threatening situations, the best defense is a cool head. That is why your ability to think calmly and respond decisively can help you steer clear of danger. Naturally, if you find yourself in a dangerous situation, your best option is to use common sense and leave.

The fact is that any home care situation can be dangerous — not only because you could be threatened but because you could be injured while caring for a patient. Whether the hazards you face stem from weapons, drugs, violence, or accidents, your awareness of possible dangers and your willingness to take simple precautions can minimize your risk and make the most of your time spent giving home care. Some of the most important safety precautions involve dressing properly, planning ahead for a visit, getting safely inside the patient's home, exiting safely after the visit, and documenting your safety concerns.

Dress properly

If your agency doesn't require you to wear a uniform, it probably has a dress code designed to help you look professional, maintain a therapeutic patient environment, and promote your safety. As specified in the dress code, choose comfortable clothing that allows you to walk briskly, move freely, and bend, stoop, stretch, and lift without undue exposure. Wearing a lab coat over your street clothes can help identify you as a health care worker. Choose shoes with nonskid soles that allow you to move quickly without slipping. Avoid earrings or other accessories that can be grasped and pulled by another person. Keep your fingernails clean and trimmed. Don't wear perfume; many people are sensitive to it, especially when ill.

Most safety experts advise against carrying a wallet or purse during home visits. Instead, keep your agency identification and driver's license in a secure pocket. Some experts suggest carrying a small amount of money, such as a ten-dollar bill, in an easily accessible pocket. This could be used in an emergency or as a distraction for a would-be attacker.

Plan ahead

Before leaving for a series of home visits, make sure you have accurate addresses and directions to each patient's home. Also, inquire about the neighborhood you'll be visiting if it's new to you. Plan the safest route to each patient's home, even if that route isn't the shortest one. Note the locations of police stations, public telephones, and other public buildings. Make sure your agency knows where you're going. Check in several times during the day so someone can track your progress, especially if you're going to a high-risk neighborhood.

Also, make sure your car is ready to go; check the fuel level, tire pressure, windshield wipers and fluid, lights, battery, and such. Before you leave, note the weather forecast and lock your purse and valuables in the trunk. Make sure that no personal items will be visible inside the car when you leave it. Carry an extra set of keys. Never enter a home that isn't posted on the schedule.

Make an entrance

When you locate the house or building where your patient lives, you'll need to find a safe parking place. In most cases, it will be the space closest to the patient's home. However, sometimes a busier, better-lit spot may make a better choice as long as it isn't too far away. When selecting a parking place, observe the neighborhood carefully and assess the approach to the patient's home. If the mood of the neighborhood seems disturbing or if you see groups of people standing around on the street, drive to a safe, well-lit place and call your supervisor. Perhaps an escort could come to your aid or a family member could escort you from an acceptable parking place into the patient's home.

If the patient lives in an apartment building, you'll need continued vigilance even after entering the building. Observe the entrance for suspicious people or activity. Quickly check the building's physical condition for immediate hazards, such as obstacles in hallways and dim lighting. Scan the stairs or elevator for potential hazards. Try to avoid using the stairs in a large building and wait for an empty elevator rather than riding with a group of people you don't know. If the elevator isn't working, ask a family member to escort you from the entrance to the apartment.

Stay alert even after you enter the patient's home. First, ask the patient or caregiver how many people and animals are present, where they are, and what they're doing. If you encounter a potentially hazardous situation, respond according to agency policy. For example, if someone is drinking in the home, consider asking him to refrain from doing it until you leave. If you see someone taking illegal drugs, ask the person to stop. If he refuses, arrange another time for the home visit and leave, according to your agency's policy. Notify your supervisor right away.

The bottom line is this: If you feel threatened for any reason when you're in a patient's home, respond proactively rather than reactively to help prevent a potential hazard from developing into a real one.

Make an exit

When leaving your patient's home, you should still be taking active safety precautions. For example, check the route to your car while still at the patient's door. Have your car keys out and ready. Use extra caution if you see unusual activity, an unusual number of people congregating, or unusual police activity. Ask a family member to escort you to your car, if necessary. As you approach the car, quickly observe the area around, under, and inside it to check for threatening people or objects, such as broken glass and sharp metal.

Document safety concerns

If you have any problems getting to a patient's home or carrying out your duties while you're there, document and report them immediately. Doing so will help prevent another staff member from encountering the same — or worse — problems and being unprepared. Your agency probably has a policy for reporting such incidents in the patient's record and for reporting them to the authorities, particularly if they involve weapons or violence.

Hazard management

Certain situations you encounter in a patient's home may create added safety concerns, such as a hostile pet, an angry patient or family member, a weapon in the home, fire hazards, mobility hazards, and other threats related to the patient's home, food, plants, products, or drugs. You also have to reduce the risks associated with mental illness, infection, and emergencies.

Hostile pets

If the patient has a dog, even if it seems to be a friendly dog, the safest course of action is to ask the patient to put the animal in another room during your visit. Even a normally calm dog may grow worried and protective during unfamiliar procedures. The dog may think that you're fighting with or harming its owner when you administer wound care, give an injection, or perform passive range-of-motion exercises, for example.

In general, it's better to avoid these possibly provocative situations by removing the dog from the room. If that isn't possible, then avoid interacting with the dog, even if it seems friendly. If you find yourself facing a hostile dog in spite of these proactive precautions, take these suggestions to help thwart — or at least control — a confrontation:

• Keep the dog in sight but don't make eye contact with him. Look down or to the side.

• Slowly move toward an exit or safe area.

• Talk to the dog in a calm, firm voice. Try giving a command. If that doesn't work, continue talking to him in a soothing but firm voice.

• Think about what object you could use to distract the dog, such as a clipboard or a box of tissues. As the dog moves toward you, drop the object in front of him. This action may distract him long enough to allow your escape.

• If a sweater or jacket is available, wrap it around your forearm. Then, if the dog lunges, push your protected arm to the back of his mouth. Use your other hand to deliver a sharp blow to his nose.

• If you get bitten despite these actions, obtain immediate treatment for the wound.

Although the risk of being bitten is much smaller if the patient has a cat instead of a dog, the risk of getting scratched is just as real. Even a scratch from a healthy cat can raise the risk of infection. Even if a patient's cat appears calm and relaxed, don't try to touch or pet it. If you do pet it and you get scratched, wash the area carefully at the patient's house, and seek medical attention after you leave. Any time you feel that a patient's pet poses a safety hazard, tell your supervisor. That way, other team members who visit the patient's home will be prepared to ask the patient to remove or contain the pet during home visits.

Hostile people

Even a seemingly safe home can be the setting for a confrontation with a threatening patient or family member. The confrontation may stem from an alcohol- or drug-induced state, a mental or physical illness, or a criminal intention. It may also represent the family's reaction to stress and anger.

No matter what creates a personal threat, the situation is still frightening and potentially dangerous. Therefore, your first goal should be to prevent a dangerous situation before it starts. Try to minimize the danger and thwart a threat by looking at the provoking situation, the people involved, their physical strength, the environment, and whether help is available. (See *Guidelines for responding to hostility,* page 66.)

If a patient or family member seems protective and hostile when you arrive, mention the patient's physician or referral source by name. Briefly explain the purpose of your visit and the assessment questions or procedures you're there to accomplish. These steps may be enough to allow the visit to proceed smoothly. If possible, defer assessment of all conditions not directly related to the need for home care until another time.

If a patient's or family member's hostility seems to stem from fear, these guidelines may help:

• Try to draw the person out.

• Find out if he ever had a frightening encounter with a stranger in the house.

Guidelines for responding to hostility

If you encounter a hostile patient or family member, use the following guidelines to help ease the situation:

• First, quickly assess the possible reason behind the hostility. Remember that behavior changes can accompany many physical and mental illnesses. Are you aware of a disorder that could be involved?

• Next, determine the level of threat involved.

• If you're facing low-level hostility, calm the person with a simple verbal intervention, such as, "You seem upset. Can we sit down and talk about your concerns?" This approach shows concern for the person's feelings.

• Try other statements as well, such as, "What can we do to make you more comfortable in this situation?" This shows caring while allowing the person to cooperate with you in reducing the threat and calming the situation. It also helps the person spend energy finding a solution rather than continuing the cycle of hostility.

• Be aware of your visible demeanor and body language.

• Find a way to look calm and confident, no matter how uneasy you may feel.

• Maintain eye contact and speak clearly and calmly.

• Be assertive but not aggressive.

• Express caring for the hostile person.

• Maintain a relaxed stance.

• Don't block the door and don't be obvious in your search for a possible escape route.

• Help him express his concerns by asking a sincere, open-ended question, such as, "What would help you feel safer in receiving home health care?"

Weapons

Weapons, especially firearms, present a real and frightening danger for home health care professionals in many home environments—from the inner city to the suburbs to rural areas. This is why it's important to know whether firearms are present in the home and what to do if they are. Your agency probably has a policy addressing these issues. In addition to this policy, other helpful guidelines include the following:

• Don't allow the patient or his family to keep a loaded firearm in the same room where you're delivering care.

• If the patient is willing to remove the gun to a safer (and preferably locked) location, make a verbal or written agreement that the patient will continue to store the gun elsewhere during home care visits.

• If the patient refuses to remove a gun from the room, stop the visit and leave, making it clear why you're leaving.

• Notify your supervisor and the patient's physician about the gun. Your agency may have an incident report on which to document the problem.

Fire hazards

Fires are a common cause of accidents in the home, and cigarettes are a common cause of household fires. A cigarette, if dropped on a sofa, a bed, or an upholstered chair, may smolder for hours before suddenly turning into a major blaze. Other fire risks include space heaters, wood- and coal-burning stoves, electrical appliances, and a lack of smoke detectors. To detect possible fire hazards in the home, check for these risk factors:

- family members who smoke
- use of ashtrays for trash
- emptying of ashtrays before cigarettes are completely out
- presence of small children in the home
- easy availability of matches and lighters
- small space heaters located near furnishings, flammable materials, or high-traffic areas
- stove installation by an unqualified person without regard for building codes
- improper storage of fuel for heaters or stoves
- electrical cords crossing the flow of traffic or stretched under furniture or carpets
- frayed or cracked electrical cords
- overloaded electrical cords
- electrical outlets and switches with cover plates that are markedly warm to the touch
- exposed wiring or overloaded electrical circuits
- no safety covers over unused electrical outlets (if small children are in the home)
- light bulbs of inappropriate size and type for lamps or fixtures
- lack of smoke detectors or lack of functional batteries in smoke detectors
- inadequate number or placement of smoke detectors.

Mobility hazards

Falls are another common cause of injury in the home. Assess the risk of falling and other injuries by checking for these risk factors:

- cluttered walkways
- loose rugs that aren't tacked down
- slippery floors, especially in the kitchen or bathroom
- poorly lit stairways
- no light switches at the top and bottom of stairs
- no night-lights
- absent, loose, or partial handrails along the stairs
- flimsy fixtures holding handrails to the walls
- insecure footing, loose treads, frayed carpet, or obstacles on stairs
- stair edges obscured by dark or deep pile carpeting
- items stored on stairs
- variation in the height of individual stairs
- poorly lit or cluttered passages and walkways
- dimly lit rooms.

Although mobility hazards can affect any patient, they're especially dangerous for elderly patients and those with problems involving gait or mentation. For example, certain types of cerebrovascular accidents and dementias can give the patient a false sense about his ability to walk. Also, patients recovering from surgery or recent injury may be unaccustomed to the temporary limitations on their mobility. In addition, many drugs cause dizziness and orthostatic hypotension, which can increase the risk of a fall. For these reasons, you'll want to make a special effort to identify and remove mobility hazards from the patient's environment, provide mobility aids and gait training if needed, ask family members to help the patient move from room to room, and have the patient's physician or pharmacist evaluate all of his drugs for their potential to contribute to falls.

Room-related risks

In most homes, the kitchen, bathroom, and bedroom pose particular risks. The kitchen holds the greatest risk of fires and burns for both adults and children. These dangers can be minimized and even avoided by ensuring the patient takes the following precautions:

• properly maintains ventilation systems and range exhausts
• keeps appliance cords and extension cords well away from the sink and stove
• uses ground fault interrupters to protect against shock and to quickly shut off the electricity before serious injury or death can occur
• has good lighting — especially over the stove, sink, and counters — to help avoid burns and cuts
• uses blinds or curtains on windows and frosted bulbs, indirect lighting, shades, or globes on light fixtures (if the patient is an older patient who complains of glare from the lights)
• stores items within arm's reach or uses a step stool.

The bathroom poses a high risk of falls, burns, accidental ingestion of poisons, and potentially serious accidents because of the close proximity of water to electricity. To minimize the patient's risk, ensure the patient takes the following precautions:

• uses a nonskid mat, abrasive strips, or another nonslip surface in the bathtub or shower
• uses a bath stool or shower chair (if the patient is frail or unsteady or can't rise from a low sitting position)
• has grab bars firmly attached to wall studs beside the toilet and in the tub

or shower (if the patient needs assistance or is unsteady) and knows how to use them safely
• has assistance with bathing (if the patient faces a high risk of falling in the bath despite safety devices)
• sets water heater at 120° F (48.8° C) or lower or uses a thermometer to check the temperature of bath water (110° F [43.3° C] or lower for small children and frail elderly patients)
• never leaves a child alone around water, including during playtime in the tub
• has a close proximity and clear pathway to the bathroom
• uses a bedside commode if necessary
• unplugs bathroom appliances when not in use
• has ground fault interrupters to protect against shock.

The patient's bedroom can also be a hazardous area. Possible hazards include:

• loose rugs and runners
• oversized bedding and bedspreads
• telephone and light switches beyond reach
• inadequate lighting, especially at night
• electrical and telephone cords
• smoking in bed
• use of a heater, hot plate, electric teapot, or coffeepot near bedding
• improper use of electric blanket or heating pad.

Food, plant, and product hazards

Foods that are handled or stored improperly can create a serious health threat, especially for very young children, frail elderly people, pregnant women, and people who are immuno-

Food safety checklist

To reduce the risk of food hazards, make sure that patients and family members take these safety precautions when working with food:

• washing their hands before handling any foods and after handling poultry, other meats, and food waste

• washing their hands after using the bathroom or blowing a nose

• defrosting frozen foods by placing them in the refrigerator, running them under cold water, or using a microwave on the defrost setting rather than defrosting at room temperature

• using one cutting board for raw meat and a different cutting board for everything else

• cleaning the food preparation area thoroughly after preparing foods

• discarding any food items that smell or look spoiled or have passed the "sell by" date on the label

• discarding any food, especially meats and mayonnaise-based items, that have been stored too long at temperatures between 45° and 140° F (7.2° and 60° C)

• cooking foods thoroughly to 140° F

• avoiding recipes that call for raw eggs

• thoroughly washing fruits and vegetables, especially if they'll be eaten unpeeled

• storing cooked foods on the top shelves of the refrigerator and raw foods on the bottom shelves

• never returning foods from a serving dish to the original container

• not storing acidic foods or drinks in chipped or damaged galvanized or leaded-crystal containers

• changing dish towels daily and whenever a towel is used to mop up spills or wipe a counter.

---

suppressed. Fortunately, following a few simple rules can increase the safety of all foods in the home. (See *Food safety checklist.*)

Plants also pose a hazard especially to families with young children. During your household assessment:

• Scan indoor and outdoor areas for toxic plants such as oleander.

• Make sure that families with young children know about common indoor plants that could harm a child if ingested, such as dieffenbachia, philodendron, and asparagus fern.

• Inform the family that the degree of harm caused by ingesting these plants depends on the age and general health of the child involved, his degree of sen-

sitivity, and the toxicity of the individual plant.

• Warn parents about harmful outdoor plants (such as tulips and firethorn) that produce flowers or berries that could be attractive to children.

• Remind patients and families that even common food plants can have poisonous parts or can be poisonous if eaten raw or prepared improperly. For example, potatoes that have turned green from exposure to light are toxic and shouldn't be eaten. All of the parts of a rhubarb plant are poisonous except a well-cooked stem. Many wild mushrooms contain powerful toxins. A good rule of thumb is to recommend that patients and their families avoid eating anything they can't positively identify as a safe food.

In addition, many household products are poisonous when ingested. To help assess the risk of poisoning in a patient's home, check to see where the patient stores cleaners, antiseptics, and any other product labeled "Keep away from children." Also, check the location of "safe" products that can do damage when used improperly or ingested in large quantities, such as vitamin and mineral supplements (which could cause iron toxicity) and mouthwashes (which could cause alcohol overdose).

When caring for a patient with dementia — especially if small children are in the home — it's even more important to assess for food, plant, and product dangers and to minimize the risk of those you find. Simply placing dangerous compounds on a high shelf may not ensure safety. Instead, find a way to secure these products behind locks or child-safe devices.

Medication risks

It may be second nature for you to assess for medication hazards, especially interactions and adverse effects. However, some medication hazards are more common in the home environment such as problems with storage and labeling. Most people tend to store medicines in the bathroom, even though the increased heat and moisture in a bathroom make it a poor choice for storage. To minimize the risk for medication hazards, the following guidelines are helpful:

• Check to make sure the patient's drugs are stored in a safe location that isn't too hot or moist and is inaccessible to children.

• Make sure the patient's drugs are in their original containers and bear legible labels.

• Urge the patient to discard outdated drugs by flushing them down the toilet.

• Determine the patient's knowledge of basic drug safety. (See *Medication safety checklist.*)

• Urge the patient to turn on a light or use a night-light to take drugs at night. If that won't work, urge the patient to keep only the drugs he needs during the night beside the bed and keep them in a very specific location.

Mental illness and dementia

A mentally ill patient or family member may pose a threat to you and deserves close evaluation. For example, watch for signs that the person is losing control; remember that verbal interventions are most effective early in the course of a conflict. Ask an upset person about his concerns and what he needs to feel better. Suggest that the person come to a quiet place with you to sit and talk. Say something like, "You seem to have concerns about this. Will you share them with me?"

Along with a confident attitude, project an expectation that the threatening person will stay in control. You may even want to say something like, "I expect you to stay in control of yourself while we talk about this." Even if you can convince a mentally ill person to talk calmly with you, remember to maintain your safety by:

• keeping a clear route to the door

• increasing your personal space slightly

• staying out of the kitchen, where potential weapons may be readily available.

If the person is delusional and believes that he is being threatened, express understanding for his feelings in a calm, soothing tone. Say something like, "What you're feeling must be very frightening. Even though I'm not seeing or hearing what you are, I understand that it's distressing to you." Then do what you can to try to increase the person's feelings of safety. For instance, tell him that it's safe to talk with you. Allow about four times your typical personal space. If the person is angry, don't try to touch him. Doing so will only increase his agitation while placing you within arm's reach of being grabbed or struck.

Although violence usually isn't a hallmark of dementia, it can occur from time to time. Most patients with dementia, such as that caused by Alzheimer's disease, don't know why they're angry and agitated. In fact, trying to get them to explain their behavior may only increase their anxiety and agitation. As with any threatening situation, the best option is to stop it before it develops. For the patient with dementia, this usually means anticipating needs and avoiding unfamiliar situations. A family member who knows the patient's routine can help determine the best time for a visit, when the patient isn't too tired or hungry.

When you arrive, ask a familiar family member to introduce you to the patient and explain the reason for your visit. When interviewing the patient, watch how your assessment questions affect him. If impaired memory makes

Medication safety checklist

To reduce a patient's risk of medication hazards, take these steps:

• Make sure the patient knows the name of each drug, how much to take, when to take it, and which adverse effects could occur.

• Tell the patient to take a list of his prescription and nonprescription drugs (or the medication containers) to every physician visit.

• Caution the patient to take his medications just as the physician prescribed them, without changing doses or timing unless he first consults the physician.

• If necessary, encourage the patient to use a daily schedule, calendar, or even an alarm to help him remember to take his drugs.

• Suggest that the patient use a compartment box to help him remember whether he took his drugs each day.

• Warn the patient not to share his drugs with someone else or take someone else's drugs.

• Encourage proper and safe storage.

• Tell the patient not to keep sleeping aids near the bed to reduce the risk of taking a dose twice.

• Warn the patient not to drink alcohol with any drug.

• Advise the patient to use one pharmacy to fill all prescriptions and talk with the physician about any bothersome reactions to drugs.

• Tell the patient to review the package insert and ask for a large-print label if necessary.

him unable to answer your questions, he may become frustrated and angry.

If a loss of language skills makes it difficult for him to communicate, he'll probably grow even more frustrated. If you see a patient becoming more and more frustrated, stop making demands on him. Invite him to sit quietly or walk with you. Be careful not to startle or repel the patient by touching him. Try changing the conversation to one that isn't threatening. For example, if you say something about an object easily visible in the room, the patient may be able to focus on it and talk about it without stress.

No matter what attempts you use to defuse the situation, the patient may remain agitated and angry if he has an unmet need. If this happens, you'll need to try to determine the nature of that need—usually a challenging task. Consider both physical and emotional problems. For example, pain, constipation, and hunger can lead to agitation. An older man with an enlarged prostate may be retaining urine and thus be increasingly uncomfortable.

Emotional needs can lead to agitation in many ways. For example, if a female patient with dementia insists she needs to pick up her children after school, she may not be comforted when you tell her that her children are grown and gone. Perhaps the underlying problem is that the patient feels unneeded. Maybe she'd feel more comforted by hearing about her importance to her children and being invited to perform a task.

Many families have trouble knowing how to handle a patient who has a mental illness or dementia. When you visit, consider gathering family members together so they can share their feelings and emotions with each other to help facilitate a plan of care. Consult

with a psychiatric nurse if possible and your agency employs or contracts with one. Today, many agencies employ a certified psychiatric home health nurse who may consult about difficult situations, work together with other nurses, or manage cases. The psychiatric nurse's focus will be largely on family dynamics and options (including community referrals) to help reduce the effects of mental illness on the patient and the family.

Infection

To prevent the transmission of infection, all members of the home health care team must comply with standard precautions and with the agency's policies and procedures concerning infection control. (See *Infection control principles.*) Keep in mind that, although infection control is second nature to you, it isn't familiar to most patients and their families. Evaluate patients and their caregivers to determine their ability to understand and apply infection control measures, such as:
- handwashing before and after giving patient care
- using individual thermometer covers and cleaning the thermometer after each use
- cleaning the diaphragm of a stethoscope with 70% alcohol after each use
- using disposable items whenever possible
- taking only items essential to care into the home
- using a 1:10 solution of household bleach and water to clean nondisposable equipment contaminated with blood or body fluids
- discarding disposable equipment that has been contaminated with blood

or body fluids in a plastic bag and securely closing it before placing it in the household trash

• pouring liquid waste, such as urine and colostomy drainage, into the toilet (after raising the seat) and then flushing and disinfecting the toilet

• disposing of solid waste, such as contaminated tissues, dressings, and disposable supplies, in a plastic bag and securing the top before placing it in the household trash

• double-bagging infectious solid waste and closing the top securely before placing it in the household trash

• disposing of used needles and syringes intact, without recapping them, into a heavy plastic container or a metal can with a lid (such as a coffee can)

• handling linen soiled with blood or body fluids carefully to avoid spreading droplets or infectious particles

• wearing gloves to fold soiled linens while trying not to shake them

• washing soiled linens with hot soapy water separate from other household wash and possibly adding bleach or Lysol disinfectant to the wash.

If you feel that a patient and family can't apply infection control procedures adequately, tell your supervisor. Your agency may need to recommend that the patient be admitted to an intermediate care facility. Also, notify your supervisor if a patient's or family member's blood or body fluids get on you or your clothing. You may want to carry an extra set of clean clothes in your car.

Emergencies

To help patients respond quickly and appropriately to an emergency, encourage your older patients to post

Infection control principles

To help protect yourself from infection and reduce the risk of transmitting infection to patients and their families, be sure to follow standard precautions, as outlined by the Centers for Disease Control and Prevention. Here are some principles to keep in mind:

• Wash your hands thoroughly before and after each home visit.

• Carry antimicrobial cleaning wipes or "waterless soap" with you in case you can't wash your hands.

• Handle all bodily substances as if they're infectious, regardless of the patient's diagnosis.

• Use barrier protections, such as gloves, gowns, face masks, and eye shields, as needed.

• Don't recap used needles unless you use a mechanical device to do so.

• Dispose of all sharps (such as disposable syringes, needles, and scalpel blades) in a puncture-resistant container.

• If you need to perform cardiopulmonary resuscitation, use a mask with a one-way valve so you don't breathe the patient's expired air.

• If your patient may have active tuberculosis, wear a high efficiency particulate air respirator, also called a HEPA mask.

• Keep your vaccinations current, including those for hepatitis B, tetanus, and possibly influenza.

• At the end of your work day, remove your clothes as soon as you get home and store them in a safe, contained area until you can wash them.

emergency numbers by the phone or program them into the phone. If the patient has impaired vision, a telephone with large numbers may be helpful. At least one telephone should be placed in a low position so the patient can reach it even if he can't stand. Some patients wear a fanny pack during the day to keep a cordless phone and other necessities readily available.

If the patient lives alone, consider recommending a telephone alert system. These systems usually require the patient to wear a device around his neck. If he needs help and can't reach a phone, he can push a button on the device. A system operator then calls the patient on the phone. If he doesn't answer, the operator activates emergency aid. Suggest that the patient contact his insurance company to see if any part of this service is reimbursable.

If your patient's condition changes dramatically or he has a serious accident, you'll need to activate the emergency response system. Usually, this means calling 911. If you do, follow these important instructions.

• Start with a short, general description of the situation.

• Give the most accurate street address you can or the closest cross streets.

• Don't rely on landmarks unless you're sure the ambulance driver can't confuse them.

• Be especially careful with the address if you're using a cellular phone. This is because the 911 caller location service may not work with a cellular phone.

• No matter what kind of phone you use, don't hang up until the ambulance arrives because the dispatcher may need more information.

Regardless of whether your home visit is routine or turns into a full-fledged emergency, it's useful—necessary, perhaps—to remember that you may be your patient's main source of safety. By being well-prepared for each visit, assessing and responding to threats calmly, and reducing the risks of common household hazards, you can help your patients return to independence and maximize the length and quality of their lives.

6

Documenting home care

Especially in the home care field, documentation forms the primary method by which you communicate with other members of the patient's home care team. Documentation also provides the only legal and medical record of the patient's condition, care, and outcomes.

Although every home care agency has its own standards and requirements for documentation, they all adhere to a similar set of documentation principles. Most use forms approved or required by the Health Care Financing Administration (HCFA). When documenting a patient's care, make sure you follow sound documentation principles and use the forms preferred by your employer. Typically, you'll use specified forms to document a patient's referral to home care, your initial patient assessment, the plan of care, medical updates and recertifications, progress notes, and discharge summaries.

Documentation principles

Accurate and complete documentation allows you to demonstrate the quality of the patient's care, show active adherence to a compliance program, judge patient outcomes, maintain consistent reimbursement for billed activities, and meet certification and accreditation requirements. Naturally, the documentation completed by each person in your agency must meet the standards, guidelines, and conditions of the payer, particularly Medicare. (See *Documentation tips to ensure reimbursement,* pages 76 and 77.)

Without documentation, you have no proof that care was given, a plan of care was followed, or a response was obtained from the patient. Documentation provides the necessary communication links between team members, the agency and the team, and the payer and the agency. It qualifies the patient for services and eventually forms the basis of the agency's and the payer's evaluations.

Documentation serves several purposes, including:
• maintenance of patient-specific data
• verification of home visits and validation that team members followed the plan of care
• demonstration of informed consent for services
• confirmation that the services are skilled

75

Documentation tips to ensure reimbursement

Medicare and other third-party payers may question your patient's eligibility for reimbursement if you use certain words and phrases listed here. Use this table to revise these problem terms and help ensure continued reimbursement.

PROBLEM TERMS	SUGGESTED REVISION
Ambulates without difficulty	Quantify where and how far the patient can ambulate without difficulty. If the patient can truly ambulate without difficulty, he may need to be discharged.
Chronic	Substitute *acute episode* or *acute exacerbation.*
Discussed	Substitute *educated* or *instructed.*
Doing well	Substitute *following instructions*, *taking medications as ordered*, or something similar.
General weakness	Substitute *cannot ambulate without assistance*, *short of breath on walking 10'*, *chairbound*, or *bedbound.*
Intake poor	Describe the patient's intake exactly, such as *no solid food* or *less than 20 oz of water ingested per day.* If you complete a calorie count, attach it to the documentation.
No change	Substitute *problem continues* or *problem remains unresolved.*
Improving	Provide objective details, such as *shortness of breath continues with walking 15'* or *wound size reduced from ¾" to ⅝" (2 cm to 1.5 cm).*
No complaints	Substitute objective details, such as *balance steady* or *patient denies dizziness.*
No problems	Substitute *no new problems.*
Observed	Change to *assessed* or *evaluated for*, and then record specific, measurable findings.
Reinforced	Substitute *instructed* or *taught* and explain why reinstruction was needed. For example, write *patient couldn't comprehend previous instructions due to recent transient ischemic attack.*
Stable	Substitute *objective assessment reveals patient responding to medical treatment.*
Noncompliant	Substitute such phrases as *patient complains of intolerable side effects* or *patient has difficulty understanding instructions.*

Documentation tips to ensure reimbursement *(continued)*

PROBLEM TERMS	SUGGESTED REVISION
No progress	Document specific findings, such as *wound size remains 2 cm,* or document how the patient's status is deteriorating.
Plateaued	Document how you reached this conclusion. Identify the plan of care that you'll use to move patient off the plateau.
Reviewed	Substitute specific details, such as *continues to need instruction because of effects of cerebrovascular accident.*

- confirmation that the patient is homebound
- coordination of services among team members
- a record of interventions and outcomes
- proof of health improvements
- demonstration that reimbursement requirements were met
- a mechanism for data retrieval
- a record for financial and legal issues
- protection for the patient
- proof that the patient received services for which he qualified
- communication tool between agency and payer
- evidence of an individualized plan of care.

Outcome tracking

In this era of cutting costs, one of the most important aspects of documentation is to allow an evaluation of the patient's outcomes. Outcomes are specific, quantifiable goals or objectives identified jointly by the home care team, the patient, and the patient's family. (See *How to write an objective,* page 78.) They provide direction for the patient's plan of care. Thus, outcome-based documentation focuses on

specific, measurable goals and the criteria used to measure the patient's progress toward achieving those goals. Consequently, outcome-based documentation should:

- help home care providers and patients to use resources more effectively
- describe the instructional outcomes of a learning session between two or more people
- modify the patient's activities of daily living when resources are diminished or inadequate
- focus on the results of care
- measure the achievement of stated objectives
- show when the patient is ready for discharge.

At each visit, concentrate on documenting the patient's progress toward his stated outcomes as specifically as possible. Remember not to leave any area of the documentation form blank. Instead, write "N/A" in areas of the form that don't apply to your patient. If you don't, whoever reviews the form may assume that you omitted care.

Homebound status requirements

To receive Medicare reimbursement for home services, your initial assess-

How to write an objective

The key to outcome-based documentation is the development of specific, precise objectives. When writing an objective, keep these guidelines in mind:

• Choose an objective that is realistic, measurable, and observable.
• Use cognitive, affective (emotional), or psychomotor domains to develop the objective.
• Include a timeline appropriate to the diagnosis.
• Identify specific subsets of activities that combine to meet the outcome, as needed.

For example, consider a patient with insulin-dependent diabetes who's referred to you for home care teaching and follow-up. An example of an outcome for this patient might read: "By the end of visit 5, the patient will demonstrate an understanding of how to monitor blood glucose as a means of managing his diabetes."

To achieve this outcome, you would develop subsets of activities to show progression toward the objective. Before the fifth visit, the patient would need to:

• list signs and symptoms of hypoglycemic and hyperglycemic reactions
• demonstrate how to test his blood glucose level by using the blood glucose monitor
• explain the importance of blood glucose monitoring and its relationship to his diabetes
• demonstrate how to set up the equipment and dispose of syringes
• demonstrate how to draw up insulin
• demonstrate how to give himself an injection
• demonstrate how to document his site selection and rotation
• relate appropriate information about his prescribed diet and insulin therapy
• state the relationship between activity, exercise, and insulin requirements
• identify measures to maintain blood glucose levels when sick.

By accomplishing all of these subset activities by the fifth visit, the patient achieves the original objective.

ment must document that your patient is homebound. In other words, it should specify that:

• Leaving home is difficult and taxing for the patient, takes considerable effort, and requires assistance from equipment or another person.
• The patient rarely leaves home and usually does so only for medical appointments.

At least once per month, you'll need to reassess the patient to confirm that he qualifies as homebound. Specifically describe the patient's difficulty in leaving home, the length he can walk without assistance or rest, and the functional limitations that make leaving home difficult or unsafe for the patient. (See *Documenting your patient's homebound status.*)

If your patient leaves home, make sure you explain the reason in your documentation. Also, note the level of assistance the patient needed from devices or people, describe the level of pain reported by the patient during the outing, and document any changes in vital signs.

Justifying skilled care

The need for intermittent skilled care is another requirement that must be evident in your documentation. Examples of tasks that support the need for skilled care include:

- teaching about new medications and their adverse effects
- administering I.V. drugs
- administering insulin
- monitoring blood glucose levels
- strengthening of legs through exercises
- evaluating and teaching swallowing techniques
- removing and changing an indwelling catheter every 4 to 6 weeks
- providing wound care for pressure ulcers or other wounds
- teaching the patient and family or caregiver about the patient's illness, special diet, energy conservation, and current status.

Setting visit frequency

Usually, a physician's order determines the skilled need and the frequency of visits. Other issues may be considered as well, however, such as:

- the patient's diagnosis
- the acuteness of the patient's condition
- the patient's or family's ability to learn
- the provider's judgment about the patient's cognitive capabilities and availability of other persons to be taught.

Your documentation should outline the visit frequency based on your agency's work week.

Documenting your patient's homebound status

To ensure accurate documentation of your patient's homebound status, consider using the descriptions that best match your patient's condition, such as:

- confined to bed and unable to bear weight on legs
- restricted to wheelchair
- unable to use stairs to leave the home
- maximum assistance of one (or two) persons needed for transfer
- maximum assistance of one (or two) persons needed to ambulate on all surfaces
- history of recent falls from delayed balance reactions
- limited activities (sitting, walking, activity intolerance) from cardiac, respiratory, or musculoskeletal problems
- loss of sensation and severe weakness in legs
- severe pain when standing, sitting, or walking for more than ___ minutes
- fractures or disabilities preventing ambulation without assistance from a person or device
- paraplegia, quadriplegia, hemiplegia, or paresis
- severe dyspnea or angina with simple activities, such as dressing or walking
- unable to tolerate prolonged activity because of cardiac or respiratory condition or pain
- unable to tolerate standing because of impaired peripheral circulation, wound, or pain
- mental confusion, extreme anxiety, or paranoia.

Orders management

Verbal orders from physicians are common in home health care. If you receive one, write it down, sign it, and date it. Place a copy in the patient's chart and send the original to the physician to be signed and dated. Only after both of you sign the order and the physician returns the original copy to the agency or sends a signed order via facsimile can the services on the order be billed and reimbursed.

Also keep in mind that documentation by all disciplines must agree with the original physician's order. If the order includes an allowance for p.r.n. visits, document the specific need for these visits if they occur.

If a patient refuses or misses a planned visit, you may not be able to carry out the physician's order completely. But you don't need another order. Simply contact the physician, explain the need for a change in visit frequency for that week, and document the reason for the change and the phone call you made to the physician. For example, write, "After calling the patient to set up a planned visit, the patient refused because she did not want the nurse to visit today. We reviewed her medications over the phone and planned the next visit for the following week. Physician notified."

Patient referrals

Home care begins when your agency receives a patient referral form, or intake form. The data on this form is used to make sure the patient is eligible for home health care and that the agency can provide the services the patient needs. (See *Referral for home care.*) Data needed to establish eligibility include the following:

• The patient is homebound.
• The patient needs skilled intermittent services.
• The patient needs reasonable and medically necessary care.
• The patient is under a physician's care.

Initial assessment record

If the referral form convinces you that the patient is most likely eligible for home care, the next step is to complete an initial assessment in the patient's home within 48 hours. If Medicare will be paying for the patient's care, you'll need to document your initial assessment on what is called an OASIS form. OASIS stands for Outcomes and Assessment Information Set. This HCFA form was designed particularly to measure outcomes for adults who receive home care. (See *Outcome and assessment information set,* pages 83 to 96.) You probably won't use it for pediatric or pregnant patients.

OASIS allows you (and HCFA) to measure and track more than 80 assessment topics involving the patient's socioeconomic, demographic, physiological, mental, emotional, environmental, support, health, function, and health service utilization characteristics. By using it at your initial assessment and again at the 60-day recertification point, you'll gain a good understanding of how the patient has improved, what services he still needs, and whether he'd be better served in

Referral for home care

Also called an intake form, this form is used to document the patient's needs when you begin your evaluation of a new patient. Use the form below as a guide.

ELECTION BENEFIT PERIOD (1) 2 3 4

Date of Referral: _05/01/00_   Branch _____   Chart#: _0001236_   H __

Info Taken By: _Victoria Mansfield_   Admit Date: _05/02/00_

Patient's Name: _Terry Elliot_

Address: _11 Second Street_

City: _Hometown_   State: _PA_   Zip: _10981_

Phone: _881-555-2937_   Date of Birth: _07/08/24_

Primary Caregiver Name & #: _Helen Elliot_   _881-555-2937_

Insurance Name: _Medicare_   Ins.#: _123-45-6789A_

Is this a managed care policy (HMO): _No_

Primary Dx: (Code _891.0_) _Open wound ankle/Complications (Onset)_ Date: _05/02/00_

(Code _250.72_) _Type 2 diabetes /Uncontrolled (Exac.)_ Date: _05/02/00_

(Code _443.89_) _Periph vascular disease (Exac)_   Date: _05/02/00_

Procedures: (Code _86.28_) _Debridement wound (Onset)_   Date: _05/02/00_

Referral Source: _Dr.'s office_   Phone: _881-555-6900_

Physician Name & Phone #: (UPIN _22222_) _Dr. Kyle Stevens_

Phone: _881-555-6900_

Physician Address: _Dr.'s Medical Center, Hometown, PA 10981_

Hospital _N/A_   Admit _N/A_   Discharge _N/A_

Functional Limitations: Pain Management, _Pain, ambulation dysfunction_

ORDERS/SERVICES (specify amount, frequency and duration):

SN: _5-7 visits/wk x 9 wks for assessment and wound care (L) ankle. Saline wet to dry drsg_

AI: _3-5 visits/wk x 9 wks for assistance with ADLs and personal care_

PT, OT, ST: _PT 1-3 visits/wk x 9 wks to assess mobility and safety, and_
develop home exercise program

MSW: _1-2 visits x 1 mo. for financial assessment and long-term planning_

Spiritual Coordinator: _N/A_   Counselor: _N/A_

Volunteer: _N/A_

Other Services Provided: _N/A_

Goals: _Wound healing without complications_

Equipment: _walker and dressing supplies_

Company & Phone #: _Best Med Equip. Co_   _881-260-1026_

Safety Measures: _Correct use of supportive devices_ Nutritional Req _20% protein, 30% fat_

FUNCTIONAL LIMITATIONS: (Circle Applicable)		**ACTIVITIES PERMITTED:** (Circle Applicable)		
(1) Amputation	5. Paralysis	9. Legally Blind	1. Complete Bedrest	5. Partial Wgt Bearing	A. Wheelchair
2. Bowel/ Bladder	(6) Endurance	A. Dyspnea With Minimal Exer	2. Bedrest BRP	6. Independent at Home	(B) Walker
3. Contracture	(7) Ambulation		3. Up as Tolerated		C. No Restriction
4. Hearing	8. Speech	B. Other	(4) Transfer Bed/Chair	7. Crutches	D. Other— specify
				8. Cane	

(continued)

Referral for home care *(continued)*

Accessibility to bath Y (N)   Shower Y (N)   Bathroom (Y) N   Exit (Y) N
Mental Status: (Circle) (Oriented) Comatose (Forgetful) Depressed Disoriented
    Lethargic   Agitated   Other

Allergies: *NKA*

- Hospice Appropriate Meds   • Med company: *N/A*

MEDICATIONS: *Humulin N 24 units SC ͡q am*   *changed*
Tylenol 325–1000 mg q4h prn pain po   *unchanged*
Darvocet N 100 one tab q4h prn pain po   *new*
MOM 30 cc qhs prn po   *unchanged*

Living Will   Yes_____   No *X*   Obtained_____   Family to mail to office_____

Guardian, POA, or Responsible Person: *wife*

Address & Phone Number: *same*

Other Family Members: *N/A*

ETOH: *∅*   Drug Use: *∅*   Smoker *1–2 ppd x 25 yrs*

HISTORY: *Chronic peripheral vascular disease with periodic open wounds of feet*
and legs. Seen by Dr. in office 04/28/00 and new wound of (L) ankle debrided.

Social History (place of birth, education, jobs, retirement, etc.): *Korean War veteran*
retired (x 18 yrs) construction worker

ADMISSION NOTES: VS: T *99°0*   AP *88*   RR *22*   BP *150/82*
Lungs: *diminished bilat. at bases*   Extremities: *(R) BKA, (L) foot pale, DP and PT pulses +.*
Wgt: *195 lb.*   Recent wgt loss/gain of *denies*

Admission Narrative: *Patient independent in Insulin administration and instruct*
ed in Insulin dosage change with good understanding. Wound of (L) ankle-outer
malleolar area = 4 cm x 5 cm x 1 cm deep; open with beefy red appearance,
wound edges pink, moderate amount serosanguineous drainage present. Wound
care performed by RN per care plan. Pain controlled with Darvocet prn.

Psychosocial Issues *Wife refuses to be involved with wound care at all.*

Environmental Concerns *Cluttered home, 2 dogs and 1 cat in house*

Are there any cultural or spiritual customs or beliefs of which we should be aware
before providing Hospice services? *N/A*

Funeral Home: *N/A*   Contact made YES____ NO____
DIRECTIONS: *1 block before intersection of Main St, on Second St.*

Agency Representative
Signature: *Victoria Mansfield, RN, BSN*   Date: *05/02/00*

---

another care setting. Your agency may also use OASIS data to drive its quality improvement program. In addition, the agency may electronically transmit OASIS data to a standard state system installed by HCFA. Eventually, OASIS

(Text continues on page 96.)

Outcome and assessment information set

Medicare Home Health Care Quality Assurance and Improvement Demonstration Outcome and Assessment Information Set (OASIS-B)

OASIS Items to Be Used at Specific Time Points

Start of Care (or Resumption of Care Following Inpatient Facility Stay): 1-69
Follow-Up: 1, 4, 9-11, 13, 16-26, 29-71
Discharge (not to inpatient facility): 1, 4, 9-11, 13, 16-26, 29-74, 78-79
Transfer to Inpatient Facility (with or without agency discharge): 1, 70-72, 75-79
Death at Home: 1, 79
Note: For items 51-67, please note special instructions at the beginning of the section.

CLINICAL RECORD ITEMS

a. (M0010) Agency ID:
   2 6 9 3 8 7 H C

b. (M0020) Patient ID Number: _SM962_

c. (M0030) Start of Care Date:
   0 5 / 0 2 / 2 0 0 0
   month   day   year

d. (M0040) Patient's Last Name:
   E L L I O T _ _ _ _ _ _

e. (M0050) Patient State of Residence:
   P A

f. (M0060) Patient Zip Code:
   1 0 9 8 1

g. (M0063) Medicare Number: (including suffix if any)
   1 2 3 4 5 6 7 8 9 A
   ☐ NA- No Medicare

h. (M0066) Birth Date:
   0 7 / 0 8 / 1 9 2 4
   month   day   year

I. (M0080) Discipline of Person Completing Assessment:
   ☒ 1-RN   ☐ 2-LPN   ☐ 3-PT
   ☐ 4-SLP/ST   ☐ 5-OT   ☐ 6-MSW

j. (M0090) Date Assessment Information Recorded: 0 5 / 0 2 / 2 0 0 0
   month   day   year

DEMOGRAPHICS AND PATIENT HISTORY

1. (M0100) This Assessment Is Currently Being Completed for the Following Reason:
   ☒ 1-Start of care
   ☐ 2-Resumption of care (after inpatient stay)
   ☐ 3-Discharge from agency — not to an inpatient facility [Go to M0150]
   ☐ 4-Transferred to an inpatient facility — discharged from agency [Go to M0830]
   ☐ 5-Transferred to an inpatient facility — not discharged from agency [Go to M0830]
   ☐ 6-Died at home [Go to M0906]
   ☐ 7-Recertification reassessment (follow-up) [Go to M0150]
   ☐ 8-Other follow-up [Go to M0150]

2. (M0130) Gender:
   ☒ 1-Male   ☐ 2-Female

3. (M0140) Race/Ethnicity (as identified by patient):
   ☒ 1-White, non-Hispanic
   ☐ 2-Black, African-American
   ☐ 3-Hispanic
   ☐ 4-Asian, Pacific Islander
   ☐ 5-American Indian, Eskimo, Aleut
   ☐ 6-Other
   ☐ UK-Unknown

(continued)

4. (M0150) Current payment sources for home care: (Mark all that apply.)
- ☐ 0-None: no charge for current services
- ☒ 1-Medicare (traditional fee-for-service)
- ☐ 2-Medicare (HMO/managed care)
- ☐ 3-Medicaid (traditional fee-for-service)
- ☐ 4-Medicaid (HMO/managed care)
- ☐ 5-Workers' compensation
- ☐ 6-Title programs (e.g., Title III, V, or XX)
- ☐ 7-Other government (e.g., CHAMPUS, VA, etc.) _____
- ☐ 8-Private insurance
- ☐ 9-Private HMO/managed care
- ☐ 10-Self-pay
- ☐ 11-Other (specify)
- ☐ UK-Unknown

5. (M0160) Financial factors limiting the ability of the patient/family to meet basic health needs: (Mark all that apply.)
- ☐ 0-None
- ☐ 1-Unable to afford medicine or medical supplies
- ☐ 2-Unable to afford medical expenses that are not covered by insurance/Medicare (e.g., copayments)
- ☐ 3-Unable to afford rent/utility bills
- ☐ 4-Unable to afford food
- ☒ 5-Other (specify) _Has PACE_

6. (M0170) From which of the following inpatient facilities was the patient discharged during the past 14 days? (Mark all that apply.)
- ☐ 1-Hospital
- ☐ 2-Rehabilitation facility
- ☐ 3-Nursing home
- ☐ 4-Other (specify)
- ☒ NA-Patient was not discharged from an inpatient facility [If NA, go to M0200]

7. (M0180) Inpatient discharge date (most recent): __ __ /__ __ /__ __ __ __
     month   day   year
- ☐ UK-Unknown

8. (M0190) Inpatient diagnoses and three-digit ICD code categories for only those conditions treated during an inpatient facility stay within the last 14 days (no surgical or V-codes):

Inpatient facility diagnosis   ICD
a. _____   (__ __ __)
b. _____   (__ __ __)

9. (M0200) Medical or treatment regimen change within past 14 days: Has this patient experienced a change in medical or treatment regimen (e.g., medication, treatment, or service change due to new or additional diagnosis, etc.) within the last 14 days?
- ☐ 0-No [If no, go to M0220]
- ☒ 1-Yes

10. (M0210) List the patient's medical diagnoses and three-digit ICD code categories for those conditions requiring changed medical or treatment regimen (no surgical or V-codes):

Changed medical regimen   ICD
diagnosis
a. _Open wound ① ankle_   (_8 9 1_)
b. _____   (__ __ __)
c. _____   (__ __ __)
d. _____   (__ __ __)

11. (M0220) Conditions prior to medical or treatment regimen change or inpatient stay within past 14 days: If this patient experienced an inpatient facility discharge or change in medical or treatment regimen within the past 14 days, indicate any conditions that existed prior to the inpatient stay or change in medical or treatment regimen. (Mark all that apply.)
- ☐ 1-Urinary incontinence
- ☐ 2-Indwelling/suprapubic catheter
- ☐ 3-Intractable pain
- ☐ 4-Impaired decision making
- ☐ 5-Disruptive or socially inappropriate behavior
- ☐ 6-Memory loss to the extent that supervision required
- ☒ 7-None of the above
- ☐ NA-No inpatient facility discharge and no change in medical or treatment regimen in past 14 days
- ☐ UK-Unknown

Outcome and assessment information set *(continued)*

12. (M0230/M0240) Diagnoses and Severity Index: List each medical diagnosis or problem for which the patient is receiving home care and ICD code category (no surgical or V-codes), and rate them using the following severity index. (Choose one value that represents the most severe rating appropriate for each diagnosis.)

0-Asymptomatic, no treatment needed at this time
1-Symptoms well controlled with current therapy
2-Symptoms controlled with difficulty, affecting daily functioning; patient needs ongoing monitoring
3-Symptoms poorly controlled, patient needs further adjustment in treatment and dose monitoring
4-Symptoms poorly controlled, history of rehospitalizations

Primary diagnosis	ICD	Severity rating	Date of onset
a. *Open wound ① ankle*	(8 9 1)	☐0 ☐1 ☒2 ☐3 ☐4	*4/28/00*
Other diagnosis	ICD	Severity rating	
b. *Type 2 diabetes*	(2 5 0)	☐0 ☐1 ☒2 ☐3 ☐4	*1984*
c. *PVD*	(4 4 3)	☐0 ☐1 ☐2 ☒3 ☐4	*1995*
d. _____	(_ _ _)	☐0 ☐1 ☐2 ☐3 ☐4	_____
e. _____	(_ _ _)	☐0 ☐1 ☐2 ☐3 ☐4	_____
f. _____	(_ _ _)	☐0 ☐1 ☐2 ☐3 ☐4	_____

Surgical procedure_____   Code_____   Date_____

13. (M0250) Therapies the patient receives at home: (Mark all that apply.)
☐ 1 - Intravenous or infusion therapy (excludes TPN)
☐ 2 - Enteral nutrition (nasogastric, gastrostomy, jejunostomy, or any other artificial entry into the alimentary canal)
☒ 4 - None of the above

14. (M0260) Overall prognosis: BEST description of patient's overall prognosis for recovery from this episode of illness
☐ 0 - Poor: little or no recovery is expected and/or further decline is imminent
☒ 1 - Good/Fair: partial to full recovery is expected
☐ UK - Unknown

15. (M0270) Rehabilitative prognosis: BEST description of patient's prognosis for functional status
☒ 0 - Guarded: minimal improvement in functional status is expected; decline is possible
☐ 1 - Good: marked improvement in functional status is expected
☐ UK - Unknown

16. (M0280) Life expectancy: (Physician documentation is not required.)
☒ 0 - Life expectancy is greater than 6 months
☐ 1 - Life expectancy is 6 months or fewer

17. (M0290) High risk factors characterizing this patient: (Mark all that apply.)
☒ 1 - Heavy smoking
☐ 2 - Obesity
☐ 3 - Alcohol dependency
☐ 4 - Drug dependency
☐ 5 - None of the above
☐ UK - Unknown

LIVING ARRANGEMENTS

18. (M0300) Current residence:
☒ 1 - Patient's owned or rented residence (house, apartment, or mobile home owned or rented by patient/couple/ significant other)
☐ 2 - Family member's residence
☐ 3 - Boarding home or rented room
☐ 4 - Board and care or assisted living facility
☐ 5 - Other (specify)

19. (M0310) Structural barriers in the patient's environment limiting independent mobility: (Mark all that apply.)
☐ 0 - None
☒ 1 - Stairs inside home that must be used by the patient (e.g., to get to toileting, sleeping, eating areas)
☐ 2 - Stairs inside the home that are used optionally (e.g., to get to laundry facilities)
☒ 3 - Stairs leading from inside house to outside
☐ 4 - Narrow or obstructed doorways

(continued)

20. (M0320) Safety hazards found in the patient's current place of residence: (Mark all that apply.)
- ☐ 0 - None
- ☐ 1 - Inadequate floor, roof, or windows
- ☐ 2 - Inadequate lighting
- ☐ 3 - Unsafe gas/electric appliance
- ☐ 4 - Inadequate heating
- ☐ 5 - Inadequate cooling
- ☒ 6 - Lack of fire safety devices
- ☐ 7 - Unsafe floor coverings
- ☐ 8 - Inadequate stair railings
- ☐ 9 - Improperly stored hazardous materials
- ☐10 - Lead-based paint
- ☐11 - Other (specify)

21. (M0330) Sanitation hazards found in the patient's current place of residence: (Mark all that apply.)
- ☒ 0 - None
- ☐ 1 - No running water
- ☐ 2 - Contaminated water
- ☐ 3 - No toileting facilities
- ☐ 4 - Outdoor toileting facilities only
- ☐ 5 - Inadequate sewage disposal
- ☐ 6 - Inadequate/improper food storage
- ☐ 7 - No food refrigeration
- ☐ 8 - No cooking facilities
- ☐ 9 - Insects/rodents present
- ☐10 - No scheduled trash pickup
- ☐11 - Cluttered/soiled living area
- ☐12 - Other (specify)

22. (M0340) Patient lives with: (Mark all that apply.)
- ☐ 1 - Lives alone
- ☒ 2 - With spouse or significant other
- ☐ 3 - With other family member
- ☐ 4 - With a friend
- ☐ 5 - With paid help (other than home care agency staff)
- ☐ 6 - With other than above

SUPPORTIVE ASSISTANCE

23. (M0350) Assisting person(s) other than home care agency staff: (Mark all that apply.)
- ☐ 1 - Relatives, friends, or neighbors living outside the home
- ☒ 2 - Person residing in the home (excluding paid help)
- ☐ 3 - Paid help
- ☐ 4 - None of the above (If none of the above, go to M0390)
- ☐UK - Unknown (If unknown, go to M0390)

24. (M0360) Primary caregiver taking lead responsibility for providing or managing the patient's care, providing the most frequent assistance, etc. (other than home care agency staff):
- ☐ 0 - No one person (If no one person, go to M0390)
- ☒ 1 - Spouse or significant other
- ☐ 2 - Daughter or son
- ☐ 3 - Other family member
- ☐ 4 - Friend or neighbor or community or church member
- ☐ 5 - Paid help
- ☐UK - Unknown (If unknown, go to M0390)

25. (M0370) How often does the patient receive assistance from the primary caregiver?
- ☒ 1 - Several times during day and night
- ☐ 2 - Several times during day
- ☐ 3 - Once daily
- ☐ 4 - Three or more times per week
- ☐ 5 - One to two times per week
- ☐ 6 - Less often than weekly
- ☐UK - Unknown

26. (M0380) Type of primary caregiver assistance: (Mark all that apply.)
- ☒ 1 - ADL assistance (bathing, dressing, toileting, bowel/bladder, eating/feeding)
- ☒ 2 - IADL assistance (meds, meals, housekeeping, laundry, telephone, shopping, finances)
- ☐ 3 - Environmental support (housing, home maintenance)
- ☒ 4 - Psychosocial support (socialization, companionship, recreation)
- ☒ 5 - Advocates or facilitates patient's participation in appropriate medical care
- ☐ 6 - Financial agent, power of attorney, or conservator of finance
- ☐ 7 - Health care agent, conservator of person, or medical power of attorney
- ☐UK - Unknown

SENSORY STATUS

27. (M0390) Vision with corrective lenses if the patient usually wears them:
- ☒ 0 - Normal vision: sees adequately in most situations; can see medication labels, newsprint
- ☐ 1 - Partially impaired: cannot see medication labels or newsprint, but can see obstacles in path and the surrounding layout; can count fingers at arm's length
- ☐ 2 - Severely impaired: cannot locate objects without hearing or touching them OR patient nonresponsive

Outcome and assessment information set *(continued)*

28. (M0400) Hearing and ability to understand spoken language in patient's own language (with hearing aids if the patient usually uses them):

☒ 0 - No observable impairment; able to hear and understand complex or detailed instructions and extended or abstract conversation

☐ 1 - With minimal difficulty, able to hear and understand most multi-step instructions and ordinary conversation; may need occasional repetition, extra time, or louder voice

☐ 2 - Has moderate difficulty hearing and understanding simple, one-step instructions and brief conversation; needs frequent prompting or assistance

☐ 3 - Has severe difficulty hearing and understanding simple greetings and short comments; requires multiple repetitions, restatements, demonstrations, additional time

☐ 4 - Unable to hear and understand familiar words or common expressions consistently OR patient nonresponsive

29. (M0410) Speech and oral (verbal) expression of language (in patient's own language):

☒ 0 - Expresses complex ideas, feelings, and needs clearly, completely, and easily in all situations with no observable impairment

☐ 1 - Minimal difficulty in expressing ideas and needs (may take extra time, makes occasional errors in word choice, grammar or speech intelligibility; needs minimal prompting or assistance)

☐ 2 - Expresses simple ideas or needs with moderate difficulty (needs prompting or assistance, errors in word choice, organization or speech intelligibility); speaks in phrases or short sentences

☐ 3 - Has severe difficulty expressing basic ideas or needs and requires maximal assistance or guessing by listener; speech limited to single words or short phrases

☐ 4 - Unable to express basic needs even with maximal prompting or assistance but is not comatose or unresponsive (e.g., speech is nonsensical or unintelligible)

☐ 5 - Patient nonresponsive or unable to speak

30. (M0420) Frequency of pain interfering with patient's activity or movement:

☐ 0 - Patient has no pain or pain does not interfere with activity or movement
☐ 1 - Less often than daily
☒ 2 - Daily, but not constantly
☐ 3 - All of the time

31. (M0430) Intractable pain: Is the patient experiencing pain that is not easily relieved, occurs at least daily, and affects his sleep, appetite, physical or emotional energy, concentration, personal relationships, emotions, or ability or desire to perform physical activity?

☒ 0 - No
☐ 1 - Yes

INTEGUMENTARY STATUS

32. (M0440) Does patient have a skin lesion or an open wound (excluding "ostomies")?

☐ 0 - No (If no, go to M0490)
☒ 1 - Yes

33. (M0450) Does patient have a pressure ulcer?

☒ 0 - No (If no, got to M0468)
☐ 1 - Yes

33a. (M0450) Current number of pressure ulcers at each stage: (Circle one response for each stage.)

Pressure ulcer stages
a) Stage 1: Nonblanchable erythema of intact skin; heralding of skin ulceration. In darker skin, warmth, edema, hardness, or discolored skin may be indicators.

Number of pressure ulcers

0	1	2	3	4 or more

b) Stage 2: Partial thickness skin loss involving epidermis and/or dermis. The ulcer is superficial and presents clinically as an abrasion, blister, or shallow crater.

Number of pressure ulcers

0	1	2	3	4 or more

c) Stage 3: Full-thickness skin loss involving damage or necrosis of subcutaneous tissue that may extend down to, but not through, underlying fascia. The ulcer presents clinically as a deep crater with or without undermining of adjacent tissue.

Number of pressure ulcers

0	1	2	3	4 or more

d) Stage 4: Full-thickness skin loss with extensive destruction, tissue, necrosis, or damage to muscle, bone, or supporting structures (e.g., tendon, joint capsule, etc.)

Number of pressure ulcers

0	1	2	3	4 or more

e) In addition to the above, is there at least one pressure ulcer that cannot be observed due to the presence of eschar or a nonremovable dressing, including casts?

☒ 0 - No   ☐   1 - Yes

(continued)

Outcome and assessment information set *(continued)*

33b. (M0460) Stage of most problematic (observable) pressure ulcer:

- ☐ 1 - Stage 1
- ☐ 2 - Stage 2
- ☐ 3 - Stage 3
- ☐ 4 - Stage 4
- ☐ NA- No observable pressure ulcer

33c. (M0464) Status of most problematic (observable) pressure ulcer:

- ☐ 1 - Fully granulating
- ☐ 2 - Early/partial granulation
- ☐ 3 - Not healing
- ☐ NA- No observable pressure ulcer

34. (M0468) Does this patient have a stasis ulcer?

- ☐ 0 - No (If no, go to M0482)
- ☒ 1 - Yes

34a. (M0470) Current number of observable stasis ulcer(s):

- ☐ 0 - Zero
- ☒ 1 - One
- ☐ 2 - Two
- ☐ 3 - Three
- ☐ 4 - Four or more

34b. (M0474) Does this patient have at least one stasis ulcer that cannot be observed due to the presence of a nonremovable dressing?

- ☒ 0 - No
- ☐ 1 - Yes

34c. (M0475) Status of most problematic (observable) stasis ulcer:

- ☐ 1 - Fully granulating
- ☒ 2 - Early/partial granulation
- ☐ 3 - Not healing
- ☐ NA- No observable stasis ulcer

35. (M0482) Does this patient have a surgical wound?

- ☒ 0 - No (If no, go to M0490)
- ☐ 1 - Yes

35a. (M0484) Current number of (observable) surgical wounds: (If a wound is partially closed but has more than one opening, consider each opening as a separate wound.)

- ☐ 0 - Zero
- ☐ 1 - One
- ☐ 2 - Two
- ☐ 3 - Three
- ☐ 4 - Four or more

35b. (M0486) Does this patient have at least one surgical wound that cannot be observed due to the presence of a nonremovable dressing?

- ☐ 0 - No
- ☐ 1 - Yes

35c. (M0488) Status of most problematic (observable) surgical wound:

- ☐ 1- Fully granulating
- ☐ 2 - Early/partial granulation
- ☐ 3 - Not healing
- ☐ NA- No observable surgical wound

RESPIRATORY STATUS

36. (M0490) When is the patient dyspneic or noticeably short of breath?

- ☐ 0 - Never; patient is not short of breath
- ☒ 1 - When walking more than 20 feet, climbing stairs
- ☐ 2 - With moderate exertion (e.g., while dressing, using commode, or bedpan, walking distances less than 20 feet)
- ☐ 3 - With minimal exertion (e.g., while eating, talking, or performing other ADLs) or with agitation
- ☐ 4 - At rest (during day or night)

37. (M0500) Respiratory treatments utilized at home: (Mark all that apply.)

- ☐ 1 - Oxygen (intermittent or continuous)
- ☐ 2 - Ventilator (continually or at night)
- ☐ 3 - Continuous positive airway pressure
- ☒ 4 - None of the above

ELIMINATION STATUS

38. (M0510) Has this patient been treated for a urinary tract infection in the past 14 days?

- ☒ 0 - No
- ☐ 1 - Yes
- ☐ NA- Patient on prophylactic treatment
- ☐ UK- Unknown

39. (M0520) Urinary incontinence or urinary catheter presence:

- ☒ 0 - No incontinence or catheter (includes anuria or ostomy for urinary drainage) (If no, go to M0540)
- ☐ 1 - Patient is incontinent
- ☐ 2 - Patient requires a urinary catheter (i.e., external, indwelling, intermittent, suprapubic) (Go to M0540)

Outcome and assessment information set *(continued)*

40. (M0530) When does urinary incontinence occur?

- ☐ 0 - Timed voiding defers incontinence
- ☐ 1 - During the night only
- ☐ 2 - During the day and night

41. (M0540) Bowel incontinence frequency:

- ☒ 0 - Very rarely or never has bowel incontinence
- ☐ 1 - Less than once weekly
- ☐ 2 - One to three times weekly
- ☐ 3 - Four to six times weekly
- ☐ 4 - On a daily basis
- ☐ 5 - More often than once daily
- ☐ NA- Patient has ostomy for bowel elimination
- ☐ UK- Unknown

42. (M0550) Ostomy for bowel elimination: Does this patient have an ostomy for bowel elimination that (within the last 14 days): a) was related to an inpatient facility stay, or b) necessitated a change in medical or treatment regimen?

- ☒ 0 - Patient does not have an ostomy for bowel elimination
- ☐ 1 - Patient's ostomy was not related to an inpatient stay and did not necessitate change in medical or treatment regimen
- ☐ 2 - Ostomy was related to an inpatient stay or did necessitate change in medical or treatment regimen

NEURO/EMOTIONAL/BEHAVIOR STATUS

43. (M0560) Cognitive functioning: (patient's current level of alertness, orientation, comprehension, concentration, and immediate memory for simple commands)

- ☐ 0 - Alert/oriented, able to focus and shift attention, comprehends and recalls task directions independently
- ☒ 1 - Requires prompting (cuing, repetition, reminders) only under stressful or unfamiliar conditions
- ☐ 2 - Requires assistance and some direction in specific situations (e.g., on all tasks involving shifting of attention), or consistently requires low stimulus environment due to distractibility
- ☐ 3 - Requires considerable assistance in routine situations; is not alert and oriented or is unable to shift attention and recall directions more than half the time
- ☐ 4 - Totally dependent due to disturbances such as constant disorientation, coma, persistent vegetative state, or delirium

44. (M0570) When confused (reported or observed):

- ☒ 0 - Never
- ☐ 1 - In new or complex situations only
- ☐ 2 - On awakening or at night only
- ☐ 3 - During the day and evening, but not constantly
- ☐ 4 - Constantly
- ☐ NA- Patient nonresponsive

45. (M0580) When anxious (reported or observed):

- ☐ 0 - None of the time
- ☐ 1 - Less often than daily
- ☒ 2 - Daily, but not constantly
- ☐ 3 - All of the time
- ☐ NA- Patient nonresponsive

46. (M0590) Depressive feelings reported or observed in patient: (Mark all that apply.)

- ☐ 1 - Depressed mood (e.g., feeling sad, tearful)
- ☐ 2 - Sense of failure or self-reproach
- ☒ 3 - Hopelessness
- ☐ 4 - Recurrent thoughts of death
- ☐ 5 - Thoughts of suicide
- ☐ 6 - None of the above feelings observed or reported

47. (M0600) Patient behaviors (reported or observed): (Mark all that apply.)

- ☐ 1 - Indecisiveness, lack of concentration
- ☐ 2 - Diminished interest in most activities
- ☐ 3 - Sleep disturbances
- ☐ 4 - Recent change in appetite or weight
- ☐ 5 - Agitation
- ☐ 6 - A suicide attempt
- ☒ 7 - None of the above behaviors observed or reported

48. (M0610) Behaviors demonstrated at least once a week (reported or observed): (Mark all that apply.)

- ☐ 1 - Memory deficit: failure to recognize familiar persons/places, inability to recall events of past 24 hours, significant memory loss so that supervision is required
- ☐ 2 - Impaired decision-making: failure to perform usual ADLs or IADLs, inability to appropriately stop activities jeopardizes safety through actions
- ☐ 3 - Verbal disruption: yelling, threatening, excessive profanity, sexual references, etc.

(continued)

Outcome and assessment information set *(continued)*

☐ 4 - Physical aggression: aggressive or combative to self and others (e.g., hits self, throws objects, punches, performs dangerous maneuvers with wheelchair or other objects)

☐ 5 - Disruptive, infantile, or socially inappropriate behavior (excludes verbal actions)

☐ 6 - Delusional, hallucinatory, or paranoid behavior

☒ 7 - None of the above behaviors demonstrated

49. (M0620) Frequency of behavior problems (reported or observed) (e.g., wandering episodes, self-abuse, verbal disruption, physical aggression, etc.):

☒ 0 - Never
☐ 1 - Less than once a month
☐ 2 - Once a month
☐ 3 - Several times each month
☐ 4 - Several times a week
☐ 5 - At least daily

50. (M0630) Is this patient receiving psychiatric nursing services at home provided by a qualified psychiatric nurse?

☒ 0 - No
☐ 1 - Yes

ADL/IADLs

For Questions 51 to 67, complete the "current" column for all patients. For these same items, complete the "prior" column at start of care or resumption of care; mark the level that corresponds to the patient's condition 14 days prior to the start of care. In all cases, record what the patient is able to do.

51. (M0640) Grooming: Ability to tend to personal hygiene needs (i.e., washing face and hands, hair care, shaving or makeup, teeth or denture care, fingernail care):

Prior Current

☒ ☐ 0 - Able to groom self unaided, with or without the use of assistive devices or adapted methods
☐ ☐ 1 - Grooming utensils must be placed within reach before able to complete grooming activities
☐ ☒ 2 - Someone must assist the patient to groom self
☐ ☐ 3 - Depends entirely upon someone else for grooming needs
☐   UK - Unknown

52. (M0650) Ability to dress upper body (with or without dressing aids), including pullovers, undergarments, front-opening shirts and blouses, managing zippers, buttons, and snaps:

Prior Current

☒ ☐ 0 - Able to get clothes out of closets and drawers, put them on, and remove them from the upper body without assistance
☐ ☒ 1 - Able to dress upper body without assistance if clothing is laid out or handed to the patient
☐ ☐ 2 - Someone must put on upper body clothing
☐ ☐ 3 - Depends entirely upon another person to dress the upper body
☐   UK - Unknown

53. (M0660) Ability to dress lower body (with or without dressing aids), including slacks, undergarments, socks or nylons, shoes:

Prior Current

☒ ☐ 0 - Able to obtain, put on, and remove clothing and shoes without assistance
☐ ☐ 1 - Able to dress lower body without assistance if clothing and shoes are laid out or handed to patient
☐ ☒ 2 - Someone must help put on undergarments, slacks, socks or nylons, and shoes
☐ ☐ 3 - Depends entirely upon another person to dress lower body
☐   UK - Unknown

Outcome and assessment information set *(continued)*

54. (M0670) Bathing: Ability to wash entire body; excludes grooming (washing face and hands only):

Prior Current

- ☑ ☐ 0 - Able to bathe self in shower or tub independently
- ☑ ☐ 1 - With the use of devices, able to bathe self in shower or tub independently
- ☐ ☐ 2 - Able to bathe in shower or tub with the assistance of another person:
  (a) for intermittent supervision or encouragement or reminders OR
  (b) to get in and out of the shower or tub OR
  (c) for washing difficult-to-reach areas
- ☐ ☑ 3 - Participates in bathing self in shower or tub, but requires presence of another person throughout the bath for assistance or supervision
- ☐ ☐ 4 - Unable to use the shower or tub and is bathed in bed or bedside chair
- ☐ ☐ 5 - Unable to effectively participate in bathing and is totally bathed by another person
- ☐ UK - Unknown

55. (M0680) Toileting: Ability to get to and from the toilet or bedside commode:

Prior Current

- ☑ ☑ 0 - Able to get to and from the toilet independently with or without a device
- ☐ ☐ 1 - When reminded, assisted, or supervised by another person, able to get to and from the toilet
- ☐ ☐ 2 - Unable to get to and from the toilet but is able to use a bedside commode (with or without assistance)
- ☐ ☐ 3 - Unable to get to and from the toilet or bedside commode but is able to use a bedpan/urinal independently
- ☐ ☐ 4 - Totally dependent in toileting
- ☐ UK - Unknown

56. (M0690) Transferring: Ability to move from bed to chair, on and off toilet or commode, into and out of tub or shower, and ability to turn and position self in bed if patient is bedfast:

Prior Current

- ☐ ☐ 0 - Able to transfer independently
- ☑ ☑ 1 - Transfers with minimal human assistance or with use of an assistive device
- ☐ ☐ 2 - Unable to transfer self but able to bear weight and pivot during the transfer process
- ☐ ☐ 3 - Unable to transfer self and unable to bear weight or pivot when transferred by another person
- ☐ ☐ 4 - Bedfast, unable to transfer but able to turn and position self in bed
- ☐ ☐ 5 - Bedfast, unable to transfer and unable to turn and position self
- ☐ UK - Unknown

57. (M0700) Ambulation/Locomotion: Ability to walk safely, once in a standing position, or use a wheelchair, once in a seated position, on a variety of surfaces:

Prior Current

- ☑ ☐ 0 - Able to walk independently on even and uneven surfaces and climb stairs with or without railings (i.e., needs no human assistance or assistive device)
- ☐ ☑ 1 - Requires use of a device (e.g., cane, walker) to walk alone or requires human supervision or assistance to negotiate stairs or steps or uneven surfaces
- ☐ ☐ 2 - Able to walk only with the supervision of assistance of another person at all times
- ☐ ☐ 3 - Chairfast, unable to ambulate but able to wheel self independently
- ☐ ☐ 4 - Chairfast, unable to ambulate and unable to wheel self
- ☐ ☐ 5 - Bedfast, unable to ambulate or be up in a chair
- ☐ UK - Unknown

(continued)

58. (M0710) Feeding or eating: Ability to feed self meals and snacks: (*Note:* This refers only to the process of eating, chewing, and swallowing, not preparing the food to be eaten.)

Prior Current

☒ ☒ 0 - Able to feed self independently

☐ ☐ 1 - Able to feed self independently but requires:
(a) meal set-up OR
(b) intermittent assistance or supervision from another person; OR
(c) a liquid, pureed, or ground meat diet

☐ ☐ 2 - Unable to feed self and must be assisted or supervised throughout the meal/snack

☐ ☐ 3 - Able to take in nutrients orally and receives supplemental nutrients through a nasogastric tube or gastrostomy

☐ ☐ 4 - Unable to take in nutrients orally and is fed nutrients through a nasogastric tube or gastrostomy

☐ ☐ 5 - Unable to take in nutrients orally or by tube feeding

☐ UK - Unknown

59. (M0720) Planning and preparing light meals (e.g., cereal, sandwich) or reheat delivered meals:

Prior Current

☒ ☐ 0 - (a) Able to independently plan and prepare all light meals for self or reheat delivered meals; OR
(b) Is physically, cognitively, and mentally able to prepare light meals on a regular basis but has not routinely performed light meal preparation in the past (i.e., prior to this home care admission)

☐ ☒ 1 - Unable to prepare light meals on a regular basis due to physical, cognitive, or mental limitations

☐ ☐ 2 - Unable to prepare any light meals or reheat any delivered meals

☐ UK - Unknown

60. (M0730) Transportation: physical and mental ability to safely use a car, taxi, or public transportation (bus, train, subway):

Prior Current

☐ ☐ 0 - Able to independently drive a regular or adapted car, OR uses a regular or handicap-accessible public bus

☒ ☒ 1 - Able to ride in a car only when driven by another person; OR able to use a bus or handicap van only when assisted or accompanied by another person

☐ ☐ 2 - Unable to ride in a car, taxi, bus, or van, and requires transportation by ambulance

☐ UK - Unknown

61. (M0740) Laundry: Ability to do own laundry—to carry laundry to and from washing machine, to use washer and dryer, to wash small items by hand:

Prior Current

☐ ☐ 0 - (a) Able to take care of all laundry tasks independently; OR
(b) Physically, cognitively, and mentally able to do laundry and access facilities, but has not routinely performed laundry tasks in the past (i.e., prior to this home care admission)

☒ ☐ 1 - Able to do only light laundry, such as minor hand wash or light washer loads; due to physical, cognitive, or mental limitations, needs assistance with heavy laundry such as carrying large loads of laundry

☐ ☒ 2 - Unable to do any laundry due to physical limitation or needs continual supervision and assistance due to cognitive or mental limitation

☐ UK - Unknown

Outcome and assessment information set *(continued)*

62. (M0750) Housekeeping: Ability to safely and effectively perform light housekeeping and heavier cleaning tasks:

Prior Current

☐ ☐ 0 - (a) Able to independently perform all housekeeping tasks; OR
(b) Physically, cognitively, and mentally able to perform all housekeeping tasks but has not routinely participated in housekeeping tasks in the past (i.e., prior to this home care admission)

☐ ☐ 1 - Able to perform only light housekeeping (e.g., dusting, wiping kitchen counters) tasks independently

☐ ☐ 2 - Able to perform housekeeping tasks with intermittent assistance or supervision from another person

☐ ☐ 3 - Unable to consistently perform any housekeeping tasks unless assisted by another person throughout the process

☒ ☒ 4 - Unable to effectively participate in any housekeeping tasks

☐ UK - Unknown

63. (M0760) Shopping: Ability to plan for, select, and purchase items in a store and to carry them home or arrange delivery:

Prior Current

☐ ☐ 0 - (a) Able to plan for shopping needs and independently perform shopping tasks, including carrying packages; OR
(b) Physically, cognitively, and mentally able to take care of shopping, but has not done shopping in the past (i.e., prior to this home care admission)

☐ ☐ 1 - Able to go shopping, but needs some assistance:
(a) By self is able to do only light shopping and carry small packages, but needs someone to do occasional major shopping; OR
(b) Unable to go shopping alone, but can go with someone to assist

☒ ☒ 2 - Unable to go shopping, but is able to identify items needed, place orders, and arrange home delivery

☐ ☐ 3 - Needs someone to do all shopping and errands

☐ UK - Unknown

64. (M0770) Ability to use telephone: Ability to answer the phone, dial numbers, and effectively use the telephone to communicate:

Prior Current

☒ ☒ 0 - Able to dial numbers and answer calls appropriately and as desired

☐ ☐ 1 - Able to use a specially adapted telephone (i.e., large numbers on the dial, teletype phone for the deaf) and call essential numbers

☐ ☐ 2 - Able to answer the telephone and carry on a normal conversation but has difficulty placing calls

☐ ☐ 3 - Able to answer the telephone only some of the time or is able to carry on only a limited conversation

☐ ☐ 4 - Unable to answer the telephone at all but can listen if assisted with equipment

☐ ☐ 5 - Totally unable to use the telephone

☐ ☐ NA - Patient does not have a telephone

☐ UK - Unknown

MEDICATIONS

65. (M0780) Management of oral medications: Patient's ability to prepare and take all prescribed oral medications reliably and safely, including administration of the correct dosage at the appropriate times/intervals; excludes injectable and IV medications: (*Note:* This refers to ability, not compliance or willingness.)

Prior Current

☒ ☒ 0 - Able to independently take the correct oral medication(s) and proper dosage(s) at the correct times

☐ ☐ 1 - Able to take medication(s) at the correct time if:
(a) individual dosages are prepared in advance by another person; OR
(b) given daily reminders; OR someone develops a drug diary or chart

☐ ☐ 2 - Unable to take medication unless administered by someone else

☐ ☐ NA - No oral medications prescribed

☐ UK - Unknown

66. (M0790) Management of inhalant/mist medications: Patient's ability to prepare and take all prescribed inhalants/mist medications (nebulizers, metered dose devices) reliably and safely, including administration of the correct dosage at the appropriate times/intervals; excludes all other forms of medication (oral tablets, injectable and I.V. medications):

Prior Current
- ☐ ☐ 0 - Able to independently take the correct medication and proper dosage at the correct times
- ☐ ☐ 1 - Able to take medication at the correct times if:
  (a) individual dosages are prepared in advance by another person; OR
  (b) given daily reminders.
- ☐ ☐ 2 - Unable to take medication unless administered by someone else
- ☒ ☒ NA - No inhalants/mist medications prescribed
- ☐ UK - Unknown

67. (M0800) Management of injectable medications: Patient's ability to prepare and take all prescribed injectable medications reliably and safely, including administration of correct dosages at appropriate times/intervals; excludes I.V. medications:

Prior Current
- ☒ ☒ 0 - Able to independently take the correct medication and proper dosage at the correct times
- ☐ ☐ 1 - Able to take injectable medication at the correct times if:
  (a) individual syringes are prepared in advance by another person, OR
  (b) given daily reminders
- ☐ ☐ 2 - Unable to take injectable medications unless administered by someone else
- ☐ ☐ NA - No injectable medications prescribed
- ☐ UK - Unknown

EQUIPMENT MANAGEMENT

68. (M0810) Patient management of equipment (includes only oxygen, I.V./infusion therapy, enteral/parenteral nutrition equipment or supplies): Patient's ability to set up, monitor and change equipment reliably and safely, to add appropriate fluids or medication, and to clean/store/dispose of equipment or supplies using proper technique: (*Note:* This refers to ability, not compliance or willingness.)

- ☐ 0 - Patient manages all tasks related to equipment completely independently.
- ☐ 1 - If someone else sets up equipment (i.e., fills portable oxygen tank, provides patient with prepared solutions), patient is able to manage all other aspects of equipment.
- ☐ 2 - Patient requires considerable assistance from another person to manage equipment, but completes portions of the task independently.
- ☐ 3 - Patient is only able to monitor equipment (e.g., liter flow, fluid in bag) and must call someone else to manage the equipment.
- ☐ 4 - Patient is completely dependent on someone else to manage all equipment.
- ☒ NA - No equipment of this type used in care (If NA, go to M0830).

69. (M0820) Caregiver management of equipment (includes only oxygen, I.V./infusion equipment, enteral/parenteral nutrition, ventilator therapy equipment or supplies): Caregiver's ability to set up, monitor, and change equipment reliably and safely, to add appropriate fluids or medication, and to clean/store/dispose of equipment or supplies using proper technique: (*Note:* This refers to ability, not compliance or willingness.)

- ☐ 0 - Caregiver manages all tasks related to equipment completely independently.
- ☐ 1 - If someone else sets up equipment, caregiver is able to manage all other aspects.
- ☐ 2 - Caregiver requires considerable assistance from another person to manage equipment, but independently completes significant portions of task.
- ☐ 3 - Caregiver is only able to complete small portions of task (e.g., administer nebulizer treatment, clean/store/dispose of equipment or supplies).
- ☐ 4 - Caregiver is completely dependent on someone else to manage all equipment.
- ☐ NA - No caregiver
- ☐ UK - Unknown

Outcome and assessment information set *(continued)*

EMERGENT CARE

70. (M0830) Emergent care: Since the last time OASIS data were collected, has the patient utilized any of the following services for emergent care (other than home care agency services)? (Mark all that apply.)

☒ 0 - No emergent care services (If no emergent care and patient discharged, go to M0855)

☐ 1 - Hospital emergency room (includes 23-hour holding)

☐ 2 - Doctor's office emergency visit/house call

☐ 3 - Outpatient department/clinic emergency (includes urgicenter sites)

☐ UK - Unknown

71. (M0840) Emergent care reason: For what reason(s) did the patient/family seek emergent care? (Mark all that apply.)

☐ 1 - Improper medication administration, medication adverse effects, toxicity, anaphylaxis

☐ 2 - Nausea, dehydration, malnutrition, constipation, impaction

☐ 3 - Injury caused by fall or accident at home

☐ 4 - Respiratory problems (e.g., shortness of breath, tracheobronchial obstruction, respiratory infection)

☐ 5 - Wound infection, deteriorating wound status, new lesion/ulcer

☐ 6 - Cardiac problems (e.g., fluid overload, exacerbation of heart failure, chest pain)

☐ 7 - Hypoglycemia/hyperglycemia, diabetes out of control

☐ 8 - GI bleeding, obstruction

☐ 9 - Other than above reasons

☐ UK - Reason unknown

DATA ITEMS COLLECTED AT INPATIENT FACILITY ADMISSION OR AGENCY DISCHARGE ONLY

72. (M0855) To which inpatient facility has the patient been admitted?

☐ 1 - Hospital (Go to M0890)

☐ 2 - Rehabilitation facility (Go to M0903)

☐ 3 - Nursing home (Go to M0900)

☐ 4 - Hospice (Go to M0903)

☐ NA - No inpatient facility admission

73. (M0870) Discharge disposition: Where is the patient after discharge from your agency? (Choose only one answer.)

☐ 1 - Patient remained in the community (not in hospital, nursing home, or rehab facility)

☐ 2 - Patient transferred to a noninstitutional hospice (Go to M0903)

☐ 3 - Unknown because patient moved to a geographic location not served by this agency (Go to M0903)

☐ UK - Other Unknown (Go to M0903)

74. (M0880) After discharge, does the patient receive health, personal, or support services or assistance? (Mark all that apply.)

☐ 1 - No assistance or services received

☐ 2 - Yes, assistance or services provided by family or friends

☐ 3 - Yes, assistance or services provided by other community resources (e.g., Meals-On-Wheels, home health services, homemaker assistance, transportation assistance, assisted living, board and care)

(Go to M0903)

75. (M0890) If the patient was admitted to an acute care hospital, for what reason was he/she admitted?

☐ 1 - Hospitalization for emergent (unscheduled) care

☐ 2 - Hospitalization for urgent (scheduled within 24 hours of admission) care

☐ 3 - Hospitalization for elective (scheduled more than 24 hours before admission) care

☐ UK - Unknown

Outcome and assessment information set *(continued)*

76. (M0895) Reason for hospitalization: (Mark all that apply.)
☐ 1 - Improper medication administration, medication side effects, toxicity, anaphylaxis
☐ 2 - Injury caused by fall or accident at home
☐ 3 - Respiratory problems (shortness of breath, infection, obstruction)
☐ 4 - Wound or tube site infection, deteriorating wound status, new lesion/ulcer
☐ 5 - Hypoglycemia/hyperglycemia, diabetes out of control
☐ 6 - GI bleeding, obstruction
☐ 7 - Exacerbation of heart failure, fluid overload, heart failure
☐ 8 - Myocardial infarction, stroke
☐ 9 - Chemotherapy
☐ 10 - Scheduled surgical procedure
☐ 11 - Urinary tract infection
☐ 12 - I.V. catheter-related infection
☐ 13 - Deep vein thrombosis, pulmonary embolus
☐ 14 - Uncontrolled pain
☐ 15 - Psychotic episode
☐ 16 - Other than above reasons
(Go to M0903)

77. (M0900) For what reason(s) was the patient admitted to a nursing home? (Mark all that apply.)
☐ 1 - Therapy services
☐ 2 - Respite care
☐ 3 - Hospice care
☐ 4 - Permanent placement
☐ 5 - Unsafe for care at home
☐ 6 - Other
☐ UK - Unknown

78. (M0903) Date of last (most recent) home visit:
_0_ _5_ / _0_ _2_ / _2_ _0_ _0_ _0_
month   day   year

79. (M0906) Discharge/transfer/death date: Enter the date of the discharge, transfer, or death (at home) of the patient.

_ _ _ / _ _ / _ _ _ _
month   day   year
☐ UK - Unknown

data may be used as the basis for HCFA's planned prepayment system.

When completing the OASIS form, follow these guidelines:
• Check at least one box for each numbered topic on the form.
• Include the patient's major diagnoses and ICD-9 codes.
• Make sure that the patient's primary diagnosis is the one that requires skilled intermittent care.
• Double-check the patient's Medicare number on the form with the number on the patient's Medicare card.
• Complete the "Current" column in the section on activities of daily living for all patients; complete the "Prior" column at the start or resumption of care using the patient's condition as it was 14 days before the start of care.

• Obtain information as needed from the patient's family or caregivers if the patient can't provide it.

Plan of care

After confirming a patient's eligibility, performing an initial assessment, and verifying a physician's order, you'll need to create a plan of care that addresses the patient's needs. Most agencies use HCFA form 485 to create the plan of care. (See *Home health certification and plan of care.*)

Each patient's plan of care should document:
• the identification of the patient and physician
• primary and secondary diagnoses and dates of onset

Home health certification and plan of care

Known as form 485, the form below includes space for assessing functional abilities and documenting plan of care. This information is required for Medicare reimbursement.

1. Patient's HI Claim No. *000491675*	2. Start of Care Date *05/02/00*	3. Certification Period From: *05/02/00* To: *07/02/00*
4. Medical Record No. *541234*		5. Provider No. *0472*

6. Patient's Name and Address
Terry Elliot
11 Second Street
Hometown, PA 10981

7. Provider's Name, Address, and Telephone Number
Very Good Home Care
Health Rd
Hometown, PA 10981

8. Date of Birth *07/08/24*	9. Sex ☒ M ☐ F

10. Medications: Dose/Frequency/Route (N)ew (C)hanged
Humulin N 24u sc qam (c)
Tylenol 325 mg-1000 mg q 4h prn pain
Darvocet-N 100 one tab q 4h prn pain PO (N)
Mom 30 cc qhs prn PO

11. IDC-9-CM *891.0*	Principal Diagnosis *Open wound ankle*	Date *05/02/00*
12. ICD-9-CM *86.28*	Surgical Procedure *Debridement wound*	Date *05/02/00*
13. ICD-9-CM *250.73* *443.89*	Other Pertinent Diagnoses *Type 2 diabetes* *Peripheral vascular disease*	Date *05/02/00* *04/01/00*

14. DME and Supplies *Walker Wound Care Supplies*	15. Safety Measures *Correct use of supportive devices*

16. Nutritional requirements *20% protein, 30% fat*	17. Allergies: *NKA*

18. a. Functional Limitations

1 ☒ Amputation	5 ☐ Paralysis	9 ☐ Legally Blind
2 ☐ Bowel/Bladder (Incontinence)	6 ☒ Endurance	A ☐ Dyspnea with Minimal Exertion
3 ☐ Contracture	7 ☒ Ambulation	B ☐ Other
4 ☐ Hearing	8 ☐ Speech	

18. b Activities Permitted

1 ☐ Complete Bedrest	6 ☒ Partial Weight Bearing	A ☐ Wheelchair
2 ☐ Bedrest BRP	7 ☐ Independent At Home	B ☒ Walker
3 ☐ Up as Tolerated	8 ☐ Crutches	C ☐ No Restrictions
4 ☐ Transfer Bed/Chair	9 ☐ Cane	D ☐ Other (Specify)
5 ☐ Exercises Prescribed		

19. Mental Status

1 ☒ Oriented	4 ☐ Depressed	7 ☐ Agitated
2 ☐ Comatose	5 ☐ Disoriented	8 ☐ Other
3 ☒ Forgetful	6 ☐ Lethargic	

20. Prognosis:

1 ☐ Poor	3 ☐ Fair	5 ☐ Excellent
2 ☒ Guarded	4 ☐ Good	

21. Orders for Discipline and Treatments (Specify Amount/Frequency/Duration)
SN: Observe/assess: Cardiopulmonary, respiratory, musculoskeletal, GI, and circulatory systems function. Assess: nutritional intake and dietary compliance related to wound healing; skin integrity and peripheral pulses; diabetic home management; and home safety. Instruct patient/caregiver in: diabetic management; signs/symptoms of wound infection; wound care; home safety; and emergency measures. SN to provide: wound care, until patient is independent: daily wound care to (L) ankle area = clean area with saline and apply wet to dry saline dressing. SN visits: 5-7/wk x 3 wks; 2-4/wk x 3 wks; 1-3/wk x 3 wks

(continued)

Home health certification and plan of care *(continued)*

---

22. Goals/Rehabilitation Potential/Discharge Plans

SN: GOALS: wound healing without infection or further complications, compliance with diabetic home management. Rehab potential to achieve goals: fair. D/C plan: to family/self when care is independent.

---

23. Nurse's Signature and Date of Verbal SOC Where Applicable	25. Date HHA Received Signed POT
Victoria Mansfield, RN 05/02/00	*05/12/00*

---

24. Physician's Name and Address

Dr. Kyle Stevens
Dr's Medical Center
Hometown, PA 10981

26. I certify/recertify that this patient is confined to his/her home and needs intermittent skilled nursing care, physical therapy and/or speech therapy or continues to need occupational therapy. The patient is under my care, and I have authorized the services on this plan of care and will periodically review the plan.

---

27. Attending Physician's Signature and Date Signed

Kyle Stevens, M.D. 05/05/00

28. Anyone who misrepresents, falsifies, or conceals essential information required for payment of Federal funds may be subject to fine, imprisonment, or civil penalty under applicable Federal laws.

FORM HCFA-485-(C-4) (0-94) (Print Aligned)   PROVIDER

- homebound status and functional limitations
- current diet and medications
- potential rehabilitation goals, if applicable
- specific orders to meet the patient's needs.

Updates and recertification

If the plan of care requires a change, such as an increase in the frequency of visits because of a change in the patient's condition, you'll need to update the plan of care to address this change. In your documentation, include:

- details of the change in the patient's condition to support the change in plan of care
- the possibility of hospitalization and return home on discharge if applicable
- changes in the patient's support system.

Even if the patient's condition does not change, you'll need to update his plan of care every 57 to 62 days if Medicare is paying for his care. Documentation for recertification must clearly support the patient's continued need for care within Medicare's (or another insurer's) guidelines. Complete a clinical summary and then send it to the patient's physician and the reimbursement agent. Commonly, you'll use HCFA form 485 for recertification. If so, follow these guidelines:

- Include all updated data, as amended by verbal orders, since the start of care.
- Record the primary diagnosis as the one that reflects the patient's current needs — not the original reason for home health care.
- Include other diagnoses, as appropriate, to demonstrate the impact on the patient's current status and need for continued care.
- Include a summary of all disciplines involved, including the home health care aide.
- Provide updated information about treatments, goals, and the frequency and duration of visits.
- Include what has already been accomplished as well as realistic goals for continued treatment.
- Review the new orders with the patient's physician and sign a verbal order for start of care as evidence of your communication and agreement with the physician about the patient's need for continued services

Sometimes, HCFA may request that you use form 486 instead of 485 for medical updates and possibly for recertification. (See *Medical update and patient information*, page 100.) On this form, you'll use a list of codes to describe the skills services provided to the patient:

A1 Skill observation and assessment
A2 Indwelling urinary catheter insertion
A3 Bladder instillation
A4 Open wound care and dressing
A5 Decubitus care (partial tissue loss with signs of infection or full tissue loss)
A6 Venipuncture
A7 Restorative nursing
A8 Postcataract care

A9 Bowel or bladder training
A10 Chest physiotherapy (percussion and postural drainage)
A11 Administration of vitamin B_{12}
A12 Administration of insulin
A13 Administration of other I.M. or subcutaneous injections
A14 Administration of I.V. clysis
A15 Teaching ostomy or ileostomy care
A16 Teaching nasogastric feeding
A17 Reinsertion of nasogastric feeding tube
A18 Teaching gastrostomy feeding
A19 Teaching parenteral nutrition
A20 Teaching care of tracheostomy
A21 Administration of tracheostomy care
A22 Teaching inhalation treatment
A23 Administration of inhalation treatment
A24 Teaching of administration of injection
A25 Teaching diabetic care
A26 Disimpaction and follow-up enema
A27 Other treatments not listed but ordered by physician
A28 Wound care and dressing (closed incision or suture line)
A29 Decubitus care (other than listed in A5)
A30 Teaching care of any indwelling catheter
A31 Management and evaluation of patient plan of care
A32 Teaching and training of other skilled nursing services ordered by physician.

The physician must specify in writing exactly what is to be done for codes A1, A4, A5, A6, A7, A22, A23, A27, A28, A29, and A32.

Other disciplines use specific codes as well with different letters to indicate the skilled service involved. For instance, physical therapists use num-

Medical update and patient information

When requested by Medicare, you will have to complete form 486, shown below. This form provides Medicare with information to support the need for skilled nursing care.

Department of Health and Human Services
Health Care Financing Administration

Form Approved
OMB No. 0938-0357

Medical Update and Patient Information

1. Patient's HI Claim No. *000491675*	2. SOC Date *05/02/00*	3. Certification Period From: *07/02/00* To: *09/02/00*

4. Medical Record No. *54/234*	5. Provider No. *0472*

6. Patient's Name and Address *Terry Elliot, 11 Second St., Hometown, PA*	7. Provider's Name *Very Good Home Care*

8. Medicare Covered: ☒ Y ☐ N	9. Date Physician Last Saw Patient: *06/30/00*

10. Date Last Contacted Physician: *06/12/00*

11. Is the Patient Receiving Care in an 1861 (J)(1) Skilled Nursing Facility or Equivalent?
☐ Y   ☒ N   ☐ Do Not Know

12. ☐ Certification   ☒ Recertification   ☐ Modified

13. Dates of Last Inpatient Stay: Admission *N/A* Discharge *N/A*	14. Type of Facility: *N/A*

15. Updated information: New Orders/Treatments/Clinical Facts/Summary from Each Discipline

SN: 06/12/00: Dr. Contacted to report temp = 101° orally, increased amt. thick, tan, foul smelling drainage. Pt. started on Cephalexin 500 mg BID po x 10 days, increase wound care to BID and increase SN visits for wound care to 12–14 x 3 wks.

PT: 06/01/00: Verbal order received to increase patient to ambulate as tolerated with walker. Continue strengthening home exercise program.

SN: 06/02/00: Decrease wound care to daily. Decrease SN visits to 5–7 x 7 wks.

16. Functional Limitations (Expand From 485 and Level of ADL) Reason Homebound/Prior Functional Status *FL: Ambulation, endurance, open, draining wound. RH: Unable to ambulate more than 15 ft. before becoming exhausted. PFS: Independent ambulation.*

17. Supplementary Plan of Care on File from Physician Other than Referring Physician: ☐ Y ☒ N (If Yes, Please Specify Giving Goals/Rehab. Potential/Discharge Plan)

18. Unusual Home/Social Environment *Cluttered home with narrow hallways*

19. Indicate Any Time When the Home Health Agency Made a Visit and Patient Was Not Home and Reason Why if Ascertainable *N/A*	20. Specify Any Known Medical and/or Non-Medical Reason the Patient Regularly Leaves Home and Frequency of Occurrence *Dr's office visits as needed.*

21. Nurse or Therapist Completing or Reviewing Form *Holly Dougherty, RN, BSN*	Date (Mo., Day, Yr.) *07/02/00*

HCFA-486 (C3) (02-94) (Print Aligned)   PROVIDER

bers that start with B, speech pathologists use C, occupational therapists use D, social workers use E, and home care aides use F. Each F code denotes a specific care activity, such as F1 for a tub or shower bath, F6 for catheter care, and F8 for assistance with ambulation.

Progress notes

At each visit, you'll need to write a progress note. This is where you document the patient's condition and any significant events that occur while you are providing care. (See *The progress note*, page 102.) When completing a progress note, record information in chronological order and make sure you include at least the following:
• any changes in the patient's condition
• skilled nursing interventions performed related to the plan of care
• patient's response to services provided
• any event or incident in the home that would affect the treatment plan
• patient's vital signs
• teaching performed with patient and caregiver, including any written materials and brochures provided and return demonstrations of any skills or procedures.

Write progress notes legibly in black ink. Avoid repetition as well as spelling and grammatical errors. Date each entry with the day, month, and year. Sign each entry and include your title. Avoid addendums. Don't erase entries or use correction fluid; instead, follow your agency's policy on correcting errors.

Provide a heading for each entry if different members of the home care team use the same form. Use only agency-approved abbreviations and symbols. Use flow sheets and checklists to record vital signs, intake and output, and nutritional data. Clearly state why the patient is homebound and continue to document his ongoing homebound status. Document conversations and care coordination among team members, including the physician. If the patient receives skilled nursing and physician visits on the same day, document the reason for each visit.

Include only pertinent medical information, keeping your statements brief, concise, consistent, and specific. Avoid using the terms "stable" and "chronic." Use objective data, such as specific dimensions and sizes, rather than subjective data. Also, reflect the patient's continuing need for care.

Also document the specific skilled care provided and how it relates to the patient's diagnosis and plan of care. Record all verbal and written instructions, return demonstrations, verbalizations of learning, and any resistance to learning. Justify the need to repeat instructions.

Finally, document the patient's progression toward desired outcomes. Outline teaching given to the patient and caregiver and their return demonstrations. Explain the patient's response to care and services provided in comparison to the goals. Detail psychological changes and pain status. Document supervision given, changes in the patient's status, and the staff's response. Record initial medications (including over-the-counter) and those added to the patient's regimen during care. Finally, complete your progress note within 24 hours of providing care and place

The progress note

Progress notes describe — in chronological order — patient problems and needs, nursing observations, reassessments, and interventions. A sample appears below.

☐ PHONE REPORT	☐ COORDINATION NOTE	☒ CLINICAL NOTE CONTINUATION

Patient Name *Terry Elliot*   ID# *541234*   Date *06/12/00*

T=101°   P=100   R=28   BP=160/94. Patient unaware of fever but complaining of increased pain at wound site. Darvocet is controlling pain but patient taking it q 4hr. while awake. Wound of Ⓛankle =4 cm x 4.5 cm x 1 cm deep. Open area appears pink with increased amounts of thick, tan drainage. Wound is foul smelling. Dr's office contacted and patient to start on Cephalexin PO. SN to increase visits for BID wound care. Pt denies other complaints. Glucometer FBS = 140 this am. Lungs with diminished breath sounds at bases. Appetite good, bowels regular – had BM today. Began instruction to patient on Cephalexin dose, schedule, and adverse effects. Patient appears quite anxious about wound condition. Explanation of signs, symptoms, and treatment of wound infection reinforced. Pt. able to repeat most explanations. Support offered. SN to return for pm wound care today and patient should have begun antibiotic therapy by then.

Holly Dougherty, RN, BSN
SERVICE BY (SIGNATURE)   TITLE

it in the patient's medical record within 7 days (per agency policy).

Clinical pathways

Clinical pathways (also known as critical paths, care maps, and care guidelines) are widely used as documentation tools and a way to manage patient outcomes in home care, long-term care,

and acute care settings. In general, clinical pathways help to decrease length of stay, decrease costs, and improve outcomes of care. Think of a clinical pathway as a road map that outlines a patient's entire course of care. Pathways have been developed for a wide range of specific diagnoses and surgical procedures, although the format may differ somewhat from agency to agency.

One of the most helpful aspects of clinical pathways is that they can be used to help spotlight trends in achieving goals. By studying reports assembled at the end of care, your agency can determine which expected outcomes weren't achieved (called variances) to see a clearer picture of how the services provided related to the outcomes obtained—and, by extension, how improvements in services might improve outcomes.

A clinical pathway offers a simple, standardized tool to organize a sometimes daunting number of care tasks. It serves as both a plan of care and a documentation system coordinated by a single professional, usually a nurse case manager. If you're that person, you'll use the pathway to coordinate the patient's care and to make sure that nothing is left out of the patient's treatment or education. A pathway also greatly improves communication among disciplines. You no longer need to wonder what goals the physical or occupational therapist is working toward: they're clearly defined and outlined on the clinical pathway.

Clinical pathways also save time by sparing you from researching and writing an entire plan of care by hand. You need only complete the appropriate pathway for the patient's primary diagnosis, and much of your work is done. You'll also find yourself spending less time documenting visit patterns, expected outcomes, and guidelines for patient teaching and treatment. This one tool can accomplish all of that by being personalized for an individual patient.

Clinical pathways are kept in patients' charts and are initialed and dated by home care team members as treatments are provided—on a per-visit basis for home care. Each home care agency determines which procedures and disorders warrant using a clinical pathway. Agencies that specialize in providing care for pediatric clients would naturally have more pathways built on pediatric diagnoses than an agency that provides care for elderly clients.

Discharge summary

When the patient no longer needs or is eligible for home care, a discharge summary is prepared. (See *Preparing a discharge summary,* page 104.)

When preparing a discharge summary, include the following topics:
• services provided
• patient's clinical and psychosocial condition at the time of discharge
• recommendations for further care and supportive services, as appropriate
• patient's response to and comprehension of teaching plan
• outcomes that are achieved and not achieved, including reasons for lack of achievement.

Electronic documentation safeguards

Using a computer to document patient care can help increase your speed and accuracy, reduce your reliance on recall, and expedite the exchange of data among care providers and third-party payers. By improving legibility, it can also reduce the risk of misinterpreta-

Preparing a discharge summary

Discharge Summary

CODE _01_

Admission Date _05/02/00_
Discharge Date _07/14/00_

Name: _Terry Elliot_   Medical Record No.: _541234_

Address: _11 Second St., Hometown, PA 10981_   Phone No.: _881-555-2937_

Primary Diagnosis: _Open wound -Ⓛ ankle_

Physician: _Dr. Kyle Stevens_   Date of Birth: _07/08/24_

Services Provided: ☒ Nursing   ☐ Occupational Therapy   ☐ Speech Therapy
                   ☐ Aide   ☒ Physical Therapy   ☐ Social Work
                   ☐ Other_____

Reason for Discharge:
      ☒ Condition Improved   ☐ Died in Hospital
      ☐ Self/Family Choice   ☐ Referred to Hospital
      ☐ Moved Out of Area   ☐ Placed in Long-Term Institution
      ☐ Referred to Another Agency ☐ Referred, Not Admitted
      ☐ Died at Home   ☐ Other_____

Physician Notified of Closure: ☒ Yes   ☐ No   Date: _07/14/00_
           Family Notified: ☒ Yes   ☐ No   Date: _07/14/00_

Able to verbalize knowledge of the etiology, signs and symptoms, and
sequelae/complications of health problem(s).
              Patient: ☐ Yes   ☒ Partially   ☐ No
      Family/Caregiver: ☒ Yes   ☐ Partially   ☐ No

Able to demonstrate knowledge and skills related to the treatment and management of
health problem(s).
              Patient: ☐ Yes   ☒ Partially   ☐ No
      Family/Caregiver: ☐ Yes   ☒ Partially   ☐ No

Patient Status:
   The patient's condition is: ☐ Stable ☐ Unstable ☒ Improving
                               ☐ Declining ☐ Other _____

ADL STATUS: ☒ Improving   ☐ Unchanged   ☐ Declining

	Dependent	Partially Independent	Independent	Functional Outcomes:	From	To
Bathing			X	Knowledge	_poor_	_fair_
Dressing			X	Skill	_fair_	_good_
Toileting			X	Psychosocial	_poor_	_fair_
Transferring			X	Health Status	_poor_	_fair_
Feeding			X			
Ambulation		X				
Activity Tolerance	(poor)	(fair)	(good)			

SUPPORT SYSTEMS: ☒ Family   ☐ Caregiver   ☐ Friends
      ☐ Community resources   ☒ Patient uses support systems appropriately
      ☐ Support systems inadequate ☐ Patient uses support systems ineffectively
      ☐ Other _____

COMMENTS: _____
_____

tion. In addition, it can help to standardize care by providing structures, input formats, and mandatory charting fields for assessment and other notes.

Many home care agencies have specific computer programs that develop the plans of care, formulate goals, monitor patients' progress, update medications, and generate visit notes. Also, many agencies have computers that are programmed to produce the exact information Medicare or another third-party payer wants — in the format they want it. In addition, some agency computer systems include algorithms for patient care, standardized plans of care, medication sheets, and disease information handouts that can be used as teaching tools.

Like manual documentation, computerized documentation provides a detailed account of the patient's clinical status, diagnostic tests, treatments, and medical history. Unlike the manual method, computerized records store all the patient's medical data in a single, easily accessible location.

Even with all of its time-saving and improvement features, computerized documentation does have some disadvantages. Patients may be less truthful about their histories if they know the information is stored in a computer. Many of the questions that patients need to answer can't always be standardized into a simple answer field. Finally, computers sometimes malfunction, resulting in lost or misplaced information.

Electronic documentation raises some legal concerns as well, particularly about patient privacy and confidentiality. A traditional chart can be safeguarded simply by locking it in a desk or chart room. This isn't so with electronic documents. In fact, you may be able to access a patient's chart from a laptop computer while you're still at the patient's home. This means that unauthorized persons may also gain access to that information.

To help keep electronic records safe, keep your password secure and confidential. Choose a password that other people would have trouble guessing. Don't write it down. If you suspect that someone else is using your password, change it and tell your supervisor about your concern.

Never leave patient information displayed on a screen unattended. Also, date and time all of your computer entries. Know your state's rules and regulations and your agency's policies and procedures regarding privileged data, confidentiality, and disclosure. Also, make sure to log off when you're finished working in a patient's record.

Whether you use paper or electronic charting, you always need to provide accurate, appropriate documentation. Keep these tips in mind:

- State the reasons for the patient's homebound status.
- Provide evidence to substantiate that the patient is using his personal strengths and resources, such as support systems, good health habits, and a safe environment, to facilitate his return to independence.
- Describe the primary caregiver, including whether this person lives with the patient, his relationship to the patient, his age and physical ability, and his willingness to help the patient.
- Document physical changes needed in the patient's home for him to be safe and receive proper care. Also, docu-

ment assistance given to the family regarding community support.

• Make sure the plan of care is comprehensive by including more than just the patient's physiological problems. Also include information about the home environment, needed resources, and the emotional states and attitudes of the patient, family, and caregivers.

• Keep a copy of the plan in the patient's home for easy reference.

• Make sure that all your documentation reflects the plan of care.

• Keep the plan updated, noting changes in the patient's condition or care needs; make note of any reports you make to the physician.

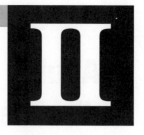

Home care standards for disorders and treatments

7 Adult disorders and treatments

Acquired immunodeficiency syndrome

Acquired immunodeficiency syndrome (AIDS) is caused by the human immunodeficiency virus (HIV) and refers to the most advanced stages of HIV infection. HIV kills or impairs cells of the immune system and progressively destroys the body's ability to fight infections and certain cancers. Patients with AIDS are susceptible to opportunistic infections that are caused by microbes and that usually don't cause illness in healthy people. HIV can be transmitted through contact with HIV-contaminated blood, sexual contact with an infected partner, or the sharing of needles or syringes contaminated with a small amount of infected blood. Women infected with HIV can transmit the virus to their fetuses and newborns during pregnancy, childbirth, and breastfeeding. There is no evidence that HIV is spread through sweat, tears, urine, or feces. Studies of families and caregivers of HIV-infected individuals have shown that HIV clearly isn't spread through casual contact such as sharing food utensils, towels, bedding, swimming pools, telephones, or toilet seats.

Because the diagnosis of HIV and its progression to AIDS is commonly surrounded by fear and misconception in regards to its transmission, education of the patient and his support system and caregiver is crucial. Poor nutrition, weight loss, dehydration, fatigue, and opportunistic respiratory infections are major concerns when treating a patient with AIDS; therefore, assessments and care should focus on these areas. Careful monitoring of respiratory status, temperature, hydration, and weight loss should be done at each visit. Because social isolation and depression are also problems a patient with AIDS may face, the patient and caregiver should be referred to appropriate support services.

Previsit checklist

Physician orders and preparation
● Medication dosage and route

- Diet orders
- Order for support services
- Activity orders and restrictions
- Durable medical equipment orders
- Oxygen orders
- Do-not-resuscitate (DNR) order

Equipment and supplies

- Supplies for standard precautions and proper sharps disposal
- Vital signs equipment
- Infusion system (preferably a needleless system)
- Nutrition and intake journal
- Scale
- Copy of advance directive and DNR order

Safety requirements

- Standard precautions for infection control, including secondary infections (such as tuberculosis), and sharps disposal
- System to assist with adherence to complex medication regimen
- Information on medications, including dosage, adverse effects, interactions, and safe storage
- Emergency plan and access to functional phone and list of emergency phone numbers
- Identification and correction of environmental hazards and patient-specific concerns (for example, not sharing razors and bleeding precautions)
- Fire evacuation plan, functional smoke detectors, and access to functional fire extinguisher
- Standard oxygen precautions as needed

Major diagnostic codes

- Cytomegaloviral disease 078.5
- Diarrhea 787.91
- Fever of unknown origin 780.6
- HIV infection without/with symptoms V08/042
- Kaposi's sarcoma 176.9
- Malaise and fatigue 780.79
- Mycobacterium, pulmonary 031.0
- *Pneumocystis carinii* pneumonia 136.3
- Pneumonia (bacterial) 482.9
- Pneumonia (viral) 480.9
- Tuberculosis (pulmonary) 011.9

(To assign a fifth digit, see appendix A, page 638.)

Defense of homebound status

- Inability to ambulate farther than 10′ (3 m) secondary to fatigue
- Continuous invasive procedure (I.V. therapy)
- Reverse isolation for severe immunosuppression
- End-of-life care
- Severe dyspnea
- Mental status impairment requiring 24-hour care and supervision
- Pain associated with movement
- Maximal assistance required with activities of daily living (ADLs)

Selected nursing diagnoses and patient outcomes

Knowledge deficit related to contagious nature of organism

The patient or caregiver will:

- detail the use of standard precautions and refrain from risky behavior

(N)

• describe the mode of transmission of the disease (N)
• demonstrate meticulous hand washing (N)
• verbalize measures to decrease the risk of bleeding, such as ways to prevent falls and the use of gloves for yard work. (N)

Fatigue related to disease process or weight loss

The patient or caregiver will:

• discuss the causes of fatigue (N)
• share feelings regarding the effects of fatigue on his life (N)
• establish priorities for daily and weekly activities (N)
• participate in activities that stimulate and balance physical, cognitive, affect, and social domains. (N, PT)

Altered nutrition: Less than body requirements related to anorexia, fatigue, nausea, and vomiting

The patient or caregiver will:

• increase oral intake as evidenced by _____ (N, D)
• describe causative factors when known. (N, D)

Altered oral mucous membrane related to dehydration and impaired ability to perform mouth care

The patient or caregiver will:

• maintain integrity of the oral cavity (N)
• be free from oral discomfort during food and fluid intake (N)
• demonstrate knowledge of oral hygiene. (N)

Ineffective management of therapeutic regimen: Individuals related to insufficient knowledge of condition, treatments, pharmacologic therapy, rest and activity balance, or signs and symptoms of complications

The patient or caregiver will:

• describe strategies to address progression or complications of his condition if they arise (N, SW)
• discuss situations that challenge his continued successful management. (N, SW)

Activity intolerance related to bed rest, immobility, or generalized weakness

The patient or caregiver will:

• identify methods for energy conservation. (N, PT)

Bathing or hygiene self-care deficit related to weakness and tiredness

The patient or caregiver will:

• identify methods to improve care. (N, PT, OT)

Risk for fluid volume deficit

The patient or caregiver will:

• maintain adequate hydration. (N, D)

Diarrhea related to adverse effects of medication, tube feedings, or infectious processes

The patient or caregiver will:

• identify causative factors (N, D)
• identify methods to reduce amount of diarrhea (N, D)
• maintain adequate hydration and nutrition. (N, D)

Ineffective airway clearance related to retained secretions, excessive mucus, or infection

The patient or caregiver will:

• maintain adequate oxygenation (N, RT)
• demonstrate effective coughing and deep-breathing exercises. (N, RT)

Risk for impaired skin integrity
The patient or caregiver will:
• maintain skin integrity   (N)
• identify methods to prevent skin breakdown.   (N)

Skilled nursing services

Care measures
• Perform a complete assessment, including the patient's weight, at each visit.
• Assess the level of care performed by the patient or caregiver.
• Assess adherence to the medical regimen.
• Assess for adverse drug effects as well as interactions with food and other drugs.
• Make sure copies of the DNR order and advance directive are in the home.
• Assess the effectiveness of pain medications.
• Perform skilled assessment of the mental and cognitive, nutrition and hydration, integumentary, cardiovascular, GI, and genitourinary systems; pay particular attention to objective and subjective data of the respiratory system and evidence of infection, such as thrush, rashes, fever, and discharge.
• Arrange for referrals to and conferences with support services.
• Coordinate support services. (This is important because patients with AIDS usually have a large number of support services, which may include financial assistance, housing, group therapies, medications, and counseling.)
• Administer I.V. medications as ordered; instruct in the maintenance of I.V. lines.
• Assess activity tolerance.

• List sources of support for significant others, particularly children, and help the patient implement wishes for meeting children's future needs.

Patient and family teaching
• Explain the AIDS disease process and the treatment plan. Allow time for the patient and family to express and discuss fears and frustrations as well as ask questions.
• Teach about adverse drug effects and reactions.
• Instruct about the plan of care and emergency plan.
• Instruct patient or caregiver to post emergency phone numbers.
• Teach safety precautions to prevent disease transmission (HIV and opportunistic diseases), including hand washing and proper care of bodily fluids and excretions.
• Review potential complications that may result from immunosuppression.
• Explain how to properly handle and prepare food. Stress the importance of frequent hand washing and of cooking all poultry, eggs, meat, and fish.
• Explain how to keep an intake and nutrition journal.
• Teach ways to avoid exposure to infectious situations.
• Teach activity restrictions or limitations.
• Explain safe sexual practices, such as latex condoms and dental dams.
• Emphasize the need for coordinating care. Keep the physician up-to-date on the patient's status; many medications can interfere with anti-HIV drugs.

Interdisciplinary actions

Dietitian
- Recommendations for increased caloric needs and for foods that minimize nausea and GI upset
- Development of 12 meal plans that adhere to the patient's food preferences

Home care aide
- Bathing and personal care
- Light housekeeping and laundry
- Respite care
- Meal preparation

Occupational therapist
- Training and education in performance of ADLs
- Instruction in techniques used to conserve energy

Physical therapist
- Instruction in home exercise program
- Instruction in safe transfer techniques
- Instruction in use of adaptive and assistive devices

Social worker
- Assessment of coping mechanisms
- Short-term counseling
- Referral to community agencies and support services

Discharge plan
- Assurance that the patient and caregiver will be able to manage the disease process in the home with a physician and community support system follow-up services
- Referral to outpatient services or hospice

- Continued home care visits for the homebound patient with skilled care needs
- Pain- and symptom-free at end of life (death with dignity)

Documentation requirements
- Variances to expected outcomes
- Skilled assessment of all systems on each visit, including respiratory, nutritional, and mental status
- Symptoms of secondary infection
- Reaction to and effectiveness of medication regimen and plan of care
- Intake and weight (each visit), vital signs, and laboratory results
- Stability of care situation
- Significant stressors affecting both the patient and caregiver
- Patient and caregiver participation in care
- Details of teaching and percentage of patient and caregiver comprehension of instructions and plan of care
- Support systems in place
- Conferences with and referrals to support services
- Patient and caregiver progress toward goals
- All infectious disease precautions taken at each visit and all instructions given regarding transmission
- Patient and caregiver compliance with transmission precautions

Reimbursement reminders
- HIV and AIDS are listed as catastrophic, incurable illnesses by reimbursement agencies. Medications are expensive. When primary insurance benefits run out or the patient doesn't have a pharmacy benefit, combination

resources need to be utilized, such as local health departments and local AIDS Alliance offices.

- The home care nurse needs to be aware of and participate in coordinating multiple reimbursement sources.

Insurance hints

- Have a complete list of all reimbursement sources currently involved with the patient (insurance, health department, AIDS Alliance) in front of you when speaking with a case manager.
- Keep an accurate record of current education needs.
- Record objective data showing disease progression, including symptoms of secondary infection, laboratory results, weight loss, medication adverse effects, and mental status changes.
- Report any changes in the plan of care and if hospice care is being considered.

Aerosol therapy

Aerosol therapy is a method of delivering medication in mist form directly to the respiratory tract, where the mucosal lining absorbs the medication almost immediately. Aerosolized medications may be used to treat a variety of respiratory disorders, including asthma, chronic obstructive pulmonary disease (COPD), and pneumonia. Examples of commonly used inhalant medications are bronchodilators (both short- and long-acting), corticosteroids, and nonsteroidal anti-inflammatory drugs (NSAIDs). Bronchodilators act by relaxing the smooth muscle of the bronchial airways and are used to prevent and treat bronchospasm in patients with reversible obstructive airway disease. Corticosteroids and NSAIDs are long-term, maintenance medications that reduce inflammation in the airways. The goal of aerosol therapy in respiratory disorders is to prevent symptoms, reduce the frequency and severity of exacerbation, control inflammation, and reverse airflow obstruction. The home care nurse should educate the patient or caregiver about the medication being used and explain how to administer aerosol therapy.

Previsit checklist

Physician orders and preparation

- Care and teaching orders for each discipline
- Medication as indicated
- Aerosol therapy as indicated
- Activity orders and restrictions

Equipment and supplies

- Vital signs equipment
- Supplies for standard precautions and proper sharps disposal
- Metered-dose inhaler as indicated
- Nebulizer equipment and supplies with prescribed medication as indicated

Safety requirements

- Standard precautions for infection control and sharps disposal
- Emergency plan and access to functional phone and list of emergency phone numbers
- Identification and correction of environmental hazards and patient-specific concerns
- Fire evacuation plan, functional smoke detectors, and access to functional fire extinguisher

- Standard oxygen precautions as indicated
- Equipment storage instructions
- Removal of expired medication
- Information on medications, including dosage, adverse effects, interactions, and safe storage
- Instructions on signs and symptoms of medical emergency and actions to take

Major diagnostic codes
- Acute bronchitis 466.0
- Asthma with/without status asthmaticus 493.90/493.91
- Chest physiotherapy 93.99
- COPD 496
- Emphysema with/without bleb (cystic dilatation) 492.0/492.8
- Nebulizer therapy 93.94
- Pneumonia 486

Defense of homebound status
- Inability to ambulate farther than 10' (3 m) due to dyspnea with minimal exertion
- Inability to ambulate farther than 10' due to fatigue and poor endurance related to severe, uncontrolled respiratory disorder
- Inability to negotiate stairs due to profound shortness of breath

Selected nursing diagnoses and patient outcomes

Ineffective breathing pattern related to hyperventilation, hypoventilation syndrome, decreased energy or fatigue, or respiratory muscle fatigue
The patient or caregiver will:

- demonstrate an effective respiratory rate and experience improved gas exchange in the lungs   (N, PT, RT)
- delete the causative factors, if known, and relate adaptive ways of coping with them.   (N, PT, OT, SW, PH)

Ineffective airway clearance related to bronchospasm and increased pulmonary secretions
The patient or caregiver will:
- demonstrate effective coughing and increased air exchange in the lungs.
(N, PT, RT)

Activity intolerance related to shortness of breath
The patient or caregiver will:
- identify factors that reduce activity intolerance   (N, PT, RT)
- exhibit a decrease in hypoxic signs of increased activity (pulse, blood pressure, respirations)   (N, PT, OT, RT)
- progress to the highest level of mobility possible.   (N, PT, OT)

Knowledge deficit related to aerosol therapy
The patient or caregiver will:
- understand appropriate use of inhalant medications (for example, correct dose and frequency of maintenance and as-needed inhalants
(N, PH, RT)
- demonstrate the correct technique for administration of aerosol therapy (metered-dose inhaler or nebulizer treatment).   (N, PH, RT)

Impaired gas exchange related to ventilation perfusion imbalance
The patient or caregiver will:
- maintain adequate gas exchange.
(N, RT)

Altered nutrition: Less than body requirements related to inability to digest or ingest food due to biological factors

The patient or caregiver will:

• maintain adequate nutritional intake (N, D)

• identify methods of increasing caloric intake. (N, D)

Fatigue related to poor physical condition

The patient or caregiver will:

• identify ways to conserve energy. (N, PT)

Anxiety related to threat to or change in health status

The patient or caregiver will:

• report a reduction in anxiety level (N, SW)

• identify methods to help alleviate anxiety and stress. (N, SW)

Skilled nursing services

Care measures

• Perform a skilled assessment of the respiratory system.

• Obtain a patient history relevant to respiratory and oxygenation status.

• Assess for normal breath sounds.

• Assess for adventitious breath sounds.

• Assess for abnormal breathing patterns, sounds, chest movements, secretions, and skin and mucous membrane color.

• Assess for signs of cerebral anoxia, activity intolerance, and chest pain.

• Perform a skilled assessment of the cardiovascular, mental and cognitive, and nutrition and hydration systems.

• Assess the level of care and compliance with use of metered-dose inhaler or nebulizer performed by the patient or caregiver.

• Assess for adverse drug effects.

Patient and family teaching

• Describe the respiratory disease process.

• Explain the aerosol medication regimen, including dosage, purpose, and potential adverse effects and interactions.

• Explain the goal of aerosol therapy (regular doses of anti-inflammatory medication prevent acute exacerbation and short-acting bronchodilator PRN to treat acute symptoms).

• Explain how to use and care for a metered-dose inhaler or a mini-nebulizer as necessary.

• Teach how to coordinate the administration of a bronchodilator and a corticosteroid.

• Emphasize the importance of rinsing the mouth thoroughly with water or saltwater to reduce the risk of fungal infection if the patient is using a corticosteroid.

• Explain how to inspect the mouth for signs of fungal infection.

• Emphasize the importance of always using a spacer with a steroid inhaler to minimize the amount of medication deposited in the mouth and throat and to prevent irritation of upper airways and development of fungal infection.

• Explain that if a metered-dose inhaler hasn't been used recently, a dose should be released into the air first to test the spraying ability.

• Explain that a metered-dose inhaler typically contains approximately 200 puffs of medication. Tell the patient or caregiver that an empty inhaler will float but one that is half-full will partially submerge in plain water.

Interdisciplinary actions

Home care aide
• Assistance with personal care and hygiene needs
• Assistance with activities of daily living (ADLs)

Occupational therapist
• Instruction on energy conservation techniques
• Training for ADLs
• Assessment of need for and instruction in the use of adaptive equipment

Physical therapist
• Development and teaching of an individualized home exercise program
• Performance and instruction of pulmonary physical therapy, such as breathing exercises and chest physiotherapy, as indicated

Respiratory therapist
• Recommendation for personalized medication and physiotherapy regimen to enhance adherence to plan of care
• Evaluation of respiratory status and effectiveness of plan of care

Social worker
• Assessment of social and emotional factors
• Referral to community resources and support groups
• Counseling and referral for stress management and reduction

Discharge plan
• Effective management of aerosol therapy in the home by the patient or caregiver with physician follow-up services
• Referral to hospice
• Pain- and symptom-free at end of life (death with dignity)

Documentation requirements
• Subjective and objective data that focuses first on respiratory system assessment and then on other systems
• Instructions on aerosol therapy and maintenance of equipment as well as phone number provided for oxygen supplier
• Performance of skilled procedures (for example, nebulizer treatment)
• Understanding of and compliance with medication regimen
• Progress of patient or caregiver toward educational goals
• Patient response to care
• Type of aerosol therapy used and times administered
• Specific deficits in initial knowledge level and then progress as evidenced by specific concepts and procedures that are verbalized or demonstrated
• Specific factors that indicate the need for home care, including variances to expected outcomes; specific barriers to learning (for example, impaired vision or impaired mental status and cognitive ability); no available, willing, and able caregiver; and a patient new to medications or aerosol therapy

Reimbursement reminders

- Indicate an expected end point of daily visits (when daily visits have been ordered).
- Obtain a physician's order for any plan of care changes and document them in the patient's record.
- Determine which supplies and durable medical equipment are covered by Medicare.
- Verify that a metered-dose inhaler alone is insufficient in treating the patient's asthma to ensure that he qualifies for a nebulizer machine.
- Determine that the patient's oxygen saturation level is 88% or less to ensure that he qualifies for oxygen.
- Verify that respiratory therapist services are usually provided by the company that supplies the durable medical equipment on a routine or as-needed basis.

Insurance hints

- Report objective data about the patient's homebound status.
- Present objective patient findings, changes in clinical condition, and changes in care since last contact (for example, new physician's orders).
- Report specifics about the patient and caregiver education process.
- Present progress toward established goals.

Amputation

Amputation is the surgical removal of a portion of an extremity, usually the leg. It can be done at several levels, including digits (toes), ankles, knees, elbows, and at the point of attachment to the torso. The most common cause of amputation is gangrene from impaired venous or arterial circulation, but it may also occur as a result of a traumatic injury. Patients who have recently undergone amputation of an extremity will require assistance with activities of daily living (ADLs) and instruction on how to care for the stump, use a prosthesis, and prevent complications.

Previsit checklist

Physician orders and preparation

- Wound care directions
- Activity and transfer orders
- Diet orders — increase protein and fluid to encourage wound healing
- Comfort measures for pain control and phantom pain
- Review of other team members' notes to coordinate care
- Consent for photographing wound if pictures will be taken

Equipment and supplies

- Vital signs equipment
- Tape
- Gauze
- Biological dressings
- Wound cremes and gels
- Biohazard bag for discarding dressings
- Wound cleaner or normal saline solution
- Camera for photographing wound per agency policy
- Film for camera and patient consent form
- Supplies for standard precautions
- Stump shrinker

Safety requirements

- Standard precautions for infection control
- Emergency plan and access to functional phone and list of emergency phone numbers
- Identification and correction of environmental hazards and patient-specific concerns
- Fire evacuation plan, functional smoke detectors, and access to functional fire extinguisher
- Clear pathways for wheelchair or other assistive devices
- Precaution against sitting for long periods of time or hanging the stump over the end of the bed or chair

Major diagnostic codes

- Amputation, arm/complicated 887.4/ 887.5
- Amputation, below knee/complicated 897.0/897.1
- Amputation, fingers (one or both hands)/complicated 886.0/886.1
- Amputation, foot/complicated 896.0/ 896.1
- Amputation, leg/complicated 897.4/ 897.5
- Amputation, leg both/complicated 897.6/897.7
- Amputation, toes 895.0
- Atherosclerosis 440.9
- Atherosclerosis with gangrene 440.24
- Gangrene, diabetic, any site 250.7
- Peripheral vascular disease 443.9
(To assign a fifth digit, see appendix A, page 638.)

Defense of homebound status

- Non-weight-bearing status prescribed

- Inability to ambulate due to adjustment to prosthesis
- Inability to ambulate farther than 10′ (3 m) or navigate stairs independently
- Inability to transfer from wheelchair to car
- Need for leg to be elevated
- Bedridden
- Weakness
- Limited mobility
- Assistance required to ambulate or transfer

Selected nursing diagnoses and patient outcomes

Knowledge deficit related to care (standard precautions for infection control, dressing technique, activity, and transfer)

The patient or caregiver will:

- demonstrate or verbalize infection-control principles   (N, PT)
- demonstrate or verbalize safe transfer technique   (N, PT)
- demonstrate correct posture while sitting.   (N, PT)

Impaired skin integrity related to surgical incision

The patient or caregiver will:

- demonstrate or verbalize correct dressing change technique   (N, PT)
- verbalize signs and symptoms of infection and hemorrhage and report them to the physician   (N, PT)
- have the wound heal without complications   (N, PT)
- verbalize or demonstrate proper skin hygiene   (N)
- demonstrate how to apply a stump sock.   (N, PT)

Impaired mobility related to amputation or the need for a prosthesis

The patient or caregiver will:

● demonstrate proper use of the prosthesis (N, PT)

● verbalize the need to provide maximum care as ordered by the physician (N, PT)

● demonstrate the use of adaptive equipment, such as a wheelchair and crutches (N, PT)

● verbalize feelings of increased strength and endurance. (N, PT)

Risk for injury related to alteration in balance and gait

The patient or caregiver will:

● verbalize appropriate safety precautions (N, PT)

● ask for assistance in transfers (N, PT)

● be free from injuries (N, PT)

● demonstrate safe transfer techniques. (N, PT)

Pain related to surgical incision or amputation

The patient or caregiver will:

● verbalize the pain-control regimen (N)

● verbalize one nonpharmacologic method of pain relief (N, PT)

● achieve pain relief (N, PT)

● express an understanding of phantom pain (N, PT)

● perform activities to minimize pain, such as early ambulation. (N, PT)

Body image disturbance related to amputation

The patient or caregiver will:

● verbalize acceptance of the change in body (N, SW)

● be able to look at the affected part of body (N)

● demonstrate ability to provide care related to amputation (N, PT)

● maintain social contact with a support system (N, SW)

● access community support groups for amputees. (N, SW)

Activity intolerance related to bed rest or immobility or generalized weakness

The patient or caregiver will:

● identify methods for increasing activity level (N, PT)

● identify methods for conserving energy (N, PT)

● demonstrate proper exercise techniques. (N, PT)

Risk for infection

The patient or caregiver will:

● show no signs of infection (N)

● demonstrate proper cleaning and care of the amputation site (N)

● demonstrate the ability to assess for signs and symptoms of infection and report them to the physician or nurse. (N)

Skilled nursing services

Care measures

● Assess the cardiovascular, integumentary, musculoskeletal, and nutrition and hydration systems.

● Assess the level of care performed by the patient or caregiver related to safe transfer.

● Assess the effectiveness of treatment regimens and wound healing and document findings.

● Assess the patient's ability to follow physical therapy instructions.

● Assess the fit of the prosthesis.

• Assess the wound site for proper healing and absence of infection, and photograph as ordered.
• Assess the patient's or caregiver's ability to perform wound care and dressing changes.
• Report any untoward changes in the patient's condition to the physician.

Patient and family teaching
• Explain the signs and symptoms of infection.
• Instruct in phantom pain control.
• Teach ways to manage stump pain and maintain pain at 3 or less on a 0-to-10 scale 80% of the time.
• Review ways to prevent falls.
• Instruct in wound care.
• Discuss an exercise program that will help the patient maximize his independence.

Interdisciplinary actions

Home care aide
• Assistance with hygiene and ADLs

Occupational therapist
• Education in energy conservation techniques
• Education and assistance in bathing and self-care

Physical therapist
• Assistance and instruction in transfer techniques
• Referral to the orthotist for stump fitting
• Instruction in safety and fall prevention
• Instruction in upper-body strength training

Social worker
• Provision of community referrals for independence
• Instruction in psychosocial support and coping strategies

Discharge plan
• Safe management of transfers in the home by the patient or caregiver
• Management of stump care in the home with appropriate physician follow-ups
• Referral to outpatient services

Documentation requirements
• Skilled assessment
• Patient's response to care, including altered body image
• Effectiveness of pain control, rating pain at 3 or less on a 0-to-10 scale 80% of the time
• Wound care
• Changes in the size and character of incision, including drainage and edema
• Patient's or caregiver's ability to provide care related to dressing change
• Interdisciplinary team communication
• Patient's ability to transfer safely
• Readiness for prosthesis, including increased strength, minimal edema, and a well-healed and nontender extremity
• Patient and family education performed and its effectiveness
• Specific factors that indicate a need for home care, including teaching wound care, the patient's response to care, wound condition and progress, and the patient's ability to perform self-care

Reimbursement reminders

• Ensure that dressing supplies are covered by Medicare; managed care plans may require that dressings be obtained from a specified provider.

• Check if wound gels are covered by the plan before ordering.

• Ensure that assistive devices are covered by Medicare, including a physical therapist to coordinate the ordering of wheelchairs, a stump mold, and an orthotist consultation.

• Provide a prosthesis fitting plan and stump changes.

Insurance hints

• Report specific, measurable progress toward goals (for example, "Wound care was b.i.d. for 7 days; now wound care is q.d. for 14 days. Anticipate that wound care will decrease to q.o.d in 3 days.")

• Assess wound healing: drainage, approximation of edges, edema, and pain at 3 or less on a 0-to-10 scale 80% of the time.

• Describe adjustment issues, such as the patient's resistance to or acceptance of providing self-care, dressing changes, and activity.

• Assess progress of goals in self-care for hygiene, dressings, and transfers.

• Describe gains in knowledge and skills and concepts that have been mastered.

• Present specific data on the homebound status, such as the patient's inability to navigate stairs from his second-floor residence.

• Emphasize the next step in care; show that there is a progressive plan for rehabilitation.

• Describe the goals and treatments of each member of the team and how long care will continue.

• Report any comorbid conditions, such as diabetes or chronic lung or heart disease, that could affect the patient's ability to provide self-care and delay wound healing.

Amyotrophic lateral sclerosis

A progressive degenerative neurologic disease of unknown cause, amyotrophic lateral sclerosis (ALS) is characterized by weakness and muscle wasting without accompanying sensory or cognitive changes. A loss of upper and lower motor neurons occurs in the spinal cord and brain stem. When upper motor neurons are affected, the muscles become spastic, leading to contractures. When lower motor neurons are affected, the muscles become flaccid, leading to paralysis. Most physical problems in the patient with ALS are focused on managing swallowing and oral secretions, communication, immobility, and respiratory muscle dysfunction. For these issues, teaching for the patient's family should focus on preventing complications, maximizing respiratory functioning, and providing care for basic needs.

Previsit checklist

Physician orders and preparation

• Order for an indwelling urinary catheter or intermittent catheterization

- Order for physical, speech, and occupational therapy
- Order for a specialty bed, a wheelchair, and other assistive devices
- Activity orders and restrictions
- Order for nutritional requirements
- Order for home oxygen therapy
- Order for home suctioning equipment
- Medication dosage and route

Equipment and supplies
- Supplies for standard precautions
- Indwelling urinary catheter or supplies for intermittent catheterization as per the physician's order
- Gloves
- Dressing equipment to change dressing around gastrostomy feeding tube, if indicated
- Irrigation kit for gastrostomy tube
- Sterile water
- Suctioning kits (nasotracheal and oropharyngeal)
- Oxygen equipment
- Leg bag or urinary bag attachment device

Safety requirements
- Standard precautions for infection control
- Home assessment for placement of grab bars and supportive devices in the bathroom as well as removal of throw rugs and carpeting
- Aspiration precautions
- Oxygen precautions, safe handling and placement of home oxygen equipment, and notification of local fire and police departments of oxygen use in the home
- Safe use of suction equipment and assessment for proper function

- Skin care and protection, including frequent position changes
- Avoidance of extremes in temperature on the skin
- Extremity supports to keep limbs in normal anatomic alignment
- Functioning communication or emergency device such as an adaptive signaling device, a home intercom system, and 911 speed dial on telephone
- Adequate lighting
- Emergency plan and access to functional phone and list of emergency phone numbers
- Identification and correction of environmental hazards and patient-specific concerns
- Fire evacuation plan, functional smoke detectors, and access to functional fire extinguisher

Major diagnostic codes
- ALS 335.20
- Apnea 786.03
- Dysphagia 787.2
- Incomplete bladder emptying 788.21
- Incontinence of feces 787.6
- Incontinence of urine 788.30
- Orthopnea 786.02
- Primary lateral sclerosis 335.24
- Progressive bulbar palsy 335.22
- Progressive muscular atrophy 335.21
- Respiratory failure, acute/chronic 518.81/518.83
- Retention of urine 788.20
- Shortness of breath 786.05
- Tachypnea 786.06

Defense of homebound status
- Inability to ambulate farther than 10′ (3 m) due to progressive debilitating neurologic status or dyspnea

- Progressive inability to maintain respiratory functioning or severe shortness of breath
- Inability to ambulate or transfer without maximum assistance
- Progressive deterioration of neurologic status
- Bedridden

Selected nursing diagnoses and patient outcomes

Risk for disuse syndrome
The patient or caregiver will:
- demonstrate proper body alignment and positioning   (N, OT, PT)
- demonstrate proper evaluation of skin status   (N)
- verbalize the need to have adequate nutrition and fluid intake to prevent complications   (N, D)
- demonstrate proper use of assistive devices to prevent skin breakdown and respiratory, GI, and genitourinary complications   (N, OT, PT)
- perform active range-of-motion (ROM) exercises as able   (N, PT)
- implement passive ROM exercises every 2 hours as tolerated   (N, PT)
- verbalize signs and symptoms of respiratory and genitourinary tract infection.   (N)

Ineffective breathing pattern related to musculoskeletal impairment or neuromuscular dysfunction
The patient or caregiver will:
- demonstrate proper use of supplemental oxygen   (N, RT)
- demonstrate use of the oropharyngeal suction apparatus   (N, RT)
- demonstrate use of nasotracheal suction equipment   (N, RT)

- verbalize why the patient should be turned and repositioned every 2 hours to prevent pooling of secretions in the lungs   (N, PT, RT)
- state why the head of the patient's bed should be elevated to 30 degrees to support ventilation and lung expansion   (N, RT)
- recognize the signs and symptoms of a respiratory infection, including fever, cough, sputum production or change in color of sputum, thickened secretions, audible wheezes, change in level of responsiveness, lethargy, and increased effort necessary to breathe.   (N)

Fatigue related to muscle weakness
The patient or caregiver will:
- recognize the need for adequate rest periods   (N, PT)
- support weakened limbs with splints or braces   (N, OT, PT)
- demonstrate measures to provide comfort.   (N)

Risk for aspiration
The patient or caregiver will:
- verbalize ways to reduce the threat of aspiration, including drinking thickened liquids, eating ground and pureed foods, and taking small bites in a non-rushed mealtime atmosphere (N, SP)
- demonstrate raising the head of the bed 30 degrees to prevent aspiration after meals   (N, SP)
- demonstrate care of a gastrostomy tube, if applicable   (N)
- recognize signs and symptoms of a gastrostomy tube problem, including a tube that is blocked, has come out, or has retracted into the abdominal cavity   (N)
- recognize signs and symptoms of a gastrostomy tube stoma infection, in-

cluding red skin, drainage, fever, and general malaise. (N)

Bathing, hygiene, feeding, dressing, and grooming self-care deficit related to neuromuscular impairment
The patient or caregiver will:
• demonstrate how to maximize the patient's energy while performing care activities, including taking frequent rest periods, focusing on one activity at a time, and taking adequate time to complete an activity (N, OT, PT)
• demonstrate care activities, including bathing, shaving, personal hygiene, and dressing. (N, OT)

Impaired verbal communication related to weakening of the musculoskeletal system
The patient or caregiver will:
• demonstrate alternative methods of communication, such as message boards, cue cards, picture boards, pointing, eye movements, blinking, and computer use with eye movement (N, SP)
• utilize alternative methods of communication to reduce feelings of isolation. (N)

Ineffective family coping: Compromised related to temporary preoccupation by a significant person who is trying to manage emotional conflicts and personal suffering and is unable to perceive or act effectively in regard to a patient's needs or a prolonged disease or disability progression that exhausts the supportive capacity of significant people
The patient or caregiver will:
• demonstrate patience and willingness to participate in patient care (N, SW)

• articulate when the responsibilities of providing care for the patient are overwhelming and determine methods to reduce home caregiver stress (N, SW)
• plan rest periods for the home caregiver to support the need for respite care. (N, SW)

Altered sexuality patterns
The patient or caregiver will:
• demonstrate patience with the physical and respiratory changes associated with the disease process (N)
• recognize alternative methods to fulfill sexuality needs. (M, MD, SW)

Impaired physical mobility related to neuromuscular impairment
The patient or caregiver will:
• demonstrate proper passive or active ROM exercises (N, PT)
• demonstrate proper use of braces and splints (OT, PT)
• verbalize the need for frequent position changes to protect skin integrity (N)
• demonstrate safe transfer techniques. (N, PT)

Skilled nursing services

Care measures
• Assess the neurologic, mental and cognitive, nutrition and hydration, respiratory, cardiovascular, GI, genitourinary, musculoskeletal, and integumentary systems.
• Administer enteral feedings and I.V. medications.
• Provide nasotracheal and oropharyngeal suctioning as needed.
• Maintain urinary drainage system.

- Assess primary caregiver's ability to perform daily care, including bathing, meals and enteral feedings, and elimination needs.
- Assess primary caregiver's ability to provide or assist with ROM, and integumentary and musculoskeletal status support.
- Assess the home situation and need for assistive devices or durable medical equipment.
- Evaluate all prescribed medications and the patient's response to them and perform ongoing assessment of patient or caregiver adherence to the medication regimen.
- Assess social and emotional functioning of the patient and family and discuss end-of-life options in collaboration with the social worker.

Patient and family teaching

- Emphasize home safety.
- Instruct in airway maintenance and emergency airway procedures.
- Explain nasotracheal and oropharyngeal suctioning.
- Teach home oxygen therapy use and safety precautions.
- Explain how to administer enteral feedings and assess for complications.
- Instruct in gastrostomy tube care and assessment of site for infection.
- Instruct in the application of splints.
- Teach proper skin care.
- Instruct in proper turning and repositioning techniques as well as frequency.
- Educate about expected activity limitations.
- Instruct in indwelling catheter care or intermittent catheterization, including looking for signs and symptoms of infection.
- Instruct in bowel elimination care.

Interdisciplinary actions

Dietitian
- Evaluation

Home care aide
- Assessment of need for home care aide, depending on the abilities of the home caregiver
- Gradual withdrawal of home care aide support as the caregiver's confidence in patient care increases
- Assistance with hygiene care and activities of daily living (ADLs)
- Provision of housekeeping tasks as needed
- Respite care

Occupational therapist
- Assessment of ADLs and prescription of assistive devices as indicated
- Education in energy conservation techniques

Physical therapist
- Initiation of prescribed rehabilitation program, including transfers and active and passive ROM exercises
- Recommendations for home exercise program
- Recommendations for home safety

Social worker
- Assessment of need for and referrals to community services
- Provision of emotional support and counseling
- Discussion of end-of-life options: tracheostomy and mechanical ventilation as support or control of respirations as disease progresses, advance directive, and do-not-resuscitate order

Speech pathologist
- Evaluation
- Recommendation of appropriate oral diet consistency to prevent aspiration
- Instructions for alternate methods of communication

Discharge plan
- Management of progressive deterioration of neurologic functioning at home by patient or caregiver
- Independent care by patient and caregiver, including ability to recognize and respond to integumentary, respiratory, GI, or genitourinary complications
- Continuation of home care visits for homebound patient with skilled care needs
- Assurance that patient will be pain- and symptom-free at end of life (death with dignity)

Documentation requirements
- Patient and caregiver response to instruction
- Patient's or caregiver's ability to care for the patient, including the ability to perform gastrostomy tube feedings, indwelling urinary catheter care, nasotracheal and oropharyngeal suctioning, use of assistive devices, maintenance of normal anatomic alignment, repositioning, and transfers
- Assessment of integumentary, respiratory, GI, genitourinary, or neurologic functioning
- Treatments or care given
- Response to care or therapy and patient progress
- Identification of specific factors that indicate the need for home care, including variances from expected outcomes and need for involvement of other members of the health care team

Reimbursement reminders
- Explain to the patient that the waiting period for individuals disabled by ALS to obtain Medicare coverage is 24 months.

Insurance hints
- Provide a review of hospitalization (if appropriate) and the current condition of the patient, home environment, and availability of a caregiver.
- Provide an objective review of systems, including physical abilities, ambulation, and the use of or need for assistive devices.
- Thoroughly assess the skin and report objective findings. In the event of open or reddened areas, provide accurate wound dimensions, prescribed dressing, and the capability of the caregiver to perform wound care.
- Provide current laboratory values.
- To promote reimbursement, document specific patient needs and tolerance of care measures. If the patient is receiving gastrostomy tube feedings, objectively document the patient's tolerance to feedings, the patency of the gastrostomy tube, and the condition of the skin surrounding the tube. If the patient is supported by oral nutrition, objectively document the patient's and caregiver's ability to maintain a patent airway.

Angina pectoris

Angina is caused by atherosclerotic heart disease. Blood flow through the coronary arteries is decreased, producing ischemia to the myocardium. This results in anginal pain. Typically, upper chest pain is the final product of the ischemic process, but pain may also radiate to the neck, jaw, shoulders, and hands. Anginal pain is considered to be a warning sign of an impending myocardial infarction (MI). Angina may be chronic (predictable, occurs on exertion, relieved by rest), unstable (progressively increases in frequency, intensity, and duration), or nocturnal (occurs during sleep and may be relieved by sitting upright). Because an MI can follow long-standing anginal episodes, the home care nurse must emphasize the importance of modifying diet, activity, and behavior to the patient.

Previsit checklist

Physician orders and preparation
- Diet restrictions
- Activity orders and restrictions
- Exercise program
- Medication dosage and route
- Oxygen therapy

Equipment and supplies
- Vital signs equipment
- Supplies for standard precautions
- Oxygen and oxygen tubing

Safety requirements
- Standard precautions for infection control
- Regulation of activities to reflect current cardiac status
- Action plan for symptoms that require immediate medical assistance

- System to assist with adherence to complex medication regimen
- Information on medications, including dosage, adverse effects, interactions, and safe storage
- Emergency plan and access to functional phone and list of emergency phone numbers
- Identification and correction of environmental hazards and patient-specific concerns
- Fire evacuation plan, functional smoke detectors, and access to functional fire extinguisher
- Oxygen precautions, safe handling and placement of home oxygen equipment, and notification of local fire and police departments of oxygen use in the home, if necessary

Major diagnostic codes
- Acute myocardial infarction 410.9
- Angina 413.9
- Angina, unstable 411.1
- Atherosclerosis (coronary) 414.00
- Atrial fibrillation/flutter 427.31/427.32
- Cardiac dysrhythmias 427.9
- Cardiomyopathy 425.4
- Chronic ischemic heart disease 414.9
- Heart failure, congestive/left 428.0/428.1
- Hypertension, without/with congestive heart failure 402.90/402.91

(To assign a fifth digit, see appendix A, page 638.)

Defense of homebound status
- Bedridden
- Maximal assistance required for ambulation

- Severe shortness of breath, decreased endurance, limited ambulation of less than 10′ (3 m) at a time
- Chest pain on exertion
- Dyspnea on exertion
- Deteriorating respiratory status
- End-stage cardiac disease

Selected nursing diagnoses and patient outcomes

Pain related to myocardial ischemia
  The patient or caregiver will:
- administer sublingual nitroglycerin at the first sign of chest discomfort (N)
- administer sublingual nitroglycerin in advance of strenuous activities to avoid pain (N)
- remain alert to adverse effects of nitroglycerin (N)
- experience relief of pain after rest or the administration of nitroglycerin (N)
- state how to contact emergency medical personnel (N)
- contact emergency medical personnel if pain isn't relieved after three doses of nitroglycerin within 10 minutes. (N)

Altered tissue perfusion (cardiopulmonary) related to interruption of arterial flow
  The patient or caregiver will:
- identify factors that increase tissue perfusion alteration (N)
- identify methods to increase tissue perfusion (N)
- state the cause of altered tissue perfusion (N)
- have a decreased incidence of angina (N)
- demonstrate proper administration of sublingual nitroglycerin. (N)

Fluid volume excess related to compromised regulatory mechanism, excess fluid intake, or excess sodium intake
  The patient or caregiver will:
- identify signs and symptoms of fluid overload (N)
- identify methods to help prevent fluid overload, such as decreased sodium intake and fluid restriction (N)
- remain normovolemic. (N)

Decreased cardiac output
  The patient or caregiver will:
- identify signs and symptoms of decreased cardiac output and notify the nurse or physician (N)
- identify ways to conserve energy (N, OT)
- maintain adequate cardiac output (N)
- state purposes of medications and adhere to the prescribed medication regimen. (N)

Activity intolerance related to generalized weakness or imbalance between oxygen supply and demand
  The patient or caregiver will:
- identify methods for conserving energy (N, OT)
- adhere to a light exercise regimen as indicated (N, PT)
- state the need for frequent rest periods. (N, PT)

Ineffective breathing pattern related to _____
  The patient or caregiver will:
- discuss methods of reducing dyspnea (N)
- discuss causative factors of dyspnea (N)
- maintain adequate oxygenation. (N)

Ineffective family coping: Compromised related to prolonged disease or disability progression that exhausts the supportive capacity of significant people

The patient or caregiver will:
- identify healthy coping strategies (N, SW)
- identify causes of stress (N, SW)
- verbalize feelings of stress and anxiety (N)
- seek assistance from supportive networks. (N, SW)

Knowledge deficit related to lack of exposure

The patient or caregiver will:
- state purposes, dosages, routes, and adverse effects of prescribed medications (N)
- state causative factors of angina as well as strategies to prevent complications (N)
- identify risk factors for heart disease. (N)

Skilled nursing services

Care measures
- Perform a comprehensive assessment of the respiratory and cardiovascular system.
- Provide the patient with home safety instructions and information related to the administration of correct medication dosages, signs of toxicity, adverse effects, and drug interactions.
- Assess vital signs on each visit.
- Assess fluid retention and evaluate lower extremities.
- Assess amount, frequency, and site of anginal pain.
- Ensure medication management.

- Assess oxygen saturation and documentation.
- Assess response to therapy.

Patient and family teaching
- Teach about foods that are low in fat, cholesterol, and sodium.
- Teach energy-conservation techniques.
- Instruct in medication purposes, administration, and adverse effects.
- Explain the need for daily weighing and when to report a fluctuation.
- Teach ways to manage angina and when to seek medical assistance.
- Review risk factors for heart disease.

Interdisciplinary actions

Dietitian
- Consultation for development of individualized low-fat, low-cholesterol, low-sodium diet

Physical therapist
- Conditioning exercises

Discharge plan
- Safe management of episodes of angina in the home by patient or caregiver with physician follow-up services
- Referral to outpatient services

Documentation requirements
- Physical assessment findings and vital sign measurements
- Frequency and duration of angina, precipitating factors, and alleviating factors
- Outcome of nitroglycerin administration

- Patient's response to skilled nursing interventions
- Patient's compliance with the medication regimen
- Patient's compliance with the self-care program
- Specific factors indicating a need for home care, including variances to expected outcomes, abnormal laboratory values, behavioral outcomes of teaching instructions, and all episodes of anginal pain as well as follow-up care delivered

Reimbursement reminders

- Report specific care and teaching instructions as well as progress toward goals.
- Communicate and document all changes in the plan of care.

Insurance hints

- Present objective patient findings, abnormal laboratory values, and changes since the last update.
- Report communications with the physician or caregiver.

Arrhythmias

Cardiac arrhythmias occur for various reasons. Patients who have been diagnosed with an arrhythmia may or may not have had the cause of the irregularity identified and treated. Symptoms and impending problems guide the home care team to early intervention and prevention of complications or to assistance that enables the patient to experience the best possible quality of life.

Previsit checklist

Physician orders and preparation

- Weight monitoring
- Intake and output
- Diet orders
- Fluid restrictions
- Activity orders and restrictions
- Antiarrhythmic drugs
- Anticoagulant drugs
- Laboratory studies to monitor drug levels

Equipment and supplies

- Scale for weighing
- Stethoscope
- Blood pressure cuff
- Thermometer
- Needle or butterfly set
- Alcohol preps
- Cotton balls or 2″ × 2″ dressing
- Tourniquet
- Syringes
- Adhesive bandages
- Laboratory tubes
- Transporting bags and requisitions or request forms
- Supplies for proper sharps disposal, including a container
- Cooler
- Holter monitor as prescribed

Safety requirements

- Standard precautions for infection control and sharps disposal
- Recognition of symptoms of complications and follow-up action plan
- Implementation of treatment protocols for complications
- Adaptation of lifestyle and activities of daily living (ADLs) due to decreased energy

- Preoperative patient teaching, if indicated
- Standard oxygen therapy safety precautions, if indicated
- Anticoagulant precautions
- Emergency plan and access to functional phone and list of emergency phone numbers
- Identification and correction of environmental hazards and patient-specific concerns
- Fire evacuation plan, functional smoke detectors, and access to functional fire extinguisher

Major diagnostic codes

- Acute myocardial infarction 410.90
- Atrial fibrillation/flutter 427.31/427.3
- Bundle branch block 426.3
- Cardiac dysrhythmia, unspecified 427.9
- Complete heart block 426.0
- Conduction disorder, unspecified 426.9
- Heart failure, congestive/left 428.0/428.1
- Ischemic heart disease (chronic) 414.9
- Pacemaker V45.0
- Palpitations 785.1
- Paroxysmal supraventricular tachycardia 427.0
- Paroxysmal ventricular tachycardia 427.1
- Percutaneous transluminal coronary angioplasty 35.96
- Premature beats, unspecified 427.60
- Unspecified tachycardia 785.0
- Valve replacement 35.2
- Ventricular fibrillation 427.41

Defense of homebound status

- Cardiac restrictions on activity
- Poor endurance related to decreased cardiac output
- Dyspnea on exertion
- Bedridden
- Inability to ambulate without maximal assistance

Selected nursing diagnoses and patient outcomes

Decreased cardiac output related to conduction disorders

The patient or caregiver will:
- verbalize or demonstrate signs and symptoms requiring emergency treatment and identify emergency care access plan   (N)
- demonstrate stable cardiovascular and respiratory state with increased mobility and endurance. (N, OT, PT)

Self-care deficit related to weakness and tiredness

The patient or caregiver will:
- have personal care needs met
                              (N, HCA, OT, PT)
- demonstrate energy conservation measures for ADLs, such as sitting in front of a mirror to shave or resting arm between strokes.   (N)

Ineffective individual coping related to inadequate level of confidence in ability to cope or situational crisis

The patient or caregiver will:
- demonstrate compliance with treatments and medications   (N, OT, PT)
- contact or use identified community support systems and resources
                             (N, OT, PT, SW)

- adapt lifestyle to relieve symptoms and improve quality of life.
(N, HCA, OT, PT, SW, D)

Altered peripheral tissue perfusion (cardiopulmonary) related to mechanical reduction of venous or arterial blood flow
The patient or caregiver will:
- identify symptoms of decreased tissue perfusion and seek medical assistance should they occur (N)
- maintain adequate tissue perfusion. (N)

Risk for activity intolerance
The patient or caregiver will:
- identify effective methods of energy conservation (N, OT, PT)
- verbalize understanding of causes of activity intolerance. (N)

Knowledge deficit related to medical regimen and health issues due to lack of exposure
The patient or caregiver will:
- verbalize an understanding of purposes, administration, and adverse effects of prescribed medications (N)
- verbalize an understanding of the disease process (N)
- identify signs and symptoms of complications related to arrhythmia and when to seek medical attention. (N)

Anxiety related to a threat to or change in health status
The patient or caregiver will:
- verbalize feelings (N, SW)
- demonstrate appropriate coping mechanisms (N, SW)
- demonstrate a reduction in anxiety level. (N, SW)

Skilled nursing services

Care measures
- Assess all body systems, especially cardiopulmonary.
- Monitor vital signs and weight.
- Assess fluid status and intake and output.
- Assess for the presence of edema.
- Observe for jugular vein distention.
- Perform auscultation for extra heart sounds and murmurs.
- Monitor the amount and type of exercise.
- Assess the emotional response to illness and the effectiveness of coping mechanisms.
- Monitor lifestyle adaptation methods.
- Monitor medication use and adverse effects.
- Implement bowel regimen.
- Assess the patient's response to the plan of care and report progress to the physician.
- Perform venipuncture per physician's orders.

Patient and family teaching
- Instruct on how to take a radial pulse.
- Explain the importance of recording daily weight using the same scale.
- Demonstrate intake and output measurement.
- Emphasize the importance of following an exercise program or ordered therapy plan.
- Teach coping mechanisms.
- Teach relaxation techniques.
- Instruct in medication administration, interactions, contraindications, and adverse effects.

- Instruct in energy conservation techniques.
- Discuss possible invasive procedures that may be necessary to correct the arrhythmia.
- Review safe use and care of home oxygen, if indicated.
- Describe signs and symptoms that should be reported to the physician.
- Discuss when to call emergency medical personnel.
- Emphasize the importance of compliance with the treatment plan.
- Instruct in the use and care of a Holter monitor, if prescribed.

Interdisciplinary actions

Dietitian
- Development of personalized meal plan to meet dietary restrictions such as stable amounts of dietary sources of vitamin K

Home care aide
- Personal care and assistance with ADLs

Occupational therapist
- Instructions in use of energy-conservation devices
- Energy-conservation techniques

Physical therapist
- Evaluation
- Cardiac exercise program for increased endurance and strength
- Development of plan for independent and safe mobility

Social worker
- Evaluation of problems
- Referrals to appropriate community resources and counseling

Discharge plan
- Return to self-care with physician follow-up
- Referral to outpatient services

Documentation requirements
- Cardiopulmonary status
- Progress toward goals
- Subjective and objective signs and symptoms, including irregular pulse changes, murmurs, arrhythmias, shortness of breath, and abnormal breath sounds
- Weight and fluid status
- Activity tolerance changes
- Specific care, treatments, and medications administered
- Instructions given, demonstrated, and provided in writing
- Response to care and instructions
- Coordination of patient care with other members of the health care team
- Notification given to physician of abnormal laboratory results and any changes in the plan of care
- Medication changes and the specific need to monitor the patient's response to changes

Reimbursement reminders
- Assess the patient for signs and symptoms beyond what the patient can assess himself, such as pulse rate and rhythm and weight.
- Verify that schedule changes by other members of the health care team discipline have an accompanying order from the physician.
- Identify barriers to learning, which require the need for ongoing visits.

- Document multidisciplinary planning and communication.
- Check that the blood-drawing supplies are considered routine to ensure they are nonbillable.

Insurance hints

- Determine initially how often to report clinical conditions, and always notify the physician immediately if patient changes affect the frequency or duration specified in the initial plan of care.
- Present objective data specific to established goals and provide routine updates that address progress.
- Note possible barriers to care and learning.

Asthma

Asthma is the most common chronic disease that affects children and young adults. It's characterized by airway inflammation, airway obstruction or narrowing, and bronchial hyperreactivity, which is an exaggerated bronchoconstrictor response to a variety of stimuli. These stimuli are commonly called asthma "triggers." Acute episodes of asthma involve wheezing, progressively worsening shortness of breath, chest tightness, and coughing. Acute episodes are recurrent, vary in intensity, and are usually reversible.

Airway inflammation is the key to the development of asthma. Although asthma is characterized by acute exacerbation, the underlying inflammation is continuous. When the asthma patient is exposed to an asthma trigger, the bronchial mucosa release histamine and leukotrienes (powerful bronchoconstrictors), resulting in increased inflammation, edema, and mucus secretion. As the airways narrow, the patient begins to wheeze and has increased difficulty breathing. If not treated quickly and effectively, an acute exacerbation of asthma may lead to severe respiratory distress.

Improvements in asthma control or the prevention of acute exacerbation can significantly enhance the asthma patient's quality of life. Patient and caregiver education is crucial in enabling the asthma patient to attain optimal control. The home care nurse can provide patient and caregiver education in the home as well as physical assessment of the patient and assessment of the patient's environment for asthma triggers.

Previsit checklist

Physician orders and preparation

- Care and teaching orders for each discipline
- Oral medication as indicated
- Aerosol therapy as indicated
- Chest physiotherapy as indicated
- Activity orders and restrictions

Equipment and supplies

- Vital signs equipment
- Supplies for standard precautions and proper sharps disposal
- Peak flow meter
- Metered-dose inhaler as indicated
- Nebulizer with prescribed medication as indicated
- Oxygen as indicated

Safety requirements

- Standard precautions for infection control and sharps disposal and storage
- Fire evacuation plan, functional smoke detectors, and access to functional fire extinguisher
- Standard oxygen precautions as needed
- Instructions for proper equipment storage
- Information on medications, including dosage, adverse effects, interactions, and safe storage
- Proper disposal of expired drugs
- Instruction regarding signs and symptoms of a medical emergency and actions to take
- Emergency plan and access to functional phone and list of emergency phone numbers
- Identification and correction of environmental hazards and patient-specific concerns
- Stepped action plan for exacerbating conditions, such as high humidity, very hot weather, and high pollen counts

Major diagnostic codes

- Asthma, without/with status asthmaticus 493.90/493.91
- Bronchitis, acute 466.0
- Chest physiotherapy 93.99
- Chronic obstructive asthma, without/with status asthmaticus 493.20/493.21
- Chronic obstructive pulmonary disease 496
- Nebulizer therapy 93.94

Defense of homebound status

- Inability to ambulate farther than 10′ (3 m) due to dyspnea with minimal exertion
- Inability to ambulate farther than 10′ due to fatigue and poor endurance related to severe and uncontrolled asthma
- Inability to negotiate stairs due to a profound shortness of breath
- Profound weakness
- Bedridden
- Oxygen therapy

Selected nursing diagnoses and patient outcomes

Ineffective breathing patterns related to hypoventilation syndrome or respiratory muscle fatigue

The patient or caregiver will:
- demonstrate an effective respiratory rate and experience improved gas exchange in the lungs   (N, PT, RT)
- relate the causative factors, if known, and adaptive ways of coping with them.
(N, OT, PH, PT, SW)

Ineffective airway clearance related to bronchospasm and increased pulmonary secretions

The patient or caregiver will:
- demonstrate effective coughing and increased air exchange in the lungs.
(N, PT, RT)

Ineffective management of therapeutic regimen: Families related to complexity of therapeutic regimen

The patient or caregiver will:
- describe the asthma disease process, causes and factors contributing to

symptoms, and the regimen for symptom control   (N, OT, PT, RT)
- verbalize feelings of stress related to care   (N, SW)
- demonstrate improved management of the therapeutic regimen as evidenced by improved asthma self-management practices, such as medications, peak flow meter, avoidance of asthma triggers, and activity.
   (N, OT, PH, PT, RT, SW)

Activity intolerance related to shortness of breath
   The patient or caregiver will:
- identify factors that reduce activity tolerance   (N, PT, RT)
- exhibit a decrease in hypoxic signs that occur with increased activity, such as increased pulse, blood pressure, respirations, and cyanotic nail beds
   (N, OT, PT, RT)
- progress to the highest level of mobility possible.   (N, OT, PT)

Knowledge deficit related to asthma management, including oral medications, aerosol therapy, peak flow meter, and asthma triggers
   The patient or caregiver will:
- state the correct dose and time for each asthma medication prescribed as well as adverse effects and precautions for each   (N, PH)
- demonstrate correct technique for administration of aerosol therapy (metered-dose inhaler or nebulizer treatment)   (N, PH, RT)
- verbalize understanding of the parameters for use of episodic oral and inhaled asthma medication as necessary   (N, PH, RT)

- demonstrate correct use of the peak flow meter as well as documentation and interpretation of the results   (N)
- verbalize knowledge of personal asthma and allergy triggers   (N)
- explain measures being taken to avoid asthma and allergy triggers (N)
- verbalize understanding of infection control measures.   (N)

Anxiety related to a threat to or change in health status
   The patient or caregiver will:
- identify appropriate coping mechanisms   (N, SW)
- verbalize feelings of anxiety   (N)
- identify causes of anxiety   (N)
- state that the level of anxiety has decreased.   (N)

Skilled nursing services

Care measures
- Monitor vital signs.
- Assess the respiratory system.
- Obtain a patient history relevant to respiratory and oxygenation status.
- Perform auscultation of breath sounds.
- Assess for abnormal breathing patterns, sounds, chest movements, secretions, and skin and mucous membrane colors.
- Assess for signs of cerebral anoxia, activity intolerance, and chest pain.
- Assess the cardiovascular, mental and cognitive, and nutrition and hydration systems.
- Assess the level of care and understanding of the patient or caregiver in the use of the peak flow meter, the metered-dose inhaler, and oral medications.

- Check the patient's peak flow meter readings chart or diary and assess for abnormal readings.
- Assess for asthma triggers in the patient's environment.
- Assess patient or caregiver compliance with avoidance of asthma triggers.
- Ask whether the patient has had any asthma attacks since the last home visit.
- Assess the patient's response to therapies.
- Administer medications.
- Collect specimens, such as sputum cultures and serum laboratory values.

Patient and family teaching

- Explain the asthma disease process.
- Provide instruction on the medication regimen (oral and aerosol), including dosage, frequency, purpose, adverse effects, and interactions.
- Instruct in the purpose and use of the peak flow meter, including documentation and interpretation of results.
- Outline ways to identify asthma triggers and emphasize the importance of avoiding them.
- Emphasize the importance of following established asthma management strategies and the treatment plan to provide optimum control of asthma symptoms.
- Instruct the patient or caregiver to consult with a physician regarding an influenza vaccine (annually) and a pneumonia vaccine (one-time dose).
- Teach safe oxygen use in the home.
- Review energy-conservation methods.
- Instruct in coughing and deep-breathing exercises.

Interdisciplinary actions

Home care aide

- Assistance with personal care and hygiene

Occupational therapist

- Instruction in energy-conservation techniques
- Training in performing activities of daily living
- Assessment of need for and instruction in use of the adaptive equipment

Physical therapist

- Development and instruction of an individualized home exercise program
- Performance and instruction in pulmonary physical therapy, such as breathing exercises and chest physiotherapy, as indicated

Social worker

- Referral to community resources and support groups
- Counseling and referral for stress management and reduction

Discharge plan

- Effective management of asthma care in the home by the patient or caregiver with physician follow-up services

Documentation requirements

- Subjective and objective data related to assessment of the respiratory system and other systems
- Asthma trigger assessment findings
- Results of peak expiratory flow rate monitoring

- Instructions given related to asthma management
- Skilled procedures performed, such as nebulizer treatment and chest physiotherapy
- Understanding of and compliance with the medication regimen
- Understanding of and compliance with peak flow meter use
- Patient compliance with avoidance of asthma triggers
- Patient and caregiver progress toward educational goals
- Patient response to care
- Laboratory results pertinent to care
- Variances to expected outcomes
- Specific barriers to learning (for example, impaired vision and impaired mental status or cognitive ability)
- Specific factors indicating a need for home care, including no available, willing, and able caregiver; patient newly diagnosed with asthma; or patient new to medications, aerosol therapy, peak flow meter use, oxygen use, or chest physiotherapy
- Specific deficits in initial knowledge level, then follow-up of progress as evidenced by specific concepts and procedures the patient has verbalized or demonstrated

Reimbursement reminders

- Indicate an expected end point of daily visits (when daily visits have been ordered).
- Obtain a physician's order for any plan of care changes and document them in the patient's record.
- Determine which supplies and durable medical equipment are covered by Medicare.
- Verify that a metered-dose inhaler alone is insufficient in treating the pa-

tient's asthma to ensure that he qualifies for a nebulizer machine.
- Determine that the patient's oxygen saturation level is 88% or less to ensure that he qualifies for oxygen.
- Verify that respiratory therapist services are usually provided by the company that supplies the durable medical equipment on a routine or as-needed basis.

Insurance hints

- Report objective data about the patient's homebound status.
- Present objective patient findings, changes in clinical condition, and changes in care since last contact (for example, new physician's orders).
- Report specifics about the patient and caregiver education process.
- Present progress toward established goals.

Asthma trigger assessment

According to the National Asthma Education Program, asthma is a lung disease characterized by airway obstruction, narrowing, or inflammation or by hyperreactivity to various stimuli. Factors that stimulate the airways to react in an exaggerated manner are referred to as *asthma triggers*. A patient may have multiple triggers, which may vary over time and with age.

Viral respiratory infection is the most common cause of acute exacerbation in children under 2 years of age. As children grow, viral infections are still a problem, but allergens become increasingly more common triggers until they are the predominant cause of asthma exacerbation in teenagers. In the elderly, viral infections are the most common asthma trigger.

Successful long-term management of asthma depends on identifying and minimizing exposure to asthma triggers. Avoidance strategies should be designed to eliminate or minimize exposure to specific allergens or irritants known to be triggers for an asthma patient. The home care nurse has an important role in identifying individual asthma triggers and teaching avoidance measures.

Previsit checklist

Physician orders and preparation

- Specific initial and ongoing physician's orders
- Care and teaching orders for each discipline
- Oral medication and aerosol therapy orders as indicated
- Activity orders and restrictions

Equipment and supplies

- Supplies for standard precautions
- Peak flow meter
- Metered-dose inhaler as indicated
- Nebulizer with prescribed medication as indicated
- Oxygen as indicated

Safety requirements

- Standard precautions for infection control
- Emergency plan and access to functional phone and list of emergency phone numbers
- Fire evacuation plan, functional smoke detectors, and access to functional fire extinguisher

- Oxygen precautions, safe handling and placement of home oxygen equipment, and notification of local fire and police departments of oxygen use in the home
- Information on medications, including dosage, adverse effects, interactions, and safe storage
- Proper disposal of expired drugs
- Instruction on signs and symptoms of medical emergency and actions to take

Major diagnostic codes

- Acute upper respiratory infection 465.9
- Allergic rhinitis due to other allergen 477.8
- Allergic rhinitis due to pollen 477.0
- Asthma 493
- Bronchitis, acute 466
- Chronic obstructive pulmonary disease 496
- Congestive heart failure 428
- Gastroesophageal reflux disease 530.81
- Influenza with other respiratory manifestations 487.1
- Influenza with pneumonia 487.0
- Nebulizer therapy 93.94
- Pneumonia 486

Defense of homebound status

- Unable to ambulate farther than 10′ (3 m) due to dyspnea with minimal exertion
- Unable to ambulate more than 10′ due to fatigue and poor endurance related to severe, uncontrolled asthma
- Unable to negotiate stairs due to profound shortness of breath

Selected nursing diagnoses and patient outcomes

Knowledge deficit related to identification and control of asthma and its triggers

The patient or caregiver will:
- describe the asthma disease process, causes and factors contributing to symptoms (triggers), and the regimen for symptom control   (N, OT, PT, RT)
- verbalize knowledge of personal asthma and allergy triggers   (N)
- identify common asthma triggers   (N)
- identify ways to avoid common asthma triggers   (N)
- demonstrate measures being taken to avoid asthma and allergy triggers.   (N, RT, HCA)

Ineffective breathing pattern

The patient or caregiver will:
- demonstrate a stable respiratory status with an effective respiratory rate and improved gas exchange in the lungs   (N, RT)
- demonstrate an adequate breathing pattern as evidenced by lack of respiratory distress.   (N)

Ineffective airway clearance related to bronchospasm and increased pulmonary secretions

The patient or caregiver will:
- demonstrate effective coughing and increased air exchange in the lungs.   (N, RT)

Ineffective management of therapeutic regimen: Individuals

The patient or caregiver will:
- demonstrate improved management of therapeutic regimen as evidenced by improved asthma self-management practices (specify: medications, peak flow meter, avoidance of asthma triggers, activity).   (N)

Activity intolerance related to shortness of breath

The patient or caregiver will:
- identify factors that reduce activity tolerance and verbalize measures to improve them   (N, OT, PT, RT, SW)
- exhibit a decrease in hypoxic signs of increased activity (pulse, blood pressure, respirations)   (N, RT)
- return to independence in activities of daily living (ADLs), exercise regimens, and all self-care.   (N, OT, PT)

Knowledge deficit related to medications

The patient or caregiver will:
- state correct dose and time for each asthma medication prescribed and adverse effects and precautions for each   (N)
- demonstrate correct technique for administration of aerosol therapy (metered-dose inhaler, nebulizer treatment)   (N, RT)
- verbalize understanding of parameters for use of as-needed oral and inhaled asthma medication   (N, RT)
- demonstrate adherence to multiple medication regimen.   (N)

Skilled nursing services

Care measures
- Perform initial full assessment of all systems, including the respiratory system (breath sounds and abnormal breathing patterns, chest movements, secretions).

- Assess skin and mucous membrane color.
- Assess for signs of cerebral anoxia, activity intolerance, and chest pain.
- Carefully assess the patient and the patient's environment for potential asthma triggers.
- Assess patient and caregiver compliance with avoidance of asthma triggers.
- Check patient's peak flow meter readings chart or diary; assess for lower than normal readings and connection between low readings and potential asthma triggers.

Patient and family teaching

- Instruct patient and caregiver about the patient's asthma triggers and assess understanding of the measures required to avoid or minimize exposure to asthma triggers, the importance of compliance with avoidance measures, and the potential effects of noncompliance.
- Emphasize the need to pretreat with physician-ordered aerosol therapy if exposure to a known trigger such as exercise is unavoidable.
- Describe how to keep an asthma diary and record factors or situations that might be triggering asthma attacks.
- Explain the need to intensify patient's asthma regimen during upper respiratory infections to avoid deterioration of asthma control.
- Discuss consulting physician regarding allergy skin testing to identify allergens and obtain appropriate treatment, annual influenza vaccine and one-time pneumonia vaccine, and treatment of allergic rhinitis, sinusitis, and gastroesophageal reflux disease if indicated.

- Review medication regimen, oral and aerosol, including dosage, frequency, purpose, potential adverse effects, and interactions.
- Emphasize importance of following established asthma management and treatment plan to provide optimum control of asthma symptoms.

Interdisciplinary services

Home care aide

- Assistance with personal care and hygiene needs
- Assistance with ADLs

Occupational therapist

- Instruction on energy conservation techniques
- Training in ADLs
- Assessment of need for and instruction in use of adaptive equipment

Physical therapist

- Development and teaching of an individualized home exercise program
- Performance of and instruction about pulmonary physical therapy — breathing exercises and chest physiotherapy as indicated

Respiratory therapist

- Recommendations on how to identify and avoid triggers
- Instruction on use of a peak flow meter and interpretation of results

Social worker

- Assessment of social and emotional factors
- Referral to community resources and support groups
- Counseling and referral for stress management and reduction

Discharge plan
- Effective management by patient and caregiver of asthma care in the home with physician follow-up services

Documentation requirements
- Findings from asthma trigger assessment
- Instructions given related to asthma management, including strategies to avoid or minimize exposure to asthma triggers
- Performance of skilled procedures; for example, nebulizer treatment and chest physiotherapy
- Patient understanding of and compliance with avoidance of asthma triggers, medication regimen, and peak flow meter use
- Patient and caregiver progress toward education goals
- Variances to expected outcomes
- Specific barriers to learning (for example, impaired vision, mental status, and cognitive ability)
- Lack of available, willing, and able caregiver
- Patient newly diagnosed with asthma
- Patient new to medications, aerosol therapy, peak flow meter use, oxygen use, chest physiotherapy
- Specific deficits in initial knowledge level, then progress as evidenced by specific concepts and procedures verbalized and demonstrated

Reimbursement reminders
- When daily visits have been ordered, indicate expected end point of daily visits.

- Obtain a physician's order for any plan of care change, and document this in the patient's record.
- Supplies and durable medical equipment covered by Medicare: nebulizer machine (Medicare part B, 80% of allowable charge, physician must indicate that metered-dose inhaler alone is insufficient to treat the patient's asthma), oxygen (Medicare part B, 80% of allowable charge, patient's oxygen saturation level must be 88% or lower).
- Respiratory therapist services are usually provided by the company supplying the durable medical equipment on a routine or as-needed basis.

Insurance hints
- Present objective data about homebound status.
- Present objective patient findings, changes in clinical condition, and changes in care since last contact (for example, new physician's orders).
- State specific asthma triggers in the patient's environment and measures being taken to instruct the patient and caregiver in avoidance or control of asthma triggers.
- Present other specifics about patient and caregiver education process.
- Document progress toward established goals.

Bedridden patient care

Being bedridden isn't a medical diagnosis but rather a state of functional limitation secondary to illness, injury, or infirmity. It pertains to adults as well as to a growing number of infants and children who require long-term care.

Bedridden patients need to be considered as thinking, functioning human beings. Although bedridden status doesn't in itself signify a loss of mental or reasoning power, developmental skills, such as walking, crawling, speech, and hand-eye coordination, can be delayed in infants and children.

Bedridden patients pose specific challenges to the home care nurse. Round-the-clock care is commonly necessary, but insurance and financial limitations can complicate this need. Extensive family and caregiver education is also required. These care situations can benefit greatly from community resources that provide additional education, support, supplies, funding, and respite. Social service involvement can be helpful in making these referrals. Nurses need to be aware of and encourage families to tap into these resources.

Previsit checklist

Physician orders and preparation
- Orders for medications, including dosages and routes
- Diet orders
- Venipuncture
- Wound care
- Catheter care
- Suctioning orders

Equipment and supplies
- Vital signs equipment
- Supplies for standard precautions
- Equipment for suctioning
- Supplies for wound care
- Venipuncture supplies

Safety requirements
- Standard precautions for infection control
- Proper technique for transferring the patient and moving the patient in bed
- Medication and dangerous equipment out of reach of bedridden children and mentally impaired adults
- Functioning call bell or intercom system
- System to assist with adherence to complex medication regimen
- Information on medications, including dosage, adverse effects, interactions, and safe storage
- Emergency plan and access to functional phone and list of emergency phone numbers
- Identification and correction of environmental hazards and patient-specific concerns

Major diagnostic codes
- Amyotrophic lateral sclerosis 335.20
- Cerebral artery occlusion with infarction 434.91
- Chronic obstructive pulmonary disease 496
- Cirrhosis of the liver 571.5
- Debility 799.3
- Decubitus ulcer 707.0
- Multiple sclerosis 340
- Paralysis 344.9
- Paraplegia, lower extremity/upper extremity 344.1/344.2
- Parkinson's disease 332.0
- Pneumonia 486
- Quadriplegia 344.00
- Respirator dependent V46.1
- Spinal cord injury, traumatic 952.9

• Ventilation continuous positive airway pressure/continuously greater than 96 hours 93.90/96.72

Defense of homebound status

• Bedridden status
• Inability to ambulate independently
• Open or draining wound
• Maximal assistance required to transfer
• Quadriplegia
• Severe dyspnea
• Respiratory dependence
• Extreme weakness
• Hemiplegia or paraplegia

Selected nursing diagnoses and patient outcomes

Activity intolerance related to deconditioning effects of bed rest
    The patient or caregiver will:
• identify factors that reduce activity tolerance   (N, OT, PT)
• exhibit a decrease in hypoxic signs of increased activity (pulse, blood pressure, respirations)   (N, PT)
• report a reduction of symptoms of activity intolerance.   (N, PT)

Risk for altered development related to compromised physical ability and dependence or related to inadequate sensory stimulation secondary to prolonged bed rest
    The patient or caregiver will:
• continue to demonstrate appropriate behavior in personal, social, language, and cognitive or motor activities.   (N, OT, PT, SW)

Risk for impaired skin integrity related to impaired mobility secondary to bed rest
    The patient or caregiver will:
• express willingness to participate in the prevention of pressure ulcers   (N, PT)
• describe causes and prevention methods   (N, PT)
• demonstrate intact skin integrity free of pressure ulcers.   (N, PT)

Caregiver role strain related to unrealistic expectations of caregiver by care receiver, other family members, or home care agency
    The caregiver will:
• share frustrations regarding caregiving responsibility   (N, SW)
• identify two changes that could be made to improve daily life   (N, SW)
• relate intent to listen without giving advice   (N, SW)
• convey empathy regarding daily responsibilities   (N, SW)
• establish a plan for weekly support or help.   (N, SW)

Impaired bed mobility related to insufficient strength and endurance for movement secondary to fatigue, decreased motivation, or pain
    The patient or caregiver will:
• demonstrate ways to increase mobility   (N, OT, PT)
• report and demonstrate an increase in mobility.   (N, OT, PT)

Bathing, hygiene, dressing, grooming, feeding, or toileting self-care deficit related to weakness and tiredness or neuromuscular or musculoskeletal impairment

The patient or caregiver will:
• identify safe performance of activities of daily living (ADLs).   (N)

Constipation related to insufficient physical activity or neurologic impairment

The patient or caregiver will:
• identify dietary changes that will help prevent constipation   (N, D)
• demonstrate understanding of the bowel regimen   (N)
• identify factors that help prevent constipation   (N)
• maintain regular bowel elimination.   (N, D)

Risk for aspiration

The patient or caregiver will:
• demonstrate proper measures for preventing aspiration   (N, SP)
• identify signs of aspiration. (N, SP)

Skilled nursing services

Care measures
• Assess the mental and cognitive, integumentary (paying close attention to high-risk areas for breakdown, such as bony prominences and the sacral area), cardiovascular, GI, genitourinary, and nutrition and hydration systems.
• Assess the performance of range-of-motion (ROM) exercises and other activities in bed.
• Assess the developmental status and risk for impaired development.

• Assess the environment and safety practices in place as well as the potential for injury.
• Assess elimination needs and practices and the need for supportive equipment, such as a bedside commode or urinal.
• Assess the caregiver's skill and competence in providing care.
• Assess wounds and provide dressing changes.
• Implement a bladder training program.
• Administer medications as ordered by the physician and assess the patient's response.
• Monitor vital signs.
• Assess for signs and symptoms of infection.
• Perform venipuncture as ordered.
• Perform urinary catheter care and change as necessary.
• Evaluate the patient's response to treatments and care.
• Provide comfort care.
• Perform nasotracheal or oropharyngeal suctioning.

Patient and family teaching
• Demonstrate ROM exercises.
• Teach how to perform ADLs safely.
• Instruct on how to render treatments and wound care.
• Explore methods of mental stimulation.
• Outline safety precautions.
• Instruct on how to assist with elimination needs and bathing.
• Teach skin care measures.
• Explain ways to prevent pneumonia.
• Teach signs and symptoms of infection and when to call a physician.
• Instruct in proper suctioning technique.

• Provide information on medication dosages, purposes, routes, and adverse effects.

Interdisciplinary actions

Dietitian
• Consultation for nutritional needs

Home care aide
• Bathing and personal care
• Light housekeeping and laundry when indicated
• Meal preparation

Occupational therapist
• Instruction on adaptive aids and assessment of use
• Instruction and assessment in performance of ADLs

Physical therapist
• Development of and instruction in the individualized home exercise program
• Chest physiotherapy
• Instruction in the use of assistive devices
• Instruction in safe transfer techniques

Social worker
• Counseling
• Exploration and referral to community agencies and support groups

Discharge plan
• Patient and caregiver independence with performance of ADLs and ROM exercises and management of elimination needs
• Safety measures in place and functioning

• Patient and caregiver comprehension of the developmental level and stimulation requirements
• Patient and caregiver comfort with the care situation
• Referral to outpatient services
• Continuation of home care visits for homebound patient with skilled care needs

Documentation requirements
• Skilled assessment of all systems
• Subjective or objective data related to the developmental status and risk for impaired development
• Current patient or caregiver skill level and any physical or mental limitations
• Risk for injury or skin breakdown
• Stressors affecting the patient or care environment
• Teaching and instruction given and responses confirmed
• Referrals to and conferences with support agencies and disciplines
• Patient or caregiver participation in care
• Patient or caregiver progress toward goals

Reimbursement reminders
• Depending on the medical diagnoses or treatments that have warranted home health involvement, the skilled nurse may have a very limited time in the home. Therefore, it's important that instruction start immediately and be documented thoroughly.
• Home care aide support services are covered by Medicare (when a skilled service is involved) but aren't covered by many other reimbursement plans.

- Registered dietitian services aren't reimbursable under current Medicare home care benefits.
- Medicare covers other nutritional solutions only when they are the only source of nutrition or if they are given by enteral tube feedings.

Insurance hints

- Report objective findings and changes that have occurred since last contact.
- Present changes to plan of care and interteam communication.
- Present objective data reflecting patient status and the need for skilled services in the home.
- Identify higher-cost alternatives considered by the health care team or patient (such as inpatient settings).
- Present objective data about the patient's progression from homebound status and the target date to end home care services.

Bowel and bladder retraining

Bowel and bladder retraining can be an option when caring for an elderly client who is dealing with incontinence and its ramifications. It may also be useful for a cancer patient suffering from spinal cord compression. If used appropriately, the interventions included as part of bowel and bladder retraining can not only restore continence but also enhance self-confidence and elevate self-esteem immeasurably. Home care patients requiring bowel and bladder retraining will need close assessment and teaching of strategies.

Previsit checklist

Physician orders and preparation
For bowel retraining:

- Order for enterostomal therapist consult for assistance with designing an individualized bowel retraining program
- Order for a high-fiber diet
- Stool softeners or laxatives
- Order for a bedside commode

For bladder retraining:

- Order for self-catheterization
- Order for diet, including foods to maintain a urine pH less than 7 and create alkaline urine

Equipment and supplies
For bowel retraining:

- Bedside commode
- Gloves
- Water-soluble lubricant

For bladder retraining:

- Urinary catheter
- Gloves
- Silicone rubber catheter that the patient can utilize for self-catheterization

Safety requirements

- Cautious use of laxatives in bowel retraining program
- Close monitoring for signs and symptoms of urinary tract infection during bladder retraining
- Maintenance of sterility during urinary catheterization
- Standard precautions for infection control
- Adequate lighting

- Fire evacuation plan, functional smoke detectors, and access to functional fire extinguisher
- System to assist with adherence to complex medication regimen
- Information on medications, including dosage, adverse effects, interactions, and safe storage
- Emergency plan and access to functional phone and list of emergency phone numbers
- Identification and correction of environmental hazards and patient-specific concerns

Major diagnostic codes
- Hematuria 599.7
- Incontinence, feces 787.6
- Incontinence, mixed (urge and stress) 788.33
- Incontinence, other 788.39
- Incontinence, stress, female/male 625.6/788.32
- Incontinence, urge 788.31
- Incontinence of urine 788.30
- Incontinence of urine with continuous leakage 788.37
- Incontinence without sensory awareness 788.34
- Indwelling urinary catheter, insertion/replacement 57.94/57.95
- Urinary tract infection 599.0
- Vaginitis 616.10

Defense of homebound status
- Incapacitating bowel incontinence
- Decubitus ulcers secondary to bowel incontinence
- Incapacitating urinary incontinence
- Bedridden

Selected nursing diagnoses and patient outcomes

Altered urinary elimination related to a urologic disorder
The patient or caregiver will:
- alter clothing and environment to promote continence   (N, ET)
- participate in a urinary training program   (N, ET)
- report decreased urinary frequency, urgency, and dribbling   (N, ET)
- report regained bladder control.
             (N, ET)

Risk for infection related to urinary incontinence
The patient or caregiver will:
- display no signs of urinary tract infection   (N)
- correctly identify signs and symptoms of urinary tract infection and when to report them   (N)
- increase fluid intake and void regularly   (N)
- demonstrate aseptic procedure for catheterization.   (N, ET)

Impaired skin integrity related to incontinence-induced skin breakdown
The patient or caregiver will:
- express an accurate understanding of skin care, including use of incontinence pads and protective skin barriers   (N)
- maintain clean, dry, intact skin (N)
- display no signs of skin infection.
             (N)

Bowel incontinence related to rectal sphincter abnormality, lower motor nerve damage, general decline in muscle tone, or loss of rectal sphincter control

The patient or caregiver will:
- identify appropriate measures for establishing continence (N)
- identify appropriate skin care measures. (N)

Functional urinary incontinence related to neuromuscular limitation or weakened supporting pelvic structures

The patient or caregiver will:
- achieve urinary continence (N)
- demonstrate proper techniques for bladder retraining. (N)

Total urinary incontinence related to neuropathy preventing transmission of nerve impulses indicating bladder fullness, trauma or disease affecting spinal cord nerves, anatomic (fistula), loss of bladder muscle control following surgery, or neurologic dysfunction causing the trigger of urination at unpredictable times

The patient or caregiver will:
- demonstrate proper bladder-training techniques. (N)

Skilled nursing services

Care measures
- Assess the mental and cognitive, GI, and genitourinary systems.
- Assess the level of care by the patient or caregiver. Observe the performance of catheterization or use of the bedside commode. Note adherence to scheduled voiding and defecation times.
- Provide skin care.
- Perform catheterization as ordered.
- Assess the effectiveness of the treatment regimen: assess for continued in-

continence or fecal impaction; palpate bladder for urine retention.
- Ensure that the patient has no history of heart problems if bowel impaction occurs and requires digital removal.

Patient and family teaching
For bowel retraining:
- Emphasize the importance of consuming 15 to 30 g of fiber per day.
- Encourage oral intake of 3,000 ml of fluid per day.
- Promote use of the bedside commode or toilet for all bowel movements.
- Advise the patient to try to move the bowels at the same time each day.
- Tell the patient to drink something hot before each scheduled bowel movement.
- Teach signs and symptoms of fecal impaction.
- Discuss stimulants, including glycerin suppositories and chemical stimulants, such as Dulcolax, castor oil, Senokot, and cascara, if laxatives are needed for defecation.

For bladder retraining:
- Review foods (such as cranberry juice and blueberries) that will decrease a urinary pH and minimize bacterial adhesion to the bladder wall.
- Tell the patient to avoid foods (such as milk and almonds) that produce alkaline urine.
- Outline a schedule of voiding times. Schedule times once every 2 to 3 hours.
- Advise the patient to palpate the bladder after voiding to evaluate urine retention.
- Emphasize the importance of limiting fluids after 7:00 p.m.
- Teach signs and symptoms of urinary tract infection.

• Teach intermittent self-catheterization procedure, emphasizing aseptic technique.

Interdisciplinary actions

Enterostomal therapist
• Assistance with designing an individualized bowel and bladder retraining program

Discharge plan
• Safe management of the bowel and bladder retraining program by the patient or caregiver in the home with physician follow-up services
• Referral to outpatient services
• Continued home care visits for the homebound patient with skilled care needs

Documentation requirements
• Assessment findings
• Subjective and objective data regarding signs and symptoms of urinary incontinence or fecal impaction
• Results of consult with the enterostomal therapist
• Patient and caregiver participation in care
• Patient and caregiver progress toward educational goals
• Patient response to care
• Teaching provided and patient and caregiver response to instruction

Reimbursement reminders
• If skin breakdown has already occurred and requires the development of a skin care regimen, make certain that the wound care performed matches the care ordered by the physician; reimbursement won't occur otherwise.
• Make certain that any wound care supplies ordered can be classified as nonroutine supplies.

Insurance hints
• Present objective data about the patient's homebound status.
• Report objective patient findings and changes that have occurred since last contact.
• Report new laboratory values and changes to the plan of care.
• Detail the progress of patient education.
• Present information and findings that show how home care mitigated the need for acute or inpatient care.

Brain tumor care

A brain tumor is an intracranial neoplasm, either benign or malignant, that causes a rise in intracranial pressure because of the space it occupies in the skull. There are several different types of brain tumors, including gliomas, adenomas, meningiomas, and neuromas. A brain tumor may originate in the central nervous system or metastasize from another site in the body. The effectiveness of treatment depends on the site, type, and size of the tumor. Each patient must be evaluated and treated individually based on the lesion. Treatment usually involves surgery, radiation, and chemotherapy. Providing care can be challenging due to the many problems the patient with a brain tumor may face.

Previsit checklist

Physician orders and preparation
- Vital signs
- Neurologic checks
- Medications, including dosage and route
- Venipuncture
- Diet orders
- Activity restrictions and limitations

Equipment and supplies
- Vital signs equipment
- Oxygen supplies as necessary
- Venipuncture supplies
- Transporting bags and requisitions or request forms
- System for sharps disposal, including container
- Dressing and wound care supplies, including sterile applicators, dressings, 4″ × 4″ gauze, gloves, ointments, solutions, toppers, gauze rolls, and nonadherent dressings

Safety requirements
- Standard precautions for infection control and sharps and medical waste disposal
- Recognition of the signs and symptoms of complications and a follow-up action plan
- Implementation of treatment protocols for complications
- Adaptation of lifestyle and activities of daily living (ADLs)
- Preoperative patient teaching as necessary
- System to assist with adherence to complex medication regimen
- Information on medications, including dosage, adverse effects, interactions, and safe storage
- Emergency plan and access to functional phone and list of emergency phone numbers
- Identification and correction of environmental hazards and patient-specific concerns

Major diagnostic codes
- Alteration in consciousness, transient/persistent 780.02/780.03
- Benign tumor of central nervous system 225.9
- Cerebral edema 348.5
- Convulsions, nonfebrile, nonepileptic 780.39
- Malignant brain neoplasm, secondary 198.3
- Metastases, bone 198.5
- Metastases, general 199.0
- Neoplasm, brain, primary 191.9
- Transient ischemic attacks 435.9

Defense of homebound status
- Unsafe mental status changes due to lesion
- Altered level of consciousness or comatose
- Limited mobility or too weak to leave home
- Requires maximum assistance in all activities
- Medical restriction due to potential for postoperative infection after recent brain surgery
- Postoperative meningitis requiring high-dose steroid therapy
- Pain and weakness
- Unsafe, unsteady gait
- Status after recent cerebrovascular accident

Selected nursing diagnoses and patient outcomes

Pain related to surgery
The patient or caregiver will:
• verbalize decreased pain and demonstrate management of discomfort, rating pain at 3 or less on a 0-to-10 scale 80% of the time (N)
• experience an improved quality of life as a result of care measures (N, HCA, OT, PT, SW)
• be comfortable through a dignified end of life. (N, HCA, SW)

Risk for infection
The patient or caregiver will:
• remain free from infection and afebrile (N)
• verbalize and demonstrate correct postoperative wound care technique (N)
• adhere to the medical regimen (N, HCA, OT, PT)
• experience a decrease in complications from chemotherapy or radiation therapy. (N)

Bathing, hygiene, dressing, grooming, feeding, and toileting self-care deficit
The patient or caregiver will:
• have personal care needs met (N, HCA, OT, PT)
• apply information related to the disease process and possible complications into ADLs. (N, HCA, OT, PT, SW)

Ineffective individual coping related to a situational crisis
The patient or caregiver will:
• demonstrate compliance with treatments and medications (N, OT, PT)

• contact or use identified community support systems and resources (N, OT, PT, SW)
• adapt the lifestyle to relieve symptoms and improve the quality of life (N, HCA, OT, PT, SW)
• verbalize and demonstrate the knowledge of complications or changes warranting notification of the nurse or physician. (N)

Altered nutrition: Less than body requirements related to the inability to ingest or digest food or absorb nutrients due to biological, psychological, or economic factors
The patient or caregiver will:
• maintain optimal nutritional status with the ingestion of high-calorie supplements and foods easy to chew and swallow (N, HCA, SP)
• demonstrate safe-swallowing technique and communication. (SP)

Skilled nursing services

Care measures
• Perform a skilled assessment of all body systems.
• Conduct neurologic checks.
• Monitor vital signs.
• Assess for signs and symptoms of infection.
• Assess fluid status and weights.
• Monitor nutrition.
• Assess skin integrity and the oral mucosa.
• Prepare for surgical intervention as indicated.
• Provide postoperative wound care as indicated and ordered.
• Monitor the patient's response to pain and medications.

- Assess emotional response to the illness and the effectiveness of coping mechanisms.
- Observe closely for seizure activity.
- Monitor medication use and adverse effects.
- Implement and monitor a bowel regimen.
- Assess the patient's response to care and report it to the physician.
- Perform venipuncture per the physician's orders.
- Assess pain.
- Weigh the patient daily.

Patient and family teaching

- Teach postoperative wound care.
- Discuss the chemotherapy or radiation therapy regimen and schedule.
- Discuss the steroid therapy regimen.
- Review potential complications that may result from an immunosuppressed state.
- Review the disease process related to seizure activity and emphasize the importance of using seizure medications.
- Teach skin care needs and methods to prevent breakdown.
- Teach coping mechanisms.
- Discuss relaxation techniques.
- Instruct in medication use, contraindications, and adverse effects.
- Plan diet changes as indicated.
- Teach energy conservation techniques.
- Instruct in the safe use and care of home oxygen as necessary.
- Describe signs and symptoms that should be reported to the physician.
- Discuss when to call emergency medical personnel.

Interdisciplinary actions

Dietitian

- Consultation

Home care aide

- Personal care and assistance with ADLs
- Home exercise program participation

Occupational therapist

- Energy-conservation techniques
- Safe performance of ADLs
- Use of adaptive or assistive devices and equipment
- Cognitive training

Physical therapist

- Home exercise program for increased endurance and safe mobility
- Bed mobility exercises
- Safe transfer, ambulation, and positioning techniques
- Caregiver and home care aide instruction and supervision of ordered and established home exercise program

Social worker

- Exploration of problems and available resources
- Eligibility for additional services or resources
- Referral to appropriate community resources
- Psychosocial counseling
- Spiritual support referrals
- Referral for hospice evaluation

Speech pathologist

- Evaluation and swallowing assessment
- Recommendation of food types and textures

- Aspiration precautions, instruction, and supervision
- Speech dysphagia plan for safe swallowing and effective communication

Discharge plan

- Safe management of tasks at home through end of life
- Trained caregiver and physician follow-up services
- Discharge from home care when goals are met
- Referral to hospice evaluation and care

Documentation requirements

- Skilled assessment, including subjective and objective signs and symptoms
- Specific care, treatments, and medications administered
- Instructions given, demonstrated, and provided in writing
- Response to care and instructions
- Coordination of patient care with other members of the health care team
- Progress toward goals as well as prevention of complications usually associated with patients receiving radiation therapy, chemotherapy, and surgical interventions
- Laboratory results and notification given to the physician with the visit note
- Medication changes and the specific need to monitor the patient's response to these changes

Reimbursement reminders

- Ensure that any schedule changes or additional services or treatments by any discipline have an accompanying order from the physician.
- Identify any barriers to learning, which could result in the need for ongoing visits.
- Document multidisciplinary planning and communication continuously.
- Note that blood drawing supplies are considered routine and as such are non-billable.
- Note that dressing and wound care supplies aren't considered routine and are billable when specifically identified in the plan of care as ordered by the physician.
- Note that if daily care is ordered (for postoperative wound care or as the patient's condition declines), a beginning and ending date must be specified.

Insurance hints

- Determine how often to initially report clinical conditions and always immediately report if patient changes affect the initial care planning frequency or duration.
- Present subjective and objective data specific to established goals.
- Report barriers to care and learning.
- Address progress toward specific goals and prevention of complications in regular updates.

Burns

A burn is a traumatic skin injury caused by heat, electrical current, chemicals, friction, shearing forces, or excessive exposure to sunlight. Burns are classified according to depth and extent of injury: first-degree (partial thickness), second-degree (superficial or deep partial thickness), and third-degree (full-thickness) burns. For the home care nurse, burns mean not only intensive acute care but extensive patient teaching and preparation for long-term patient management.

Previsit checklist

Physician orders and preparation
- Vital signs
- Activity orders and restrictions
- Medication dosage and route
- Order for specific wound care
- Order for nutritional consultation for comprehensive nutritional assessment and design of individualized high-protein diet for wound healing

Equipment and supplies
- Specific dressing change supplies as specified by physician
- Supplies for standard precautions
- Vital signs equipment
- Medication information

Safety requirements
- Standard precautions for infection control
- Information on medications, including dosage, adverse effects, interactions, and safe storage
- Medical identification bracelet
- System to assist with adherence to complex medication regimen
- Emergency plan and access to functional phone and list of emergency phone numbers
- Identification and correction of environmental hazards and patient-specific concerns

Major diagnostic codes
- Burn, unspecified 949.0
- Burn of face and head, unspecified degree 941.0
- Burn of lower limbs, unspecified degree 945.0
- Burn of trunk, unspecified degree 942.0
- Burn of upper extremity except wrist or hand, unspecified degree 945.0
- Burn of wrist or hand, unspecified degree 944.0
- Burns (classified according to extent of body surface involved — refer to a coding manual for specific codes) 948

(To assign a fifth digit, see appendix A, page 638.)

Defense of homebound status
- Bedridden
- Poor respiratory status due to smoke inhalation
- Assistance required for ambulation
- Severe functional limitations because of pain or contracture
- Edema of lower extremities

Selected nursing diagnoses and patient outcomes

Impaired skin integrity related to traumatic injury
   The patient will:
- remain free from infection throughout the recovery period   (N)
- demonstrate notable wound healing
                                        (N)
- exhibit a minimal amount of scar tissue.   (N)

Knowledge deficit related to the recovery from burn injury

The patient or caregiver will:

- verbalize an understanding of the need for adequate nutrition (N, D)
- verbalize an understanding of the degree and severity of injury, procedures, and progress (N)
- verbalize and correctly demonstrate the dressing change procedure for prevention of sepsis (N)
- verbalize understanding of the need for debridement or grafting procedures. (N)

Risk for infection

The patient or caregiver will:

- remain free from infection (N)
- identify signs and symptoms of infection (N)
- demonstrate proper infection control measures. (N)

Altered nutrition: Less than body requirements related to increased caloric needs secondary to wound healing

The patient or caregiver will:

- follow a proper diet (N, D)
- receive adequate nutrition (N, D)
- verbalize an understanding of nutritional needs. (N, D)

Impaired physical mobility related to pain, musculoskeletal impairment, intolerance to activity, or decreased strength and endurance

The patient or caregiver will:

- demonstrate proper range-of-motion exercises (N, PT)
- increase activity level gradually (N, PT)
- rate pain at 3 or less on a 0-to-10 scale 80% of the time. (N)

Body image disturbance related to trauma or injury

The patient or caregiver will:

- verbalize feelings and emotions (N, SW)
- demonstrate acceptance of body changes. (N, SW)

Skilled nursing services

Care measures

- Assess the integumentary and nutrition and hydration systems.
- Ensure adequate fluid intake.
- Monitor urine output.
- Monitor metabolic needs and ensure adequate nutrition.
- Provide wound management.
- Prepare the patient for debridement and escharotomy.
- Ensure aseptic technique in all procedures.
- Provide emotional support.
- Prepare the patient for rehabilitation.

Patient and family teaching

- Educate regarding the degree and severity of injury, procedures, and progress.
- Explain the grafting procedure.
- Educate regarding debridement and escharotomy.

Interdisciplinary actions

Dietitian

- Consultation regarding the need for nutritional assessment and development of an individualized, high-protein diet for wound healing

Home care aide
- Assistance with hygiene needs and activities of daily living

Physical therapist
- Consultation for prevention of contractures and loss of function

Discharge plan
- Ability of the patient or caregiver to manage the disease process in the home with physician and community support system follow-up services
- Referral to outpatient services
- Continuation of home care visits for homebound patient with skilled care needs

Documentation requirements
- Physical assessment findings
- Patient and caregiver teaching as well as the response
- Effects of medications
- Variances to expected outcomes
- Wound care provided
- Specific care provided
- Progress toward goals
- Abnormal laboratory values as well as when the physician was notified and any changes to the plan of care

Reimbursement reminders
- Record changes in the plan of care.
- Report measurable data on the patient's progress and goals. Include a time frame for ending home care visits.

Insurance hints
- Provide objective patient findings and changes since the last update.

- Report new symptoms and changes in the plan of care.
- Report measurable changes and information that communicate the status of the patient and the need for skilled home care services.

Cancer

A group of diseases characterized by the uncontrolled growth and spread of abnormal cells, cancer is the second leading cause of death in the United States (exceeded only by heart disease). It may be caused by internal (hormones, immune conditions, and inherited mutations) or external (chemicals, radiation, and viruses) factors.

Screening examinations conducted by a health care professional or regular self-examinations can result in early detection of many types of cancer. The earlier cancer is treated, the more likely it is that treatment will succeed. Many treatment options exist; the treatment chosen will depend on such factors as the type, stage, location, and degree of metastasis of the cancer.

In addition to providing physical care to the patient, the nurse must provide support and education. Home care needs vary greatly from one patient to the next, depending on the type, stage, and location of the cancer and the mode of treatment; basic guidelines follow.

Previsit checklist

Physician orders and preparation
- Frequency of visits

- Type of laboratory work and frequency
- Diet orders
- Activity orders and restrictions
- Medication orders
- Wound care, when applicable

Equipment and supplies

- Vital signs equipment
- Nutritional tools, such as total parenteral nutrition administration pump, nasogastric pump set, and supplemental feeding solutions
- Medication information sheets, including adverse effects and interactions
- Wound care supplies
- Scale
- Sharps disposal system, including container
- Medication administration supplies for I.M. or I.V. medications
- Occupational Safety and Health Administration (OSHA)-approved cleanup kit for in-home chemotherapy

Safety requirements

- Standard precautions for infection control and sharps disposal
- OSHA precautions for the use of in-home chemotherapy
- Action plan for drug interactions or infection
- System to assist with adherence to complex medication regimen
- Information on medications, including dosage, adverse effects, interactions, and safe storage
- Emergency plan and access to functional phone and list of emergency phone numbers
- Identification and correction of environmental hazards and patient-specific concerns

Major diagnostic codes

- Adrenal cancer 194.0
- Bladder cancer 188.9
- Brain cancer 191.9
- Breast cancer 174.9
- Cervix, cancer of 180.9
- Colon cancer 153.9
- Esophagus, cancer of 150.9
- Gastric cancer 151.9
- Head or neck, cancer of 195.0
- Leukemia, acute 208.0
- Leukopenia 288.0
- Liver, metastatic cancer of 197.7
- Lung cancer 162.9
- Mastectomy, simple/radical 85.42/85.46
- Metastases, general/bone 199.1/198.5
- Multiple myeloma 203.0
- Ovarian cancer 183.0
- Pancreatic cancer 157.9
- Pleural effusion 197.2
- Prostate cancer 185
- Spinal cord tumor 239.7
- Uterus, cancer of the 179

Defense of homebound status

- Inability to ambulate farther than 10′ (3 m) due to excessive weakness
- Continuous invasive procedure
- Severe pain (specify site)
- Weakness or dizziness
- Severe functional limitations
- Severely restricted mobility due to

- Impending death

Selected nursing diagnoses and patient outcomes

Knowledge deficit related to new diagnosis of cancer or a change in treatment

The patient or caregiver will:
• verbalize comprehension of the disease, potential adverse effects and benefits of treatments, treatment procedure, and goals and plan of care (N)
• describe care measures to manage common adverse effects of the proposed treatment regimen (N, D, PH)
• demonstrate the ability to perform necessary care measures. (N, OT, PT)

Nausea related to the effects of chemotherapy

The patient or caregiver will:
• report decreased nausea (N, D, PH)
• name foods and beverages that don't increase nausea (N, D)
• verbalize correct use of medications to decrease nausea. (N)

Risk for infection related to decreased white blood cell count

The patient or caregiver will:
• list signs and symptoms of infection (N)
• perform excellent personal hygiene (N, HCA)
• take precautions to decrease the chance of injury or infection (for example, avoiding dental work, eliminating uncooked foods, avoiding people who are ill or infected) (N)
• remain free from infection throughout treatment (N)
• demonstrate appropriate sterile (touch-free) technique for care of invasive lines. (N)

Altered nutrition: Less than body requirements related to decreased oral intake secondary to the adverse effects of chemotherapy or radiation therapy

The patient or caregiver will:
• increase oral intake as evidenced by _____ (N, D)
• list foods high in calories and protein that are part of the patient's regular diet (N, D)
• name foods or beverages that increase adverse effects of treatment (N, D)
• demonstrate correct use of nutritional supplements when indicated (N)
• identify caloric intake required and meal plans that meet needs. (N, D)

Body image disturbance related to changes in appearance secondary to adverse effects of chemotherapy or radiation therapy

The patient or caregiver will:
• verbalize knowledge of prosthetic devices and items available (N, PT, SW)
• demonstrate understanding of need for alteration in activities of daily living (N)
• verbalize understanding of change in body image (N)
• demonstrate an understanding and ability to resume care responsibilities (N, OT, PT)
• initiate new or reestablish existing support systems. (N)

Skilled nursing services

Care measures
• Assess the mental and cognitive, integumentary, cardiovascular, GI, genitourinary, and nutrition and hydration systems.

- Assess for pain or weakness
- Assess the patient's ability to perform self-care.
- Assess for signs and symptoms of infection or bleeding.
- Administer prescribed medications.
- Administer or instruct the patient or caregiver to administer pain medications 30 minutes prior to painful procedures.
- Assess bowel function. If constipation occurs, institute measures, such as increasing fluids, fiber, and activity and using stool softeners and laxatives, to return the patient to normal bowel function as quickly as possible.
- Assess the home environment to ensure safety and instruct the patient and caregiver on measures to be taken to prevent injury and infection.
- Assess patient and caregiver knowledge on the disease and treatment regimen.
- Monitor blood counts as ordered.
- Assess patient and caregiver anxiety level, feelings of hopelessness, and fear.
- Encourage the use of support services.

Patient and family teaching

- Instruct on how to monitor for signs and symptoms of infection, when to report them, and the use of standard precautions.
- Instruct in pain management.
- Information on medications, including dosage, adverse effects, interactions, and safe storage
- Explain the disease process and the treatment plan.
- Advise to avoid foods that may increase adverse effects of medications.

Interdisciplinary actions

Dietitian
- Consultation for complete nutritional needs and an individualized plan of care

Home care aide
- Bathing and personal care as well as light housekeeping, laundry, and meal preparation, if necessary

Social worker
- Counseling and referral to community support services for stress management and reduction, financial assistance, and respite services

Discharge plan
- Ability of patient and caregiver to manage the disease process in the home with physician and community support system follow-up services
- Referral to outpatient services or hospice
- Continuation of home care visits for the homebound patient with skilled care needs

Documentation requirements
- Skilled assessment
- Subjective and objective data on the level of pain and resolution of pain (Document using the same criteria on each visit.)
- Subjective and objective data on the signs and symptoms of infection
- Patient's reaction to treatment and the onset of adverse effects as well as methods used to treat or alleviate them
- Results of blood work

- Records of nutrition, hydration, and weekly weight
- Records of all instructions and the reinforcement of previously given instructions
- Patient and caregiver comprehension and response to teaching
- Patient and caregiver participation in care
- Referral to and conferences with support services
- Patient and caregiver progress toward educational goals
- Patient response to care
- Complications due to treatment, which are helpful in demonstrating the need for skilled services (for example, constipation, mouth sores, skin breakdown, nausea, and vomiting)
- Barriers to learning or performance of care (for example, physical, mental, or cognitive impairment or lack of a caregiver)

Reimbursement reminders
- Note that registered dietitian services at home aren't reimbursable under Medicare.

Insurance hints
- Present objective data regarding homebound status.
- Make a list of all objective patient findings and changes since last contact before interaction with case manager.
- Know new laboratory values and any new change in clinical condition.
- Give specifics regarding the patient and caregiver education progress.

Cardiac care

Patients with common degenerative cardiovascular disorders — hypertension, coronary artery disease, myocardial infarction, heart failure, and cardiomyopathy — can receive home care. Other patients eligible for in-home cardiac care include individuals with less common inflammatory cardiac ailments that can cause debilitating damage and those with valvular conditions, which can result in stenosis or insufficiency.

Home care for all these patients includes basic safety information, dietary instruction, and medical regimen instruction. The patient and caregiver must be clear about the components of an individualized action plan for dangerous cardiac signs and symptoms. Dates and times of scheduled visits should be emphasized and left in writing in the home setting.

Previsit checklist

Physician orders and preparation
- Medication orders
- Activity orders and restrictions
- Cardiac diet orders

Equipment and supplies
- Vital signs equipment
- Supplies for standard precautions
- Sharps disposal system

Safety requirements
- Standard precautions for infection control and sharps disposal
- Supervised medication administration
- Safety precautions to prevent falls

• Information on medications, including dosage, adverse effects, interactions, and safe storage

• Knowledge of symptoms that require immediate contact with emergency personnel; knowledge of phone numbers for reaching emergency personnel who are available 24 hours per day, 7 days per week

• System to assist with adherence to complex medication regimen

• Emergency plan and access to functional phone and list of emergency phone numbers

• Identification and correction of environmental hazards and patient-specific concerns

Major diagnostic codes

• Abdominal aortic aneurysm 441.4
• Angina 413.9
• Angina, unstable 411.1
• Angioplasty, coronary/other 36.09/39.50
• Atrial fibrillation/flutter 427.31/427.32
• Cardiac dysrhythmia 427.9
• Chronic obstructive pulmonary disease 496
• Coronary atherosclerosis 414.00
• Heart block 426.9
• Left heart failure/congestive heart failure 428.1/428.0
• Myocardial infarction 410.92
• Obesity/morbid obesity 278.00/278.01
• Peripheral vascular disease 443.9
• Venous thrombosis 453.9

Defense of homebound status

• Bedridden
• Restriction of activity

• Diminished respiratory capacity or severe shortness of breath

• Maximal assistance required for transfer or ambulation

• Angina with activity

• Lower-extremity edema impairing ambulation

Selected nursing diagnoses and patient outcomes

Risk for injury related to difficulty ambulating, shortness of breath, or anginal episodes

The patient or caregiver will:

• remain free from injury (N, OT, PT)
• verbalize the importance of avoiding obstacles, such as climbing stairs, wearing shoes without nonskid soles, and attempting to extricate self from the tub without assistance. (N, OT, PT)

Fatigue related to decreased cardiac output

The patient or caregiver will:

• verbalize the importance of frequent rest periods throughout the day
(N, OT, PT)
• verbalize a decrease in episodes of shortness of breath (N, OT, PT)
• schedule rest periods before meals and morning care (N, OT, PT)
• demonstrate energy conservation techniques. (N, OT, PT)

Knowledge deficit related to modified lifestyle

The patient or caregiver will:

• verbalize the importance of a cardiac diet, a cardiac rehabilitation and exercise program, smoking cessation, and adherence to the medication regimen (N, D, OT, PT)

• verbalize food choices in accordance with the cardiac diet (N, D)
• demonstrate physical activities in accordance with cardiac rehabilitation and exercise program.

(N, OT, PT)

Skilled nursing services

Care measures
• Assess the mental and cognitive, cardiovascular, respiratory, integumentary, and nutrition and hydration systems.
• Assess daily weight and fluid retention.
• Assess throughout episodes of chest pain.

Patient and family teaching
• Provide home safety information.
• Teach energy conservation techniques.
• Explain oxygen precautions for safe home use.
• Instruct in the medication regimen, adverse effects, and interactions.
• Teach specifics of the cardiac diet.
• Demonstrate the procedure for applying antiembolic stockings.
• Discuss signs and symptoms to report to the physician.
• Discuss signs and symptoms that necessitate consultation with emergency medical personnel.

Interdisciplinary actions

Dietitian
• Development of an individualized cardiac diet
• Nutritional assessment

Occupational therapist
• Energy-conservation techniques, when applicable

Physical therapist
• Referral as part of cardiac rehabilitation program

Social worker
• Referral to educational and support groups

Discharge plan
• Management of cardiac care in the home with physician and community support system follow-up services
• Referral to outpatient services
• Continuation of home care visits for homebound patient with skilled care needs

Documentation requirements
• Variances to expected outcomes
• Specific care rendered and instruction provided
• Progress toward goals
• Abnormal laboratory values
• Medication changes
• Barriers to learning

Reimbursement reminders
• Ensure that coordination occurs among team members based on the plan of care.
• Document if an ordered service must be placed on hold temporarily due to patient illness and obtain a physician's order to reflect this; otherwise, it may appear that the ordered discipline isn't making scheduled visits.

Insurance hints
* Present objective patient findings and report new changes.
* Report mental status changes.
* Provide updates regarding the patient's continued homebound status.

Cardiomyopathy

Cardiomyopathy refers to a group of diseases characterized by the destruction of heart tissue, particularly the myocardium. Although the specific cause is unclear, conditions commonly associated with cardiomyopathy include diabetes, hypertension, alcohol abuse, and thyroid disease. Among the most frequently affected population are black males ages 40 to 60.

Cardiomyopathy results in ineffective pumping of the heart, which commonly leads to fluid backup and symptoms of heart failure. Nursing care focuses on relieving symptoms and teaching the patient about living with the condition.

Previsit checklist

Physician orders and preparation
* Oral medications as indicated
* Activity orders and restrictions
* Dietary restrictions (for a cardiac diet)

Equipment and supplies
* Vital signs equipment
* Medication information

Safety requirements
* Standard precautions for infection control
* Information on medications, including dosage, adverse effects, interactions, and safe storage
* Disposal of I.V. and I.M. administration supplies and sharps
* Medical identification bracelet
* Restriction of activities
* System to assist with adherence to complex medication regimen
* Emergency plan and access to functional phone and list of emergency phone numbers
* Identification and correction of environmental hazards and patient-specific concerns

Major diagnostic codes
* Angina 413.9
* Cardiomyopathy:
  – alcoholic 425.5
  – congestive, constrictive, familial 425.4
  – hypertrophic, obstructive 425.1

Defense of homebound status
* Bedridden
* Poor or limited energy and endurance
* Dyspnea on exertion
* Cardiac restrictions on activity
* Severe functional limitations
* Lower-extremity edema that impairs ambulation

Selected nursing diagnoses and patient outcomes

Decreased cardiac output related to mechanical heart problems
The patient or caregiver will:
• comply with the medication regimen (as demonstrated by maintenance of normal pulse and blood pressure)
(N, PH)
• be free from dizziness and chest pain
(N, PH)
• demonstrate clear breath sounds upon auscultation (N)
• report stable weight. (N)

Knowledge deficit related to the disease process and the effect on the patient's lifestyle
The patient or caregiver will:
• state the importance of adhering to the treatment regimen, including dietary restrictions, activity restrictions, and the medication regimen
(N, D, PH, OT, PT)
• state importance of resting before mealtimes and activities of daily living
(N, OT)
• demonstrate improved tolerance of physical activity without fatigue, weakness, or chest discomfort.
(N, OT, PT)

Skilled nursing services

Care measures
• Assess the mental and cognitive, cardiopulmonary, and nutrition and hydration systems.
• Assess the level of care of the patient or caregiver.
• Assess the effectiveness of the treatment regimen, including vital signs and breath sounds; check the apical pulse for irregularities; and assess for anginal symptoms, dyspnea, and the stability of weight and fluid overload.
• Evaluate the patient's compliance with the activity restrictions, the medication regimen, and dietary restrictions.

Patient and family teaching
• Stress the need for activity restriction.
• Teach how to measure a pulse rate and assess blood pressure.
• Instruct about medications, including actions, interactions, and therapeutic and adverse effects.
• Review foods found on a cardiac diet.
• Instruct in signs and symptoms to report to the physician.
• Instruct in signs and symptoms which necessitate contacting emergency medical personnel.

Interdisciplinary actions

Dietitian
• Comprehensive nutritional assessment and design of an individualized cardiac diet

Discharge plan
• Management of cardiomyopathy in the home with physician and community support system follow-up services
• Referral to outpatient services
• Continuation of home care visits for the homebound patient with skilled care needs

Documentation requirements

- Skilled assessment, including subjective and objective data related to signs and symptoms of decreased cardiac output
- Variances to expected outcomes
- Specific care provided, particularly teaching instructions
- Changes in the plan of care
- Barriers to learning
- Measurable progress toward goals
- Abnormal laboratory values
- Medication changes
- Changes in vital signs and action taken
- Episodes of distress and interventions utilized to alleviate distress

Reimbursement reminders

- Be sure to follow up on changes in the patient's condition, communicating status and changes in the plan of care to healthcare team members.

Insurance hints

- Present objective patient findings and new changes.
- List direct interventions.
- Provide measurable changes and information that communicate the status of the patient and the need for skilled home care services.

Cast care

Casts are used to promote the healing of fractures or connective tissue by immobilizing the broken bone or soft tissue to prevent further injury. They also allow fractures to maintain normal bone alignment during healing. Casts are made from various materials, most commonly fiberglass.

Because a cast alters the patient's ability to ambulate, the nurse must clearly document the patient's functional limitations. The presence of a cast isn't sufficient to justify that the patient is homebound, and skilled services will be of short duration unless the patient has other functional limitations. To be independent, the patient must be able to ambulate 30′ (9 m) and ascend and descend a flight of stairs (about 13 steps) without sitting.

The focus of home care for this patient is safety and education. In some cases, the patient may need rehabilitation services only.

Previsit checklist

Physician orders and preparation

- Rehabilitation team notes
- Activity orders and restrictions
- Orders for any additional needs such as wound or pin care supplies

Equipment and supplies

- Wound or pin care supplies, if necessary

Safety requirements

- Clear walkways
- Plastic trash bags or commercial products to keep the cast dry (for when it is exposed to moisture)
- System to assist with adherence to complex medication regimen
- Information on medications, including dosage, adverse effects, interactions, and safe storage

- Emergency plan and access to functional phone and list of emergency phone numbers
- Identification and correction of environmental hazards and patient-specific concerns

Major diagnostic codes

- Ankle fracture, closed/open 824.8/ 824.9
- Arm fracture, closed/open 818.0/ 818.1
- Femur fracture 821.0
- Forearm fracture, closed/open 813.20/813.30
- Multiple fractures, closed/open 829.0/ 829.1
- Tibia or fibula fracture 823.8

Defense of homebound status

- Activity intolerance — inability to ambulate farther than 10' (3 m) at one time
- Fatigue — inability to ambulate farther than 10' without an increase in symptoms of pain or shortness of breath
- Imposed activity restriction by physician _____

Selected nursing diagnoses and patient outcomes

Knowledge deficit related to care of cast
The patient or caregiver will:
- verbalize knowledge of cast care (N)
- demonstrate proper cast cleaning technique (N)
- verbalize complications to report to the physician. (N)

Risk for peripheral neurovascular dysfunction
The patient or caregiver will:
- verbalize signs and symptoms of neuromuscular dysfunction to report to the physician (N, PT)
- verbalize or demonstrate methods to decrease swelling of the affected extremity (N, PT)
- remain free from nerve injury (N)
- demonstrate the appropriate use of assistive devices (N, PT)
- demonstrate proper massage technique distal to the cast. (N, PT)

Risk for impaired skin integrity related to pressure from the cast or surgical incision
The patient or caregiver will:
- verbalize how to detect signs and symptoms of an infection or drainage beneath the cast (N)
- demonstrate proper skin care (N)
- describe skin care after cast removal. (N)

Impaired skin integrity related to surgical incision
The patient or caregiver will:
- verbalize signs and symptoms of infection to report to the physician (N)
- verbalize an understanding of proper nutrition, which will aid in wound healing. (N, D)

Altered health maintenance related to cast care and personal cleanliness
The patient or caregiver will:
- demonstrate proper use of crutches (N, PT)
- be free from body odor (N, HCA)
- explain and use methods to bathe without affecting the cast (N, PT)
- be free from injury. (N, PT)

Pain related to fracture, surgery, or trauma to soft tissue

The patient or caregiver will:

• verbalize proper use of analgesia and rate pain at 3 or less on a 0-to-10 scale 80% of the time   (N, PH)

• demonstrate optimal movement related to proper pain control   (N)

• report satisfaction with sleep pattern.   (N)

Impaired physical mobility related to immobilization of the extremity or pain

The patient or caregiver will:

• remain free from muscle spasms and contractions   (N, PT)

• perform at the expected level of independent care   (N, PT, OT)

• demonstrate proper use of adaptive devices, such as crutches, a wheelchair, a cane, a walker, and a trapeze
                                                 (N, PT)

• maintain functional mobility and range of motion in the affected limb
                                                 (N, PT)

• complete a home exercise program
                                                 (N, PT)

• express satisfaction with mobility.
                                                 (N, PT)

Risk for injury related to an unsteady gait caused by the cast

The patient or caregiver will:

• remain free from injury   (N, PT)

• verbalize knowledge of a home safety plan to prevent falls   (N, PT)

• rearrange the home to accommodate adaptive equipment such as a wheelchair.   (N, PT)

Skilled nursing services

Care measures

• Complete initial evaluation and identify comorbidities (for example, dementia, advanced age, neurologic dysfunction, and heart and lung disease) that decrease the patient's ability to learn and perform self-care.

• Assess for complications of treatment, including neurovascular compromise, constipation, pain, and debilitation.

• Assess the mental and cognitive, musculoskeletal, cardiopulmonary, and integumentary systems at each visit.

• Weigh the patient at each visit.

Patient and family teaching

• Provide education regarding injury prevention.

• Instruct in wound and incision care.

Interdisciplinary actions

Home care aide

• Hygiene

Occupational therapist

• Assistance with management of activities of daily living

• Energy conservation

Physical therapist

• Home exercise program

• Safety planning

Social worker

• Assistance in obtaining community resources such as transportation and home support services

Discharge plan
- Patient return to normal routine following cast removal
- Referral to outpatient services

Documentation requirements
- Description of functional losses or gains in clear terms, such as distance walked with and without crutches and self-care ability, including dressing, feeding, bathing, toileting, and grooming
- Effectiveness of pain control regimen
- Stages of healing wounds or incisions in centimeters
- Description of plan to improve patient function if progress stalls

Reimbursement reminders
- Remember that the presence of a cast, even a long leg cast, doesn't make a patient homebound; be clear about functional limitations and the patient's ability to use adaptive equipment; note especially upper-body strength that is needed to use equipment such as crutches.
- If rehabilitation services are required, they should be used only for a brief time and focus on patient and caregiver education that is needed to develop a home exercise and safety program.
- A brief course of physical therapy after the cast is removed is indicated for many patients.
- Request occupational therapy if the patient needs energy conservation or assistance with self-care for an upper-extremity fracture.

Insurance hints
- Describe progressive levels of self-care, including dressing, feeding, bathing, toileting, grooming, and using adaptive equipment.
- Describe progress toward rehabilitation goals, such as safe transfers from bed to chair, sitting to standing, and wheelchair to car as well as bathroom transfers.
- List the collaborative plan of care for all team members providing services.
- Compare and contrast the roles of each rehabilitation team member.
- Describe care that will be needed after cast removal.
- Describe the cast treatment plan from the physician. (The patient may need a series of casts before recovery.)
- Describe other conditions, such as chronic lung disease, and how they affect the patient's use of assistive devices.

Cellulitis

Cellulitis is an inflammation that spreads into tissues of an affected area. It commonly affects elderly homebound patients and may accompany diabetes, osteomyelitis, and peripheral vascular disease. Cellulitis is often initiated by a puncture wound and spreads to the surrounding tissues, which become painful and exhibit warmth and erythema. The condition must be treated immediately after the first possible symptom to prevent the infection from developing into gangrene or sepsis in immunocompromised patients.

Previsit checklist

Physician orders and preparation
- Wound care orders
- Diet orders
- Medications such as antibiotics
- Laboratory tests and wound cultures
- Activity restrictions
- Social work services consultation
- Medication orders

Equipment and supplies
- Vital signs equipment, including thermometer
- Wound care supplies (vary depending on the location of the wound and the physician's preferred regimen)
- Culturette swabs for obtaining culture and sensitivity of wound
- Supplies for obtaining blood specimens for laboratory tests, including syringes, Vacutainers, alcohol wipes, and a tourniquet
- Supplies for initiating home antibiotic therapy
- I.V. bag of antibiotic per physician's orders
- I.V. tubing
- I.V. start kit
- Angiocaths
- Supplies for standard precautions and sharps disposal, including container

Safety requirements
- Standard precautions for infection control, sharps disposal, and I.V. solution disposal
- Observance for symptoms of allergic reaction to antibiotics
- Observance for adverse effects from administration of multiple medications

- Sterile technique in performing wound care
- Standard precautions in drawing blood and collecting wound specimens
- System to assist with adherence to complex medication regimen
- Information on medications, including dosage, adverse effects, interactions, and safe storage
- Emergency plan and access to functional phone and list of emergency phone numbers
- Identification and correction of environmental hazards and patient-specific concerns

Major diagnostic codes
- Arterial graft, recent 39.58
- Cellulitis, general (refer to exact location of the infection for specific code) 682.9
- Cellulitis of the arm 682.3
- Cellulitis of the leg/foot 682.6/682.7
- Cellulitis of the trunk 682.2
- Decubitus ulcer 707.0
- Diabetes mellitus, with complications 250.90
- Femoral-popliteal bypass 39.29
- Osteomyelitis, acute/chronic 730.0/730.1
- Skin graft 86.60
- Staph infection 041.1
- Vascular insufficiency 459.81

Defense of homebound status
- Difficulty ambulating related to infection of the lower extremity
- Maximum assistance required to ambulate or transfer
- Weakness and decreased weight-bearing ability
- Bedridden

- Open, infected wound
- Confined to home due to I.V. antibiotic therapy

Selected nursing diagnoses and patient outcomes

Pain related to inflamed extremity
The patient or caregiver will:
- verbalize an acceptable level of pain relief (N)
- demonstrate compliance with the medication regimen (N, PH)
- state the importance of adhering to the treatment regimen to prevent systemic spread of infection. (N)

Impaired skin integrity related to infection
The patient or caregiver will:
- demonstrate signs and symptoms of healing of the localized infection (ET, N)
- demonstrate an increased ability to perform care (N, PT)
- consume at least 1,800 calories per day for adequate wound healing (D)
- describe three ways to prevent injury to the extremities and the recurrence of infection (N)
- list three signs and symptoms of localized infection and indicate when to contact medical personnel (N)
- verbally contract to participate in an individualized exercise program designed to prevent loss of function and increase circulation to the affected limb to promote wound healing. (N, PT)

Skilled nursing services

Care measures
- Assess the mental and cognitive, nutrition and hydration, integumentary (particularly extremities), cardiovascular, and neurologic systems.
- Assess the level of comprehension of the patient or caregiver regarding the importance of maintaining an adequate nutritional status and activity level (as tolerated).
- Assess the level of comprehension of the patient or caregiver regarding the possibility of performing dressing changes after the certification period ends.
- Assess the effectiveness of the treatment regimen by monitoring wound healing. Document and photograph the wound periodically. Document the size, color, temperature, and exudate of the wound and assess for signs and symptoms of nutritional depletion.
- Treat the wound according to the physician's orders.
- Obtain laboratory tests and wound cultures as ordered.

Patient and family teaching
- Review dietary instructions to promote nutritional adequacy.
- Emphasize the need to protect the affected limb.
- Explain the medication regimen, stressing the importance of compliance.
- Describe possible adverse reactions.
- Instruct in the use of standard precautions.
- Explain the potential for disease transmission.

- Emphasize the expected level of physical activity to promote full range-of-motion (ROM).

Interdisciplinary actions

Dietitian
- Maintenance of adequate nutritional status to promote wound healing

Enterostomal nurse
- Recommendations for individualized wound care regimen

Physical therapist
- Development of an individualized exercise program to prevent loss of function to affected limb and increase circulation to the wound area

Social worker
- Information on assistance with meals (Meals On Wheels) and contact with appropriate suppliers of dressing supplies and I.V. antibiotics

Discharge plan
- Management of wound-care regimen in the home with physician and community support system follow-up services
- Referral to outpatient services
- Continuation of home care visits for homebound patient with skilled care needs

Documentation requirements
- Vital sign measurements
- Condition of wound site (current photograph of wound, size in centimeters, color, temperature, exudate, and culture results)
- Treatment in exact detail
- Patient's response to treatment and plan of care
- Results of laboratory testing
- Findings from nutritional assessment
- Findings from physical therapy evaluation
- Patient and caregiver participation in care, including maintenance of nutritional status, participation in the physical therapy program, willingness to perform dressing changes, and willingness to learn to initiate I.V. therapy
- Care coordination between disciplines
- Verbal and written instructions, return demonstrations, verbalization of learning, and resistance to learning
- Patient and caregiver progress toward educational goals

Reimbursement reminders
- All nonroutine supplies must be specifically ordered by the physician and entered into Locator 14 (supplies) of the Health Care Financing Administration Form 485 or ordered by the physician within the specific order for treatment of a surgical wound requiring the use of certain supplies and entered into Locator 21 (Orders for Treatment).
- Ensure that the wound care provided exactly matches the orders from the physician for enterostomal therapy to ensure reimbursement from Medicare.
- Sometimes, physical therapy services aren't authorized. In those cases, the nurse must also bear responsibility for teaching ROM exercises.

• Note that registered dietitian services at home aren't reimbursable under Medicare.

• Note that registered physical therapist services at home are reimbursable under Medicare; for services to be reimbursable under Blue Cross/Blue Shield, a registered physical therapist (not a licensed physical therapy assistant) must follow the patient throughout the course of therapy.

• Note the following information when billing for medical supplies: name of supply item, date supply was used, number of units used, and charge per unit.

• Record the treatment that required the supplies in the clinical notes.

• Note that supplies that are billed but not documented will be denied.

• Indicate in goals when daily visits are expected to end, if daily care has been ordered.

Insurance hints

• Present objective data about homebound status.

• Present objective patient findings and changes since last contact.

• Report new laboratory values and any changes in clinical condition.

Cerebrovascular accident

A cerebrovascular accident (CVA), or stroke, occurs when blood flow to the cerebral tissues is interrupted, either by a clot or by hemorrhage. Lack of oxygen produces tissue death or injury in the region of the brain affected by the CVA, ultimately resulting in neurologic deficits that may improve with re-

habilitation. Predisposing factors for CVA include hypertension, carotid artery disease, diabetes mellitus, and smoking. Home care for the patient and family focuses on maximizing physical functioning to achieve the highest level of independence possible. This can be accomplished through an intensive multidisciplinary approach.

Previsit checklist

Physician orders and preparation

• Medication orders
• Bladder and bowel regimen
• Physical, speech, and occupational therapy
• Specialty bed, wheelchair, and other assistive devices
• Activity orders and restrictions
• Nutritional supplementation and dietary orders

Equipment and supplies

• Vital signs equipment
• Intermittent urinary catheter kit, if applicable
• Gastrostomy feeding tube care supplies and durable medical equipment, if applicable
• Suctioning kits (nasotracheal and oropharyngeal)
• Extremity supports to keep limbs in normal anatomic alignment

Safety requirements

• Standard precautions for infection control and sharps disposal
• Home assessment for placement of grab bars and supportive devices in the bathroom as well as removal of obstacles and hazards to aid patient mobility

- Aspiration precautions
- Safe use of suctioning equipment
- Avoidance of extremes in temperature on the skin
- Functioning communication and emergency device (bell, home intercom system, 911 speed dial on telephone)
- Emergency plan and access to functional phone and list of emergency phone numbers
- System to assist with adherence to complex medication regimen
- Information on medications, including dosage, adverse effects, interactions, and safe storage
- Identification and correction of environmental hazards and patient-specific concerns
- Safe disposal of incontinence pads

Major diagnostic codes

- Apraxia 438.81
- Artery, basilar/carotid/vertebral/multiple and bilateral 433.0/433.1/433.2/433.3
- Cerebral artery occlusion, unspecified 434.9
- Cerebral atherosclerosis 437.0
- Cerebral embolism 434.1
- Cerebral thrombosis 434.0
- CVA 436
- CVA with cognitive deficits 438.0
- CVA with speech and language deficits 438.10
- Hemiplegia affecting unspecified side 438.20
- Incontinence of feces 787.6
- Incontinence of urine 788.30
- Incontinence without sensory awareness 788.34
- Intracerebral hemorrhage 431
- Monoplegia of lower limb 438.40
- Monoplegia of upper limb 438.30

- Occlusion and stenosis of precerebral arteries 433
- Retention of urine 788.20
- Subarachnoid hemorrhage 430
- Subdural hemorrhage 432.1
- Transient cerebral ischemia 435
- Unspecified intracranial hemorrhage 432.9

Defense of homebound status

- Status recent CVA with paralysis
- Right or left hemiplegia or hemiparesis
- Quadriplegia
- Assistance needed for all activities
- Maximum assistance required to ambulate
- Inability to ambulate
- Wheelchair-dependent
- Possible inability to maintain airway with food and fluid due to dysphagia
- Inability to verbally communicate needs
- Questionable cognitive status due to interruption in blood flow to cerebral tissues

Selected nursing diagnoses and patient outcomes

Altered cerebral tissue perfusion
   The patient or caregiver will:
- recognize that changes in cognitive functioning are a result of the CVA
                                        (N)
- verbalize action plan to recognize change in mental status, including restlessness, drowsiness, lethargy, inability to follow commands or to do a previous activity, or unresponsiveness (N)

• contact the physician for changes including increased weakness or paralysis, choking, or respiratory distress (N)

• recognize abnormal body posturing or movements indicating seizure activity due to cerebral hypoxia. (N)

Impaired physical mobility

The patient or caregiver will:

• recognize ways to maintain and improve functional abilities (N, OT, PT)

• demonstrate how to place the body in normal anatomic alignment (N, OT, PT)

• demonstrate passive range-of-motion (ROM) exercises to the affected side, supporting major joints and soft tissue (N, PT)

• demonstrate active ROM exercises to the unaffected side (N, PT)

• demonstrate the correct method to turn and reposition the patient every 2 hours and support the body in normal anatomic alignment (N, PT)

• recognize ways to reduce lower-extremity edema with the use of splints and pillows (N, PT)

• demonstrate how to assess for thrombophlebitis of the lower extremities to include calf measurement and assessing for Homans' sign (N, PT)

• demonstrate position changes from bed to chair, chair to chair, chair to standing, and bed to standing using correct body mechanics while supporting weak, uncontrollable limbs. (N, OT, PT)

Self-care deficit related to bathing, grooming, toileting, and eating

The patient or caregiver will:

• recognize and demonstrate ways to use the unaffected side to perform care activities (N, OT, PT)

• demonstrate first dressing the affected extremities and then dressing the unaffected extremities to maximize dressing with minimal assistance (N, OT, PT)

• demonstrate use of assistive devices to maximize independence with toileting, grooming, and meals. (N, OT, PT)

Impaired verbal communication

The patient or caregiver will:

• recognize that impaired verbal communication doesn't reduce thinking or comprehension in the individual who had a stroke (N, SP)

• recognize the cause of speech impairment and utilize techniques obtained by speech therapy to maximize speech recovery (SP)

• recognize that speech impairment doesn't mean the patient can't hear (N, SP)

• demonstrate waiting an adequate time for a response from the patient when communicating (N, SP)

• demonstrate facing the patient when communicating and speaking slowly (N, SP)

• demonstrate use of short, simple statements and questions to permit the processing of information (N, SP)

• recognize frustration and anger as a normal response to the loss of functioning (N, SP)

• determine alternative methods to enhance communication, including writing tablets, flash cards, and computerized talking boards. (N, SP)

Sensory or perceptual alterations

The patient or caregiver will:

• keep a neat, well-lit, uncluttered home environment to reduce the chance of injury (N, HCA)

• demonstrate teaching of complex activities as a series of small steps, each to be achieved to complete the one activity (N, OT)

• demonstrate placing care items within the patient's field of vision or on the unaffected side to promote independence (N, OT, PT)

• demonstrate scanning the environment by head movements or eye movements to reduce the chance of injury and facilitate mobility. (N, OT)

Altered urinary elimination related to neurogenic bladder

The patient or caregiver will:

• recognize the pattern for urinary frequency or incontinence (N)

• demonstrate a bladder retraining program. (N)

Impaired swallowing

The patient or caregiver will:

• recognize that dysphagia can lead to choking, drooling, aspiration, or regurgitation (N, SP)

• demonstrate proper physical alignment while eating and drinking, including sitting upright, minimizing distractions, keeping the neck slightly flexed, eating pureed or soft foods, and swallowing food one bite at a time (N, SP)

• demonstrate how to inspect the mouth for food "pocketing" (N, SP)

• demonstrate correct use of an oropharyngeal suction apparatus to prevent aspiration. (N, SP)

Ineffective airway clearance

The patient or caregiver will:

• demonstrate use of the home oropharyngeal suction machine (N)

• recognize signs of a blocked airway. (N)

Impaired skin integrity

The patient or caregiver will:

• recognize normal skin integrity and ways to prevent skin breakdown (N)

• demonstrate proper body alignment and use of splints to support limbs and prevent skin breakdown (N, OT, PT)

• determine a turning and repositioning schedule to reduce skin breakdown. (N, PT)

Altered thought processes

The patient or caregiver will:

• recognize impulsive behavior as being a part of the CVA (N)

• demonstrate reorienting the patient to person, time, and place. (N)

Risk for injury

The patient or caregiver will:

• recognize hazards in the home that might cause injuries (N)

• demonstrate head scanning to view the environment before ambulating (N, PT)

• demonstrate use of assistive devices to promote independence with ambulation. (N, OT, PT)

Ineffective individual coping

The patient or caregiver will:

• recognize how the sudden change in physical status and independence affects feelings of self-worth (N)

• demonstrate supportive behavior while the patient exhibits frustration or anxiety. (N)

Social isolation

The caregiver will:

• recognize that the patient's inability to communicate at the previous level of functioning leads to feeling "left out" of conversations and communication (N)

• encourage the patient to participate in family and group communication activities with the use of communication devices. (N, OT)

Powerlessness

The patient or caregiver will:

• recognize how the change in physical status and functioning hinders the patient's ability to be independent, which can affect income and feeling like a functioning member of society (N)

• demonstrate supportive, encouraging behavior to assist the patient with finding a new role within the home and family unit. (N)

Skilled nursing services

Care measures

• Assess the heart rate, skin integrity, swallowing function, bowel and bladder continence, and speech and motor function, including balance.

• Maintain blood pressure control.

• Assess nutritional status.

• Provide dietary instruction and offer the use of supplemental feedings, if indicated.

• Assess medication compliance and need as well as knowledge of medications, including common adverse effects.

Patient and family teaching

• Teach safety.

• Instruct in activity limitations and the exercise regimen.

• Introduce bowel and bladder retraining programs.

• Teach the causes, complications, and prevention of a CVA.

• Teach how to evaluate the social and emotional functioning of the patient and caregiver, including recognizing depression.

• Present options for reintegration into the community after rehabilitation.

• Teach nasotracheal and oropharyngeal suctioning.

• Instruct in enteral feedings, if applicable.

• Teach gastrostomy tube care, if applicable.

• Teach proper application of splints.

• Teach skin care.

• Instruct in repositioning and turning.

Interdisciplinary actions

Home care aide

• Assessment of caregiver's ability to provide patient care

• Encouragement of patient and caregiver to provide care

• Reduction of frequency of home care aide interventions as the patient and caregiver gain confidence in providing care

• Assistance with activities of daily living (ADLs)

Occupational therapist

• Assessment of ADLs

• Provision of adaptive devices as indicated

• Provision of therapies addressing fine motor skills

• Energy-conservation techniques

Physical therapist
- Initiation of rehabilitation program, including transferring, standing, and walking
- Assessment of equipment needs, functional features, and safety factors at home
- Continuation of rehabilitation program as prescribed

Social worker
- Assessment of the need for community resources
- Provision of emotional support and counseling

Speech pathologist
- Assessment of swallowing ability
- Provision of therapy according to speech deficit
- Instruction of caregiver on speech therapy techniques

Discharge plan
- Patient will safely function at all levels to the best of his ability after CVA
- Patient and caregiver will be able to manage physical deficits related to CVA in the home with physician and community support system follow-up services
- Referral to outpatient services
- Continuation of home care visits for homebound patient with skilled care needs

Documentation requirements
- Assessment, including subjective and objective data with regards to physical alterations related to CVA
- Patient and caregiver response to instruction

- Observation of patient's and caregiver's ability to perform oropharyngeal suctioning and gastrostomy tube feedings (if applicable), use assistive devices, and maintain normal anatomic alignment, reposition, and transfer
- Changes in integumentary, respiratory, GI, genitourinary, or neurologic functioning
- Ability of caregiver to care for the patient

Reimbursement reminders
- Schedule the date of the onset of services for shortly after the CVA. If the CVA occurred months before home care services, additional documentation for justification of need will be necessary.
- Focus rehabilitation efforts on restoring function and a home exercise regimen for maintenance of function.
- Ensure coordination among health care team members and communicate changes in the plan of care to all members.

Insurance hints
- Provide a review of hospitalization, as necessary, and the current condition of the patient, the home environment, and availability of the caregiver.
- Provide an objective review of current status, including physical abilities, ambulation, and use or need for assistive devices.
- Provide thorough skin assessment and report objective findings. In the event of open or reddened areas, provide accurate wound dimensions, prescribed dressing, and capabilities of caregiver to perform wound care.
- Provide current laboratory values.
- Provide an objective evaluation of the respiratory and nutritional status.

If the patient is receiving gastrostomy tube feedings, provide information on the patient's tolerance of feedings, the patency of the gastrostomy tube, and the condition of the skin surrounding the tube. If the patient can be supported by oral nutrition, objectively evaluate the patient and caregiver's ability to maintain a patent airway.

• Provide an objective review of the communication pattern, cognitive level, and ability to comprehend instructions.

Chest physiotherapy

Chest physiotherapy is beneficial in respiratory conditions characterized by excessive accumulation of secretions in the lungs. Chest physiotherapy techniques aid in the removal of secretions from the airways, help prevent or treat atelectasis, and may help prevent pneumonia. Included in chest physiotherapy are chest assessment, effective breathing and coughing exercises, postural drainage, percussion, and vibration. Nurses, physical therapists, and respiratory therapists may perform chest physiotherapy. Patients and caregivers may also be taught to perform these techniques.

Previsit checklist

Physician orders and preparation
• Care and teaching orders for each discipline
• Oral medication orders as indicated
• Aerosol therapy as indicated
• Chest physiotherapy orders
• Activity orders and restrictions

Equipment and supplies
• Vital signs equipment
• Supplies for standard precautions and proper sharps disposal
• Tilt board, adjustable bed, bed blocks, and pillows to increase postural drainage
• Metered-dose inhaler as indicated
• Nebulizer with prescribed medication as indicated
• Oxygen as indicated

Safety requirements
• Standard precautions for infection control and sharps disposal
• Oxygen precautions as necessary
• Equipment storage instructions
• Disposal of expired medication
• Information on medications, including dosage, adverse effects, interactions, and safe storage
• Instruction regarding signs and symptoms of medical emergency and actions to take
• System to assist with adherence to complex medication regimen
• Emergency plan and access to functional phone and list of emergency phone numbers
• Identification and correction of environmental hazards and patient-specific concerns

Major diagnostic codes
• Acute bronchitis 466.0
• Asthma 493.9
• Cancer of the larynx 161.9
• Cancer of the trachea 162.0
• Chest physiotherapy 93.99
• Chronic obstructive pulmonary disease 496
• Nebulizer therapy 93.94

- Pneumonia 486
- Tracheostomy, mediastinal/other 31.2/31.29

Defense of homebound status

- Inability to ambulate farther than 10′ (3 m) due to dyspnea with minimal exertion
- Inability to ambulate farther than 10′ due to fatigue and poor endurance related to severe, uncontrolled respiratory disorder
- Inability to negotiate stairs due to profound shortness of breath
- Maximum assistance required for transfers

Selected nursing diagnoses and patient outcomes

Ineffective breathing pattern
The patient or caregiver will:
- demonstrate an effective respiratory rate and experience improved gas exchange in the lungs (N, PT, RT)
- verbalize the causative factors, if known, and relate adaptive ways of coping with them. (N, PT, OT, PH, SW)

Ineffective airway clearance related to bronchospasm and increased pulmonary secretions
The patient or caregiver will:
- demonstrate effective coughing and increased air exchange in the lungs. (N, PT, RT)

Activity intolerance related to shortness of breath
The patient or caregiver will:
- identify factors that reduce activity tolerance (N, PT, RT)
- exhibit a decrease in hypoxic signs with increased activity (elevated pulse, blood pressure, respirations) (N, OT, PT, RT)
- progress to the highest level of mobility possible. (N, PT, OT)

Knowledge deficit related to chest physiotherapy
The patient or caregiver will:
- verbalize and demonstrate an understanding of and compliance with chest physiotherapy techniques and when to perform them. (N, PT, RT)

Skilled nursing services

Care measures
- Assess the respiratory system, including breath sounds, oxygenation status, breathing patterns, and activity intolerance.
- Obtain a patient history relevant to the respiratory and oxygenation status.
- Assess the cardiovascular, mental and cognitive, and nutrition and hydration systems.
- Assess the level of care and compliance of the patient or caregiver with use of the metered-dose inhaler or nebulizer (if applicable).
- Assess the level of care and compliance of the patient or caregiver with chest physiotherapy techniques.

Patient and family teaching
- Review the respiratory disease process.

- Instruct in the oral and aerosol medication regimen, including dosage, frequency, purpose, potential adverse effects, and interactions.
- Demonstrate chest physiotherapy techniques, including breathing exercises; controlled, effective coughing; and percussion, vibration, and postural drainage.
- Teach when to perform chest physiotherapy.
- Instruct in signs and symptoms of respiratory complications.
- Encourage high fluid intake (2 to 2.5 L of fluid daily unless contraindicated) to keep secretions liquid.
- Instruct the patient or caregiver to consult with the physician about receiving an influenza vaccine (annually) and a pneumonia vaccine (one-time dose).

Interdisciplinary actions

Home care aide
- Assistance with personal care and hygiene needs

Occupational therapist
- Instruction in energy-conservation techniques
- Training in activities of daily living
- Assessment of the need for and instruct in use of adaptive equipment

Physical therapist
- Development and teaching of an individualized home exercise program
- Performance and instruction in pulmonary physical therapy, including breathing exercises and chest physiotherapy, as indicated

Social worker
- Referral to community resources and support groups, such as counseling for stress management and reduction

Discharge plan
- Management of chest physiotherapy in the home by the patient or caregiver with physician follow-up services
- Continuation of home care visits for the homebound patient with skilled care needs

Documentation requirements
- Subjective and objective data related to assessment of the respiratory and other systems
- Skilled procedures performed, such as nebulizer treatment and chest physiotherapy
- Understanding of and compliance with the chest physiotherapy regimen
- Understanding of and compliance with the medication regimen
- Patient response to care
- Variances to expected outcomes
- Specific barriers to learning (for example, impaired vision and mental status and cognitive ability)
- Availability of willing and able caregiver
- Patient's previous experience with medications, aerosol therapy, or chest physiotherapy
- Specific deficits in initial knowledge level, then progress toward goals as evidenced by specific concepts and procedures that are verbalized or demonstrated

Reimbursement reminders

- Indicate the expected end point of daily visits (when daily visits have been ordered).
- Obtain a physician's order for any plan of care change and document it in the patient's record.
- Determine which supplies and durable medical equipment are covered by Medicare.
- Note that the physician must indicate that a metered-dose inhaler alone is insufficient in treating the patient's respiratory disorder to ensure Medicare coverage of the nebulizer machine. (Medicare part B covers 80% of the allowable durable medical equipment charge; the patient or a secondary provider is responsible for the remaining 20%.)
- Note that the patient's oxygen saturation level must be 88% or less to ensure Medicare coverage of oxygen. (This must be reevaluated every 3 weeks.)
- Note that respiratory therapist services are usually provided by the company supplying the durable medical equipment on a routine or as-needed basis.

Insurance hints

- Present objective data about the patient's homebound status.
- Present objective patient findings, changes in clinical condition, and new changes in care (for example, new physician's orders).
- Present specifics about the patient and caregiver education process.
- Present progress toward established goals.

Chronic obstructive pulmonary disease

Chronic obstructive pulmonary disease (COPD) refers to a group of respiratory conditions characterized by persistent, progressive airflow obstruction and dyspnea. Included within the classification of COPD are chronic bronchitis, asthma, and emphysema.

Causative factors for COPD include cigarette smoking, pollution, occupational exposure, allergy, autoimmunity, and respiratory infection. The goals of COPD management are to maximize airflow, prevent and manage complications (such as infection and hypoxemia), and improve the quality of life.

Previsit checklist

Physician orders and preparation

- Care and teaching orders for each discipline
- Oral medication as indicated
- Aerosol therapy as indicated
- Chest physiotherapy as indicated
- Oxygen instructions as indicated
- Activity orders and restrictions

Equipment and supplies

- Vital signs equipment
- Supplies for standard precautions
- Metered-dose inhaler as indicated
- Nebulizer with prescribed medication as indicated
- Oxygen as indicated

Safety requirements

- Standard precautions for infection control and sharps disposal
- Oxygen precautions, if indicated
- Equipment storage instructions
- Disposal of expired medication
- Instruction regarding signs and symptoms of a medical emergency and actions to take
- System to assist with adherence to complex medication regimen
- Information on medications, including dosage, adverse effects, interactions, and safe storage
- Emergency plan and access to functional phone and list of emergency phone numbers
- Identification and correction of environmental hazards and patient-specific concerns

Major diagnostic codes

- Acute bronchitis 466.0
- Chest physiotherapy and postural drainage 93.99
- Chronic airway obstruction, not elsewhere classified 496
- Chronic bronchitis without/with mention of acute exacerbation 491.20/491.21
- Emphysema with bleb (cystic dilatation)/without bleb 492.0/492.8
- Nebulizer therapy 93.94

Defense of homebound status

- Inability to ambulate farther than 10′ (3 m) due to dyspnea with minimal exertion
- Inability to ambulate farther than 10′ due to fatigue and poor endurance related to severe, uncontrolled COPD
- Inability to negotiate stairs due to profound shortness of breath
- Oxygen dependence

Selected nursing diagnoses and patient outcomes

Ineffective breathing pattern
The patient or caregiver will:
- demonstrate an effective respiratory rate and experience improved gas exchange in the lungs   (N, PT, RT)
- relate the causative factors, if known, and relate adaptive ways of coping with them.   (N, OT, PH, PT, SW)

Ineffective airway clearance related to bronchospasm and increased pulmonary secretions
The patient or caregiver will:
- demonstrate effective coughing and increased air exchange in the lungs.   (N, PT, RT)

Ineffective management of therapeutic regimen: Individuals
The patient or caregiver will:
- describe the COPD disease process as well as causes, factors contributing to symptoms, and the regimen for symptom control   (N, OT, PT, RT)
- demonstrate improved management of the therapeutic regimen as evidenced by improved COPD management of such practices as medication regimen, inhalation therapy, oxygen therapy, chest physiotherapy, and activity.   (N, OT, PH, PT, RT, SW)

Activity intolerance related to short-ness of breath

The patient or caregiver will:
• identify factors that reduce activity intolerance (N, PT, RT)
• verbalize and demonstrate an understanding of and compliance with energy-conservation measures (N, OT, PT)
• exhibit a decrease in hypoxic signs with increased activity, such as increased pulse, blood pressure, and respirations (N, PT, OT, RT)
• participate in a pulmonary rehabilitation program (N, OT, PT, RT)
• demonstrate progress to the highest level of mobility possible. (N, OT, PT)

Knowledge deficit related to COPD management, including oral medications, aerosol therapy, and oxygen therapy

The patient or caregiver will:
• state the correct dose and time for each medication prescribed as well as the adverse effects and precautions for each (N, PH)
• demonstrate correct technique for administration of aerosol therapy (metered-dose inhaler or nebulizer treatment) (N, PH, RT)
• verbalize an understanding of parameters for use of oral and inhaled medication (N, PH, RT)
• demonstrate correct use of oxygen (N, RT)
• verbalize an understanding of infection-control measures. (N)

Altered nutrition: Less than body requirements related to decreased oral intake

The patient or caregiver will:
• tolerate small, frequent meals (N, D)
• reach an acceptable baseline weight. (N, D)

Skilled nursing services

Care measures
• Assess the respiratory system, including breath sounds, breathing patterns, secretions, oxygenation status, and patient history relevant to the respiratory and oxygenation status.
• Assess the cardiovascular, mental and cognitive, and nutrition and hydration systems.
• Assess the level of care and compliance of the patient or caregiver with use of the metered-dose inhaler, nebulizer, oral medications, oxygen therapy, and chest physiotherapy.
• Perform chest physiotherapy, if indicated.

Patient and family teaching
• Review the respiratory disease process.
• Instruct on the medication regimen, both oral and aerosol, including dosage, frequency, purpose, potential adverse effects, and interactions.
• Emphasize the importance of following established COPD management and treatment plans to provide optimum control of COPD symptoms.
• Instruct on the importance of eliminating all pulmonary irritants, particularly cigarette smoke.

- Encourage the patient to participate in a smoking-cessation program.
- Review low rate of oxygen flow and adverse effects associated with oxygen administration above prescribed levels, if indicated.
- Instruct on oxygen safety measures.
- Teach breathing retraining exercises to strengthen and coordinate respiratory muscles, decrease the effort of breathing, and help empty the lungs more completely.
- Instruct the caregiver in chest physiotherapy and postural drainage to aid in the clearance of secretions.
- Encourage high fluid intake (2 to 2.5 L of fluid daily unless contraindicated) to keep secretions liquid.
- Promote small, frequent meals (even a small increase in the abdominal contents may press on the diaphragm and hinder breathing).
- Teach use of liquid nutritional supplements to improve caloric intake.
- Refer to community resources, such as Meals On Wheels, to provide assistance with meal preparation.
- Teach early signs and symptoms of respiratory infection, including increased dyspnea or fatigue; change in the color, amount, and character of sputum; and low-grade fever.
- Teach the importance of taking antibiotics exactly as prescribed and finishing the prescription.
- Instruct the patient or caregiver to consult with a physician about receiving an influenza vaccine (annually) and a pneumonia vaccine (one-time dose).
- Teach pulmonary rehabilitation (exercise and physical conditioning enhance oxygenation of tissues and allow a higher level of functioning).
- Teach energy-conservation techniques.

Interdisciplinary actions

Dietitian
- Assessment of nutritional status
- Instruction in proper diet

Home care aide
- Assistance with personal care and hygiene needs

Occupational therapist
- Instruction in energy-conservation techniques
- Training in activities of daily living
- Assessment of the need for and instruction in the use of adaptive equipment

Physical therapist
- Development and teaching of an individualized home exercise program
- Performance and instruction in pulmonary physical therapy, such as breathing exercises and chest physiotherapy, as indicated

Social worker
- Referral to community resources and support groups, such as counseling for stress management and reduction

Discharge plan
- Management of COPD in the home by the patient or caregiver with physician and community support system follow-up services
- Referral to outpatient services

• Continuation of home care visits for the homebound patient with skilled care needs

Documentation requirements

• Subjective and objective data related to respiratory assessment and signs and symptoms related to the respiratory disease process
• Instructions given related to COPD management
• Skilled procedures performed, such as nebulizer treatment and chest physiotherapy
• Understanding of and compliance with the medication regimen
• Understanding of and compliance with oxygen use
• Patient and caregiver progress toward educational goals
• Patient response to care
• Variances to expected outcomes
• Specific barriers to learning, such as impaired vision or mental status and cognitive ability
• Availability of a willing and able caregiver
• COPD as a new diagnosis for patient
• Patient's previous experience with medications, aerosol therapy, oxygen use, and chest physiotherapy
• Specific deficits in initial knowledge level, then progress as evidenced by specific concepts and procedures that are verbalized or demonstrated

Reimbursement reminders

• Indicate an expected end point of daily visits (when daily visits have been ordered).

• Obtain a physician's order for any plan of care change and document it in the patient's record.
• Determine which supplies and durable medical equipment are covered by Medicare.
• Note that the physician must indicate that a metered-dose inhaler alone is insufficient in treating the patient's COPD to ensure Medicare coverage of the nebulizer machine. (Medicare part B covers 80% of the allowable durable medical equipment charge; the patient or a secondary provider is responsible for the remaining 20%.)
• Note that the patient's oxygen saturation level must be 88% or less to ensure Medicare coverage of oxygen. (This must be reevaluated every 3 weeks.)
• Schedule respiratory therapy.
• Note that respiratory therapist services are usually provided by the company supplying the durable medical equipment on a routine or as-needed basis.

Insurance hints

• Present objective data about the patient's homebound status.
• Present objective patient findings, changes in clinical condition, and new changes in care (for example, new physician's orders).
• Present specifics about the patient and caregiver education process.
• Present progress toward established goals.

Cirrhosis

Cirrhosis is a chronic, progressive liver disorder characterized by degenerative and anatomic changes that may lead to liver dysfunction and liver failure. Cirrhosis is an irreversible reaction to hepatic necrosis and inflammation. Changes in blood flow cause numerous complications, which can eventually lead to bleeding esophageal varices.

The four major types are Laënnec's cirrhosis (alcohol-induced, nutritional, or portal cirrhosis), postnecrotic cirrhosis (acute viral hepatitis or exposure to hepatotoxins), biliary cirrhosis (chronic biliary obstruction), and cardiac cirrhosis (severe right-sided heart failure). Home care focuses on frequently assessing symptoms to monitor the disorder's progress and teaching the patient and caregiver about health promotion and prevention of further complications.

Previsit checklist

Physician orders and preparation
- Dietary restrictions
- Fluid allowance
- Sodium restrictions
- Laboratory tests, including liver enzyme, serum bilirubin, serum protein, and serum ammonia levels
- Prothrombin time
- Activity orders and restrictions

Equipment and supplies
- Tape measure
- Hospital bed
- Toilet extender, bedside commode, urinal, or bedpan
- Appropriate Vacutainer and needles for blood draws
- System for sharps disposal, including a container
- Vital signs equipment
- Supplies for standard precautions

Safety requirements
- Standard precautions for infection control and sharps disposal
- Bleeding precautions
- Appropriate plan of action for dangerous symptoms of hepatic coma and portal-systemic encephalopathy
- System to assist with adherence to complex medication regimen
- Information on medications, including dosage, adverse effects, interactions, and safe storage
- Emergency plan and access to functional phone and list of emergency phone numbers
- Identification and correction of environmental hazards and patient-specific concerns

Major diagnostic codes
- Alcoholic cirrhosis 571.2
- Ascites 789.5
- Cirrhosis, non-alcohol-related 571.5
- Hepatitis, chronic 571.40

Defense of homebound status
- Inability to ambulate farther than 10′ (3 m) due to shortness of breath from ascites

- Non-weight-bearing status due to chronic pain from fluid volume excess in lower extremities
- Inability to ambulate farther than 10' due to chronic abdominal pain
- Mental impairment due to toxic accumulations in the blood stream, requiring the assistance of another person to leave home

Selected nursing diagnoses and patient outcomes

Fluid volume excess
The patient or caregiver will:
- verbalize an understanding of health problem (N)
- verbalize an understanding of the cause of fluid retention (N)
- maintain or decrease abdominal girth (N)
- maintain or decrease the amount of peripheral edema (N)
- maintain a comfortable breathing pattern (N)
- demonstrate clear breath sounds (N)
- demonstrate and verbalize the knowledge and management of a sodium- and fluid-restricted diet (N, D)
- state the correct dose and time for each medication and vitamin supplement as well as adverse effects and precautions for each. (N, PH)

Risk for injury related to hemorrhage
The patient or caregiver will:
- verbalize an understanding of the need to avoid sharp objects (N)
- verbalize an understanding of early signs of bleeding (N)
- exhibit no signs of active bleeding (N, HCA)

- have a stable blood pressure and heart rate (N)
- avoid constrictive clothing (N, HCA, OT)
- verbalize an understanding of how to protect vulnerable areas from injury (N, HCA)
- verbalize understanding of partial thromboplastin time levels and the need to maintain an acceptable level. (N)

Altered thought processes
The patient or caregiver will:
- verbalize an understanding of neurologic changes and when to report these changes (N)
- demonstrate and verbalize the knowledge and management of a protein-restricted diet (N, D)
- state the correct dose and time for each medication (to decrease ammonia levels) as well as adverse effects and precautions for each (N, PH)
- remain safe and protected from injury (N, HCA, PT)
- remain oriented to person, place, and time (N, HCA)
- verbalize an awareness of any need for assistance (N, HCA, PT, SW)

Altered nutrition: Less than body requirements
The patient or caregiver will:
- maintain optimal nutritional status (N, D)
- maintain optimal fluid balance (N, D)
- eliminate alcohol from the diet (N, D)
- maintain body weight (N, D)
- demonstrate and verbalize the knowledge and management of all aspects of the diet (N, D)

• keep a dietary log as a teaching tool for an appropriate diet (N, D)
• not experience nausea, vomiting, or a decrease in appetite (N, D)
• rest before each meal (N, D)
• maintain a weight log (N, D, HCA)
• state the correct dose and time for each medication (antiemetic) as well as adverse effects and precautions for each. (N, PH)

Activity intolerance
The patient or caregiver will:
• maintain an optimal level of functioning (N, HCA, PT)
• allow for frequent rest periods (N, HCA)
• allow for rest periods between simple activities (N, HCA, PT)
• maintain vital signs within a predetermined range during activity. (N, PT)

Risk for infection
The patient or caregiver will:
• avoid scratching the skin (N, PH)
• keep fingernails and toenails clipped short (N)
• verbalize how to care for dry, itchy skin (N, PH)
• report any cough or elevated temperature immediately (N, HCA)
• avoid persons with infections. (N)

Body image disturbance
The patient or caregiver will:
• express concerns over body image (N, HCA, SW)
• report changes in behavior and emotional needs (N, HCA, PT, SW)
• use referral to a support group, if needed. (N, SW)

Skilled nursing services

Care measures
• Assess the cardiovascular, pulmonary, mental and cognitive, nutrition, integumentary, and GI systems.
• Continually assess patient and caregiver ability to provide care as the condition changes.
• Assess the effectiveness of the medication regimen.
• Assess dietary compliance.
• Assess vital signs, abdominal girth, peripheral edema, weight, and mental status.
• Assess respiratory status for dyspnea with or without exertion, shortness of breath, and breath sounds.
• Assess for activity intolerance.
• Maintain skin integrity and provide appropriate care for reddened or open areas.
• Assess for signs and symptoms of GI bleeding.
• Assess for bleeding as evidenced by petechiae, ecchymoses, and bleeding from the mouth, gums, nose, vagina, or rectum.
• Assess patient and caregiver coping abilities.
• Assess the patient's mental and cognitive functioning.
• Assess and discuss the patient's changes in body image.
• Assess for alcohol use.

Patient and family teaching
• Teach about medications, including dosage, action, interactions, reason for administration, and adverse effects.
• Inform to avoid over-the-counter drugs, especially those metabolized in the liver, such as acetaminophen and

analgesics, and other medications, such as sedatives and antianxiety drugs.

- Instruct on appropriate diet.
- Warn to avoid raw shellfish and activities that might increase the risk of viral hepatitis such as I.V. drug use.
- Instruct in the need to avoid alcohol.
- Review the need for frequent rest periods.
- Emphasize the need to keep lower extremities elevated and instruct in sitting and lying positions that provide optimum breathing.
- Outline how to pace activities to allow for energy conservation.
- Indicate that hard toothbrushes and straight-edged razors should be avoided.
- Instruct on adverse effects to report, including weight gain, fever, bleeding, mental status deterioration, change in skin color or abdominal girth, and shortness of breath.

Interdisciplinary actions

Dietitian
- Consultation regarding nutritional status and development of menu plans that meet prescribed dietary restrictions

Home care aide
- Provision of personal care needs

Pharmacist
- Consultation regarding medication regimen

Physical therapist
- Instruction in the appropriate use of assistive devices and transfers

Social worker
- Referral to community resources and support groups

Discharge plan
- Management of cirrhosis in the home by the patient or caregiver with physician and community support system follow-up services
- Referral to outpatient services
- Continuation of home care visits for the homebound patient with skilled care needs

Documentation requirements
- Vital signs
- Weight log
- Abdominal girth
- Edema
- Shortness of breath with or without exertion
- Skin color
- Signs and symptoms of bleeding
- Mental and cognitive status
- Dietary and fluid compliance
- Changes in the patient's condition
- Significant stressors
- Laboratory results and specification of changes from previous results
- Teaching provided regarding the patient's condition and the response to teaching
- Patient response to the plan of care
- Changes in the plan of care and reasons for doing so
- Ability and willingness of the caregiver to care for the patient

Reimbursement reminders
- Ensure changes in status or the plan of care are communicated to all team

members and that all orders or changes in the plan of care are noted.

Insurance hints

- Present objective data about the patient's homebound status.
- Present objective patient findings and new changes.
- Report new laboratory values.
- Report changes in the clinical condition since last contact.
- Present specifics about the patient and caregiver education process.

Coronary artery bypass grafting

Coronary artery bypass grafting (CABG) is the treatment of choice for severe atherosclerosis, which isn't amenable to alternative nonsurgical treatments. Numerous complications can occur during the postoperative period, including respiratory complications related to hypoventilation and atelectasis, anemia from surgical blood loss, and cardiac arrhythmias caused by edema in cardiac tissue, fluid overload, or electrolyte imbalance. Furthermore, if the surgical incision site becomes infected, the possibility of dehiscence, sepsis, and evisceration arises. The home care nurse must not only provide scrupulous wound care but must also offer intensive patient and family teaching to prevent more serious complications.

Previsit checklist

Physician orders and preparation

- Wound care as appropriate
- Oral medications
- Activity orders and restrictions
- Nutritional consultation for individualized diet to promote wound healing or lower cholesterol and fat intake

Equipment and supplies

- Supplies for standard precautions
- Vital signs equipment
- Dressing change supplies as specified by physician
- Medication information

Safety requirements

- Standard precautions for infection control and sharps disposal
- Proper disposal of soiled dressings, sharps, and I.V. administration supplies
- Safety precautions to prevent falls
- Information on medications, including dosage, adverse effects, interactions, and safe storage
- Identification of symptoms that necessitate immediate reporting and assistance
- System to assist with adherence to complex medication regimen
- Emergency plan and access to functional phone and list of emergency phone numbers
- Identification and correction of environmental hazards and patient-specific concerns

Major diagnostic codes

- Abdominal dissecting aortic aneurysm 441.02
- Anemia 285.9
- Angina 413.9
- Atrial fibrillation/flutter 427.31/427.32
- CABG, involving artery 1/2/3/4 36.11/36.12/36.13/36.14

- Cerebrovascular accident 436
- Chronic obstructive pulmonary disease 496
- Congestive heart failure 428.0
- Constipation 564.0
- Hypertension 401.9
- Obesity/morbid obesity 278.00/278.01
- Pacemaker postinsertion care V45.0
- Postsurgical status, aortocoronary bypass status V45.81
- Substernal wound infection, seroma/ other 998.51/998.59

Defense of homebound status

- Patient on cardiac restrictions after CABG surgery
- Shortness of breath or weakness after surgery
- Extensive, infected postoperative chest wound or venous leg site
- Minimal ambulation possible due to postoperative discomfort or pain

Selected nursing diagnoses and patient outcomes

Risk for infection related to surgical incision

The patient or caregiver will:
- show no signs of infection, including redness, drainage, warmth, tenderness, inflammation at the site, and fever (N)
- verbalize an understanding of symptoms that should be reported to the physician   (N)
- observe the incision for signs and symptoms of infection   (N)
- assist with incisional care to the extent of ability.   (N)

Pain related to surgical incision

The patient or caregiver will:
- rate pain at 3 or less on a 0-to-10 scale 80% of the time   (N)
- administer pain medication as ordered   (N, PH)
- consistently verbalize when each episode of discomfort occurs.   (N)

Knowledge deficit related to cardiac-prudent lifestyle

The patient or caregiver will:
- verbalize the importance of maintaining a cardiac diet and compliance with the medication and exercise regimens   (N, D, PH, PT)
- verbalize foods to avoid on a cardiac diet   (N, D)
- demonstrate the prescribed exercise and physical activity plan.   (N, PT)

Skilled nursing services

Care measures
- Assess the mental and cognitive, integumentary, cardiovascular, respiratory, nutritional, and GI systems.
- Assess for signs and symptoms of infection.
- Assess the wound site and change the dressing according to orders.
- Monitor intake and output and weight and report weight gain or ankle edema.

Patient and family teaching
- Teach how to assess and record the patient's pulse.
- Teach how to assess the incision.
- Urge use of stool softeners and compliance with diet orders to avoid constipation.
- Review the adverse effects, functions, and schedule of all medications.

• Instruct on symptoms that necessitate calling emergency medical services.

• Instruct on correct use of antiembolic stockings.

• Emphasize the importance of medical follow-ups.

• Emphasize the importance of adhering to the cardiac diet, following the exercise regimen, and quitting smoking.

Interdisciplinary actions

Dietitian

• Comprehensive nutritional assessment of the patient, education, and planning of the cardiac diet

Occupational therapist

• Instruction in energy conservation as necessary

Physical therapist

• Development of an appropriate exercise and activity regimen as part of the cardiac rehabilitation program

Social worker

• Referral to support groups

Discharge plan

• Management of postoperative care in the home by the patient or caregiver after CABG with physician and community support system follow-up services

• Referral to outpatient services

• Continuation of home care visits for the homebound patient with skilled care needs

Documentation requirements

• Subjective and objective data on signs and symptoms of infection or healing

• Results of the nutritionist's evaluation

• Patient response to care

• Patient participation in self-care

• Patient and caregiver progress toward educational goals

• Education barriers and progress

• Variances to expected outcomes

• Care provided and the continued homebound status of the patient

Reimbursement reminders

• Note that observation and evaluation may be appropriate for longer than 3 weeks.

• Ensure that changes in status and the plan of care are communicated to team members and noted in the chart.

Insurance hints

• Present objective patient findings and new changes.

• Present updated laboratory values since last visit.

• Update about the patient's homebound status and inability to leave the home.

Coronary artery disease

Coronary artery disease (CAD) refers to a group of conditions in which blood flow through the coronary arteries is obstructed by atherosclerosis. Risk factors include a family history of CAD, old age, hypertension, diabetes mellitus, hypercholesterolemia, smoking, and obesity. Incidence is higher in men than in women, although CAD is the number one killer of women in the United States. African Americans are at a higher risk than Caucasians.

The goals of controlling risk factors are to reduce the risk of heart attack and increase the chance of survival for patients with CAD. The home care nurse must provide the necessary education to help patients manage their risk factors for this potentially fatal condition.

Previsit checklist

Physician orders and preparation
- Oral medication orders
- Dietitian consultation for comprehensive nutritional assessment
- Order for nicotine patches as part of smoking-cessation program, if necessary

Equipment and supplies
- Vital signs equipment

Safety requirements
- Standard precautions for infection control
- Monitoring for cardiac and neurologic symptoms that would necessitate contact with emergency medical services
- System to assist with adherence to complex medication regimen
- Information on medications, including dosage, adverse effects, interactions, and safe storage
- Emergency plan and access to functional phone and list of emergency phone numbers
- Identification and correction of environmental hazards and patient-specific concerns

Major diagnostic codes
- Angina 413.9
- Cardiac dysrhythmias 427.9
- Chronic ischemic heart disease 414.9
- Coronary atherosclerosis 414.00
- Diabetes (type 2), controlled/uncontrolled 250.00/250.01
- Hypertension with heart involvement without/with congestive heart failure 402.90/402.91
- Myocardial infarction (MI) 410.9
- Obesity/morbid obesity 278.00/278.01

Defense of homebound status
- Angina with activity
- Poor endurance
- Cardiac restrictions on activity
- Ambulation impaired by lower-extremity edema
- Oxygen dependence
- Status of postacute MI
- Severe functional limitations
- Poor respiratory status or severe shortness of breath
- Limited energy and endurance or dyspnea on exertion

Selected nursing diagnoses and patient outcomes

Decreased cardiac output related to obstructed blood flow through the coronary arteries

The patient or caregiver will:

• verbally contract to exhibit a weight loss that correlates with the patient's ideal weight (N, D)
• demonstrate an ability to follow the physician-supervised exercise program (N, PT)
• maintain control of diabetes and correctly monitor blood glucose levels, if applicable (N)
• exhibit blood pressure that is within normal limits (N)
• verbally contract to enter a smoking-cessation program (N)
• verbalize symptoms that should be reported to the physician (N)
• verbalize symptoms that necessitate contact with emergency medical services. (N)

Knowledge deficit related to modifiable risk factors for developing coronary atherosclerotic heart disease
The patient or caregiver will:
• verbalize the importance of quitting smoking (N)
• verbalize the importance of maintaining control of diabetes (N, D)
• verbalize the importance of achieving an ideal weight (N, D)
• verbalize the importance of maintaining a near-normal blood pressure (N)
• verbalize foods appropriate on a diet that is low in calories, total fats, cholesterol, sodium, and refined carbohydrates (N, D)
• verbalize the importance of adhering to the prescribed medication regimen. (N)

Activity intolerance related to the disease process
The patient or caregiver will:
• adhere to the prescribed activity and exercise regimen (N, PT)
• verbalize the importance of remaining active within limits of tolerance (N, PT)
• verbalize symptoms that should be reported to the physician (N)
• verbalize symptoms that necessitate contact with emergency medical services (N)
• state the necessary actions to take when activity has exceeded limitations, including medications. (N)

Skilled nursing services

Care measures
• Assess the mental and cognitive, nutrition and hydration, and cardiopulmonary systems.
• Assess for risk factors, including family history of CAD, smoking, hypertension, diabetes mellitus, obesity, and age.
• Assess the patient's typical daily diet.
• Assess vital signs on each visit, especially blood pressure.
• Check the blood glucose level if the patient is diabetic; refer to the patient's log book or use the memory function of the patient's meter to assess the patient's control over these levels.

Patient and family teaching
• Instruct in medication adverse effects and interactions.
• Provide dietary instruction and nutritional assessment.
• Instruct in the relationship between smoking, hypertension, diabetes mellitus, and obesity and CAD.
• Emphasize the far-reaching effects of untreated CAD.
• Instruct in symptoms that must be reported to the physician.

• Instruct in symptoms that necessitate contact with emergency medical services.

Interdisciplinary actions

Dietitian
• Comprehensive nutritional assessment
• Nutrition education

Physical therapist
• Development and teaching of exercise program

Occupational therapist
• Recommendation of adaptive equipment and instruction in use, including glucose monitoring devices

Social worker
• Referral to community resources and support groups, focusing particularly on risk factor modification

Discharge plan
• Management of CAD in the home by the patient or caregiver with physician and community support system follow-up services
• Referral to outpatient services
• Continuation of home care visits for the homebound patient with skilled care needs

Documentation requirements
• Subjective and objective data on signs and symptoms of CAD
• Results of blood pressure and blood glucose monitoring, if applicable

• Patient's adherence to risk modification recommendations, including smoking cessation and weight control
• Variances to expected outcomes
• Specific care rendered and teaching instructions provided
• Changes in the plan of care
• Progress toward goals
• Specific care and teaching instructions rendered
• Abnormal laboratory values
• Medication changes
• Irregularity in vital signs
• Chest pain or adverse respiratory or neurologic changes

Reimbursement reminders
• Note any change in status, action taken, change in the plan of care, and communication with team members.

Insurance hints
• Present objective patient findings and new changes.
• Report updated laboratory values and cardiac and neurologic symptoms since the last update.
• Record communication with the physician, the caregiver, and therapy team members.
• Report changes to the plan of care.
• Update regarding the patient's continuing homebound status.

Crutch walking

Ambulation aids, such as crutches, can eliminate all or partial weight bearing on an affected extremity, allowing the injured area to heal. Made of wood or lightweight metals such as aluminum, these aids typically have one or more extensions that can be adjusted to accommodate the patient's height. Although most patients use crutches for just a short time, some patients require crutches throughout their lives because of permanent functional limitations imposed by severe injuries, chronic disease, or congenital defects.

Services will be of short duration unless the patient has other functional limitations; crutch walking instruction isn't a skilled nursing need beyond education. The patient may need rehabilitation services only.

Previsit checklist

Physician orders and preparation
- Review of rehabilitation team notes
- Activity orders and restrictions

Equipment and supplies
- Crutches, appropriate to the patient's size and disability
- Wound or pin care supplies, if ordered
- Supplies for standard precautions

Safety requirements
- Removal of furniture as necessary to accommodate crutches
- Functioning communication system, such as a bell, baby monitor, or cordless phone, to summon assistance
- System to assist with adherence to complex medication regimen
- Information on medications, including dosage, adverse effects, interactions, and safe storage
- Emergency plan and access to functional phone and list of emergency phone numbers

- Identification and correction of environmental hazards and patient-specific concerns

Major diagnostic codes
For fractures:
- Ankle, closed/open 824.8/824.9
- Femur, closed/open 821.00/821.10
- Fibula 823.81
- Foot 825.20
- Tibia 823.80

For sprains and strains:
- Ankle 845.00
- Foot 845.10
- Knee/leg 844.9
- Torn meniscus 836.2

Defense of homebound status
- Inability to ambulate farther than 10′ (3 m)
- Inability to ambulate farther than 10′ without an increase in symptoms of pain or shortness of breath
- Imposed activity restriction as ordered by the physician _____
- Multiple fractures

Selected nursing diagnoses and patient outcomes

Knowledge deficit related to crutch use
The patient or caregiver will:
- verbalize a knowledge of how to use crutches   (N, PT, OT)
- demonstrate proper crutch gait (two, three, four point)   (N, PT, OT)
- demonstrate proper posture when using crutches   (N, PT, OT)

- demonstrate proper distribution of weight (on hands) while using crutches (N, PT, OT)
- maintain crutch tips in proper condition. (N, PT, OT)

Altered health maintenance related to unsteady gait and use of crutches
The patient or caregiver will:
- demonstrate proper use of crutches (N, PT, OT)
- demonstrate good personal hygiene (N)
- explain and use bathing methods that include using crutches to get in and out of the shower or bathtub (N, PT, OT)
- remain free from injury related to crutch use. (N, PT, OT)

Pain related to fracture, surgery, or trauma to soft tissue
The patient or caregiver will:
- verbalize proper analgesia use and rate pain at 3 or less on a 0-to-10 scale 80% of the time (N)
- demonstrate optimal movement related to proper pain control (N)
- report satisfaction with the sleep pattern. (N)

Impaired physical mobility related to immobilization of the extremity or pain
The patient or caregiver will:
- exhibit no joint contractures (N, PT)
- remain free from muscle spasms (N, PT)
- perform at expected level of independent care (N, PT, OT)
- demonstrate proper use of crutches (N, PT, OT)
- maintain functional mobility and range of motion in the affected limb (N, PT)

- maintain functional independence (N, PT, OT)
- complete a home exercise program (N, PT)
- express satisfaction with mobility (N, PT, OT)
- maintain activity within the prescribed limitations (N, PT, OT)
- demonstrate proper posture while using crutches. (N, PT, OT)

Risk for injury related to unsteady gait from crutches
The patient or caregiver will:
- be free from injury (N, PT, OT)
- verbalize knowledge of the home safety plan to prevent falls (N, PT, OT)
- rearrange the home for the use of crutches (N, PT, OT)
- demonstrate proper crutch storage when not in use. (N, PT, OT)

Skilled nursing services

Care measures
- Complete an initial assessment and identification of complicating factors.
- Assess safety in the patient's home.
- Perform gait training.
- Assess the mental and cognitive, cardiopulmonary, integumentary, and musculoskeletal systems.
- Assess the level of self-care ability of the patient.

Patient and family teaching
- Teach use of crutches.
- Teach safety for injury prevention.

Interdisciplinary actions

Occupational therapist
• Assistance with management of activities of daily living
• Energy conservation

Physical therapist
• Home exercise program
• Safety planning

Social worker
• Assistance in obtaining community resources, such as transportation and in-home support services

Discharge plan
• Patient return to normal routine after recovering from fracture or soft tissue injury
• Patient return to normal routine following mastery of crutch use
• Referral to outpatient services

Documentation requirements
• Description of functional losses or gains in clear terms, such as distance walked (in feet) with and without crutches and self-care ability, including dressing, feeding, bathing, toileting, and grooming
• Evaluation of the effectiveness of the pain control regimen
• Description of plan to improve patient function whenever progress stalls
• Variances to expected outcomes

Reimbursement reminders
• Remember that the need for crutches doesn't make a patient homebound; be clear about functional limitations, the patient's ability to use the crutches, upper body strength, the presence of other injuries, paresis, and chronic lung or heart disease that limits the patient's ability to use adaptive equipment.
• Note that if rehabilitation services are required, they should be used only for a brief period of time and focus on patient and caregiver education needed to develop the home exercise and safety program.
• Note that occupational therapy can be ordered if the patient needs help with energy conservation.

Insurance hints
• Describe progressive levels of self-care (dressing, toileting, bathing, grooming) and ability, including the use of adaptive equipment.
• Describe progress toward rehabilitation goals, such as safe use of stairs and transfer from sitting to standing.
• List the collaborative plan of care for all team members providing services.
• Compare and contrast the roles of each rehabilitation team member.
• Explain what care will be needed long term.
• Describe any other conditions, such as chronic lung disease, and how they affect the patient's use of crutches.
• Project any other care that may be required for the patient, such as casts and other corrective devices.

Deep vein thrombosis

Deep vein thrombosis (DVT), the formation of a clot in a deep vein, is associated with venous stasis, vessel wall injury, hypercoagulability, and local inflammation. Although more common in the calf veins, the incidence of thrombosis in the subclavian vein has increased with the use of central venous catheterization. DVT is dangerous because the deep veins carry most of the blood from the legs and accompany major arteries. Complications such as pulmonary embolism are life-threatening. Care of the patient with DVT focuses on anticoagulation therapy and its adverse effects, activity levels, and reducing the risk of recurrences.

Previsit checklist

Physician orders and preparation
- Blood studies, including prothrombin time (PT) and international normalized ratio (INR)
- Medications and administration schedule
- Activity orders and restrictions
- Comfort and pain-control measures
- Physical therapy evaluation for therapeutic exercise, range-of-motion (ROM) exercises, device application, and ambulation after cessation of prescribed bed rest
- Home care aide assistance with activities of daily living (ADLs) and personal care

Equipment and supplies
- Supplies for standard precautions and proper sharps disposal
- Phlebotomy supplies
- Measuring tape
- Moist-heat application device such as a heating pad
- Intermittent sequential compression device or antiembolism stockings
- Bedside commode

Safety requirements
- System to assist with adherence to a complex medication regimen
- Emergency plan and access to functional phone and list of emergency phone numbers
- Identification and correction of environmental hazards and patient-specific concerns related to bed rest and activity restrictions
- Standard precautions for infection control and sharps disposal
- Avoidance of sitting for long periods with extremity dependent
- Signs and symptoms of embolism to immediately report to the physician
- Instructions on signs and symptoms of medical emergency and actions to take
- Bleeding precautions
- Allergies verified and documented

Major diagnostic codes
- Arterial embolism, lower extremity 444.22
- Crushing injury, lower/upper extremity 928.*/927.*
- Deep or specified vessels (femoro-popliteal or tibial) 451.19
- Femoral vein 451.11
- Thrombophlebitis, leg or lower extremity 451.2
- Unspecified 451.9

(*Note:* The fourth digit specifies the exact location. Refer to a coding manual for more information.)

Defense of homebound status

- Bedridden or assistance of one or two persons needed for ambulation
- Required elevation of affected extremity for majority of hours during the day or non-weight-bearing status of affected leg
- Unable to ambulate farther than 10′ (3 m) because of imposed activity restriction or pain in or swelling of affected extremity

Selected nursing diagnoses and patient outcomes

Altered tissue perfusion related to diminished blood flow from thrombus

The patient or caregiver will:
- exhibit palpable pulses that are equal bilaterally   (N, PT)
- report a decrease in pain as evidenced by a rating of 3 or less on a 0-to-10 scale   (N, HCA, PT)
- verbalize an understanding of the treatment program and the need for elevation of the affected extremity   (N, MD)
- exhibit a reduction in swelling evidenced by decreased calf circumference and redness of affected extremity with return to pre-illness appearance by discharge   (N, HCA, PT)
- report an absence of numbness, tingling, and loss of motor function in affected extremity   (N, HCA, PT)
- achieve therapeutic anticoagulant blood levels (PT at 35 to 60 seconds or prescribed level; INR at 2.0 to 3.0 or prescribed level)   (N, MD)
- maintain muscle strength in affected extremity.   (N, PT)

Knowledge deficit related to planned therapy regimen

The patient or caregiver will:
- keep the affected extremity elevated   (N, HCA, PT)
- demonstrate adherence to bed rest and activity restrictions (N, HCA, PT)
- wear nonrestrictive clothing   (N, HCA)
- verbalize the major action and possible adverse effects of anticoagulation therapy   (N, PH)
- take prescribed anticoagulants   (N, MD, PH)
- maintain a consistent intake of foods containing vitamin K, including green, leafy vegetables (such as spinach and broccoli) and eggs   (N, D)
- maintain a normal pattern of elimination without report of straining during bowel movements   (N, HCA)
- apply moist heat as directed   (N, HCA, PT)
- demonstrate use of antiembolism stockings or intermittent sequential compression device as appropriate   (N, HCA, PT)
- verbalize measures to reduce the risk of embolus formation and recurrence.   (N)

Risk for injury related to anticoagulation therapy or possible embolus formation

The patient or caregiver will:
- display no evidence of altered mental status, chest pain, anxiety, or tachycardia   (N)
- exhibit no signs of excessive bleeding or bruising   (N)

- demonstrate measures to reduce the risk of bleeding such as the use of an electric razor (N)
- verbalize emergency first-aid measures for bleeding (N, HCA)
- verbalize signs and symptoms to immediately report to the physician (N)
- maintain follow-up visits with the physician and for laboratory testing. (N, MD)

Risk for impaired skin integrity related to ischemia

The patient or caregiver will:
- verbalize signs and symptoms of infection to report to the physician (N, HCA, PT)
- exhibit no evidence of skin breakdown, especially on the affected extremity (N, PT, HCA)
- demonstrate proper skin care measures (N, HCA)
- verbalize the importance of not massaging the affected area. (N)

Impaired mobility related to imposed medical activity restrictions

The patient or caregiver will:
- demonstrate correct limitation of activity and use of bedside commode (N, HCA, PT)
- verbalize feelings of maintaining strength and endurance (N, PT)
- demonstrate the use of ROM and deep-breathing exercises to maintain functional capacity (N, PT)
- participate in a home exercise program as appropriate. (N, HCA, PT)

Pain related to ischemia

The patient or caregiver will:
- verbalize the pain-control regimen (N, HCA, MD, PT)

- demonstrate one nonpharmacologic method of pain relief such as relaxation (N)
- report a decrease in pain as evidenced by a rating of 3 or less on a 0-to-10 scale (N, HCA)
- express understanding of the cause of pain related to ischemia (N)
- perform activities to minimize pain, such as ROM exercises, as ordered by the physician. (N, PT)

Diversional activity deficit related to imposed activity restrictions

The patient or caregiver will:
- describe appropriate recreational activities within mobility restrictions (N, HCA, PT)
- participate in chosen activities (N, PT)
- express satisfaction with chosen activities (N, PT)
- use appropriate community support groups, such as visiting pet therapy, church outreach, and programs for shut-ins. (N)

Skilled nursing services

Care measures
- Perform initial full assessment of all systems, including vascular, respiratory, neurologic, integumentary, and musculoskeletal systems. Reassess with each visit.
- Measure calf circumference, inspect affected extremity, and palpate pedal pulses at each visit.
- Assess care by patient and family related to limited ambulation.
- Assess the effectiveness of the treatment regimen, including anticoagulation therapy and ROM exercises.

- Evaluate the patient's adherence to the treatment regimen.
- Obtain or arrange for follow-up laboratory studies to monitor PT and INR.

Patient and family teaching
- Emphasize the importance of following activity restrictions, elevating extremities, and maintaining ROM and the home exercise program.
- Demonstrate use of a moist-heat application device, antiembolism stockings, or an intermittent sequential compression device.
- Teach signs and symptoms of adverse reactions to medications, such as bleeding, as well as signs and symptoms of embolism.
- Explain the need to maintain consistent intake of green, leafy vegetables (such as spinach and broccoli) and eggs while on anticoagulants.
- Review pain-control basics, bleeding precautions, proper skin care, and necessary safety measures.
- Describe ways to prevent constipation and recurrence of DVT.

Interdisciplinary actions

Home care aide
- Personal care and hygiene
- Assistance with ADLs

Physical therapist
- Home exercise program, therapeutic exercise, ROM, and device application and use
- Ambulation after cessation of activity restrictions

Discharge plan
- Management of disease process in home with physician and community support systems
- Discharged to self-care with return to independent status after elimination of thrombus
- Maintenance of anticoagulation therapy
- Follow-up appointments for blood studies in an authorized laboratory
- Follow-up appointments with physician at recommended intervals

Documentation requirements
- Skilled assessment, including patient's response to care; pain-control measures and the effectiveness of each used; effectiveness of anticoagulation therapy; results of blood studies; titration of anticoagulation therapy based on results of blood studies; elimination pattern; activity restrictions; adherence to exercise program and muscle strength maintenance; objective evidence of changes in extremity, including presence of pedal pulses, calf circumference measurements, and degree of redness and warmth; and evidence of complications (or lack thereof)
- Patient's or caregiver's independence with care and therapy regimen
- Patient and caregiver instruction relating to medication therapy, including drug, dose, frequency, adverse effects, and signs and symptoms to report; bleeding precautions; constipation prevention and control; activity restrictions; device application (moist heat, antiembolism stockings, or intermittent sequential compression device); safety measures associated with device

application; signs and symptoms to be reported; knowledge of preventive measures; and signs and symptoms of recurrence

• Phlebotomy (regular blood studies for PT and INR and results)

• Interdisciplinary team communication: physical therapy evaluation and need for services; plan of home exercise program, device application, or both; changes in plan of care, including adjustments in medication dosages based on the results of blood studies, and patient or caregiver understanding of those changes

• Patient's ability to transfer safely within limited activity

• Patient's adherence to instructions and therapy regimen

Reimbursement reminders

• Medicare covers phlebotomy supplies.

• Many insurance companies have contracts with specific laboratories to perform blood studies. Check for an authorized laboratory.

Insurance hints

• Report specific progress toward goals (for example, INR has been maintained at ___ level for ___ number of days); changes in calf circumference, measured in centimeters; adjustment issues, such as patient's resistance to or acceptance of imposed activity restrictions; and complications, such as constipation, skin breakdown, and infection.

• Describe gains in knowledge, such as skills and concepts mastered for relaxation and prevention of recurrence.

• Present specific data on homebound status, such as continued bed rest, changes in muscle strength related to bed rest, and activity restrictions.

• Emphasize the next step in care to show a progressive plan for independence.

• Stress comorbid conditions (such as diabetes and chronic lung or heart disease) that would affect the patient's ability to provide self-care.

Dehydration

Dehydration is a condition that results from excessive water loss from the body. Typically, this loss is in the form of extracellular fluid (interstitial and intravascular fluid), but a severe loss of extracellular fluid may result in intracellular fluid loss as well. Patients, especially those who are elderly, easily become dehydrated when they experience physiologic stressors from fluid restriction, fever, vomiting, diarrhea, infection, and diuretics. Difficulty swallowing or a diminished sense of thirst may reduce a patient's ability to notice this loss of body water. An incontinent patient may deliberately limit fluids to avoid incontinence. Water loss is accompanied by the loss of electrolytes, which can result in permanent damage or even death if not detected early and treated. Dehydration is also a common sign of impending death. Supportive care focuses on preserving the integrity of oral mucous membranes. Care also focuses on supporting the patient's right to terminate artificial hydration.

Previsit checklist

Physician orders and preparation

- Serum osmolality and electrolyte levels
- Record of weights
- Fluid intake and output
- Baseline vital signs
- I.V. replacement therapy
- Nutritional intake and calorie and fluid allotment
- History of diuretic use and orders to discontinue if previously used
- Precipitating factors, including history of incontinence, vomiting, diarrhea, infection, and difficulty swallowing
- Nutritional evaluation of dietary and fluid intake
- Enterostomal therapy evaluation (if incontinence or diarrhea is present)
- Antibiotic therapy (if infection is the underlying cause)
- Speech therapy evaluation for difficulty swallowing
- Home care aide assistance with personal care, nutrition, and ambulation
- Hospice consult

Equipment and supplies

- Supplies for standard precautions and proper sharps disposal
- Phlebotomy and I.V. replacement therapy supplies
- Bedside commode and graduated container for urine measurement
- Scale for weighing patient
- Intake and output form
- Protective underpads for use if incontinence occurs
- Oral care supplies (including mouthwash, sponge-tip applicators, artificial saliva, and water-soluble lubricant)

Safety requirements

- Standard precautions for infection control and sharps disposal
- System to assist with adherence to a complex medication regimen, including I.V. therapy, allergy notation, and drug interactions
- Emergency plan and access to functional phone and list of emergency phone numbers
- Home safety measures to prevent falls and injuries
- Identification and correction of environmental hazards and patient-specific concerns (for example, working electricity with grounded electrical receptacle for I.V. pump)
- Availability and access to foods and fluids
- Signs and symptoms of adverse effects of medication and I.V. replacement therapy to report to the physician
- Aspiration precautions if ability to swallow is impaired

Major diagnostic codes

- Dehydration (cachexia) 276.5
- Hyperosmolality dehydration 276.0
- Hypo-osmolality dehydration 276.1

Defense of homebound status

- Unable to ambulate farther than 10′ (3 m) because of extreme fatigue secondary to dehydration
- Assistance of one or two persons required to rise from sitting position and ambulate to bathroom
- Urinary incontinence that interferes with ability to leave home

Selected nursing diagnoses and patient outcomes

Fluid volume deficit related to contributing factors (such as dysphagia, heart failure, medications, dementia, depression, cerebrovascular accident, hypertension, use of diuretics, inability to obtain fluids, fear of incontinence, fever, diarrhea, renal failure, and impending death)

The patient or caregiver will:
• demonstrate an intake of 2,000 ml of fluid over a 24-hour period (N, D, HCA)
• achieve a greater intake than output for 48 hours (N, HCA)
• manifest intact and moist skin and mucous membranes (N, HCA)
• produce clear, light amber – colored urine (N, HCA)
• demonstrate good skin turgor by quick return of skin to normal configuration after being pinched and released. (N, HCA)

Knowledge deficit related to underlying factors contributing to dehydration

The patient or caregiver will:
• verbalize factors contributing to the development of dehydration (N)
• identify the role of diuretic therapy, infection, vomiting, and impending death as contributory factors (N)
• demonstrate steps to measure fluid intake and output (N, HCA)
• verbalize measures to maintain adequate fluid intake and output. (N, D, HCA)

Knowledge deficit related to administration of I.V. replacement therapy

The patient or caregiver will:

• state the rationale for I.V. replacement therapy (N)
• demonstrate the procedure for proper administration, including rate, frequency, and amount of fluid replacement, with minimal assistance (N)
• verbalize the signs and symptoms of complications, including infiltration, phlebitis, and fluid overload (N, MD)
• demonstrate adherence to regimen for follow-up blood studies. (N, MD)

Risk for injury related to extreme fatigue, alteration in fluid and electrolyte balance and, possibly, swallowing difficulties secondary to dehydration

The patient or caregiver will:
• remain free from injury (N, HCA, MD, SP)
• identify potential safety hazards (N, HCA)
• institute measures to maintain safety in the home (N, HCA)
• change positions slowly (N, HCA)
• use the bedside commode for elimination (N, HCA)
• use energy conservation measures (N, HCA)
• demonstrate measures to prevent aspiration secondary to swallowing difficulties (N, HCA, SP)
• demonstrate a plan to balance rest and activities (N, HCA)
• verbalize signs and symptoms that require immediate notification of the physician (N, HCA, SP)
• maintain appointments for follow-up blood studies and physician visits. (N)

Risk for impaired skin integrity related to fluid volume deficit, activity intolerance and, possibly, incontinence

The patient or caregiver will:
• verbalize signs and symptoms of skin problems to report to the physician (N, HCA)
• exhibit no evidence of skin breakdown, especially on bony prominences (N, ET, HCA)
• demonstrate proper skin hygiene and pressure-relieving measures (N, ET, HCA)
• demonstrate measures to control incontinence. (N, ET, HCA)

Skilled nursing services

Care measures
• Perform initial full assessment of all systems, including neurologic, integumentary, genitourinary, and GI systems.
• Assess vital signs and compare with baseline.
• Assess patient's level of self-care and level of fatigue.
• Observe the patient as he attempts to feed himself, and assess his swallowing ability.
• Obtain or arrange for blood studies, including serum osmolality and electrolyte levels, and evaluate them for changes that indicate effective therapy or deterioration in the patient's condition.
• Assess effectiveness of the treatment regimen.
• Institute I.V. replacement therapy, if ordered, and evaluate its effectiveness.
• Assess daily fluid intake and output.
• Inspect skin, including mucous membranes and areas over bony prominences, and assess skin turgor.
• Assess weight trends or measure arm circumference if bedridden.

• Assess frequency of vomiting and diarrhea episodes.
• Evaluate for changes in swallowing ability.

Patient and family teaching
• Teach the patient and family how to monitor vital signs, weight, and fluid intake and output.
• Review energy conservation techniques and safety measures.
• Emphasize the importance of frequent repositioning to prevent skin breakdown.
• Discuss signs and symptoms to report to the physician, including increased episodes of incontinence, vomiting, diarrhea, or difficulty swallowing.
• Teach signs and symptoms of I.V. infiltration, phlebitis, and fluid overload.
• Discuss I.V. replacement therapy regimen and care.
• Advise the patient to avoid diuretics (if a contributing factor) and discuss techniques to aid in swallowing without aspiration.
• Review measures to prevent recurrence.

Interdisciplinary actions

Dietitian
• Oral fluid intake planning
• Oral rehydration measures

Enterostomal therapist
• Skin care measures
• Incontinence management

Home care aide
• Personal care (emphasizing mouth care)

- Assistance with activities of daily living
- Oral rehydration measures
- Assistance with feeding
- Energy conservation activities

Speech pathologist
- Techniques to aid in swallowing
- Aspiration prevention

Discharge plan
- Patient or caregiver management of dehydration and prevention of recurrence in the home environment in conjunction with physician
- Follow-up appointments for blood studies in an authorized laboratory
- Follow-up appointments with physician at recommended intervals
- Patient understanding and control of contributing factors
- Patient knowledge of preventive measures and signs of recurrence
- Minimal complications and death with dignity achieved

Documentation requirements
- Skilled assessment, including subjective and objective indicators of dehydration; level of orientation; swallowing ability; pattern of fluid consumption and daily fluid intake; fluid preferences; ability to meet own fluid requirements and handle fluid containers; use of laxatives or diuretics; skin integrity, turgor, texture, fragility, and temperature; condition of mucous membranes; patient's response to care; measures instituted and the effectiveness of each; changes in fluid requirements or I.V. replacement therapy orders based on results of blood studies;

elimination pattern; energy level and improvement in activity tolerance; evidence of complications (or lack thereof); patient's or caregiver's independence with care and therapy regimen, including I.V. replacement therapy; patient and caregiver instructions; safety precautions; and signs and symptoms to be reported
- Regular blood studies for serum osmolality and electrolyte levels performed and their results
- Interdisciplinary team communication
- Enterostomal therapy evaluation, need for services, and plan for treatment, including skin care measures and incontinence management
- Speech therapy evaluation, need for services, and the plan for a swallowing program in the home
- Changes in plan of care, including those directly related to results of blood studies, and the patient's understanding of those changes
- Patient's ability to maintain safety within level of fatigue
- Patient's adherence to instructions and the therapy regimen
- Patient's advance directive to withhold artificial hydration

Reimbursement reminders
- Medicare covers phlebotomy supplies.
- Many insurance companies have contracts with specific laboratories to perform blood studies; check for an authorized laboratory.
- All nonroutine supplies must be specifically ordered by the physician and entered into Locator 14 (Supplies) of Health Care Financing Administration Form 485 or ordered by the physi-

cian within the specific order for treatment requiring the use of certain supplies and entered into Locator 21 (Orders for Treatment).

• When billing for medical supplies, always include the name of the supply item, the date it was used, the number of units used, and the charge per unit.

• If skin breakdown is present, wound care performed must follow the physician orders exactly for reimbursement to occur.

• If the patient has a private insurance plan, check the requirements for in-home specialty care such as speech therapy.

Insurance hints

• Report specific progress toward goals (for example, serum electrolyte levels have been maintained at ___ for ___ number of days); changes in weight, skin turgor, mucous membranes; fluid intake and output; adjustment issues, such as patient's resistance to or acceptance of I.V. replacement therapy or instructions; and complications, such as I.V. infiltration or fluid overload, skin breakdown, or aspiration.

• Describe gains in knowledge, such as skills and concepts mastered in oral rehydration measures, swallowing, and I.V. replacement therapy.

• Present specific data on the patient's homebound status, including inability to ambulate because of severe fatigue, number of persons needed to assist patient out of a chair, continued limitation in ambulation distance, and use of a bedside commode.

• Present objective patient findings and changes since previous contacts, specifically, return of serum electrolyte levels to within normal parameters, cessation of vomiting and diarrhea, gradual weight gain, and improved skin turgor.

• Report new laboratory values and any change in clinical condition since previous contact.

• Emphasize that the next step in care is to show a progressive plan for independence, including degree of independence with I.V. replacement therapy and oral rehydration measures being used.

• Stress comorbid conditions (such as increasing age, diabetes, and chronic lung or heart disease) that would affect the patient's ability to provide self-care.

Diabetes mellitus

A metabolic disorder, diabetes mellitus (DM) is characterized by a lack of the hormone insulin or insulin resistance, which elevates the blood glucose level. In DM, the liver also inappropriately produces glucose. DM alters metabolism and can lead to abnormalities in the structure of blood vessels and nerves — conditions that cause serious complications. DM is classified into two major types: type 1 (formerly known as insulin-dependent) and type 2 (formerly known as non-insulin-dependent). Destruction of beta cells in the pancreas causes an insulin deficiency that leads to type 1. Persons with this type of DM require insulin injections. Type 2 results from the decreased ability of insulin to bind to insulin receptors on the surfaces of cells or from impaired insulin secretion. Persons with this type may be able to maintain target blood glucose levels with diet and oral medication.

Perhaps more than any other chronic disease, DM requires substantial care activity on the part of the patient or caregiver for daily management. Thus, the goal of home care is to enable the patient or caregiver to reach an optimal level of independence.

When people with DM are able to maintain nearly normal blood glucose levels, the risk of chronic complications is greatly reduced. Nutritional management is the foundation of therapy for all types of DM, although pharmacologic treatment with oral medications or insulin is indicated in most cases. Regulation of physical activity and stress management are also important components of care.

Patients receiving home care for DM can have numerous comorbid conditions and complications that impact their ability to care for themselves. Vision impairment and the effects of sensory and motor neuropathy may result in functional limitations that interfere with their ability to leave the home. Many homebound patients with DM suffer from chronic, poorly healing ulcers of the lower extremities that require aggressive treatment by a skilled nurse. (See "Diabetic foot ulcers," page 215.) In addition, the higher incidence of cardiovascular and cerebrovascular disease in this population results in more cases of cerebrovascular accident and myocardial infarction, which can further affect the ability for self-care.

Previsit checklist

Physician orders and preparation
- Dietary restrictions
- Oral medication and insulin orders as indicated
- Blood glucose monitoring, including frequency and target ranges for fasting and random results
- Laboratory blood studies, including glycosylated hemoglobin (Hb A_{1C}), chemistry panel, lipid panel, and renal function studies
- Activity orders and restrictions
- Dietitian evaluation of diet and assistance with developing meal plans
- Enterostomal therapy evaluation for wound care, if appropriate
- Podiatrist for foot and nail care
- Physical therapy evaluation for activity and exercise program
- Occupational therapy evaluation for assistance and adaptation secondary to vision impairment and functional limitations
- Social work evaluation for community resources and financial assistance for equipment, medications, and supplies
- Home care aide assistance with personal care and activities of daily living (ADLs)

Equipment and supplies
- Supplies for standard precautions and proper sharps disposal
- Blood glucose monitoring supplies, including glucose meter, test strips, lancing device and lancets, and patient logbook or diary
- Phlebotomy supplies
- Wound care supplies, if appropriate

Safety requirements
- Standard precautions for infection control and sharps disposal
- System to assist with adherence to a complex medical regimen, including insulin injections as appropriate

• Emergency plan and access to functional phone and list of emergency phone numbers

• Signs and symptoms of hyperglycemia, hypoglycemia, diabetic ketoacidosis, and hyperosmolar hyperglycemic nonketotic syndrome

• Emergency treatment measures for hypoglycemia and hyperglycemia

• Foot and skin care and sick-day measures

• Allergies verified and documented

Major diagnostic codes

• Diabetes, gestational 648.8

• Diabetes mellitus, uncomplicated 250.0

• Diabetes with:
  – hyperosmolarity 250.2
  – ketoacidosis 250.1
  – neurological complications 250.6
  – ophthalmic manifestations 250.5
  – other coma 250.3
  – other specified manifestations including hypoglycemia 250.8
  – peripheral circulatory disorders 250.7
  – renal manifestations 250.4
  – unspecified complications 250.9

(To assign a fifth digit, see appendix A, page 638.)

Defense of homebound status

• Vision impairment requiring the assistance of another person to leave the home

• Non-weight-bearing status because of neuropathic foot ulcer

• Unable to ambulate farther than 10′ (3 m) because of chronic lower extremity wound or ulcer

• Unable to ambulate farther than 10′ because of foot deformities related to diabetic neuropathy

• Erratic blood glucose levels with frequent or severe episodes of hypoglycemia, causing dizziness and syncope

Selected nursing diagnoses and patient outcomes

Knowledge deficit related to diabetes management

The patient or caregiver will:

• demonstrate or verbalize knowledge and management of diet (N, D)

• state the correct dose and time as well as adverse effects and precautions for each diabetic medication prescribed (N, PH)

• demonstrate the correct technique for drawing up insulin and administering insulin injection, including site selection and safe reuse or disposal of sharps (N, OT, PH)

• verbalize or demonstrate measures to prevent and treat hypoglycemia (N, PH, PT)

• demonstrate blood glucose monitoring and logbook technique (N, OT)

• verbalize plan for obtaining supplies after discharge (N, SW)

• perform a daily examination of feet and identify and report problems. (N, HCA, PT, PO)

Altered nutrition: More (or Less) than than body requirements related to elevated blood glucose levels

The patient or caregiver will:

• describe an appropriate meal plan for weight gain or loss (N, D)

• remain free from signs and symptoms of hypoglycemic and hyperglycemic episodes (N, D, PH)

● maintain blood glucose level within individual target range.

(N, D, PH)

Ineffective management of therapeutic regimen related to complex diabetes management program

The patient or caregiver will:

● demonstrate management of therapeutic regimen as evidenced by improved management practices (such as diet, medications, blood glucose monitoring, activity, and stress management)   (N, D, OT, PH, PT, SW)

● establish a stable body weight within acceptable parameters (N, D, HCA)

● demonstrate positive coping mechanisms to adjust to chronic nature of the disease   (N, HCA, SW)

● use available resources for support and guidance   (N, SW)

● comply with prescribed regimen as evidenced by a normal to nearly normal Hb A_{1C} level

(N, D, MD, PH)

● remain free from signs and symptoms of complications associated with uncontrolled DM.   (N, D, MD, PH)

Risk for injury related to complications associated with DM

The patient or caregiver will:

● state an understanding of the importance of keeping blood glucose level within target range

(N, D, MD, PH)

● recognize signs and symptoms of hypoglycemia and hyperglycemia quickly and take appropriate action or seek emergency treatment

(N, D, MD, PH, PT)

● demonstrate preventive care measures to use in daily living to minimize injury caused by long-term complications   (N, HCA, PT, OT)

● use services of podiatrist for foot and nail care   (N, PO, PT)

● identify potential hazards resulting from possible complications. (N, MD)

Skilled nursing services

Care measures

● Perform initial full assessment of the neurologic, integumentary (including feet), cardiovascular, GI, and genitourinary systems. Also assess nutrition and hydration status.

● Assess the level of care of the patient or caregiver.

● Observe patient techniques, such as blood glucose monitoring and insulin injection.

● Assess effectiveness of the treatment regimen by checking the patient's blood glucose level and weight, referring to the patient's logbook, or using the memory function of patient's glucose meter.

● Assess for signs and symptoms of hypoglycemia and hyperglycemia.

● Obtain or arrange for blood studies, including serum chemistry panel, lipid panel, renal studies, and Hb A_{1C}.

● Investigate complaints surrounding the signs and symptoms of hypoglycemia and hyperglycemia and measures taken.

● Monitor changes in weight.

● Perform a dietary recall (24-hour and 3-day).

● Administer insulin injections if patient and caregiver are unable to do so.

● Institute dosage adjustments based on recorded blood glucose levels as ordered.

Patient and family teaching

- Teach the patient and family about DM as a disease process.
- Discuss nutritional management for DM, including specific dietary instructions that incorporate the patient's food preferences.
- Review oral medications, including the name, purpose, dose, time, precautions, and possible adverse effects.
- Review insulin type, onset of action, dose, time, precautions, and possible adverse effects.
- Demonstrate insulin and syringe preparation, storage, and administration, including drawing single and mixed doses, injection technique, site selection, reuse and disposal of syringes, and blood glucose monitoring.
- Discuss blood testing procedures, including fingerstick and phlebotomy techniques, application of blood to test strip, and interpretation of results.
- Teach how to clean and maintain the glucose meter and how to troubleshoot technical problems.
- Discuss how to access supplies after discharge and how to safely reuse or dispose of lancets.
- Advise the patient about home safety measures, such as how to recognize and prevent hyperglycemia and hypoglycemia, injury, and infection.
- Discuss care during minor illnesses, such as cold, flu, or GI upset.
- Review foot care, including daily foot inspection, use of supportive and well-fitting socks and shoes, and the importance of identifying and attending to problems promptly.
- Review skin care, including the need to avoid temperature extremes and electric blankets.
- Promote a home exercise program and the use of assistive or adaptive devices as needed.
- Identify signs and symptoms of complications as well as signs to report to the physician.

Interdisciplinary actions

Dietitian

- Development of 12 meal plans that are acceptable to the patient and meet the patient's nutritional needs.
- Consultation for complex nutritional needs, such as carbohydrate gram counting, managing the tube-fed patient with DM, renal diets, and impaired wound healing
- Development of a weight management program

Home care aide

- Personal care and hygiene
- Assistance with ADLs
- Use of adaptive devices
- Reinforcement of teaching related to skin and foot care

Occupational therapist

- Evaluation for assistive devices
- Instruction in use of adaptive aids for self-care as indicated

Physical therapist

- Evaluation and plan for individualized home exercise program
- Muscle strengthening and improvement in endurance and functional ability secondary to peripheral neuropathy

Podiatrist

- Evaluation and management of foot problems

- Preventive care in the patient with loss of protective sensation

Social worker
- Referral to community resources and support groups for diabetics
- Counseling and referral for stress management and reduction
- Evaluation of financial status and referral for assistance with securing supplies and equipment

Discharge plan
- Self-management of disease process in home with physician and community support systems follow-up
- Discharged to self-care with return to pre-illness status
- Maintenance of Hb A_{1C} level at less than 8 on antidiabetic medication therapy and lifestyle changes
- Understanding of measures to minimize the risk of short- and long-term complications of DM
- Follow-up appointments for blood studies in an authorized laboratory
- Follow-up appointments with physician at recommended intervals
- Referral to outpatient physical therapy if indicated

Documentation requirements
- Skilled assessment, including subjective and objective data with regard to signs and symptoms of hypoglycemia or hyperglycemia; results of blood glucose monitoring; findings from nutritional assessment; significant stressors experienced by the patient; insulin administration, if applicable (type, dose, time, and site of injection); patient or caregiver participation in care; degree of independence; areas of concern or difficulty with management
- Patient or caregiver progress toward educational goals, including ability to inject insulin and monitor blood glucose level
- Demonstration and return demonstration of skills, including syringe preparation, mixing, site selection, site rotation, and use of glucose meter
- Patient response to care and comprehension of reported laboratory values and any changes in medication orders
- Evaluation of hypoglycemia and hyperglycemia, including measures to treat episodes
- Patient and caregiver instructions
- Abnormal blood glucose levels, actions taken, follow-up, and outcomes

Reimbursement reminders
- The American Diabetes Association states that the reuse of insulin syringes by people with DM is safe and practical with no significant increase in rate of infection or other complication related to syringe reuse for people who are able to self-inject and are capable of safely recapping their own needles after each use. This practice may benefit some patients financially while reducing medical waste.
- Medicare coverage for diabetes supplies is as follows: glucose monitor, one every 5 years; glucose monitor with voice synthesizer, if physician documents visual acuity of 20/200 or worse; 25 test strips every month for non-insulin-dependent patients and 100 test strips every 30 days for insulin-dependent patients (Medicare will pay for more test strips if ordered by physician; supplier may ask for copy of blood

glucose log for billing purposes); lancing device, one every 6 months; control solution to check the integrity of test strips; and battery required to operate glucose meter.

• When daily care has been ordered, goals should indicate when daily visits are expected to end (for example: "Daily visits × 2 weeks to instruct patient in blood glucose monitoring and insulin injection").

• The following services *alone* aren't considered reimbursable skilled nursing services: blood glucose monitoring, insulin injection, teaching for prevention of long-term complications and for foot care, and prefilling insulin syringes for a patient or caregiver to administer at a later time.

• Registered dietitian services aren't reimbursable under the Medicare home care benefit.

• Home visits by a podiatrist are reimbursable under Medicare if certain conditions are met.

• If the patient has a private insurance plan, clarify before the visit whether the plan will reimburse for specialty in-home services, such as visits by a dietitian and podiatrist.

• Medicare will pay for daily insulin injections as a skilled nursing service if the patient is unable to self-inject and there is no willing or able caregiver. Clear documentation is necessary as to why the patient is incapable of self-injecting and efforts made to find and teach a willing caregiver.

Insurance hints

• Note whether the patient is newly diagnosed with DM or new to insulin therapy.

• Report improved glucose control using blood glucose monitoring results and blood studies.

• Describe the patient's progress toward self-management, emphasizing both positive aspects and areas needing additional teaching or instruction. Include adjustment issues (such as patient resistance to or acceptance of insulin injections or diet) and complications (such as episodes of hypoglycemia, blood glucose still out of target range, skin breakdown, and infection).

• Describe gains in knowledge, such as skills and concepts mastered in self-management and wound care techniques (if applicable).

• Present specific data on homebound status, such as episodes of hyperglycemia or hypoglycemia decreasing (for example, to less than two times per day) and foot ulcer showing signs of granulation tissue and decreased size from _____ cm on admission to _____ cm.

• Stress comorbid conditions (such as advanced age and vision or neurosensory impairment) that would affect the patient's ability to provide self-care.

Diabetic foot ulcers

The development of most diabetic foot ulcers can be linked to distal peripheral neuropathy. Frequently, an ulcer results from minor trauma to a foot that lacks protective sensation. When unnoticed trauma occurs in the presence of impaired peripheral circulation, lesions are prevented from healing. Impaired host defenses in the person with diabetes can further complicate this sequence by greatly increasing the risk of infection.

Patients with diabetic foot ulcers that don't heal well are prevalent in the home care setting. A variety of wound care treatments, from the simple to the advanced, are available for use in the home. Protocols, guidelines, and wound care teams are frequently used by home care agencies to guide the selection of a wound care regimen.

Because skilled home nursing visits are generally periodic and intermittent, patients and their caregivers must play an active role in the management and treatment of these chronic wounds. They require instruction on the prevention of future ulcer development as well as the development of osteomyelitis. Because wound care is dynamic, treatments and visit frequency necessitate regular evaluation and adjustment. In cases where osteomyelitis has been diagnosed, the patient may begin a regimen of I.V. antibiotics in the home.

Previsit checklist

Physician orders and preparation
- Wound care and treatment orders (type of dressing, cleaning method, and frequency of change)
- Medication orders (oral agents or insulin)
- Diet orders
- Treatment of infection (if applicable), including antibiotics and blood cultures
- Blood glucose monitoring, including frequency and timing, target range, sliding scale insulin orders, and parameters for notifying physician of test results

- Laboratory blood studies, including glycosylated hemoglobin (Hb A_{1C})
- Activity orders and restrictions
- Enterostomal therapy evaluation for wound care
- Podiatrist for foot and nail care and wound care consultation
- Nutritional evaluation for diet and teaching about possible increased protein and calorie needs because of ulcer
- Physical therapy evaluation for exercise program incorporating weight-bearing limitations
- Occupational therapy evaluation for activities of daily living (ADLs) training and adaptations secondary to functional limitations imposed by ulcer
- Social work evaluation for community resources and financial assistance for equipment and supplies
- Home care aide assistance with ADLs and personal care

Equipment and supplies
- Supplies for standard precautions and proper sharps disposal
- Wound treatment and dressing supplies, including irrigating solutions, dressings, packing, and topical debridement agents
- Blood glucose monitoring supplies, including glucose meter, lancing device and lancets, and patient logbook or diary
- Phlebotomy supplies
- Camera and supplies to document wound appearance as ordered

Safety requirements
- Standard precautions for wound care, infection control, and sharps disposal

- System to assist with adherence to a complex medical regimen, including insulin injections (sliding scale) as appropriate
- Emergency plan and access to functional phone and list of emergency phone numbers
- Signs and symptoms of infection, circulatory impairment, and wound healing
- Emergency treatment measures for hyperglycemia and hypoglycemia
- Foot care and sick-day measures
- Allergies verified and documented

Major diagnostic codes

- Diabetes, type 1, uncontrolled 250.03
- Diabetes, type 2, uncontrolled 250.02
- Diabetes with peripheral circulatory disorders 250.7

(To assign a fifth digit, see appendix A, page 638.)

Defense of homebound status

- Non-weight-bearing status on lower extremity because of diabetic foot ulcer requiring restricted activities
- Vision impairment requiring the assistance of another person to leave the home
- Unable to ambulate farther than 10' (3 m) because of chronic, open lower-extremity wound or ulcer

Selected nursing diagnoses and patient outcomes

Impaired skin integrity related to the development of diabetic ulcer
The patient or caregiver will:

- exhibit signs of ulcer healing in _____ visits or weeks (N, ET, MD, PT)
- demonstrate measures to maintain skin integrity of the other extremity
  (N, ET, HCA, MD, PO, PT)
- identify nutritional needs related to ulcer (N, D, MD)
- remain free from signs and symptoms of infection and circulatory impairment on each visit (N, ET, MD, PT)
- demonstrate procedure for independent wound care by discharge.
  (N, ET)

Risk for injury related to loss of sensation to lower extremities
The patient or caregiver will:

- demonstrate measures to prevent further injury to lower extremities by discharge (N, HCA, OT, PT)
- demonstrate ability to perform examination of feet and identify reportable problems.
  (N, HCA, OT, PO, PT)

Risk for infection related to ulcer development and complications associated with diabetes mellitus
The patient or caregiver will:

- remain free from signs and symptoms of infection throughout the duration of care (N, ET, HCA, MD, PT)
- exhibit vital signs within acceptable parameters (N, ET, HCA, PT)
- demonstrate appropriate measures to prevent infection (N, ET, HCA, PT)
- identify early signs and symptoms of infection that require notification of the physician. (N, ET, HCA, PT)

Knowledge deficit related to diabetes management and ulcer care
The patient or caregiver will:

- verbalize understanding of diabetic management (N, D, MD)

- demonstrate measures to control blood glucose levels   (N, D, MD, PH)
- perform ulcer care treatment independently by discharge   (N, ET, MD)
- identify signs and symptoms to report to the physician

(N, ET, HCA, PT)
- demonstrate adherence to the plan of care and proper follow-up.

(N, D, ET, HCA, MD, OT, PO, PT, SW)

Skilled nursing services

Care measures
- Perform initial assessment of the wound, including information on location, size, and depth; presence of necrosis, sinus tracts, and odor; presence and type of exudate; condition and color of wound base; condition of surrounding tissue (warmth, erythema, crepitus, induration); and signs and symptoms of localized infection.
- Perform assessment of neurovascular status of lower extremities: extent and amount of edema, including circumference measurements and degree of pitting; skin color and temperature; capillary refill; complaints of pain, including type, onset, duration, frequency, and relief measures; presence of pulses; complaints of numbness or tingling; and evidence of muscular weakness.
- Assess for signs and symptoms of systemic infection, such as fever, chills, and generalized malaise.
- Assess blood glucose control, including patient techniques, such as blood glucose monitoring and insulin injection.
- Assess the effectiveness of the treatment regimen; check patient's blood glucose level, refer to patient's logbook,

or use memory function on the patient's glucose meter.
- Investigate complaints regarding signs and symptoms of hypoglycemia and hyperglycemia and actions taken.
- Obtain or arrange for blood studies, including a chemistry panel, complete blood count with differential, and Hb A_{1C} level.
- Perform wound care as ordered, including cleaning with normal saline solution or other nontoxic agent, applying dressing to protect the wound, keeping ulcer tissue moist and surrounding tissue dry, filling wound cavities and not putting pressure on the wound bed, and observing the patient's and caregiver's ability to perform prescribed wound care.

Patient and family teaching
- Teach the patient and family about the need to completely rest the injured part as a component for healing.
- Review signs and symptoms of infection to report promptly.
- Stress that management of blood glucose levels is essential for wound healing.
- Provide education to assist in meeting blood glucose target range.
- Discuss the importance of adequate nutrition and hydration in wound healing.
- Demonstrate wound care and treatment, if applicable.
- Teach infection-control measures, including proper disposal of soiled dressings.
- Discuss how to observe and report wound characteristics.
- Review measures to prevent future ulceration, including daily examination of feet, prompt attention to problems, selection of proper footwear, and

the need for special attention to scar tissue from healed ulcer (which may be prone to breakdown).
● Encourage regular visits to a podiatrist.

Interdisciplinary actions

Dietitian
● Evaluation for appropriate diet plan
● Consultation for complex nutritional needs and optimal diet for wound healing (may include increased fluid, protein, and calorie intake)

Enterostomal therapist
● Evaluation of wound
● Consultation for wound care regimen, including specialized products and equipment

Home care aide
● Personal care, hygiene, and nutrition assistance
● Infection-control measures
● Ambulation assistance

Occupational therapist
● Evaluation for assistive devices
● Instruction in use of adaptive aids for self-care (including foot and wound care) as indicated
● Instruction and assistance for activities of daily living with non-weight-bearing status

Physical therapist
● Mobility assessment
● Exercise program to maintain physical condition while preventing weight bearing to affected area

Podiatrist
● Evaluation for foot deformities that could predispose to ulceration
● Preventive care in the patient with loss of protective sensation
● Prescription for therapeutic footwear
● Referral to footwear specialist for construction of custom-fit shoes when prescribed

Social worker
● Referral to community resources and support groups for diabetics
● Counseling and referral for stress management and reduction
● Evaluation of financial status and referral for assistance with securing supplies and equipment
● Resources to assist with disability issues related to injury

Discharge plan
● Self-management of disease process in home with physician and community support system follow-ups
● Discharge to self-care with demonstration of independence in wound care and evidence of wound healing
● Maintenance on antidiabetic medication therapy with blood glucose levels within targeted parameters
● Understanding of measures to prevent recurrence of ulcers and further injury
● Follow-up appointments for blood studies in an authorized laboratory on own
● Follow-up appointments with physician at recommended intervals
● Referral to outpatient physical therapy if indicated

Documentation requirements

• Skilled assessment, including wound care diagnosis and any supporting diagnosis

• Wound assessment, including location (using proper anatomic terms, such as plantar or flexor, distal or proximal, and medial or lateral), dimensions (in centimeters), condition of surrounding tissue (macerated, erythematous, or indurated), condition of wound base (color and presence of slough and eschar), presence or absence of signs and symptoms of infection, and progress of healing

• Successive photographs (*Note:* The patient must sign a consent form for the wound to be photographed.)

• Current treatment and progress toward healing (if the wound isn't responding to treatment, an alternative treatment must be tried)

• Patient's or caregiver's ability or inability to perform the procedures

• Recent blood glucose results and adherence to diabetic regimen

• Patient and caregiver instructions, including procedure for wound care, signs and symptoms of healing, signs and symptoms (indicating infection or circulatory impairment) to report to the physician, dietary plan, home exercise program, infection-control and safety measures, measures to reduce the risk of complications, signs and symptoms of complications, and use of assistive or adaptive devices

Reimbursement reminders

• Long-term wound care is reimbursable under Medicare if the following is documented: The wound is complex and requires the skills of a nurse; there is regular contact with the physician regarding treatment, orders, and wound progress; and new procedures have been attempted if the wound isn't responsive to current treatment.

• Daily wound care is reimbursable under Medicare if the following is documented: Daily services are medically necessary, care can't be performed less frequently without jeopardizing the medical outcome, and there is a predictable and realistic date for ending daily services.

• Medicare reimburses the home care agency for most wound care supplies. Gloves are *not* reimbursable. Check with an agency billing department for coverage benefits of specific supplies.

• Medicare reimburses some in-home podiatry services and prescription footwear. Medicare part B covers 80% of the reasonable cost for special shoes and orthoses for patients who meet the following criteria: history of partial or complete foot amputation, history of previous foot ulcer, history of preulcerative callus, peripheral neuropathy with callus formation, foot deformity, and peripheral vascular impairment.

• For coverage of special footwear, the physician certifies that the patient has one or more of the conditions above and is being treated for diabetes. The physician or podiatrist writes a footwear prescription and a qualified dispenser (podiatrist or orthotist) constructs and fits the prescribed footwear and files the appropriate claim forms.

Insurance hints

• Present objective findings as well as changes in wound status since previous contact, including dimensions. Describe the color of the wound base and the amount of exudate being produced because these characteristics dictate the choice of treatment. Note if eschar or signs of infection are present.

• Report recent blood glucose levels and patient's adherence to the diabetic regimen.

• Describe patient adherence to mobility restrictions and non-weight-bearing status.

• Report patient's or caregiver's level of participation in wound care and treatment.

• Discuss eligibility for prescription footwear and plan for obtaining it after wound has healed.

• Stress comorbid conditions (such as advanced age and vision or neurosensory impairment) that would affect the patient's ability to provide self-care.

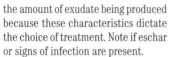

Dialysis

Dialysis is used to treat renal failure that results from a chronic, sustained loss of renal function. It involves the use of an external filter to clean the blood of by-products and to maintain blood components within normal ranges. Most symptoms of end-stage renal disease can be controlled with dialysis. However, the nurse and interdisciplinary team must continually assess the patient for signs of complications, such as infection, fluid overload, and electrolyte imbalance.

Previsit checklist

Physician orders and preparation
• Medication schedule
• Dialysis schedule, including type and frequency

• Activity orders and restrictions
• Comfort measures, including orders for analgesics
• Laboratory studies, including blood urea nitrogen (BUN) and serum electrolyte and creatinine levels as well as complete blood count (CBC)
• Wound care, including dressing type and frequency
• Physical therapy evaluation for muscle strengthening, home exercise program, and transfer training
• Medical social services evaluation for community referrals and counseling
• Home care aide assistance with activities of daily living (ADLs) and personal care

Equipment and supplies
• Supplies for standard precautions and proper sharps disposal
• Wound care supplies
• Dialysis catheter site care supplies
• Scale for weighing patient
• Dialysis equipment, including dialysate, I.V. administration set, dialyzer, sterile gloves, syringes, specimen containers, additional medications, and gauze dressings
• Phlebotomy supplies

Safety requirements
• Standard precautions for infection control and sharps disposal
• System to assist with adherence to a complex medication regimen and treatment plan
• Signs and symptoms of fluid overload and electrolyte imbalances to immediately report to the physician
• Emergency plan and access to functional phone and list of emergency phone numbers

- Instructions on signs and symptoms of medical emergency and actions to take
- Allergies verified and documented

Major diagnostic codes

- Cerebrovascular accident 436
- Decubitus ulcer 707.0
- Diabetic nephropathy 250.4
- Kidney, cystic 753.10
- Nephropathy 583.9
- Nephrosclerosis 403.9
- Renal failure, acute tubular necrosis/chronic 584.5/585
- Wound, limb lower 894.0

Defense of homebound status

- Bedridden; able to transfer from bed to chair only with assistance of two persons
- Unable to ambulate farther than 10′ (3 m) because of extreme fatigue
- Unable to ambulate because of imposed physical restrictions

Selected nursing diagnoses and patient outcomes

Fluid volume excess related to renal disease with minimal to no urine output

The patient or caregiver will:
- exhibit clear breath sounds   (N)
- demonstrate weight within acceptable parameters   (N, HCA)
- identify measures to prevent and manage fluid excess.   (N)

Risk for infection related to exposure to blood products and decreased mobility

The patient or caregiver will:
- verbalize signs and symptoms of infection to report to the physician   (N, HCA)
- state methods to prevent infection   (N, HCA)
- demonstrate a white blood cell count and differential within acceptable parameters   (N)
- demonstrate proper hand-washing and infection-control techniques.   (N, HCA)

Chronic sorrow related to progression of disease and disability

The patient or caregiver will:
- verbalize feelings of loss and sadness   (N, HCA, SW)
- focus on accomplishments of each day   (N, HCA, PT, SW)
- seek and obtain spiritual support   (N, SW)
- demonstrate optimal participation in care   (N, HCA, PT, SW)
- allow time for crying or sitting in silence and grieving over the loss of health.   (N, HCA, SW)

Death anxiety related to life-threatening complications

The patient or caregiver will:
- express concerns about dying   (N, HCA, SW)
- participate in anticipatory grieving activities such as life review (N, SW)
- consider alternatives to continued curative care in addition to hospice (when appropriate).   (N, HCA, SW)

Powerlessness related to treatment regimen and complications

The patient or caregiver will:
- participate in care planning   (N, HCA, PT)

- verbalize positive feelings about the future (N, SW)
- verbalize frustrations and anger appropriately. (N, HCA, SW)

Risk for injury related to chronic pathologic changes in all organ systems

The patient or caregiver will:
- verbalize signs and symptoms to report to the physician (N, HCA, PT)
- modify home to clear walkways and increase lighting (N, HCA, PT)
- exhibit improved strength and endurance (N, HCA, PT)
- demonstrate deep-breathing and range-of-motion exercises to maintain functional capacity. (N, HCA, PT)

Diversional activity deficit related to poor endurance and inability to maintain social contacts

The patient or caregiver will:
- describe appropriate recreational activities within mobility restrictions (N, HCA, PT)
- participate in chosen activities (N, HCA, PT)
- use community support groups, such as visiting pet therapy, church outreach, and programs for shut-ins. (N, SW)

Skilled nursing services

Care measures
- Perform initial full assessment of the cardiovascular, pulmonary, musculoskeletal, and integumentary systems; nutrition and hydration; and elimination.
- Assess care by patient and family related to dialysis procedure, ambulation, and activity.

- Assess knowledge of dangerous signs and symptoms.
- Assess the effectiveness of the treatment regimen, including trends in vital signs and weights, changes in laboratory studies, and skin integrity.
- Assess patient's coping measures and social supports that are currently in place and are effective.
- Institute dialysis as ordered.

Patient and family teaching
- Teach the patient and family the signs and symptoms of infection, fluid overload, and other complications.
- Review the medication and dialysis regimens.
- Demonstrate how to monitor vital signs, weight, and fluid intake and output.
- Discuss energy conservation and safety measures.
- Teach signs and symptoms to report to the physician.

Interdisciplinary actions

Home care aide
- Personal care
- Assistance with ADLs

Physical therapist
- Home exercise program
- Muscle strengthening
- Transfer training

Social worker
- Community referrals for independence
- Psychosocial support and coping

Discharge plan
- Return to previous level of functioning or prior status after resolution of complication
- Maintenance on dialysis with demonstrated independence with the procedure
- Follow-up appointments for blood studies in an authorized laboratory
- Follow-up appointments with physician at recommended intervals
- Complications minimized and death with dignity achieved

Documentation requirements
- Skilled assessment, including appearance, vital signs, skin and mucous membrane integrity, GI function, urine output, weight, results of blood studies, dialysis site placement and patency, site care measures, activity level, dialysis administration (type, amount, timing, dwell, and return), effectiveness of the medication regimen, evidence of complications (or lack thereof), patient's or caregiver's independence with dialysis and therapy regimen, patient's tolerance to dialysis procedure, and patient and caregiver participation in care
- Patient and caregiver instruction and progress toward educational goals
- Safety precautions, including signs and symptoms to be reported, patient's ability to maintain safety within level of fatigue, patient's adherence to instructions and therapy regimen, and patient's ability to transfer safely within limited activity
- Results of blood studies, including CBC and BUN, serum creatinine, and electrolyte levels

- Changes in plan of care, including those directly related to the results of blood studies, and the patient's or caregiver's understanding of those changes

Reimbursement reminders
- Care beyond dialysis must be clearly documented because dialysis related services aren't covered under the Medicare home care benefit.
- Don't submit a plan of care with renal disease as a primary diagnosis.

Insurance hints
- Document progress toward such goals as rehabilitation, strength, and transfer training (for example, serum electrolyte and blood glucose levels have been maintained at ___ level for ___ days). Report changes in the patient's weight, skin turgor, mucous membranes, and intake and output; adjustment issues, such as the patient's resistance to or acceptance of enteral nutrition therapy or instructions; and complications, such as nausea, vomiting, diarrhea, infection, fluid overload, and skin breakdown.
- Present specific data on homebound status, including inability to ambulate because of severe fatigue from malnutrition or cachexia, number of persons needed to assist patient out of bed, and continued limitation in ambulation distance.
- Present objective patient findings and changes since previous contact, including maintenance of BUN, serum creatinine, and electrolyte levels within normal parameters; fluid intake and output measurements; and trends in weight.
- Describe coping behaviors and mental outlook.

- Describe gains in knowledge, such as increasing independence with dialysis procedure, weight monitoring, injury prevention, and signs and symptoms of complications.
- Report new laboratory findings that change the plan of care.
- Stress comorbid conditions (such as increasing age, diabetes, and chronic lung or heart disease) that would affect the patient's ability to provide self-care.

Elder care

With the steady increase in population, there are more and more older adults who need care. The elderly are the most common population serviced through home care. Elder care in the home typically involves providing care for the patient with a range of diagnoses resulting from the increased incidence of chronic disease coupled with age-related changes. The home care needs also span a wide range, depending on a patient's individual needs. Commonly, diagnoses include such disorders as osteoporosis, osteoarthritis, cancer, heart disease, and hypertension as well as cognitive disorders such as Alzheimer's disease. Skilled care typically addresses such situations as impaired mobility, altered nutrition, safety, and medications.

Previsit checklist

Physician orders and preparation
- Medications, including pain medications and cardiotonics, and schedule as indicated
- Activity orders and restrictions

- Diet
- Physical therapy evaluation for therapeutic exercise, range of motion (ROM), and ambulation (gait training)
- Occupational therapy evaluation for activities of daily living (ADLs) and assistive devices
- Medical social work evaluation for financial assistance, placement, and community resources
- Home care aide assistance with personal care and ADLs

Equipment and supplies
- Supplies for standard precautions and proper sharps disposal
- Pulse oximeter for patients with alterations in cardiopulmonary function
- Bedside commode
- Ambulation aids

Safety requirements
- System to assist with adherence to a complex medication regimen
- Information on medications, including dosage, adverse effects, interactions, allergies, and safe storage
- Emergency plan and access to functional phone and list of emergency phone numbers
- Emergency response system (if patient lives alone)
- Identification and correction of environmental hazards and patient-specific concerns (for example, adequate lighting, bath rails and grab bars, and no loose scatter rugs)
- Standard precautions for infection control and sharps disposal
- Availability of support people in case of emergency
- Signs and symptoms to immediately report to the physician

Major diagnostic codes
- Alzheimer's disease 331.0
- Cardiovascular disease, unspecified 429.2
- Chronic ischemic heart disease, unspecified 414.9
- Congestive heart failure 428.0
- Dementia of the Alzheimer's type:
  - uncomplicated 290.0
  - with delirium 290.3
  - with delusions 290.20
- Hypertension with congestive heart failure 402.01
- Left-sided heart failure 428.1
- Osteoarthritis 715.9
- Osteoporosis, generalized 733.00
- Osteoporosis, postmenopausal 733.01
- Senile dementia, not otherwise specified 290.0
- Senile osteoporosis 733.01

(See also specific types of cancer for appropriate diagnostic codes.)

Defense of homebound status
- Delusions and propensity for violent outbursts
- Weakness and fatigue from progressive malnutrition and skin breakdown
- Unable to ambulate farther than 6' (1.8 m) due to range of joint motion limitation, loss of bone mass, and wasting of muscles and connective tissues
- Unable to ambulate farther than 6' because of kyphosis, lordosis, and spinal compression
- Unable to ambulate farther than 10' (3 m) because of fatigue, dyspnea, or unsteady gait
- Bedridden or out-of-bed assistance required

Selected nursing diagnoses and patient outcomes

Altered thought processes related to memory loss, brain dysfunction, sleep deprivation, and cognitive impairment

The patient or caregiver will:
- comply with medication regimen (N)
- respond to name and family members (N, HCA)
- discuss increasing forgetfulness (N)
- participate in care to extent possible. (N, HCA, OT, PT)

Impaired physical mobility related to pain and swelling of joints caused by disease process (or dyspnea)

The patient or caregiver will:
- rest affected joints during periods of inflammation by splinting and cushioning (N, HCA, PT)
- relieve affected joints by using raised toilet seats, wheeled carts, built-up handles on utensils, and long-handled shoe horns and pick-up forceps (N, HCA, OT, PT)
- apply ice or heat to relieve pain and swelling as ordered (N, HCA, PT)
- continue prescribed medication regimen (N, MD, PH)
- demonstrate energy conservation measures (N, HCA, OT, PT)
- demonstrate an increase in ambulation distance by 1' to 2' (0.3 to 0.6 m) with reports of less fatigue each week (N, HCA, PT)
- institute safety measures to prevent injury related to falling and impaired mobility. (N, HCA, PT)

Chronic pain related to degenerative changes in joints, bones, and muscles

The patient or caregiver will:

• use medication, positioning, braces or other supports and other pain management techniques to achieve relief
(N, HCA, OT, PT)
• verbalize a decrease in pain to tolerable levels as evidenced by rating pain at 3 or less on a 0-to-10 scale 80% of the time   (N, OT, PT)
• demonstrate improved tolerance of physical activity with minimal fatigue, weakness, or discomfort each week.
(N, HCA, OT, PT)

Self-care deficit (specify) related to current condition and age-related changes impacting functional ability
The patient or caregiver will:
• participate in care activities with assistance from support people and community resources as appropriate
(N, HCA, SW)
• return to pre-illness level of functioning with minimal limitations.
(N, OT, PT)

Impaired home maintenance management related to illness and decrease in functional ability
The patient or caregiver will:
• identify areas of deficiencies and appropriate resources for assistance
(N, SW)
• use additional support and community resources   (N, SW)
• demonstrate ability to manage home situation with minimal assistance before discharge.   (N, OT, PT, SW)

Knowledge deficit related to new medication regimen and prescribed dietary and activity restrictions
The patient or caregiver will:
• demonstrate understanding of medication regimen as evidenced by adherence to the schedule   (N, PH)

• verbalize potential adverse effects related to medication therapy (N, PH)
• state signs and symptoms to report to the physician   (N, PH)
• identify areas of imposed restrictions
(N, OT, PT)
• demonstrate adherence to imposed restrictions.   (N, D, OT, PH, PT)

Caregiver role strain related to increased demands of patient care and patient's decreased functional level
The caregiver will:
• identify times when extra assistance is needed   (N, SW)
• use appropriate resources for additional help   (N, SW)
• demonstrate a plan for respite care
(N, SW)
• verbalize a decrease in episodes of feeling overwhelmed by discharge.
(N, SW)

Skilled nursing services

Care measures
• Perform initial assessment of all systems, focusing on the neurologic (including mental and cognitive status), GI (including nutrition and hydration), musculoskeletal, integumentary, and genitourinary systems.
• Assess level of care ability of patient or caregiver for dressing and grooming, measures to minimize socially unacceptable behavior and wandering, adherence to medication regimen, and appropriate dietary regimen.
• Assess the effectiveness of the treatment regimen, including nutrient and fluid intake, ROM, cognitive status, and signs and symptoms of adverse reactions to medications.

Patient and family teaching

- Teach the patient and family strategies for coping with wandering, delusions, dementia, and agitation for patient with cognitive problems.
- Review measures for care and reorientation.
- Discuss the medication regimen, including purpose, actions, adverse effects, precautions, dosage, food and drug interaction, and safe storage.
- Explain pain-management techniques, joint and skin protection measures, fluid intake needs, and safety precautions in the home.
- Identify signs and symptoms to report to the physician.
- Promote use of assistive devices, if indicated.
- Encourage use of community resources, if indicated.

Interdisciplinary actions

Home care aide

- Personal care and hygiene
- Assistance with ADLs
- Use of adaptive devices

Occupational therapist

- Evaluation for assistive devices
- Instruction in use of adaptive and assistive devices for self-care as indicated
- Instruction in ADLs and energy conservation

Physical therapist

- Home exercise program and therapeutic and ROM exercises
- Gait training and ambulation
- Safety measures in ambulation
- Pain-management techniques
- Muscle strengthening and improvement in endurance and functional ability secondary to peripheral neuropathy
- Transfer techniques

Psychiatric clinical nurse specialist

- Evaluation of cognitive status
- Instruction in measures to decrease incidence of anxiety, depression, and frustration in patients with Alzheimer's disease

Social worker

- Referral to community resources and support groups for people with dementia (such as Alzheimer's) as appropriate
- Counseling and referral for stress management or reduction and respite care
- Financial evaluation and referral for assistance

Discharge plan

- Maintenance of maximum functional capacity within limits of disease safely in the home with community resources and physician follow-up
- Referral to community resources such as adult day-care services
- Pain- and symptom-free until death (death with dignity)

Documentation requirements

- Medication regimen compliance and titration results, including clinical effectiveness in improving patient's condition
- Safety concerns and interventions
- Family and patient interactions and teaching

- Physical assessment findings
- Cognitive status, including short and long-term memory loss, disorientation, and coping strategies
- Vital signs
- Medication and dietary adjustments and response to treatment
- Hydration and nutrition status
- Location, frequency, and intensity of pain and measures used for relief
- Condition of skin, including areas around braces or devices, skin changes, including objective description of color and turgor as well as size, appearance, and location of any breakdown; and measures to prevent or treat breakdown
- Changes in medication orders, including dose, route, and frequency
- Pain-management techniques and their effectiveness
- ROM exercise, body alignment, and lifting or pulling restrictions

Reimbursement reminders

- Emergency telephone response systems aren't covered by Medicare, even though they're usually warranted for the elderly, especially those who live alone.
- Keep in mind that documentation must reflect the patient's condition; all interventions and instructions provided to the patient; the patient's and family's response to and understanding of interventions, instructions, and notifications; coordination among the disciplines providing patient care through the agency; and plan for follow-up care or discharge from the agency. Medicare doesn't pay for ongoing debilitation; progress toward goals must be demonstrated.

- Emphasize exacerbation of a chronic illness or recent changes, such as a new medication regimen or dramatic change in functional level, that causes the patient to require care.
- Reflect the patient's continuing need for care.
- Document specific skilled care provided and how it relates to the diagnosis and plan of care.
- Justify the need to repeat instructions or reinstruct the patient.
- Refer to the plan of care and the patient's progress toward outcomes identified in the plan.
- Stress comorbid conditions (such as advanced age, diabetes, and chronic lung or heart disease) that would affect the patient's ability to provide self-care.

Insurance hints

- Present objective data about homebound status and patient findings. Use quantifiable terms, such as the distance the patient is able to ambulate, a pain rating, muscle strength measurements, or specific safety hazards. Specify how skilled care is needed.
- Objectively describe changes in the patient, both positive and negative, since previous contact.
- Report new laboratory values and changes in clinical condition since previous contact.
- Present specifics about the patient education process; identify specific barriers that interfere with teaching.

Enema administration

Enemas are commonly used to clean the lower bowel in preparation for diagnostic or surgical procedures, to relieve distention and promote expulsion of flatus, to lubricate the rectum and colon, and to soften hardened stool for removal. They shouldn't be administered to patients who have recently undergone rectal or colon surgery or experienced a myocardial infarction or to those who have abdominal conditions of unknown cause. Enemas should be administered cautiously to homebound patients with arrhythmias.

Administration of an enema involves instilling a solution into the rectum and colon; peristalsis is stimulated by mechanical distention of the colon and stimulation of rectal wall nerves. In a retention enema, the patient holds the solution within the rectum or colon for 30 minutes to 1 hour. In an irrigating enema, the patient expels the solution almost completely within 15 minutes. Typically, a home care patient requires an enema because of poor nutrition or hydration, decreased GI mobility, or a decrease in mobility.

Previsit checklist

Physician orders and preparation
- Specific type of enema to be administered
- Frequency of enema administration

Equipment and supplies
- Supplies for standard precautions
- Prescribed solution and enema administration bag with attached rectal

tube and clamp or prepackaged disposable enema set
- Bath thermometer
- Gloves
- Disposable underpads or bath towel and plastic trash bag
- Blanket
- Bedside commode or covered bedpan
- Water-soluble lubricant
- Toilet tissue
- Plastic bag for equipment disposal
- Soap and water
- Washcloth

Safety requirements
- Standard precautions for infection control
- Safety measures to prevent falls
- Prearranged signal for displaying evidence of distress
- For tap-water enema, warm (rather than hot) solution
- Allergies verified and documented

Major diagnostic codes
- Enema, transanal, for cause other than impacted feces 96.39
- Enema for removal of impacted feces 96.38

Disorders possibly warranting an order for an enema:
- Constipation 564.0
- Impaction of the intestine, unspecified 560.30

Defense of homebound status
- Unable to ambulate farther than 10′ (3 m) because of prescribed or functional immobility
- Bedridden or confined to wheelchair

- Assistance of one or two persons needed to ambulate

Selected nursing diagnoses and patient outcomes

Constipation related to immobility
The patient will:
- tolerate enema administration without difficulty and retain the solution for the time indicated (N)
- exhibit positive results such as immediate evacuation (N)
- regain and maintain normal bowel elimination pattern. (N)

Knowledge deficit related to management of long-term constipation
The patient or caregiver will:
- verbalize the importance of a high-fiber diet (N)
- verbally contract to drink at least 2,000 ml of fluid daily (N)
- ambulate to the extent of his ability (N)
- identify factors that resulted in the need for an enema (N)
- state measures to prevent future need for enema administration. (N)

Skilled nursing services

Care measures
- Perform initial full assessment of all systems, focusing on the cardiovascular, GI, and musculoskeletal systems; identify bowel elimination patterns.
- Assess level of care of patient or caregiver related to adherence to high-fiber diet, level of mobility, and food and fluid intake.
- Record time of last bowel movement and stool characteristics.

- Administer enema as ordered.
- Assess the effectiveness of the treatment regimen.
- Note amount, consistency, and color of stool returned.
- Monitor for signs and symptoms of continuing constipation.
- Note the patient's tolerance of the procedure, including any relaxation techniques used.

Patient and family teaching
- Teach the patient and family the type of enema required and the steps involved in administering it.
- Discuss ways in which the patient can express discomfort during the procedure.
- Teach the patient and family how to prepare and administer an enema using Sims' position.
- Discuss relaxation techniques that can be used to enhance the enema's effectiveness.
- Review measures to prevent constipation, including regular exercise, dietary modification, and adequate fluid intake.

Interdisciplinary actions

Home care aide
- Personal care and hygiene
- Assistance with activities of daily living
- Assistance with nutrition

Discharge plan
- Safe management of constipation or enema administration in the home with physician follow-up services
- Independence with enema administration

Documentation requirements

- Skilled assessment
- Subjective and objective data with regard to signs and symptoms of constipation, date and time of enema administration, special equipment used, type and amount of solution and retention time, approximate amount returned and characteristics of return (color, consistency, abnormalities), patient's tolerance of procedure, and patient's and caregiver's response
- Communication with the physician
- Patient and caregiver instructions, including diet, fluid, and activity requirements to prevent recurrence and the procedure for enema self-administration or caregiver administration

Reimbursement reminders

- Disposable underpads and teaching for prevention of constipation aren't reimbursable by Medicare.
- Document any variance to expected outcomes, such as inadequate return of stool and excessive discomfort.
- Document the time of the patient's last bowel movement and specific factors that contributed to the need for enema administration.

Insurance hints

- Present objective data about homebound status.
- Report objective patient findings and changes since last contact.
- Describe the condition of the patient before and after enema administration.
- Report any difficulties with retaining enema or using bathroom, commode, or bedpan.

Enteral nutrition therapy

Enteral feedings (synonymous with tube feedings) may provide a patient with all or part of his nutritional intake. Many medical conditions — such as cancer of the mouth, throat, stomach, or intestines; amyotrophic lateral sclerosis; or the patient's inability to chew or swallow from disease conditions — may necessitate enteral nutrition therapy. Maintenance of skin and mucous membrane integrity, meeting energy demands, and other body system functions depend on nutritional intake. Various enteral feeding solutions are available to assist with special needs or body demands. The enteral feeding can be administered through various tubes, such as nasogastric or percutaneous endoscopy gastrostomy (PEG), to meet the client's needs. Patient teaching and support are most important with successful administration of enteral nutrition therapy in the home.

Previsit checklist

Physician orders and preparation

- Blood glucose and serum electrolyte levels
- Record of weights
- Calorie needs
- Enteral feeding: type (bolus, gravity, or continuous), solution, amount, and frequency
- Medications and administration schedule
- Activity orders and restrictions

- Dietitian evaluation of patient's dietary and fluid intake, including calorie allotment
- Enterostomal therapy evaluation for enteral tube site care, if indicated
- Speech therapy evaluation for difficulty swallowing
- Medical social worker evaluation for financial assistance and equipment securement
- Home care aide assistance with personal care, nutrition, and ambulation
- Order for skilled nursing visits to evaluate tube problems as needed

Equipment and supplies

- Supplies for standard precautions and proper sharps disposal
- Enteral feeding supplies, including pump, syringe, solution, and mixing container
- Phlebotomy supplies
- Scale
- Feeding site care supplies, including dressings, peroxide, and tape

Safety requirements

- Standard precautions for infection control and sharps disposal
- System to assist with adherence to a complex medication regimen, including enteral nutrition therapy
- Activity restrictions
- Information on medications, including dosage, adverse effects, interactions, and safe storage
- Action plan for assessing and managing intolerance and tube dislodgment
- Emergency plan and access to functional phone and list of emergency phone numbers
- Identification and correction of environmental hazards and patient-specific concerns (for example, working electricity with grounded electrical receptacle for pump)
- Availability and access to other foods and fluids
- Information on signs and symptoms of adverse effects of enteral feedings
- Aspiration precautions (if swallowing difficulties are present)

Major diagnostic codes

- Enteral infusion of concentrated nutrition (includes nasogastric tube insertion) 96.6
- Gastrostomy (other than PEG) 43.19
- PEG tube insertion 43.11

Other diagnostic codes for conditions possibly warranting enteral nutrition therapy:
- Cachexia 799.4
- Dehydration 276.5
- Malnutrition, mild/moderate 263.1/ 263.0
- Nutrition, deficient:
  – due to insufficient food 994.2
  – due to lack of care (neglect) 995.84
  – unspecified 269.9
- Swallowing difficulty 787.2

Defense of homebound status

- Unable to transfer without maximum assistance
- Unable to ambulate farther than 10′ (3 m) because of weakness or fatigue from impaired nutritional status
- Unable to leave home because of need for continuous tube feedings

Selected nursing diagnoses and outcomes

Altered nutrition: Less than body requirements related to need for enteral feedings to meet nutritional requirements

The patient or caregiver will:
• describe appropriate technique for delivering enteral feedings   (N, D)
• remain free from diarrhea, nausea, vomiting, abdominal discomfort and distention, and high residual returns
(N, HCA)
• demonstrate an absence of signs and symptoms of aspiration, electrolyte imbalance, and hyperglycemia
(N, HCA, SP)
• maintain prescribed nutritional requirements   (N, D)
• achieve a target weight of __ lb
(N, D, HCA)
• demonstrate measures to minimize risk of aspiration.   (N, D, HCA, SP)

Risk for infection related to changes in the immune system and different osmotic concentration enteral feedings

The patient or caregiver will:
• remain free from signs and symptoms of infection, including temperature elevation, chills, malaise, erythema, and leukocytosis   (N, HCA)
• verbalize understanding of handwashing and clean techniques with enteral feeding administration.   (N)

Risk for fluid volume excess or deficit related to rate of enteral feeding

The patient or caregiver will:
• exhibit moist, pink mucous membranes; continued level of consciousness; and electrolyte levels within normal limits   (N, MD)
• maintain weight and urine output balance consistent with intake of enteral feeding.   (N, D, HCA, MD)

Risk for impaired skin integrity related to changes in nutritional intake and enteral tube insertion

The patient or caregiver will:
• remain free from skin breakdown
(N, ET, HCA)
• demonstrate measures to prevent skin breakdown   (N, ET, HCA)
• exhibit a clean, dry enteral tube insertion site.   (N, ET, HCA)

Knowledge deficit related to unfamiliarity with enteral feeding administration

The patient or caregiver will:
• demonstrate proper procedure for enteral feeding: preparing and storing solutions, adding to feeding tube, managing infusion pump, and caring for the feeding tube and site   (N)
• identify measures to assess, interpret, and adjust the regimen per the patient's status (such as high residual volumes or a dislodged tube)   (N)
• verbalize understanding of how to obtain enteral feedings and supplies
(N, SW)
• identify a resource person who is available to assist with the management of enteral feedings.   (N, SW)

Skilled nursing services

Care measures
• Perform initial full assessment of the integumentary (including mucous membranes), neurologic (including mental and cognitive status), GI (including nutrition and hydration), gen-

itourinary, cardiovascular, and respiratory systems.

• Assess the ability of the patient or caregiver to prepare and administer enteral feedings and properly store and dispose of supplies.

• Assess for signs and symptoms of absorption alterations, including residuals, tolerance of medications through tube, stool patterns, weight changes, and skin and hair changes.

• Institute enteral nutrition therapy as ordered and evaluate for effectiveness.

• Assess daily intake and output.

• Inspect skin, including mucous membranes and areas over bony prominences and at tube insertion site, and assess skin turgor.

• Evaluate weight trends weekly or as prescribed.

• Assess frequency of vomiting and diarrhea episodes.

• Evaluate for changes in swallowing ability.

• Obtain or arrange for measurement of blood glucose and serum electrolyte levels as ordered.

Patient and family teaching

• Teach the patient and family how to monitor and record vital signs, weight, and intake and output.

• Review energy conservation and safety measures.

• Discuss the signs and symptoms to report to the physician, such as vomiting, diarrhea, abdominal distention, high residuals, and difficulty swallowing or breathing.

• Demonstrate skin care at site of tube entry.

• Discuss the signs and symptoms of enteral tube feeding problems, including possible fluid overload, tube

dislodgement, infection, and electrolyte imbalance.

• Review the enteral nutrition therapy regimen and associated care.

• Teach the patient and family about measures to maintain the patient's weight.

Interdisciplinary actions

Dietitian
• Calorie allotment
• Menu planning

Enterostomal therapist
• Tube site care measures
• Site management

Home care aide
• Personal care
• Assistance with activities of daily living
• Oral intake measures and oral care
• Assistance with oral feeding, if appropriate
• Energy conservation activities

Social worker
• Evaluation for financial assistance
• Assistance with supply and equipment securement

Speech pathologist
• Techniques to aid in swallowing
• Aspiration prevention

Discharge plan
• Safe management of administration of enteral feedings in the home with physician follow-up services
• Follow-up appointments for blood studies in an authorized laboratory

• Follow-up appointments with physician at recommended intervals

Documentation requirements

• Skilled assessment, including appearance; vital signs; skin and mucous membrane integrity; GI function, including bowel sounds and bowel elimination patterns; adequate urine output; weights; tube site placement and patency; tube site care measures; and activity level
• Enteral feeding administration (type, amount, timing, residuals, and tube type)
• Patient and caregiver participation in care
• Patient and caregiver instructions and progress toward educational goals
• Patient's tolerance of enteral nutrition therapy and response to care
• Evidence of complications (or lack thereof)
• Patient's or caregiver's independence with care and therapy regimen
• Safety precautions, particularly signs and symptoms to be reported
• Blood studies, particularly blood glucose and serum electrolyte levels
• Interdisciplinary team communication
• Enterostomal therapy evaluation, need for services, and plan for treatment, including site care measures and management
• Speech pathologist evaluation and need for services; plan for swallowing program in home
• Changes in plan of care, including those directly related to results of blood studies and patient or caregiver understanding of those changes

• Patient's ability to maintain safety within level of fatigue
• Patient's adherence to instructions and therapy regimen
• Variances to expected outcomes, such as fluid overload and high residuals
• Barriers to learning, such as physical deformities, vision impairment, and unavailability of support person

Reimbursement reminders

• Nutritional solutions are usually covered only if they're the patient's sole source of nutrition.
• Coverage of enteral feeding pumps depends on the individual patient's diagnosis, but they're usually covered for feedings that are administered by way of gastrostomy or nasogastric tubes.
• Registered dietitian services aren't reimbursable under Medicare except for certain conditions.
• If patient has a private insurance plan, all care must be preauthorized. In-home specialty services, such as those of a speech pathologist and dietitian, may not be covered.
• Obtain a telephone order for any plan of care change and document in chart.

Insurance hints

• Report specific progress toward goals (for example, serum electrolyte and blood glucose levels have been maintained at ___ levels for ___ days). Identify changes in weight, skin turgor, mucous membranes, and intake and output; adjustment issues, such patient resistance to and acceptance of enteral nutrition therapy and instructions; and complications, such as nausea, vomiting, diarrhea, fluid overload, skin breakdown, and aspiration.

- Describe gains in knowledge, specifically skills and concepts mastered in enteral feeding measures and swallowing.
- Present specific data on homebound status, such as inability to ambulate because of severe fatigue from malnutrition or cachexia.
- Present objective patient findings and changes since last contact: return of blood glucose or serum electrolyte levels to within normal parameters, decrease in high residual amounts, improved skin turgor, weight gains since home care, projected weight gain, and percentage of ideal body weight.
- Report any new laboratory findings that change the plan of care.
- Stress any comorbid conditions (such as advanced age, diabetes, and chronic lung or heart disease) that would affect the patient's ability to provide self-care.

Exercises, range-of-motion

Range-of-motion (ROM) exercises are a comprehensive set of movements aimed at maintaining joint flexibility and mobility. They're an essential component of a patient's rehabilitation plan because they significantly contribute to the quality of life by maintaining joint function. Generally, each motion is repeated a minimum of five times. ROM can be done on all joints of the body, including the neck, shoulders, elbows, wrists, forearms, fingers, toes, hips, knees, and ankles. ROM exercise therapy isn't usually considered a skilled nursing or rehabilitative service. It would be a covered benefit only

in conjunction with a more comprehensive plan of care.

Previsit checklist

Physician orders and preparation
- Rehabilitation orders and team notes
- Mobility and activity restrictions
- Physical therapy evaluation for rehabilitation potential, therapeutic exercises, gait retraining, and restoration of function
- Home care aide assistance with personal care and activities of daily living (ADLs)

Equipment and supplies
- Supplies for standard precautions
- Adaptive or assistive equipment as indicated

Safety requirements
- Emergency plan and access to functional phone and list of emergency phone numbers
- Identification and correction of environmental hazards and patient-specific concerns related to functional limitations and activity restrictions (for example, clear walkways, nightlight, and removal of some furniture to accommodate adaptive equipment)
- Standard precautions for infection control

Major diagnostic codes
Note: Home care nurses should be aware of the need to clarify the patient's primary diagnosis for each episode of home care. The diagnosis on the plan of care should reflect the care being given to the patient. The diagnosis must

support rehabilitative or skilled nursing care needs.

- Arthritis, rheumatoid/unspecified 714.0/716.9
- Contracture, ankle or foot 718.47
- Effusion or swelling of joint, unspecified 719.00
- Osteoporosis:
  - generalized, unspecified 733.00
  - idiopathic 733.02
  - postmenopausal 733.01
- Pain, thoracic spine/low back 724.1/724.2
- Pain in multiple joints 719.49
- Pain with radicular and visceral spine 724.4

(To assign a fifth digit, see appendix A, page 638.)

Defense of homebound status

- Activity intolerance as evidenced by inability to ambulate farther than 10′ (3 m) without assistance or difficulty
- Unable to ambulate farther than 10′ without increased pain or fatigue
- Bedridden or confined to wheelchair
- Unsafe ambulation unless assisted by two persons
- Unable to transfer from bed to chair without significant worsening of pain and fatigue

Selected nursing diagnoses and patient outcomes

Knowledge deficit related to restorative exercise program

The patient or caregiver will:
- verbalize knowledge of how to use a walker or wheelchair   (N, HCA, PT)
- demonstrate full ROM in affected extremities   (N, HCA, PT)

- demonstrate proper posture when ambulating.   (N, HCA, PT)

Chronic pain related to degenerative changes in joints

The patient or caregiver will:
- verbalize measures for relief of pain   (N, PH, PT)
- exhibit optimal movement after institution of pain-relief measures   (N, HCA, PT)
- use adjuvant pain therapy properly for bone pain, including anti-inflammatory medication   (N, PH, PT)
- verbalize methods of preventing effects of analgesic use   (N, PT)
- report satisfaction with sleep pattern   (N, HCA)
- identify a nonpharmacologic method of pain relief   (N, PT)
- participate in home exercise program   (N, HCA, PT)
- verbalize understanding that rehabilitative exercises, such as ROM exercises, can decrease pain.   (N, PT)

Impaired physical mobility related to pain and limited motion because of inflamed joints

The patient or caregiver will:
- remain free from joint contractures   (N, HCA, PT)
- display no evidence of muscle spasms   (N, HCA, PT)
- perform at expected level of independent care   (N, HCA, PT)
- maintain functional mobility and ROM   (N, HCA, PT)
- achieve optimal functional independence   (N, HCA, PT)
- complete a home exercise program   (N, HCA, PT)
- express satisfaction with improvement in mobility   (N, HCA, PT)

• maintain activity within prescribed limitations.   (N, HCA, PT)

Activity intolerance related to prolonged bed rest and subsequent fatigue
  The patient or caregiver will:
• participate in the prescribed activity program   (N, HCA, PT)
• verbalize the need to increase activity gradually   (N, HCA, PT)
• demonstrate progressive tolerance to activity.   (N, HCA, PT)

Self-care deficit related to limited joint mobility and decreased muscle strength
  The patient or caregiver will:
• exhibit evidence of personal hygiene and cleanliness   (N, HCA)
• participate in care measures with assistance   (N, HCA, PT)
• return to pre-illness level of care functioning by discharge. (N, HCA, PT)

Skilled nursing services

Care measures
• Perform initial full assessment of all systems with emphasis on musculoskeletal system.
• Assess degree of joint limitations and muscle strength.
• Evaluate level of activity tolerance.
• Assess care for patient and family related to limited mobility and function.
• Assess the effectiveness of and adherence to the treatment regimen.

Patient and family teaching
• Teach the patient and family ways to prevent patient injury.
• Review safety measures and pain-control techniques.

• Promote performance of ROM exercises.
• Encourage use of assistive devices, if needed.

Interdisciplinary actions

Home care aide
• Personal care and hygiene
• Assistance with ADLs

Physical therapist
• Home exercise program
• Gait training
• Muscle strengthening
• Restoration of functional capacity

Discharge plan
• Return to pre-illness functional level and routine after recovery from acute exacerbation of current condition
• Follow-up appointments with physician at recommended intervals
• Referral for continuation of physical therapy on outpatient basis

Documentation requirements
• Skilled assessment, including the patient's response to care; pain-control measures and effectiveness of each used; functional losses or gains in objective terms, such as distance walked with walker or wheelchair; plan to improve patient function when progress stalls; patient's motivation for improved joint flexibility; and long-term needs of the patient, including suitability of residence and presence of a caregiver
• Patient and caregiver instructions, including exercise program, ambula-

tion, muscle strengthening, safety measures, and assistive devices

Reimbursement reminders

• The need for ROM exercises doesn't make a patient homebound; be clear about functional limitations and the patient's ability to benefit from a rehabilitative plan of care.
• Demonstrate coordination of care with rehabilitation services.
• Medicare doesn't cover conditions that are essentially "debilitation"; patient must show continued progress toward goals. When progress has plateaued, patient is custodial and should be discharged.
• If osteoporosis is the primary diagnosis, care episode should be brief.

Insurance hints

• Describe progressive levels of care (dressing, toileting, bathing, and grooming) and ability, including use of adaptive equipment.
• Describe adjustment issues, such as the patient's resistance to or acceptance of imposed activity restrictions.
• Identify rehabilitation potential.
• Describe progress toward rehabilitation goals, such as safe use of stairs and transfers from sitting to standing.
• List collaborative plan of care for all team members who provide services.
• Compare and contrast the role of each rehabilitation team member, including the need for each member's care.
• Discuss long-term needs, including possible placement issues.
• Describe comorbid conditions (such as diabetes and chronic lung or heart disease) that would affect the patient's

ability to provide self-care or achieve maximum functional level.

Fall prevention

Although a fall can occur at any age, falling and the resulting injury is one of the leading causes of death in the elderly. Because the environment is less controlled in the home setting than in an acute or long-term care facility, the patient's risk of falling increases, especially if he or she is elderly, frail, or lives alone. Safety in the home environment is key.

Conditions that predispose a patient to falls include neurosensory deficits (including mental and cognitive problems), unsteady gait, poor posture, vertigo, weakness, orthostatic hypotension, and history of a fall. These conditions result from specific disorders, age-related changes, or both. In addition, episodes of near falling — when balance is lost but no fall has occurred — increase the patient's risk of falling. Many patients also have a fear of falling.

Previsit checklist

Physician orders and preparation

• Durable medical equipment orders
• Activity orders and restrictions
• Medications and administration schedule
• Physical therapy evaluation for therapeutic exercise, range of motion (ROM), transfer and ambulation (gait training), and assistive devices
• Occupational therapy evaluation for activities of daily living (ADLs) and assistive devices

• Social work evaluation for financial assistance and community resources
• Home care aide assistance with personal care and ADLs

Equipment and supplies
• Supplies for standard precautions and proper sharps disposal
• Penlight or flashlight for neuro-checks
• Pulse oximetry if poor oxygenation is a possibility
• Phlebotomy supplies
• Assistive or adaptive devices

Safety requirements
• Correct and safe use of adaptive devices (cane, walker, or wheelchair)
• System to assist with adherence to a complex medication regimen
• Allergies verified and documented
• Emergency plan and access to functional phone and list of emergency phone numbers
• Emergency response system if patient lives alone
• Identification and correction of environmental hazards and patient-specific concerns (for example, adequate lighting in the home, including night-lights in bedroom and bathroom; safe flooring [no throw rugs or loose tiles]; walkways free from clutter; secure handrails and grab bars; nonskid mat in the bathtub; stairways well lit and in good condition)
• Standard precautions for infection control and sharps disposal
• Signs and symptoms to immediately report to the physician

Major diagnostic codes
• Injury not otherwise specified (NOS), multiple 959.8
• Medication, adverse effects, unspecified 995.2
• Orthostatic hypotension 458.0
• Osteoarthritis 715.9
• Osteoporosis, generalized 733.00
• Syncope and collapse 780.2
• Trauma, complication (early) other specified 958.8
• Tremors NOS 781.0
• Vertigo NOS 780.4
• Visual disturbance, unspecified 368.10
• Visual loss, unspecified 369.9
• Walking difficulty 781.9
• Weakness, generalized 780.7

Defense of homebound status
• Severely restricted activity (restricted to one floor of the home)
• Unsafe for ambulation without assistance of support person
• Usual activity level restricted because of constant severe pain
• Limited activity level due to orthopedic device; assistance required to transfer from bed to chair; or confined to wheelchair
• Unable to ambulate farther than 10′ (3 m) or perform ADLs because of generalized weakness or vertigo

Selected nursing diagnoses and patient outcomes

Knowledge deficit related to fall risk factors
    The patient or caregiver will:

• identify possible patient-related risk factors for falling   (N, HCA, OT, PT)
• demonstrate measures to maintain a safe home environment
(N, HCA, OT, PT)
• demonstrate safe ambulatory technique using assistive devices, a support person, or both   (N, OT, PT)
• describe techniques to avoid orthostatic hypotension, for example, dangling legs at bedside before standing up and rising slowly   (N)
• correctly identify the medications that can put patient at risk for falls, such as pain medications and antihypertensives.   (N, PH)

Impaired physical mobility related to weakness

The patient or caregiver will:
• exhibit increased activity levels and strength   (N, HCA, OT, PT)
• demonstrate ability to perform ADLs safely and without complications
(N, HCA, OT, PT)
• use assistive or adaptive devices appropriately.   (N, HCA, OT, PT)

Risk for injury related to weakness, reduced mobility, incorrect use of assistive devices, or unsafe environment

The patient or caregiver will:
• remain free from signs and symptoms of injury   (N, HCA, OT, PT)
• experience no falls or trauma
(N, HCA, OT, PT)
• demonstrate increased ease and degree of mobility, including transfers and use of assistive devices
(N, HCA, OT, PT)
• institute corrective measures to maintain a safe home environment.
(N, HCA, OT, PT)

Skilled nursing services

Care measures

• Perform an initial full assessment of all body systems with specific emphasis on the musculoskeletal, neurologic (including mental and cognitive status), cardiovascular, pulmonary, integumentary, and genitourinary systems; assess nutrition and hydration.
• Assess level of care of patient or caregiver.
• Use safe ambulatory and transfer techniques.
• Assess nutrition and hydration status and patient or caregiver ability to obtain adequate nutrition and fluids.
• Obtain or arrange for laboratory studies (serum electrolyte levels, urinalysis, a complete blood count) as ordered.
• Assess the effectiveness of the treatment regimen, including nutrient and fluid intake; ROM; ability to perform ADLs and care; episodes of near falling; cognitive status changes, especially short- and long-term memory loss and disorientation; medication compliance; signs and symptoms of adverse reactions to medications; ambulation status; and use of assistive or adaptive devices.

Patient and family teaching

• Teach the patient and family strategies for coping with limited mobility and decreased activity level.
• Review measures for care and reorientation.
• Discuss medication management, including purpose, actions, adverse effects, precautions, dosage, food and drug interaction, and safe storage.

• Describe joint protection measures, pain management techniques, fluid intake needs, and safety precautions in the home.

• Identify signs and symptoms to report to the physician (dizziness, unsteady gait, loss of balance, weakness, decreased cognition, and confusion).

• Promote use of assistive devices if indicated.

• Encourage use of community resources if indicated.

Interdisciplinary actions

Home care aide
• Assistance with personal care and hygiene
• Reporting safety hazards or unsafe activities to nurse
• Assistance with ADLs
• Use of adaptive devices

Occupational therapist
• Evaluation for assistive devices
• Instruction in use of adaptive and assistive devices for care as indicated
• Instruction in performing ADLs, using adaptive devices, and conserving energy

Physical therapist
• Home exercise program, therapeutic exercise, and ROM exercise
• Gait training and ambulation
• Safety measures in ambulation
• Pain-management techniques
• Muscle strengthening and improvement in endurance and functional ability secondary to peripheral neuropathy
• Transfer techniques

Discharge plan
• Management of disease process and safe home environment by patient or caregiver without fall or injury
• Return to optimal levels of care and activity
• Referral for continued physical therapy on an outpatient basis

Documentation requirements
• Skilled assessment, including information on the patient's home environment and identification of fall risk factors; physical assessment, with focus on findings that put patient at risk for falls; patient adherence to prescribed regimen; medication management and adverse effects and drug interactions increasing patient's risk for falls; and activity level and use of assistive devices
• Patient response to safety instructions and progress toward goals
• Stressors placing patient at risk for falls, such as anxiety, fear of falling, and lack of support systems
• Family and patient interactions and teaching of family or caregivers
• Vital signs, especially blood pressure variations with position changes
• Location, frequency, and intensity of pain and measures used for relief

Reimbursement reminders
• Durable medical equipment is covered under Medicare part B.
• Emergency telephone response systems aren't covered by Medicare, even though they're usually warranted for the elderly, especially those who live alone.

• Five or more visits per week are considered "daily" visits and must have a finite and predictable end.

• All nonroutine supplies must be specifically ordered by the physician and entered into Locator 14 (Supplies) of the Health Care Financing Administration Form 485 or ordered by the physician within the specific order for treatment requiring the use of certain supplies and entered into Locator 21 (Orders for Treatment).

• When billing for medical supplies, include the following information: name of the supply item, date the supply was used, number of units used, and charge per unit.

Insurance hints

• If care is solely to prevent falls, it must be of short duration for instruction of patient or caregiver.

• Present objective data regarding falls or risk for falls, including injuries, physical findings, coping ability, and safety hazards; describe any near falls, including response to near falling episode.

• Identify variations in blood pressure that occur with position changes.

• Report objective data regarding limitations in mobility or activity, both positive and negative, since last contact as related to homebound status.

• Present details of patient education needs and goals, including details about the patient education process; identify specific barriers that interfere with teaching.

Fracture care

A fracture, or broken bone, occurs when a bone is stressed beyond its strength by trauma, pressure, or disease. Frac-tures are classified according to the type of break, for example, *complete* (through the entire bone), *incomplete* (a partial break), *compound* (a broken bone protrudes through the skin), and *simple* (no protrusion). The surrounding tissue and nerves can be damaged as well, resulting in edema, hemorrhage, or joint damage. Treatment of bone fractures includes stabilization by open or closed reduction procedures and immobilization through splinting, casting, or traction. Home care of the patient with a fracture focuses on patient education involving care of the fracture, measures to promote healing, and prevention of complications. Patients who suffer from osteoporosis are subject to compression fractures of the spine due to loss of bone matter. (Refer to the sections on spinal cord injury, spinal stenosis, and spinal muscle atrophy for information about care of the patient with spinal compression fractures.)

Previsit checklist

Physician orders and preparation

• Cast or appliance care frequency and instructions

• Splint or brace instructions

• Wound care frequency and instructions (in cases of open reduction)

• Activity, mobility, and weight-bearing orders and restrictions

• Medication orders

• Laboratory test orders

• Physical therapy evaluation for therapeutic exercise, range of motion (ROM), and ambulation (gait training)

• Occupational therapy evaluation for activities of daily living (ADLs) and assistive devices

• Home care aide assistance with personal care and ADLs

Equipment and supplies

• Supplies for standard precautions and proper sharps disposal
• Dressing supplies
• Wound measurement device
• Camera to photograph wound and consent form
• Laboratory studies
• Durable medical equipment as ordered (such as a splint or crutches)

Safety requirements

• Emergency plan and access to functional phone and list of emergency phone numbers
• Correct and safe use of adaptive devices (immobilizer brace, splints, walker, or wheelchair)
• Identification and correction of environmental hazards and patient-specific concerns, particularly adequate lighting in the home, safe flooring (no throw rugs or loose tiles), and secure handrails and grab bars
• Standard precautions for infection control and sharps disposal
• System to assist with adherence to a complex medication regimen
• Information on medications, including dosage, adverse effects, interactions, allergies, and safe storage
• Signs and symptoms to immediately report to the physician

Major diagnostic codes

Note: The assigned code must be specific to the affected body part as designated by the fifth digit in the ICD-9 code. Dislocation is included in the fracture code. Use "closed" to designate a simple fracture and "open" to designate a compound fracture.

• Ankle not otherwise specified (NOS), closed/open 824.8/824.9
• Arm, upper NOS, closed/open 812.20/812.30
• Bone NOS, closed/open 829.0/829.1
• Cervical without spinal cord injury, closed/open 805.0/805.1
• Clavicle, open/closed 810.0/810.1
• Deep vein thrombosis 451.19
• Femur, unspecified, closed/open 821.00/821.10
• Foot (except toes), closed/open 825.2/825.3
• Hip, unspecified, closed/open 820.8/820.9
• Leg, lower NOS, closed/open 823.8/823.9
• Osteoporosis 733.00
• Pelvis, unspecified, closed/open 808.8/808.9
• Radius NOS, closed/open 813.81/813.9
• Ribs, closed/open 807.0/807.1
• Sacrum and coccyx, closed/open 805.6/805.7
• Shoulder, closed/open 812.00/812.10
• Ulna NOS, closed/open 813.82/813.93
• Vertebra, multiple, closed/open 809.0/809.1
• Wrist, unspecified, closed/open 814.00/814.01

Defense of homebound status

• Ambulation and activity restricted to one floor of home because of (specify orthopedic appliance, device, cast, or brace)
• Unable to manage stairs to outside and second floor of home because of (specify orthopedic appliance, device, cast, or brace)

• Weight bearing restricted or prohibited to (specify full or partial) on (specify affected body part)
• Activity restricted (or requires assist of one or two persons) to transfer from bed to chair and bathroom because of pain or (specify orthopedic appliance, device, cast, or brace)

Selected nursing diagnoses and patient outcomes

Knowledge deficit related to fracture care
The patient or caregiver will:
• demonstrate correct use of prescribed orthopedic appliance, such as a brace, a sling, a cast, or an immobilizer   (N, OT, PT)
• state correct dose and time for prescribed pain medications or antibiotics and the adverse effects and precautions for each   (N, PH)
• consistently adhere to prescribed activity restrictions such as limitations in weight bearing or ROM (N, OT, PT)
• demonstrate the ability to perform care for the surgical wound using correct technique   (N)
• state signs and symptoms of fracture and wound complications (pain, edema, increased redness or drainage, and fever) to report to the physician
                                               (N, PT)
• demonstrate correct technique in performing prescribed exercises.
                                               (N, PT)

Impaired physical mobility related to fracture
The patient or caregiver will:
• exhibit optimal physical mobility as evidenced by increased activity and ROM   (N, HCA, OT, PT)

• demonstrate ability to perform ADLs safely and without complications
                                        (N, HCA, OT, PT)
• participate in a home exercise program to maintain strength of the unaffected extremities.   (HCA, OT, PT)

Risk for impaired skin integrity related to use of orthopedic appliance (cast or brace) or surgical procedure for open reduction fracture
The patient or caregiver will:
• achieve or maintain skin integrity as evidenced by a well-approximated incision without redness, swelling, or drainage from the incision (N, HCA)
• report absence of pain at the fracture site   (N, HCA)
• exhibit no signs and symptoms of skin breakdown at the cast or brace site   (N, HCA, OT, PT)
• be free from complaints of pain or irritation at the cast or brace site.
                                        (N, HCA, OT, PT)

Risk for peripheral neurovascular dysfunction related to (specify fracture or use of orthopedic appliance)
The patient or caregiver will:
• exhibit warm, pink areas with intact sensation distal to fracture or appliance   (N, OT, PT)
• demonstrate brisk capillary refill with positive peripheral pulses bilaterally   (N, PT)
• state signs and symptoms of neurovascular impairment to report to the physician.   (N, PT)

Pain related to fracture
The patient or caregiver will:
• use medication as ordered for pain relief   (N, PH)

• report a decrease in pain as evidenced by a rating of 3 or less on a 0-to-10 scale   (N, HCA, PT)
• state a decreased need for pain medications   (N, HCA, PH)
• demonstrate a return to optimal activity levels with minimal complaints of pain.   (N, HCA, OT, PT)

Risk for injury related to weakness, reduced mobility, or incorrect use of assistive devices
The patient or caregiver will:
• remain free from signs and symptoms of falls or trauma   (N, HCA, OT, PT)
• demonstrate an increased ease of mobility   (N, HCA, OT, PT)
• use assistive devices correctly.
                (N, OT, PT)

Skilled nursing services

Care measures
• Perform an initial full assessment of all body systems with emphasis on the musculoskeletal, integumentary, genitourinary, cardiopulmonary, and neurologic systems; assess mental and cognitive status as well as nutrition and hydration.
• Assess the level of care of the patient or caregiver, including ability to apply orthopedic devices, wound care, medication compliance, and adherence to activity restrictions and weight-bearing restrictions.
• Assess the effectiveness of the treatment regimen, including signs and symptoms of fracture or healing, pain management, activity level, ROM, ability to perform ADLs and self-care, use of orthopedic appliance, and ambulation status and use of assistive or adaptive devices.

• Obtain or arrange for laboratory tests (prothrombin time and wound culture) as ordered.

Patient and family teaching
• Teach the patient and family skin care at the cast or brace site.
• Review safety precautions related to impaired mobility (unsteadiness of gait, potential for muscle strain, fatigue, and weakness).
• Discuss signs and symptoms to report to the physician (pain at appliance, fracture, or cast site; swelling; warmth or coldness; pallor; and numbness).
• Provide home safety instructions, including adequate lighting, uncluttered floors, easy access to telephone, and emergency numbers on hand.
• Review medication management, including indications, dosages, and adverse effects for all medications.
• Instruct on wound care as specified by physician, including type of supplies needed and where to obtain them, instructions on technique (clean or sterile) of wound care and step-by-step procedure, disposal of infectious materials, and signs and symptoms of wound complications to report to the physician.

Interdisciplinary actions

Home care aide
• Assistance with personal care and hygiene
• Report of safety hazards or unsafe activities to nurse
• Assistance with ADLs
• Use of adaptive devices

Occupational therapist

- Home safety evaluation
- ADLs retraining and modification for energy conservation and safety
- Education regarding adaptive techniques and devices for increased self-care in ADLs

Physical therapist

- Home exercise program
- Transfer and ambulation training within weight-bearing restrictions on level areas and stairs
- Home safety evaluation
- Safe use of ambulation devices

Discharge plan

- Safe management of condition by patient or caregiver in the home with follow-up with physician.
- Return to prefracture level of care and activity
- Removal of orthopedic appliance or cast with return to full weight-bearing status; referral for continued physical therapy on an outpatient basis

Documentation requirements

- Skilled assessment of peripheral neurovascular status, including signs and symptoms of compromise; dislocation; patient adherence to prescribed regimen; wound site, including measurements and description; photographs (patient must sign a consent form for wound to be photographed); and specific signs and symptoms of complications
- Patient or caregiver participation in fracture or wound care
- Activity level as well as safe use of and ongoing need for adaptive equipment

- Medication management, including pain control measures and relief
- Patient response to treatment and progress toward goals
- Stressors (such as being the caregiver to an infant or toddler, advanced age, and vision impairment or sensory-motor impairment) impacting patient adherence to the therapeutic regimen
- Patient and caregiver instructions and progress toward educational goals

Reimbursement reminders

- Durable medical equipment is covered under Medicare part B.
- Only dressing supplies for which there is a physician's order are covered.
- All nonroutine supplies must be specifically ordered by the physician and entered into Locator 14 (Supplies) of the Health Care Financing Administration Form 485 or ordered by the physician within the specific order for treatment requiring the use of certain supplies and entered into Locator 21 (Orders for Treatment).
- When billing for medical supplies, include the name of the supply item, date the supply was used, number of units used, and charge per unit.

Insurance hints

- Present objective data regarding wound condition, including pertinent laboratory studies, wound measurements, and any changes.
- Report objective data regarding limitations in mobility or activity as related to homebound status, including use of crutches, assistive devices, improvement or deterioration in transfer ability.
- Report any changes in peripheral neurovascular status or skin.

- Describe details of patient education needs and goals, including measure to maintain safety within weight-bearing limitations.
- Discuss plan and suggested date for removal of orthopedic device.
- A fracture doesn't meet homebound criteria by itself—what makes the patient homebound must be clearly documented, especially if the fracture is on an upper extremity. Stress comorbid conditions (such as advanced age or cognitive impairment, osteoporosis, and chronic lung or heart conditions) that would affect the patient's learning and ability to provide self-care.

Glucose monitoring, blood

Blood glucose monitoring provides data about how well diabetes treatment goals are being met and can guide adjustments in diet and medications. It can also be used to identify and treat hypoglycemia.

Blood glucose monitoring uses capillary whole blood to provide an immediate blood glucose value. Self-monitoring of blood glucose is recommended for all patients who use insulin or antidiabetic medications as well as for many of those who are treated with diet alone. The frequency and timing of blood glucose monitoring are dictated by the needs and goals of the individual patient.

Many home care patients with diabetes already have their own glucose meter and demonstrate various levels of experience in using it. When a patient has had experience with a glucose meter, the patient's or caregiver's ability to properly perform this procedure should be assessed. Patients with diabetes who are new to blood glucose monitoring require assistance in obtaining a glucose meter and instruction on how to use it. They also need assistance with developing a plan for obtaining blood glucose monitoring supplies on an ongoing basis. Glucose meters and supplies are available in most full-service pharmacies, through nationwide mail order distributors, and through local home medical equipment suppliers.

Selection of a glucose meter depends on the individual patient's needs. Manual dexterity and visual acuity are important factors to consider when selecting a glucose meter. If the patient has a cognitive impairment that limits his or her ability to learn new material, a caregiver who can master this skill must be identified and taught on the patient's behalf. (See "Diabetes mellitus," page 209, for more information.)

Previsit checklist

Physician orders and preparation
- Blood glucose monitoring, including frequency and timing; target range; sliding-scale insulin orders based on blood glucose monitoring results, if appropriate; and indications for notifying physician of blood glucose monitoring results
- Calorie allowance
- Oral medication and insulin orders
- Laboratory blood studies, including glycosylated hemoglobin (Hb A_{1C}), chemistry panel, lipid panel, and renal studies
- Activity orders and restrictions

• Social work evaluation for community resources and financial assistance for equipment

• Home care aide assistance with personal care and activities of daily living (ADLs)

Equipment and supplies

• Supplies for standard precautions and proper sharps disposal
• Glucose meter with instruction booklet
• Glucose meter test strips
• Lancing device and lancets
• Alcohol wipes (if needed)
• Logbook or diary
• Phlebotomy supplies

Safety requirements

• Standard precautions for infection control and sharps disposal
• System to assist with adherence to a complex medical regimen, including diet, medications, insulin injections, and blood glucose monitoring as appropriate
• Allergies verified and documented
• Emergency plan and access to functional phone and list of emergency phone numbers
• Signs and symptoms of hyperglycemia, hypoglycemia, diabetic ketoacidosis, and hyperosmolar hyperglycemic nonketotic syndrome
• Emergency treatment measures for hypoglycemia
• Foot care and sick-day measures

Major diagnostic codes

• Diabetes mellitus, uncomplicated 250.0
• Diabetes mellitus, with complications 250.9

• Diabetes, uncontrolled/gestational 250.0/648.8
• Diabetic ketoacidosis 250.1
• Hypoglycemia, diabetic 250.8
(To assign a fifth digit, see appendix A, page 638.)

Defense of homebound status

• Vision impairment that requires the assistance of another person to leave the home
• Recent history of frequent or severe hypoglycemia
• Non-weight-bearing status due to neuropathic foot ulcer
• Unable to ambulate farther than 10′ (3 m) because of complications of diabetes

Selected nursing diagnoses and patient outcomes

Knowledge deficit related to diabetes management and blood glucose monitoring

The patient or caregiver will:
• demonstrate correct technique for monitoring blood glucose levels and interpreting results (N)
• demonstrate ability to recognize and treat hypoglycemia, using blood glucose monitoring (N)
• verbalize appropriate plan for obtaining blood glucose monitoring supplies after discharge. (N, SW)

Ineffective management of therapeutic regimen related to complexity of diabetic management program

The patient or caregiver will:

• demonstrate ability to monitor blood glucose levels with minimal assistance
(N)

• remain free from signs and symptoms of hypoglycemia and hyperglycemia
(N)

• maintain blood glucose level within individual target range   (N)

• verbalize or demonstrate measures to prevent and treat hypoglycemia
(N)

• demonstrate blood glucose monitoring and logbook technique   (N)

• use available resources for support and guidance   (N, SW)

• exhibit adherence to prescribed regimen as evidenced by an Hb A_{1C} level of less than 8%   (N, MD)

• remain free from signs and symptoms of complications associated with uncontrolled diabetes.   (N, MD)

Skilled nursing services

Care measures

• Perform initial assessment of the neurologic, integumentary (including feet), cardiovascular, GI, and genitourinary systems; assess nutrition and hydration status.

• Assess the level of care of the patient or caregiver, including observation of the patient's ability to perform blood glucose monitoring and the condition of the glucose meter currently in use, including cleanliness, appropriateness for patient's functional ability, and control check using meter test strip.

• Assess the effectiveness of the treatment regimen, using the patient's logbook or the memory function on the patient's meter.

• Assess for signs and symptoms of hypoglycemia and hyperglycemia.

• Investigate complaints surrounding signs and symptoms of hypoglycemia and hyperglycemia and measures taken to treat episodes.

• Obtain or arrange for blood studies, including lipid panel, renal studies, and Hb A_{1C}.

• Institute dosage adjustments based on recorded blood glucose levels as ordered.

Patient and family teaching

• Teach the patient and family glucose meter operation (inserting strip and applying blood to test strip, reading results, changing batteries, and calibrating equipment).

• Demonstrate fingerstick and phlebotomy techniques and safe reuse or disposal of lancets.

• Review reading, recording, and interpreting results and recognizing values that are out of target range.

• Explain sliding scale use.

• Discuss management of hyperglycemia and hypoglycemia.

• Outline troubleshooting techniques and advise about technical support.

• Review health promotion and complication prevention, such as care during minor illness (cold, flu, and GI upset), foot care, and prevention of long-term complications.

• Identify signs and symptoms to report to the physician.

Interdisciplinary actions

Home care aide

• Personal care and hygiene
• Assistance with ADLs

Social worker

- Referral to community resources and support groups for people with diabetes
- Counseling and referral for stress management and reduction
- Financial evaluation and referral for assistance with securing supplies and equipment

Discharge plan

- Independence with blood glucose monitoring
- Management of disease process in home with physician and community support systems follow-up
- Discharged to self-care with return to pre-illness status
- Maintenance on antidiabetic medication therapy
- Understanding of measures to minimize risk of short- and long-term complications of diabetes
- Follow-up appointments for blood studies in an authorized laboratory on own
- Follow-up appointments with physician at recommended intervals

Documentation requirements

- Skilled assessment, including subjective and objective data with regard to signs and symptoms of hypoglycemia or hyperglycemia, results of blood glucose monitoring, possible relation of certain factors (food intake, medication administration, activity level, and physical and emotional stressors) to out-of-range results, insulin administration if applicable (type, dose, time, and site of injection), patient or caregiver participation in monitoring, de-

gree of independence, and areas of concern or difficulty with management
- Patient or caregiver progress toward educational goals
- Chemistry panel, lipid panel, renal studies, and Hb A_{1C} levels as well as changes in medication orders
- Episodes of hypoglycemia and hyperglycemia, including measures to treat episodes
- Patient and caregiver instructions

Reimbursement reminders

- Diabetes supplies covered by Medicare include blood glucose meter, one every 5 years; blood glucose meter with voice synthesizer, if physician documents visual acuity of 20/200 or worse; 25 test strips every month days for non-insulin-dependent patient and 100 test strips every 30 days for insulin-dependent patients (Medicare will pay for more test strips if ordered by physician; supplier may ask for copy of blood glucose log for billing purposes); lancing device, one every 6 months; control solution to check the integrity of test strips; and battery required to operate the glucose meter.
- Some insurers only reimburse for certain glucose meters and strips.
- Blood glucose monitoring performed by a nurse without any other skilled service being rendered is *not* considered a reimbursable skilled nursing service.
- The Joint Commission on Accreditation of Healthcare Organizations and Health Care Financing Administration require that home care agencies have quality assurance programs for blood glucose monitoring. This includes proficiency testing, use of control solutions, and staff training.

Insurance hints

- Present objective and specific data on homebound status, such as episodes of hypoglycemia decreasing, for example, to less than two per day.
- Present recent blood glucose level ranges for each time of day that blood glucose level is checked.
- Report factors that may be responsible for out-of-range results (food intake, medication administration, and monitoring technique).
- Describe patient's or caregiver's progress in monitoring of blood glucose, including such complications as episodes of hypoglycemia, blood glucose still out of target range, skin breakdown, and infection.
- Describe plan for obtaining supplies after discharge.
- Stress comorbid conditions (such as vision or neurosensory impairment, cognitive status changes, and chronic lung and cardiac disorders) that would affect the patient's ability to learn or provide self-care.

Heart failure

Caused by damage to the myocardium, heart failure (previously called congestive heart failure) prevents the heart from pumping blood effectively. It may result from various cardiac disorders as well as other conditions that increase the heart's workload. Heart failure can affect the left or right side of the heart or both. Left-sided heart failure occurs when the left ventricular end-diastolic pressure is elevated for a prolonged time. This increases left atrial pressure, which adversely affects the pulmonary system. Right-sided heart failure results from prolonged or severe left-sided heart failure, which causes venous congestion. Heart failure is now considered a chronic illness that requires case management over an extended period. The home care nurse plays an important role as teacher in the prevention of repeated exacerbations that will lead to more frequent hospitalizations and, eventually, death.

The home care nurse is generally the first health care provider to suggest transfer to hospice after the patient has an ejection fraction of less than 20% or resting tachycardia or tachypnea.

Previsit checklist

Physician orders and preparation

- Medication therapy, possibly including I.V. inotropic agents
- Cardiac activity restrictions
- Acceptable parameters for vital signs
- Dietary restrictions, such as a low-sodium diet
- Oxygen administration, including arterial blood gas (ABG) analysis, pulse oximetry, or both
- Physical therapy evaluation for home exercise program, transfer training, and endurance training
- Occupational therapy evaluation for energy conservation and assistance with functional ability, including adaptive devices as necessary
- Nutritional evaluation for prescribed dietary restrictions
- Social worker evaluation for community referrals, financial assistance, and counseling
- Home care aide assistance with personal care and activities of daily living (ADLs)

- Laboratory studies including serum electrolyte and therapeutic drug levels

Equipment and supplies
- Supplies for standard precautions and proper sharps disposal
- Scale
- Oxygen
- Bedside commode
- I.V. supplies and equipment for administration of inotropic agents
- Phlebotomy supplies, including equipment for obtaining arterial blood sample
- Pulse oximeter

Safety requirements
- System to assist with adherence to a complex medication regimen, including I.V. therapy
- Allergies verified and documented
- Emergency plan and access to functional phone and list of emergency phone numbers
- Home safety measures to prevent falls and injury, including handrail, grab bars, shower seat, and nonskid bathmat for bathroom safety as well as shoes with nonskid soles
- Oxygen therapy precautions as appropriate
- Functional smoke detector and night-light in home
- Signs and symptoms to report to the physician or emergency personnel

Major diagnostic codes
- Angina 413.9
- Angina, unstable 411.1
- Atrial fibrillation 427.31
- Atrial flutter 427.32
- Cardiac dysrhythmia 427.9

- Cardiovascular disease, unspecified 429.2
- Congestive (left- and right-sided) heart failure 428.0
- Coronary atherosclerosis 414.00
- Heart failure, unspecified 428.9
- Left-sided heart failure 428.1
- Obesity 278.00
- Peripheral vascular disease 443.9

Defense of homebound status
- Bedridden; maximum assistance required to transfer from bed to chair twice per day
- Confined to chair
- Unable to ambulate farther than 10′ (3 m) without extreme dyspnea
- Unable to climb stairs; confined to first floor of home

Selected nursing diagnoses and patient outcomes

Decreased cardiac output related to reduced stroke volume

The patient or caregiver will:
- demonstrate a pulse rate and blood pressure within acceptable parameters (N, HCA)
- report a decrease in episodes of dyspnea (N, MD)
- experience no dizziness, syncope, or chest pain (N, MD)
- exhibit pulse oximetry of at least 90%. (N)

Fluid volume excess related to blood pooling

The patient or caregiver will:

- exhibit a urine output greater than fluid intake initially followed by maintenance of output equaling intake
(N, HCA)
- demonstrate a decrease in lower-extremity edema   (N)
- display a decrease in weight initially, with gradual maintenance of weight within acceptable parameters
(N, HCA)
- report a decrease in episodes of dyspnea.   (N)

Activity intolerance related to disease process and fluid excess
The patient or caregiver will:
- demonstrate energy conservation measures   (N, HCA, OT, PT)
- use oxygen therapy as necessary and ordered to enhance functional ability
(N, PT, OT, RT)
- perform ADLs and personal care with assistance   (N, HCA, OT)
- exhibit ability to increase ambulation distance gradually throughout plan of care   (N, HCA, MD, OT, PT)
- participate in home exercise program.   (N, HCA, PT)

Noncompliance with medical regimen related to lifelong medication administration and lifestyle changes
The patient or caregiver will:
- state the importance of adhering to the treatment regimen   (N, PH)
- demonstrate compliance with the medication regimen and lifestyle changes   (N, D, HCA, OT, PT, SW)
- exhibit signs and symptoms indicating a stable cardiovascular and respiratory status   (N, MD, PT)
- use appropriate community resources for assistance   (N, SW)

- tolerate physical activity with minimal to no fatigue, weakness, discomfort, or decrease in oxygen saturation
(N, HCA, OT, PT)
- identify signs and symptoms to report to the physician.   (N, HCA, MD)

Skilled nursing services

Care measures
- Perform full nursing assessment of all systems, with emphasis on the cardiopulmonary, neurologic, genitourinary, and peripheral vascular systems, as well as an assessment of nutrition, hydration, and mobility.
- Assess vital signs, weights, and complaints of shortness of breath, dyspnea, and chest pain at each visit.
- Monitor oxygen therapy use, if ordered. Obtain or arrange for ABG analysis as ordered.
- Measure calf circumference to assess for lower-extremity edema; note amount and degree of pitting.
- Assess breath sounds for changes that indicate improvement or continued fluid retention.
- Evaluate intake and output for trends that indicate improvement or deterioration in patient's condition.
- Assess medication compliance, and monitor for signs and symptoms of possible adverse effects. Administer I.V. medications, if ordered.

Patient and family teaching
- Teach the patient and family about patient's medication regimen, adverse effects and potential drug interactions.
- Demonstrate how to record intake and output and daily weight measurements.

- Review oxygen therapy use, safety precautions, energy conservation measures, and dietary restrictions such as a low-sodium diet.
- Instruct on measures to reduce and prevent edema.
- Discuss signs and symptoms, such as increased shortness of breath and chest pain, weight gain over 2 lb (0.9 kg) in 1 day, and adverse drug reactions, to report to the physician.
- Teach assessment of pulse rate and blood pressure.
- Emphasize the importance of adherence to the medical regimen and follow-up.
- Review activity restrictions and exercise plans.

Interdisciplinary actions

Dietitian
- Comprehensive nutritional assessment
- Instruction in low-sodium diet
- Weight management

Home care aide
- Personal care
- Assistance with ADLs
- Energy conservation measures

Occupational therapist
- Energy conservation measures
- Assistive or adaptive equipment to increase functional ability

Physical therapist
- Home exercise program
- Transfer training
- Endurance training

Social worker
- Community referrals

- Assistance with finances to aid compliance
- Supportive counseling for chronic long-term disease

Discharge plan
- Management of heart failure in home with physician and community support system follow-ups
- Follow-up appointments for blood studies in an authorized laboratory
- Follow-up appointments with physician at recommended intervals
- Patient or caregiver understanding and control of disease process; knowledge of preventive measures and signs and symptoms of recurrence

Documentation requirements
- Skilled assessment, including patient's response to care; results of blood studies, including ABG analysis (if ordered); titration of medications, including oxygen needs, based on blood studies; activity restrictions and adherence to exercise program and endurance and transfer training; lower-extremity calf circumference measurements, including amount and degree of pitting edema; breath sounds; evidence of complications (or lack thereof); the patient's or caregiver's independence with care and therapy regimen
- Patient and caregiver instruction and progress toward educational goals
- Interdisciplinary team communication, including physical therapist, occupational therapist, social worker evaluation and need for services; plan for home program; and changes in the plan of care, including changes in med-

ication dosages based on blood studies; and patient and caregiver understanding of those changes
• Patient's ability to transfer safely within limited activity
• Patient's adherence to instructions and therapy regimen

Reimbursement reminders
• For oxygen therapy to be covered, pulse oximetry or ABG analysis results are required to substantiate the patient's medical need for this therapy. Also needed are skilled observation and evaluation of the patient's response to this therapy and patient and family teaching about when and how to initiate oxygen therapy appropriately.
• Patients receiving home oxygen therapy who had an initial partial pressure of oxygen of 56 or higher or an initial arterial oxygen saturation at 89% or higher must repeat laboratory testing within 60 to 90 days after the start of therapy to demonstrate a continued need and therefore continued coverage of the therapy. Additionally, the physician must see the patient and confirm the continued need for this service.
• Medicare won't reimburse for oxygen therapy ordered "p.r.n."
• Specific teaching instructions related to oxygen therapy, medications, and safety measures should be given to the patient.
• Document progress toward goals, including changes in weight, actual measurements that indicate a decrease in edema, and distance the patient is able to ambulate without complaints.
• Document abnormal laboratory values, including ABG values and serum electrolyte levels.

• Document medication changes, including reason for change.

Insurance hints
• Report specific progress toward goals (for example, pulse rate has been maintained within range of ___ beats per minute for ___ days). Identify changes in calf circumference and weight; adjustment issues, such as patient's resistance or acceptance of therapy; and complications, such as medication adverse reactions, increased shortness of breath, and chest pain.
• Describe gains in knowledge, such as skills and concepts mastered in increasing endurance, transfers, medication compliance, and measures to prevent recurrence.
• Present specific data on homebound status, such as bedridden or confined to chair; distance patient is able to ambulate, including use of stairs; and changes in muscle strength.
• Emphasize that the next step in care is to show a progressive plan for independence.
• Stress comorbid conditions (such as diabetes and chronic lung disease) that would affect the patient's ability to provide self-care.

Hepatitis

Patients living at home with hepatitis need to make lifestyle changes to decrease their symptoms, prevent recurrence, and prevent transmission of the virus. They may require skilled nursing care for complications and for teaching about managing the disease and preventing its transmission. Teaching may vary according to patient needs, symptoms, and the type and cause of the hepatitis. Depending on the severity of the illness, the patient or the caregiver may be the target audience for teaching. Close contacts of the patient must be taught proper infection control and be referred for possible prophylactic medications.

Previsit checklist

Physician orders and preparation
- Diet (may include tube feeding or parenteral nutrition)
- Medications and administration schedule
- Laboratory tests, including serum electrolyte levels and liver function tests
- Vaccine for close contacts of patient (may need to refer contacts to their own physicians)
- Activity orders and restrictions
- Physical therapy evaluation for home exercise program and muscle strengthening
- Nutritional evaluation for dietary recommendations and nutritional therapy program (enteral or parenteral nutrition therapy)
- Home care aide assistance with personal care and activities of daily living (ADLs)

Equipment and supplies
- Supplies for standard precautions and proper sharps disposal
- Phlebotomy supplies
- Enteral or parenteral nutrition supplies, such as syringes, dressings, tube feeding bag, and irrigation kit for gastrostomy tube, if needed
- Fecal occult blood test

Safety requirements
- Standard precautions for infection control and sharps disposal
- System to assist with adherence to a complex medication regimen
- Allergies verified and documented
- Emergency plan and access to functional phone and list of emergency phone numbers
- Identification and correction of environmental hazards and patient-specific concerns, such as vision impairment and the need for a night-light

Major diagnostic codes
- Hepatitis, acute:
  - alcoholic 571.1
  - infective 070.1
- Hepatitis, chemical or septic 573.3
- Hepatitis, chronic 571.40
- Hepatitis, lupoid 571.49
- Hepatitis, postnecrotic 571.49
- Hepatitis, recurrent 571.49
- Hepatitis, viral:
  - A with/without hepatic coma 070.0/070.1
  - B with/without hepatic coma 070.2/070.3
- Hepatitis, other viral specified with hepatic coma:
  - C, acute or unspecified 070.41
  - C, chronic 070.44
  - delta without mention of active hepatitis B disease 070.42
  - E 070.43
  - other specified viral hepatitis 070.49
- Hepatitis, other viral unspecified without mention of hepatic coma 070.5
  - acute or unspecified hepatitis C 070.51
  - C, chronic 070.54

–delta without mention of active hepatitis B 070.52

– E 070.53

–other specified viral hepatitis 070.59

● Unspecified viral hepatitis with/without hepatic coma 070.6/070.9

(To assign a fifth digit, see appendix A, page 638.)

Defense of homebound status

● Unable to ambulate farther than 10′ (3 m) because of weakness and malaise

● Unable to leave home because of nausea, vomiting, and diarrhea

● Unsafe to ambulate any distance because of mental status changes

● Need for continuous administration of total parenteral nutrition

● Potential to infect others secondary to weeping or draining wounds

● Bedridden because of weakness and malaise

Selected nursing diagnoses and patient outcomes

Altered nutrition: Less than body requirements related to nausea and vomiting

The patient or caregiver will:

● verbalize importance of nutrition and eating small, frequent, low-fat, high-carbohydrate meals   (N, D, HCA)

● state measures to prevent or decrease nausea   (N, D, HCA)

● demonstrate administration of tube feedings and parenteral nutrition, if indicated.   (N, D)

Risk for injury related to bleeding

The patient or caregiver will:

● verbalize reasons why hepatitis may predispose the patient to bleeding episodes   (N)

● identify signs and symptoms of bleeding and actions to take   (N)

● demonstrate understanding of importance for having blood tests at regular intervals to determine changes in coagulation profile and liver function   (N, MD)

● demonstrate safety measures to prevent injury that could lead to bleeding, including fall prevention, use of safety razor, avoidance of injections and needle sticks, the use of a soft toothbrush.   (N, HCA, PT)

Fluid volume deficit related to prolonged vomiting and diarrhea

The patient or caregiver will:

● monitor weight and intake and output and verbalize changes to report   (N, HCA)

● verbalize the importance of having blood drawn to monitor fluid and electrolyte balance   (N, MD)

● identify conditions that predispose the patient to dehydration (such as vomiting and diarrhea) and the importance of encouraging fluid intake during these times   (N, D, HCA)

● verbalize the importance of notifying the physician when prolonged nausea and vomiting occur.   (N)

Activity intolerance related to disease condition and fatigue level

The patient or caregiver will:

● remain on bed rest during acute stages of illness   (N, HCA, PT)

● verbalize scheduling daily activities to allow for rest periods   (N, PT)

- state use of medications to prevent pain from interfering with daily activities (N, PH)
- verbalize correct choice of over-the-counter (OTC) analgesics (aspirin is discouraged) (N, PH)
- participate in exercise program to regain strength after acute stage of illness (N, HCA, PT)
- demonstrate exercises to maintain strength. (N, PT)

Knowledge deficit related to disease process, recovery, treatment, and prevention

The patient or caregiver will:
- describe the disease process and transmission (N)
- state the need to avoid alcohol and OTC medications (N, MD, PH)
- identify appropriate food choices to enhance nutritional status, including components of diet (low in fat and high in carbohydrates), to be eaten in small, frequent meals to help prevent nausea (N, D, HCA)
- demonstrate appropriate skin care and infection-control measures (N, HCA)
- identify signs and symptoms of complications, including plan for emergencies (N, HCA)
- demonstrate understanding of medication regimen (N, PH)
- identify close contacts and encourage them to see their physicians for possible prophylactic medications (N)
- verbalize understanding of not donating blood. (N)

Skilled nursing services

Care measures
- Perform initial full assessment of all systems with emphasis on mental status, nutritional status, and activity level.
- Assess fluid balance, including intake and output and weight, and review laboratory studies.
- Evaluate skin condition, including signs and symptoms of pruritus and jaundice.
- Assess for signs and symptoms of bleeding.
- Assess level of activity; institute bed rest during acute periods.
- Administer I.V. or subcutaneous medications, if indicated.
- Administer tube feeding or parenteral nutrition, if indicated.
- Obtain or arrange for blood studies as ordered.

Patient and family teaching
- Teach the patient and family how to prevent disease transmission through exchanging body fluids or donating blood.
- Help identify patient contacts for prophylactic medications, if needed.
- Review nutritional needs.
- Describe measures to prevent nausea and vomiting.
- Identify signs and symptoms of bleeding and infection.
- Discuss signs and symptoms to report, such as hepatic coma, bleeding, fulminant hepatitis, and encephalopathy.

Interdisciplinary actions

Dietitian
* Nutritional evaluation
* Recommendations for nutritional therapy, including enteral or parenteral nutrition therapy

Home care aide
* Personal care
* Assistance with ADLs
* Instruction of caregivers on bathing

Physical therapist
* Home exercise program
* Muscle strengthening

Discharge plan
* Management of hepatitis infection at home with physician and community support system follow-ups
* Demonstration of measures to prevent viral transmission
* Follow-up appointments for blood studies in an authorized laboratory on own
* Follow-up appointments with physician at recommended intervals
* Knowledge of preventive measures and signs and symptoms of progression
* Completion of advance directive

Documentation requirements
* Skilled assessment, including subjective and objective data with regard to appetite and percentage of meals eaten; daily weight measurement; intake and output; evidence of patient's or caretaker's knowledge about transmission of disease and methods of prevention; mental status; evidence of skin breakdown; indicators of complications, such as signs and symptoms of bleeding and encephalopathy; activity level; changes in muscle strength; mobility status; abdominal pain; and effectiveness of analgesia
* Administration of medications and patient response
* Administration of tube feedings or parenteral nutrition
* Initial knowledge and skill level with regard to care
* Patient and caregiver instructions and progress toward educational goals, including safety precautions and signs and symptoms to be reported
* Changes in plan of care, including those directly related to results of blood studies; and the patient's or caregiver's understanding of those changes
* Patient's ability to accommodate changes in self-care within level of fatigue
* Patient's adherence to instructions and therapy regimen
* New diagnosis, recent hospitalization, significant changes or complications related to condition, or variances to expected outcomes

Reimbursement reminders
* Dietitian services aren't reimbursable under the Medicare home care benefit.
* For private insurance, check coverage before obtaining in-home specialty services.
* Medicare covers phlebotomy supplies.
* Many insurance companies have contracts with specific laboratories for processing specimens. Check for an authorized laboratory.

• Obtain a physician order for changes in the plan of care.

Insurance hints

• Report progress toward goals, including changes in weight, skin integrity, intake and output, and adjustment issues, such as the patient's resistance to or acceptance of therapy, the disease, or instructions.

• Describe gains in knowledge, such as skills and concepts mastered in maintaining nutritional status, muscle strengthening, and understanding of the disease, including treatment and prevention of transmission.

• Present objective data about homebound status, including changes in muscle strength, inability to ambulate because of severe fatigue, number of persons needed to assist patient out of chair, and continued limitation or improvement in ambulation distance.

• Stress comorbid conditions (such as diabetes and chronic heart or lung disease) that would affect the patient's ability to provide self-care.

• Describe the discharge plan.

• Project the need for future visits, including frequency and duration.

Hip fracture

The term *hip fracture* includes fractures of the head, neck, and trochanter parts of the femur. Treatment typically involves the subsequent open reduction and internal fixation (pinning) or hemiarthroplasty (replacement) procedure. Hip fracture is common in the elderly. It can pose serious health threats beyond the initial episode to the home care patient as well as special challenges to the home care team.

Such complications as the development of deep vein thrombosis, wound infection, incisional pain, and the myriad physical and psychosocial affects of decreased mobility can make the recovery period difficult for the patient with a hip fracture. Patient education to promote adherence to the therapeutic regimen and prevent future fractures is the focus of care provided by the home care team.

Previsit checklist

Physician orders and preparation

• Wound care frequency and instructions

• Activity, mobility, and weight-bearing restrictions

• Medication orders

• Laboratory test orders

• Physical therapy evaluation for home exercise program, weight bearing, ambulatory aids, and progressive gait training

• Occupational therapy evaluation for assistive and adaptive devices to promote functional ability

• Home care aide assistance with personal care and activities of daily living (ADLs)

Equipment and supplies

• Supplies for standard precautions and proper sharps disposal

• Dressing supplies

• Wound measurement device

• Camera to photograph wound and consent form for photography

• Phlebotomy supplies

• Assistive device, such as a walker, wheelchair, or cane

• Bedside commode

Safety requirements

- Standard precautions for infection control and sharps disposal
- Emergency plan and access to functional phone and list of emergency phone numbers
- Correct and safe use of adaptive devices (walker or wheelchair)
- Identification and correction of environmental hazards and patient-specific concerns (for example, adequate lighting, uncluttered floors, safe flooring without throw rugs or loose tiles, and secure handrails and grab bars)
- Availability of support people in case of emergency
- Signs and symptoms to immediately report to the physician
- Instructions on signs and symptoms of medical emergency and actions to take

Major diagnostic codes

- Fracture femur head, closed/open 820.09/820.19
- Fracture femur neck, closed/open 820.8/820.9
- Fracture femur trochanter, closed/open 820.20/820.30

Other possible diagnostic codes:
- Anticoagulation 99.19
- Arthritis 716.90
- Hip dislocation, closed/open 835.00/835.10
- Joint pain, pelvic region and thigh 719.45
- Osteoarthritis, pelvic region and thigh 715.15
- Osteomyelitis, pelvic region and thigh (chronic) 730.15
- Osteoporosis 733.00

- Rheumatoid arthritis 714.0
- Thrombosis, deep vein 451.19

Defense of homebound status

- Activity restricted to transfer from bed to chair
- Confined to first floor of home; unable to climb stairs
- Non-weight-bearing status for lower extremity with inability to ambulate
- Activity restricted by complaints of pain on movement
- Unable to ambulate farther than 10′ (3 m) because of postoperative fatigue or dyspnea

Selected nursing diagnoses and patient outcomes

Knowledge deficit related to postoperative care and treatment
   The patient or caregiver will:
- state correct dose and time for prescribed pain medications or antibiotics and the adverse effects and precautions for each   (N, PH)
- consistently adhere to prescribed activity restrictions, such as weight-bearing limits and hip restrictions on range of motion (ROM)   (N, OT, PT)
- demonstrate ability to perform care to surgical wound, using correct technique   (N, OT)
- state signs and symptoms of wound complications (pain, increased redness or drainage, and fever) to report to the physician   (N)
- demonstrate correct technique for performing prescribed exercises
          (N, HCA, PT)

• utilize adaptive equipment (such as raised toilet seat and grab bars) in bathroom.   (N, PT, OT, HCA)

Impaired physical mobility related to hip fracture and surgery
The patient or caregiver will:
• demonstrate increased ambulation, activity, and ROM   (N, HCA, OT, PT)
• participate in ADLs safely and without complications. (N, HCA, OT, PT)

Impaired skin integrity related to surgical incision
The patient or caregiver will:
• exhibit an incision that is well approximated without redness, swelling, or drainage   (N)
• report lack of pain at the incision site.   (N)

Constipation related to decreased mobility and use of analgesics
The patient or caregiver will:
• report regular bowel elimination with return to pre-illness pattern by discharge   (N, HCA, PH, PT)
• demonstrate measures to promote bowel elimination   (N, HCA, PH, PT)
• increase fluid intake and dietary fiber.   (N, HCA)

Pain related to hip fracture and surgery
The patient or caregiver will:
• report a decrease in pain weekly
                    (N, HCA, PH, PT)
• demonstrate the appropriate use of prescribed analgesics appropriately
                    (N, MD, PH)
• verbalize use of nonpharmacologic pain-relief measures   (N, HCA, PT)
• return to optimal activity levels within prescribed restrictions.
                    (N, HCA, OT, PT)

Skilled nursing services

Care measures
• Perform initial full assessment of all body systems, with emphasis on the musculoskeletal, integumentary, genitourinary, and cardiopulmonary systems; nutrition and hydration; and mental status.
• Assess level of care of patient or caregiver, for example, ability to perform wound care, medication compliance, and adherence to activity restrictions and exercise program.
• Obtain or arrange for laboratory studies as ordered.
• Assess the effectiveness of the treatment regimen, including signs and symptoms of fracture or incision healing, pain management, activity level, ROM, and weight bearing.
• Assess ability to perform ADLs and self-care.

Patient and family teaching
• Teach the patient and family wound care as specified by physician, including type of supplies needed and where to obtain; instructions on technique (clean or sterile) and step-by-step procedure; proper disposal of infectious materials; and signs and symptoms of complications to report to the physician.
• Review medication management, including indications, dosages, and adverse effects for all medications.
• Review home safety instructions, including adequate lighting, uncluttered floors, easy access to telephone, and readily available emergency numbers.
• Encourage use of assistive devices, if needed.
• Discuss signs and symptoms to report to the physician (pain at fracture

or surgical site, swelling, warmth or coldness, pallor, and numbness).

Interdisciplinary actions

Home care aide
- Personal care
- Assistance with ADLs

Occupational therapist
- Adaptive techniques and devices for increased self-care in ADLs
- Energy conservation

Physical therapist
- Home exercise program
- Safe use of assistive ambulation devices
- Home safety measures
- Progressive gait training with weight bearing
- Stair training

Discharge plan
- Safe management of hip fracture and surgical site by patient or caregiver with physician follow-ups
- Return to prefracture level of self-care and activity
- Return to full weight-bearing status; referral for continued physical therapy on an outpatient basis

Documentation requirements
- Skilled assessment of incision and wound site, including measurements, description, photographs, and specific signs and symptoms of complications (patient must sign a consent form for wound to be photographed); patient or caregiver participation in wound care; activity level; and safe use of adaptive equipment
- Patient adherence to the prescribed regimen
- Specific signs and symptoms of complications
- Activity level and the safe use of and ongoing need for adaptive equipment
- Medication management, including pain-control measures and relief
- Patient response to treatment and progress toward goals
- Stressors that impact patient adherence to therapeutic regimen
- Patient and caregiver instructions, including signs and symptoms to report to the physician; exercise program; weight-bearing restrictions; use of adaptive devices, such as walker or cane; safety measures, including skin care; and pain-relief strategies

Reimbursement reminders
- Durable medical equipment is covered under Medicare part B.
- Medicare covers phlebotomy supplies.
- Many insurance companies have contracts with specific laboratories for processing specimens. Check for an authorized laboratory.
- If the patient was discharged from a hospital to a skilled nursing facility for rehabilitation, the insurance case manager will expect that the home care plan is a continuation of previous physical rehabilitation and that the duration of home care will be short. If lengthy nursing services are needed, be very clear about the scope of service and differentiate between nursing and physical therapist services. Many patients in home care following hip surgery won't need nursing care be-

cause physical therapists can remove staples and supervise home care aides.

• Registered physical therapist services are reimbursable under the Medicare home benefit. Under Blue Cross and Blue Shield, a registered physical therapist, not a licensed physical therapy assistant, must follow the patient throughout the course of therapy.

Insurance hints

• Present objective data regarding wound condition, including pertinent laboratory studies, wound measurements, and changes.

• Report objective data regarding limitations in mobility or activity as related to homebound status, including use of assistive devices and improvement or deterioration in transfer ability.

• Report changes in peripheral neurovascular status or skin.

• Describe details of patient education needs and goals, including measures to maintain safety within weight-bearing limitations.

• Discuss plan and suggested date for discharge with follow-up with outpatient physical therapy.

• Stress comorbid conditions (such as advanced age, osteoporosis, diabetes, multiple falls, and vision or other sensory impairment) that would affect the patient's ability to provide self-care.

Hypertension

Hypertension, a sustained increase in systolic or diastolic blood pressure, is a major cause of cardiac disease, cerebrovascular accident, and renal failure. A diagnosis of hypertension is usually based on two or more incidents of systolic blood pressure being greater than 140 mm Hg or diastolic blood pressure being greater than 90 mm Hg. Because certain risk factors are known to contribute to the development of primary hypertension, both primary and secondary prevention on the part of the home care nurse is essential during case management.

Previsit checklist

Physician orders and preparation

• Oral medication orders
• Acceptable blood pressure parameters
• Activity restrictions and limitations
• Low-fat, low-cholesterol diet
• Social worker evaluation for financial assistance and referral to community resources
• Laboratory studies including sodium, potassium, blood urea nitrogen, and creatinine

Equipment and supplies

• Phlebotomy supplies
• Scale

Safety requirements

• System to assist with adherence to a complex medication regimen, including I.V. therapy
• Emergency plan and access to functional phone and list of emergency phone numbers
• Home safety measures to prevent falls and injury
• Adherence to low-fat, low-cholesterol diet
• Signs and symptoms to report to the physician

Major diagnostic codes

- Hypertension 401.9
- Hypertension, accelerated 401.0
- Hypertensive heart disease, benign/unspecified 402.1/402.9
- Hypertensive heart disease, malignant without/with congestive heart failure 402.00/402.01
- Hypertensive nephrosclerosis 403.90
- Secondary hypertension, malignant 405.0

Defense of homebound status

- Unable to ambulate farther than 10′ (3 m) because of shortness of breath on exertion and complaints of severe headache interfering with activities of daily living (ADLs)
- Impaired safe ambulation because of orthostatic hypotension

Selected nursing diagnoses and patient outcomes

Risk for injury related to increased cerebrovascular pressure

The patient or caregiver will:
- verbalize reduction or elimination of headache (N, HCA)
- exhibit alert level of responsiveness (N, HCA)
- demonstrate reduction or elimination of nausea and vomiting. (N, HCA)

Altered tissue perfusion (cerebral, cardiopulmonary, peripheral) related to increased peripheral vascular resistance

The patient or caregiver will:

- attain and maintain blood pressure within established parameters (N, HCA)
- experience no dizziness, chest pain, epistaxis, palpitations, vision changes, or hematuria (N, HCA)
- exhibit no signs of organ dysfunction. (N, MD)

Noncompliance with medical regimen related to adverse effects of prescribed treatment and conflict with sociocultural influences

The patient or caregiver will:
- state the importance of compliance with prescribed antihypertensive therapy (N, PH)
- demonstrate adherence to the prescribed regimen, including medication and diet, as evidenced by normal blood pressure measurements (N, HCA, SW)
- exhibit healthy lifestyle changes (N, HCA, MD)
- maintain weight within normal limits (N, HCA)
- engage in an appropriate exercise program. (N, HCA)

Skilled nursing services

Care measures

- Perform initial full assessment of all body systems with emphasis on cardiovascular system as well as nutritional and mental status and activity level.
- Provide home safety information and instruction.
- Measure baseline vital signs and evaluate cardiovascular status, breath sounds, and activity level.
- Measure blood pressure while patient is sitting and standing for orthostatic changes.

• Assess for signs and symptoms of adverse effects to medication therapy, such as diuresis and electrolyte imbalances.

• Assess neurologic status for changes indicative of diminished cerebral perfusion.

• Evaluate for and measure degree of lower-extremity edema.

Patient and family teaching needs

• Teach the patient and family safety measures, especially those relating to position changes (if orthostatic hypotension is present).

• Discuss appropriate food choices, including low-sodium, high-potassium foods. (Potassium is found in bananas, milk, turkey, oranges, and many salt substitutes.)

• Review monitoring of blood pressure.

• Discuss the medication regimen, including desired and adverse effects, such as fatigue and orthostatic hypotension.

• Identify signs and symptoms to report to the physician, including neurologic changes and signs and symptoms of hypokalemia.

• Emphasize the need for regular medical follow-up.

• Encourage lifestyle modifications, such as smoking cessation and the importance of nutrition, exercise, relaxation, and weight loss as appropriate.

Interdisciplinary actions

Social worker

• Community referral

• Financial assistance to enhance adherence to therapy regimen

Discharge plan

• Safe management of hypertension in the home with physician follow-up services

• Independence in ADLs

Documentation requirements

• Skilled assessment, including blood pressure measurements taken in both arms while lying down, sitting, and standing; complaints of dizziness, vision changes, headache, epistaxis, or hematuria, including frequency and degree of severity; and tolerance to changed physical activity status, especially if weakness or dyspnea occurs

• Assessment of adherence to medication regimen and presence of adverse reactions; success of dietary changes, including weight loss and serum cholesterol and lipid values; and calf circumference measurements, including degree of pitting edema

• Evidence of complications (or lack thereof); patient's or caregiver's independence with care and therapy regimen; and the patient's response to treatment, including trends in blood pressure measurements

• Patient and caregiver instructions, such as medication therapy, including drug, dosage, frequency, and adverse effects; how to take blood pressure; lifestyle modifications and effectiveness; and signs and symptoms to report to the physician

Reimbursement reminders

• Most of the skilled care surrounding the patient with hypertension involves teaching. Be sure to document the teaching plan thoroughly.

• If hypertension is the primary and exclusive diagnosis, it isn't enough to justify more than one visit.

• Identify and document variances to expected outcomes, such as elevated blood pressure, increase in peripheral edema, and difficulty adhering to medication regimen because of adverse effects or lack of finances, to justify the need for continued care.

• Identify progress toward goals, including lowering blood pressure to acceptable parameters and plan for discharge.

• Identify medication changes, including additions or deletions from therapy, rationales for changes, and contacts with physician necessitating changes.

• Use additional diagnostic codes to supplement and justify skilled care needs, including episodes of dehydration and orthostatic hypotension.

Insurance hints

• Present objective patient findings and changes since previous update; include specific blood pressure measurements.

• Report symptoms and changes since previous communication, including new or increased episodes of shortness of breath, headache, neurologic changes, and inability to comply with medication therapy, including the reason why.

• Stress comorbid conditions (such as diabetes and chronic lung or heart disease) that would affect the patient's ability to provide self-care.

• Report regarding continuing homebound status and factors affecting status.

Impaction, fecal

Fecal impaction may occur when stool is allowed to remain in the colon until it hardens and blocks the rectum. It may result from immobility, dehydration, poor bowel habits, improper diet, medications that cause constipation, and inadequate bowel cleansing after a barium enema or barium swallow. Initial interventions for relief include administration of oil retention and cleansing enemas, suppositories, and laxatives. When these measures fail, the impaction needs to be digitally removed with the physician's approval because stimulation of vagal nerve endings in the rectum may cause the heart to slow. To avoid the need for such measures, prevention is the key to managing fecal impaction.

Previsit checklist

Physician orders and preparation

• Order for digital removal of fecal impaction

• Order to begin patient on oral laxative regimen (bulk laxative or stool softener)

• Physical therapy evaluation (unless contraindicated) to increase level of mobility

• Nutritional evaluation to assess dietary intake and instruct patient or caregiver regarding dietary prevention of fecal impaction

• Home care aide assistance with personal care and activities of daily living (ADLs)

Equipment and supplies

• Supplies for standard precautions

- Gloves (two pairs)
- Linen-saver pad
- Bedpan or commode
- Plastic bag for disposal of soiled supplies
- Water-soluble lubricant
- Washcloth or cleansing wipes

Safety requirements
- Standard precautions for infection control
- Safety measures to prevent falls
- Prearranged signal for displaying evidence of distress
- Safety rails on bed so patient can be placed in Sims' position
- Walker or three-pronged cane to enhance mobility if patient can be out of bed
- Avoidance of routine laxative use apart from occasional stool softeners or bulk laxatives
- Avoidance of routine digital disimpaction by caregivers

Major diagnostic codes
- Enema for removal of impacted feces 96.38
- Fecal impaction 560.39
- Impaction, bowel, colon, or rectum 560.30

Defense of homebound status
- Bedridden or confined to chair because of (specify injury)
- Unsafe to ambulate farther than 15′ (4.5 m) because of decreased mobility due to confusion or disorientation

Selected nursing diagnoses and patient outcomes

Constipation related to immobility and lack of knowledge related to management of constipation
The patient or caregiver will:
- obtain relief from impaction   (N)
- remain free from complications associated with long-term constipation, such as nausea, pain, colonic irritation, and bowel perforation   (N, HCA)
- regain and maintain a normal bowel pattern   (N, HCA, PT)
- state when to initiate additional interventions to stimulate bowel elimination.   (N)

Knowledge deficit related to measures to promote bowel elimination
The patient or caregiver will:
- name at least three foods included in a high-fiber diet   (N, D)
- state the importance of using supplemental bran in diet   (N, D)
- verbalize the importance of drinking 2,500 to 3,000 ml of fluid daily unless contraindicated   (N, D)
- verbally contract to participate willingly in home exercise and activity program   (N, PT)
- agree to set aside a regular time each day for patient to attempt defecation   (N, HCA)
- state the importance of avoiding routine laxative use.   (N, D, PT)

Skilled nursing services

Care measures
- Perform initial full assessment of all body systems with emphasis on the neurologic (including mental and cog-

nitive status), GI (including nutrition and hydration status), integumentary (rectal tissue), and cardiovascular systems.

● Assess level of comprehension of patient or caregiver regarding importance of increasing fluid and fiber intake and activity level.

● Administer oil retention or cleansing enemas; perform manual disimpaction as ordered.

● Assess the effectiveness of the treatment regimen. Monitor number of stools per day and document stool color, consistency, and odor.

● Assess for signs and symptoms of dehydration and nutritional depletion.

Patient and family teaching

● Teach the patient and family measures to promote regular bowel elimination, including use of high-fiber diet, activity, establishing regular times for elimination, and stool softeners or bulk laxatives for occasional constipation.

● Review activity guidelines.

● Review dietary recommendations and fluid requirements.

● Identify signs and symptoms of constipation and early treatment measures.

● Discuss signs and symptoms to immediately report to the physician.

● Teach about the effect of medication regimen on bowel function, if appropriate.

Interdisciplinary actions

Dietitian
● Dietary recommendations
● Meal planning

Home care aide
● Personal care
● Assistance with ADLs

Physical therapist
● Home exercise program
● Activity instructions

Discharge plan
● Safe management of bowel regimen with no further episodes of fecal impaction with physician follow-up services

Documentation requirements
● Skilled assessment, including objective data supporting signs and symptoms of constipation and fecal impaction; results of monitoring number of stools per day, including stool characteristics; findings from nutritional assessment and physical therapy evaluation; administration of enemas, including type administered, results obtained, and patient tolerance; and use of manual disimpaction technique and results

● Patient or caregiver participation in care, such as increasing fluids, using high-fiber diet, and increasing activity

● Patient or caregiver progress toward educational goals and response to care, including any further episodes of impaction

● All verbal and written instructions, return demonstrations, verbalization of learning, and any resistance to learning

● Ways in which care helps achieve patient goals and steps taken to decrease the frequency of visits as goals are met

• Changes in the patient's condition that require continued skilled care or physician contact

Reimbursement reminders

• Dietitian services aren't reimbursable under the Medicare home care benefit.

• Registered physical therapist services are reimbursable under the Medicare home care benefit; under Blue Cross and Blue Shield, a registered physical therapist must follow the patient throughout the course of therapy, and the patient can't be followed by a licensed physical therapy assistant for services to be reimbursable.

• Teaching prevention of fecal impaction isn't a reimbursable skilled nursing service and constipation, by itself, doesn't justify homebound status. Be clear about justifying homebound status reason (such as recent or severe vomiting or diarrhea). Fecal disimpaction and bowel training are covered in some circumstances.

• Identify variances to expected outcomes and specific barriers to learning to support the need for skilled services, such as, "Caregiver is unable to demonstrate procedure for administering enema to patient because of extreme difficulty hearing. Instructions to be written down for future reference."

• Identify specific deficits in initial knowledge level and then progress as evidenced by specific concepts and information demonstrated and verbalized.

• Provide documentation that shows interdisciplinary communication.

Insurance hints

• Present objective data about homebound status, including underlying factors that contributed to impaction as interventions to prevent future occurrences.

• Present objective patient findings and changes since previous contact.

• Present specifics about patient education progress, including patient's or caregiver's ability to follow through with instructions and procedure.

Infusion therapy

Today, home care nurses see patients who receive chemotherapy, pain management, fluid replacement therapy, immunosuppressive drug therapy, thalasemia treatment with deferoxamine mesylate (Desferal), inotropic therapy, and blood and platelet transfusions in their homes. Small ambulatory pumps can be attached to a belt and programmed off site or at the patient's home via computer modem. Vascular access device technology has also improved the ability of nurses to infuse these therapies through peripheral catheters, which they can insert in the patient's home. Peripheral catheters include both midline catheters, which terminate in the proximal portion of the extremity and remain in place for about 1 month, and midclavicular catheters, which terminate in the proximal axillary or subclavian veins and can remain in place for 3 months. Tunneled and nontunneled central venous catheters, implanted ports, and implanted pumps are frequently used routes for infusion therapies.

As therapies and technology have advanced, reimbursement has become tighter. Today, patients don't begin home infusion therapy without preauthorization from the insurance carrier. Failure to obtain authorization can result in nonpayment for services provided.

Previsit checklist

Physician orders and preparation
- Medication dosage, rate, route, and site change frequency
- I.V. insertion

Equipment and supplies
For the patient receiving total parenteral nutrition (TPN) through tunneled catheter via ambulatory pump:
- Pump
- Pump tubing and filter
- TPN solution and lipids
- Multivitamins
- 10-ml syringes
- Proper sharps disposal system, including container
- Batteries for pump
- Injection caps
- Central line dressing kits
- Alcohol swabs
- Silk tape (1″ wide)
- Catheter clamp
- Saline flush
- Heparin flush (100 u/cc)

For the patient receiving medications I.V. push through peripheral I.V. catheter:
- Tourniquet
- Prefilled medication syringes
- Proper sharps disposal system, including container
- 10-ml syringes
- I.V. start kits

- Short extension tubing (microbore)
- I.V. catheter (22G and 24G)
- Injection cap
- Alcohol swab
- Heparin flush (10 u/cc)
- Saline flush (if drugs are incompatible)
- Anaphylaxis kit
- Scale

Safety requirements
- Safety of nurse traveling at night— may require an escort for protection
- Additional I.V. poles and pumps for a multilevel home
- Emergency plan and access to functional phone and list of emergency phone numbers
- All pumps plugged into a 3-prong grounded outlet to maintain proper grounding of the machine
- Adequate refrigeration capacity to store chemical spill kit in the home
- Notification of the fire and police departments and telephone and electric companies of patient on life support equipment or medically necessary oxygen or infusions
- System to assist with adherence to a complex medication regimen
- Information on medications, including dosage, adverse effects, interactions, and safe storage
- Identification and correction of environmental hazards and patient-specific concerns
- Fire evacuation plan, functional smoke detectors, and access to functional fire extinguisher

Major diagnostic codes
- Abscess or cellulitis, unspecified site 682.9

- Bacteremia 790.7
- Complication of transplanted heart/bone marrow 996.83/996.85
- Cystic fibrosis without/with meconium ileus 277.00/277.01
- Dehydration 276.5
- Drug-induced neutropenia 288.0
- Heart failure, congestive/left 428.0/428.1
- Hyperemesis 536.2
- Infusion therapy with antineoplastic agent/electrolytes/platelet inhibitor 99.25/99.18/99.20
- Lyme disease 088.81
- Noninfectious enteritis 558.9
- Osteomyelitis 730.2
- Postoperative infection, seroma/other 998.51/998.59
- Regional enteritis, unspecified site 555.9
- Unspecified deficiency anemia 281.9
(To assign a fifth digit, see appendix A, page 638.)

Defense of homebound status

- Immunosuppression secondary to disease or medication
- Maximal assistance required due to weakness
- Physician-ordered activity restriction (such as leg elevation)
- Activity restricted by weakness or shortness of breath
- Unable to ambulate or leave home without assistance

Selected nursing diagnoses and patient outcomes

Altered nutrition: Less than body requirements related to inability to ingest or digest food or absorb nutrients due to biological, psychological, or economic factors
The patient or caregiver will:
- maintain adequate nutrition.
(N, D)

Risk for infection
The patient or caregiver will:
- remain free from infection (N)
- demonstrate proper aseptic technique when administering I.V. medications and performing line care. (N)

Decreased cardiac output
The patient or caregiver will:
- show evidence of improved cardiac output (N)
- identify energy conservation techniques. (N)

Knowledge deficit related to lack of exposure
The patient or caregiver will:
- demonstrate ability to care for I.V. catheter (N)
- verbalize an understanding of procedures (N)
- verbalize an understanding of purposes of medications. (N, PH)

Altered protection related to treatments
The patient or caregiver will:
- remain free from complications related to I.V. therapy. (N)

Risk for caregiver role strain
The caregiver will:
- identify methods for relieving stress (N)
- effectively reduce stress level. (N)

Ineffective management of therapeutic regimen: Families related to the complexity of the therapeutic regimen or excessive demands on the individual or family

The patient or caregiver will:
- demonstrate proper technique for care of I.V. catheter (N)
- demonstrate proper technique for administration of I.V. medications (N)
- identify appropriate support resources. (N)

Risk for impaired skin integrity

The patient or caregiver will:
- identify ways to reduce the risk of skin breakdown (N)
- maintain skin integrity (N)
- demonstrate ability to assess vascular catheter insertion site for signs of complications. (N)

Anxiety

The patient or caregiver will:
- identify methods to decrease anxiety level (N)
- verbalize feelings (N)
- demonstrate healthy coping techniques. (N)

Skilled nursing services

Care measures
- Perform full assessment including intake and output, weight, and signs of reactions to therapy.
- Assess I.V. site.
- Administer and maintain I.V. drugs.
- Operate infusion pumps.
- Care for the vascular access site.
- Assess the patient for signs of infection, allergic response, fluid overload, or dehydration and other signs of complications.
- Restart I.V. peripherally every (specific order) day and as needed.
- Venipuncture as ordered.
- Assess the patient's response to therapy.

Patient and family teaching
- Teach proper technique for medication infusion and techniques for solving common problems related to I.V. therapy.
- Teach proper I.V. site care.
- Explain how to use the infusion pump.
- Instruct in the purpose, route, and dosage of medications.
- Demonstrate how to document the date and time of all infusions.
- Teach proper technique for heparin and saline flushing of intravascular access device.
- Describe the symptoms of I.V. infiltration and infection.
- Instruct as to when the nurse or physician on call needs to be notified.

Interdisciplinary actions

Dietitian
- Assessment of calorie needs for patients receiving TPN

Home care aide
- Assistance with activities of daily living

Social services
- Assistance with securing supportive services such as respite and hospice care
- Assessment of financial resources and exploration of personal and community resources

Discharge plan
- Completion of medication regimen

- Removal of the vascular access device
- Effective administration of medications and care of the catheter by patient or caregiver

Documentation requirements

- Medication administration, including the drug, dosage, site, and time
- Patient and caregiver teaching and the response to it
- Type of catheter used and the reason as well as insertion and dressing change dates
- Patient's response to medication and treatments, including any adverse effects or reactions
- Changes in the patient's condition, including laboratory results
- Assessment of the vascular access site
- Patient or caregiver participation in care
- Plan of treatment
- Any telephone contact

Reimbursement reminders

- Obtain preauthorization for therapy and specify the number of nursing visits, including visits as needed for catheter-related reasons.
- Ensure that all appropriate forms are signed.
- For the catheter supplies and skilled nursing care to be covered, the infused medication must be authorized by the insurer.
- The catheter must be used at least every 4 weeks for maintenance care to be covered.
- Ensure that the required immunosuppressive drugs are used to prevent or treat the rejection of a heart, liver, kidney, or bone marrow transplant.
- Use I.V. immunosuppressive drugs only when there is documented intolerance or malabsorption of oral medications.
- Ensure that the patient must have invasive hemodynamic monitoring before and after the I.V. inotropic therapy regimen is started.
- Administer chemotherapy by a pump.
- Chemotherapy, antispasmodics, and pain medication that is administered by an external or implantable pump are covered if they meet specific criteria.
- Recognize that reimbursement doesn't cover meperidine administration.
- Ensure that I.V. pain management is covered for intractable cancer pain, as it is with Medicare.
- Recognize that experimental and off-label drugs aren't covered by most insurance carriers.

Insurance hints

- Report objective findings and changes in the patient's status or plan of care.
- Report laboratory results, such as peaks and troughs, creatinine, international normalized ratio, and white blood cell count.
- Report progressive independence of the patient or caregiver with infusion therapy.

Irritable bowel syndrome

Also known as spastic colon, functional colitis, and mucous colitis, irritable bowel syndrome involves a change in bowel motility. Seen as a functional syndrome, irritable bowel is characterized by alternating periods of constipation and diarrhea with abdominal pain. The pain of this disease is relieved with defecation and a change in bowel habits.

Although there is no organic cause for this syndrome, factors that can contribute to it include type of food ingested, stress, the gastric hormones gastrin and cholecystokinin, and drugs that affect the autonomic nervous system. Small-bowel motility is increased in patients with diarrhea and decreased in patients with constipation. Stress exaggerates the bowel abnormality along with a low-fiber, low-residue diet and the ingestion of lactose or fructose. Most of the physical problems in the patient with irritable bowel syndrome are focused on nutrition and fluid and electrolyte balance. Teaching is needed for the family and patient with this condition and should focus on believing the patient's complaints (often the patient is led to believe that the symptoms are imagined) and instructing on diet adjustments, stress reduction, and changing bowel pattern signs that might indicate the need for medical intervention.

Previsit checklist

Physician orders and preparation
- Order for stool specimens
- Nutritional therapy
- Diagnostic test preparation
- Activity orders and restrictions
- Social worker evaluation for community referral and counseling

Equipment and supplies
- Supplies for standard precautions
- Stool specimen containers
- Diet and nutritional therapy patient education information
- Stress-reduction patient education information

Safety requirements
- Standard precautions for infection control
- Skin care to the perianal region in the event of diarrhea
- Emergency plan and access to functional phone and list of emergency phone numbers
- Identification and correction of environmental hazards and patient-specific concerns
- Allergies verified and documented

Major diagnostic codes
- Chronic hypotension 458.1
- Constipation 564.0
- Electrolyte and fluid disorders 276.9
- Functional diarrhea 564.5
- Irritable colon 564.1
- Orthostatic hypotension 458.0
- Volume depletion 276.5

Defense of homebound status
- Unable to leave home environment because of unpredictable bowel patterns

- Potential for hypotensive episodes due to fluid imbalance
- Unpredictable pattern of abdominal pain interfering with ability to ambulate outside the home
- Fatigue and inability to ambulate farther than 10′ (3 m) caused by fluid and electrolyte imbalance

Selected nursing diagnosis and patient outcomes

Constipation related to impaired motility of the GI tract

The patient or caregiver will:
- recognize the pattern of diarrhea and constipation (N, HCA)
- demonstrate dietary changes to reduce the frequency of constipation episodes (N, D, HCA)
- state the rationale for a high-residue, high-bulk diet with increased fluid intake (N, D)
- recognize the role of daily activity and exercise with regular elimination patterns (N, HCA)
- recognize a pending constipation episode by measuring abdominal girth and noting abdominal tenderness and audible bowel sounds. (N)

Diarrhea related to impaired motility of the GI tract

The patient or caregiver will:
- recognize the frequency of diarrhea alternating with episodes of constipation (N, HCA)
- demonstrate dietary changes to reduce the frequency of diarrhea episodes (N, HCA)
- state the rationale for a high-residue, high-bulk diet (N, D)

- state the reason for increased fluid intake to replace fluids lost during episodes of diarrhea (N)
- examine the stool, noting changes from other diarrhea episodes (N, HCA)
- state the reason for keeping a stool count, including stool characteristics. (N)

Risk for fluid volume deficit related to prolonged episodes of diarrhea

The patient or caregiver will:
- weigh self daily and verbalize the need for daily weights as an indicator of a stable fluid volume (N, HCA)
- demonstrate assessment of fluid status to include skin turgor, mucous membranes, and urine output (N)
- recognize the possibility of experiencing a drop in blood pressure with position changes (orthostatic hypotension) (N)
- state the types of fluids appropriate to replace fluids lost through the GI tract. (N)

Risk for impaired skin integrity related to irritation from episodes of diarrhea

The patient or caregiver will:
- demonstrate good skin care as evidenced by intact perianal skin (N, HCA)
- demonstrate the use of protective lubricants to facilitate intact perianal skin. (N, HCA)

Altered nutrition: Less than body requirements

The patient or caregiver will:
- maintain balanced diet within dietary restrictions (N, D)

• recognize the need to increase calorie intake to supplement nutrients lost through episodes of diarrhea
(N, D, HCA)
• demonstrate a stabilization of body weight.   (N, HCA)

Anxiety related to situational stress
The patient or caregiver will:
• recognize the role stress plays with irritable bowel syndrome   (N, SW)
• demonstrate stress-reduction techniques   (N, HCA, SW)
• state the outcome of using stress-reduction techniques on bowel patterns
(N, SW)
• recognize that the stress of having irritable bowel syndrome can increase the frequency of erratic bowel patterns
(N, SW)
• demonstrate mechanisms used to cope with the unpredictable pattern of the disease process.   (N, SW)

Skilled nursing services

Care measures
• Perform initial full assessment of all body systems with emphasis on the abdomen for tenderness, rigidity, and bowel sounds.
• Assess integumentary status and mucous membranes for fluid balance.
• Obtain or arrange for the collection of laboratory and stool specimens.
• Assess adherence to the medical regimen, need for medication, and knowledge level.
• Ensure that the patient has all prescribed medications, knows how to take them, and understands common adverse effects.

Patient and family teaching
• Teach the patient and family about home safety issues.
• Demonstrate good hand-washing techniques.
• Instruct on signs and symptoms of dehydration.
• Provide information on the causes of irritable bowel disease and when to contact the physician.
• Review diet and nutrition therapy and ways to reduce stress and anxiety.
• Discuss proper perianal skin care.
• Instruct how to promote proper fluid balance and activity level.
• Discuss dangerous signs and symptoms, such as those of dehydration.

Interdisciplinary actions

Social worker
• Community services
• Emotional support and counseling

Home care aide
• Assist with physical care
• Support skin care needs

Discharge plan
• Safe management of bowel elimination patterns with physician follow-up and verbalization of the importance of maintaining contact with the physician
• Reduction in episodes of constipation and diarrhea
• Referral for possible outpatient counseling for continued stress reduction or recommendation for stress-relief support groups

Documentation requirements

- Skilled assessment, including bowel elimination patterns (number of episodes of diarrhea and constipation, and stool characteristics); assessment of vital signs, weight, and hydration status; abdominal assessment (bowel sounds, distention, and complaints of pain); blood pressure and presence or absence of orthostatic changes; factors contributing to episodes and the patient's attempts to control them; and perianal skin integrity and measures used to enhance it, including observations of patient's or caregiver's ability to perform skin care
- Patient and caregiver instructions and response to them
- Ability of caregiver to care for the patient

Reimbursement reminders

- Medicare doesn't reimburse for disposable underpants or underpads or teaching about the prevention of constipation.
- Identify any variance to expected outcomes, such as altered bowel sounds and excessive discomfort.
- Identify the time of the patient's last bowel movement and specific factors that have contributed to the episode of irritable bowel.

Insurance hints

- Review hospitalization (if appropriate) and current condition of the patient, home environment, and availability of caregivers.
- Provide objective review of systems to include physical abilities, ambulation, use of or need for assistive devices, and any appropriate laboratory studies.
- Describe skin assessment and report objective findings. If open or reddened areas exist, provide accurate wound dimensions, prescribed dressing, and capability of caregiver to perform wound care.
- Include an objective evaluation of nutritional status, including weight and height.
- Provide an objective evaluation of unpredictable bowel patterns.
- Emphasize the strategies used to promote self-care and independence.
- Describe the progress toward goals in measurable terms: daily weight, results of serial laboratory studies, and the number of episodes of diarrhea and constipation as well as changes in frequency.
- Differentiate between home care and care provided by the primary care provider.
- Recommend additional care, such as psychotherapy or a support group, for stress control.

Knee replacement care

Knee replacement may be indicated for patients who suffer from degenerative or rheumatoid arthritis, fracture, or functional disabilities. It involves the surgical insertion of a metal or acrylic prosthesis to provide increased stability and mobility. In home care, the focus is on patient education in regard to the therapeutic regimen, including pain management, wound care (as well as monitoring the wound for healing) and the prescribed exercise program.

Physical therapy may be the primary skilled service.

Previsit checklist

Physician orders and preparation

- Wound care frequency and instructions
- Activity, mobility, and weight-bearing restrictions
- Brace, immobilizer, or other device, such as continuous passive motion device, and instructions
- Medication therapy including analgesics
- Laboratory studies
- Physical therapy evaluation for therapeutic exercise, range of motion (ROM), and ambulation (gait training)
- Occupational therapy evaluation for activities of daily living (ADLs) and assistive devices
- Home care aide assistance with personal care and ADLs

Equipment and supplies

- Supplies for standard precautions and proper sharps disposal
- Brace, immobilizer, or other device, if indicated
- Dressing supplies
- Wound measurement device
- Camera to photograph wound and consent form for photography
- Vital signs monitoring equipment
- Phlebotomy supplies
- Wound culture equipment, if indicated

Safety requirements

- Standard precautions for infection control and sharps disposal

- Emergency plan and access to functional phone and list of emergency phone numbers
- Correct and safe use of adaptive device (walker, wheelchair, or immobilizer brace)
- Home safety measures, including adequate lighting, safe flooring (no throw rugs or loose tiles), secure handrails, and grab bars
- Emergency medical plan
- Availability of support people in case of emergency
- Signs and symptoms to immediately report to the physician
- Medication information, including interactions, schedule, and notation of allergies

Major diagnostic codes

- Arthritis 716.90
- Joint disorder, lower leg 719.96
- Joint instability, lower leg 718.86
- Joint pain, lower leg 719.46
- Knee replacement, right or left (surgical) 81.54
- Osteoarthritis (degenerative joint disease), knee 715.96
- Osteomyelitis, lower leg, chronic 730.16
- Revision of knee replacement (surgical) 81.55
- Rheumatoid arthritis 714.0
- Total knee replacement 81.54

Defense of homebound status

- Bedridden or confined to chair related to non-weight-bearing restrictions
- Unable to ambulate farther than 10′ (3 m) because of pain in lower ex-

tremity, weight-bearing restrictions, or muscle weakness and fatigue
• Confined to first floor of home because of brace or immobilizer (specify device) interfering with stair climbing
• Assistance of at least one person required to transfer from sitting to standing position
• Assistance required to perform ADLs

Selected nursing diagnoses and patient outcomes

Knowledge deficit related to postoperative care after knee replacement
The patient or caregiver will:
• state the correct dose and time for prescribed pain medications, antibiotics, or both and the adverse effects and precautions for each   (N, PH)
• consistently adhere to prescribed activity restrictions, such as weight-bearing limits   (N, HCA, OT, PT)
• demonstrate the ability to perform care of surgical wound using correct technique   (N)
• state signs and symptoms of wound complications (pain, increased redness or drainage, or fever) to report to the physician   (N, HCA)
• demonstrate correct technique for performing prescribed exercises and using supportive and adaptive equipment (braces, immobilizers, or walker).   (OT, PT)

Impaired physical mobility related to knee replacement and weight-bearing restrictions
The patient or caregiver will:
• demonstrate an increase in ambulation, activity, and ROM
      (N, HCA, OT, PT)

• perform ADLs safely and without complications.   (N, HCA, OT, PT)

Impaired skin integrity related to surgical incision
The patient or caregiver will:
• exhibit a healing, well-approximated incision without redness, swelling, or drainage   (N, HCA)
• report gradual reduction in complaints of pain at incision site.
      (N, HCA)

Risk for constipation related to immobility and use of analgesics
The patient or caregiver will:
• demonstrate a return to usual bowel elimination patterns by discharge
      (N, PH, PT)
• verbalize an absence of pain with defecation   (N, PH, PT)
• report passage of soft, formed stool
      (N, PH, PT)
• demonstrate measures to improve and maintain bowel elimination.
      (N, HCA, PH, PT)

Pain related to tissue injury secondary to knee replacement surgery
The patient or caregiver will:
• demonstrate appropriate use of analgesics for pain relief   (N, PH, PT)
• identify appropriate nonpharmacologic methods of pain relief
      (N, HCA, MD, OT, PT)
• report a decrease in the level of pain with each visit   (N, HCA, PT)
• verbalize a decreased need for pain medications   (N, PH)
• return to optimal activity levels with minimal or no complaints of pain.
      (N, HCA, OT, PT)

Risk for injury related to weakness, reduced mobility, or incorrect use of assistive devices

The patient or caregiver will:

- remain free from signs and symptoms of injury   (N, HCA, OT, PT)
- exhibit increased ease of mobility (N, HCA, OT, PT)
- demonstrate correct use of assistive devices.   (N, HCA, OT, PT)

Skilled nursing services

Care measures

- Perform initial full assessment of all body systems with emphasis on the musculoskeletal, integumentary, genitourinary, and cardiopulmonary systems as well as nutrition and hydration and mental and cognitive status.
- Assess the level of care of patient or caregiver, including ability to perform wound care, medication compliance, and adherence to activity and weight-bearing restrictions.
- Assess the effectiveness of the treatment regimen (signs and symptoms of wound healing, pain management and relief measures, activity level, ROM, and ability to perform ADLs).
- Obtain or arrange for laboratory tests, including blood tests and wound culture as ordered.

Patient and family teaching

- Teach the patient and family wound care as specified by the physician, including type of supplies needed and where to obtain; technique (clean or sterile) of wound care and step-by-step procedure; proper disposal of contaminated materials; and signs and symptoms of wound complications to report to the physician.

- Review proper use of brace, immobilizer, or other device.
- Instruct on medication management, including indications, dosages, and adverse effects for all medications.
- Provide home safety instructions, including adequate lighting, uncluttered floors, easy access to telephone, and readily available emergency numbers.

Interdisciplinary actions

Home care aide
- Personal care
- Assistance with ADLs
- Assistance with ambulation as indicated

Occupational therapist
- Home safety evaluation
- ADL training
- Education regarding adaptive techniques and devices for increased self-care in ADLs

Physical therapist
- Home exercise program
- Instructions on weight-bearing restrictions
- Transfer and ambulation training within weight-bearing restrictions
- Correct application of brace or immobilizer
- Safe use of ambulation equipment

Discharge plan
- Safe management of knee replacement in the home with follow-up by physician
- Return to optimal levels of care and activity
- Removal of brace, immobilizer, or other device with return to full weight-

bearing status; referral for continued physical therapy on an outpatient basis

Documentation requirements

• Skilled assessment, including vital signs; changes indicating possible infection; wound site, including measurements, description, photographs, and specific signs and symptoms of complication (patient must sign a consent form for the wound to be photographed); patient or caregiver participation in wound care; activity level; safe use of and ongoing need for adaptive equipment; bowel elimination patterns, including constipation and measures to prevent and manage; medication management, including pain-control measures and relief; stressors that impact patient adherence to the therapeutic regimen; patient response to treatment and progress toward goals
• Patient and caregiver instructions, including signs and symptoms to report to the physician; exercise program; weight-bearing restrictions; use of adaptive or assistive devices; safety measures, including wound care; measures to prevent and manage constipation; and pain-relief strategies

Reimbursement reminders

• Durable medical equipment is covered under Medicare part B.
• Continuous passive motion device is covered under Medicare (80%) for up to 21 days after surgery.
• Only dressing supplies for which there is a physician order are covered.
• All nonroutine supplies must be specifically ordered by the physician

and entered into Locator 14 (Supplies) of the Health Care Financing Administration Form 485 or ordered by the physician within the specific order for treatment requiring the use of certain supplies and entered into Locator 21 (Orders for Treatment).
• When billing for medical supplies, include the name of the supply item, date supply was used, number of units used, and charge per unit.
• Physical therapy may be the primary skilled service involved with the patient's care because the patient's need for skilled nursing care may be minimal and physical therapists can remove staples and supervise health care aides. If so, reimbursement for skilled nursing visits may be denied unless documentation reflects the exact need for skilled nursing care.

Insurance hints

• Present objective data regarding wound condition, including pertinent laboratory studies, wound measurements, and any changes (positive or negative).
• Report objective data regarding limitations in mobility or activity as related to homebound status, including use of brace, immobilizer, continuous passive motion device, or assistive devices, and improvement or deterioration in transfer ability.
• Report changes in vital signs, unexpected wound appearance, or complaints of pain.
• Describe details of patient education needs and goals, including measures to maintain safety within weight-bearing limitations and progress with ambulation.
• Discuss plan and suggested date for removal of brace, immobilizer, or oth-

er device and return to full weight-bearing status.

Laryngectomy care

Laryngectomy, the removal of the larynx, is most frequently performed to eliminate cancerous growths. Postoperative complications include airway obstruction, dehydration, inadequate nutritional intake, impaired communication, and depression. Care for a postlaryngectomy patient in the home setting focuses on preventing complications, teaching behaviors that maximize independent functioning (particularly communication), and addressing the underlying disorder.

Previsit checklist

Physician orders and preparation

- Medications as indicated
- Aerosol therapy
- Chest physiotherapy, if indicated
- Oxygen therapy, as indicated, including orders for pulse oximetry and arterial blood gas (ABG) analysis
- Activity orders and restrictions
- Dietary and nutritional orders
- Laboratory studies
- Physical therapy evaluation for home exercise program, endurance training, and chest physiotherapy
- Respiratory therapy evaluation and instruction in respiratory equipment
- Occupational therapy evaluation for energy conservation and activities of daily living (ADL) training
- Speech therapy evaluation for communication and swallowing techniques

- Social worker evaluation for community resources, counseling, and support groups
- Home care aide assistance with personal care and ADLs

Equipment and supplies

- Supplies for standard precautions and proper sharps disposal
- Oxygen, including backup oxygen tank in case of power failure as indicated
- Tracheostomy care supplies
- Suction kits
- Portable suction machine with connecting tubing and sterile water or normal saline solution
- Handheld resuscitation bag connected to oxygen source, if indicated
- Disposable inner cannula or spare nondisposable inner cannula the same size as currently in use
- Sterile gloves
- Extra tracheostomy tube of same size and type as one currently in place
- Obturator
- Nutritional supplies, such as enteral feeding solutions or supplements, if indicated
- Phlebotomy supplies, including equipment for obtaining arterial blood sample

Safety requirements

- Standard precautions for infection control and sharps disposal
- System to assist with adherence to a complex medication regimen, including I.V. therapy
- Emergency plan and access to functional phone and list of emergency phone numbers
- Oxygen precautions, if indicated

- Medication and equipment storage instructions
- Allergies verified and documented
- Functional smoke detector and night-light in the home
- Signs and symptoms to report to the physician or emergency personnel
- Medical alert bracelet
- Avoidance of respiratory irritants, such as sawdust and smoke, and bathing and shaving precautions

Major diagnostic codes
- Acute laryngotracheitis with obstruction 464.21
- Acute tracheitis with obstruction 464.11
- Bronchitis, acute 466.0
- Cancer of the esophagus, unspecified 150.9
- Cancer of the head and neck 195
- Cancer of the larynx, unspecified 161
- Cancer of the trachea, unspecified 162.0
- Laryngectomy, radical 30.4
- Permanent tracheostomy 31.29

Defense of homebound status
- Unable to ambulate farther than 10′ (3 m) because of dyspnea with minimal exertion
- Unable to ambulate more than 10′ because of fatigue and poor endurance related to surgery
- Bedridden, requiring total care
- Unable to ambulate, requiring maximum assistance to transfer from bed to chair
- Dyspnea on exertion and requires continuous oxygen administration

Selected nursing diagnoses and patient outcomes

Ineffective airway clearance related to increased pulmonary secretions and difficulty clearing secretions
The patient or caregiver will:
- demonstrate effective coughing and increased air exchange in the lungs
(N, PT, RT)
- exhibit stable physiologic status and signs and symptoms of optimal respirations (N, PT, RT)
- demonstrate measures to manage increased secretions. (N, PT, RT)

Pain related to surgical procedure
Patient or caregiver will:
- adhere to medication plan and report a decrease in pain as evidenced by rating pain at 3 or less on a 0-to-10 scale 80% of the time
(N, HCA)
- demonstrate use of nonpharmacologic methods of pain control.
(N, HCA)

Risk for infection related to tracheostomy
The patient or caregiver will:
- remain free from signs and symptoms of acute respiratory tract infection
(N, HCA)
- demonstrate measures to prevent infection. (N, HCA, RT)

Knowledge deficit related to laryngectomy care and disease process
The patient or caregiver will:
- verbalize understanding of disease process related to laryngectomy and purpose of laryngectomy (N, PT, RT)
- demonstrate methods of alternative speech, such as esophageal speech, ar-

tificial larynges, and implanted prosthesis (N, SP)
• demonstrate the ability to perform all aspects of tracheostomy care, including suctioning, dressing change, inner cannula change, and care of equipment (N, RT)
• demonstrate appropriate use of oxygen therapy, aerosol therapy, and chest physiotherapy as indicated.
(N, PT, RT)

Risk for impaired skin integrity around tracheostomy tube insertion site related to surgery and creation of permanent tracheostomy

The patient or caregiver will:
• exhibit intact peritracheal skin, free from signs and symptoms of infection
(N, HCA, RT)
• state the signs and symptoms of infection to report to the physician
(N, RT)
• perform tracheostomy site care independently. (N, RT)

Impaired verbal communication related to laryngectomy

The patient or caregiver will:
• demonstrate the ability to communicate using alternate forms of communication. (N, OT, SP)

Body image disturbance related to creation of permanent tracheostomy and inability to communicate

The patient or caregiver will:
• demonstrate effective coping mechanisms (N, HCA, SW)
• demonstrate appropriate measures for managing changes in body image and lifestyle (N, HCA, SW)
• identify appropriate community resources. (N, SW)

Altered nutrition: Less than body requirements related to decreased oral intake, altered taste sensation, and swallowing difficulty

The patient or caregiver will:
• exhibit signs and symptoms of adequate nutrition and hydration status
(N, D, HCA)
• maintain weight within planned parameters (N, D, HCA)
• demonstrate correct use of enteral feedings, if indicated (N, D, HCA)
• demonstrate methods for correct swallowing. (N, SP)

Pain related to surgical procedure

The patient or caregiver will:
• report a decrease in pain as evidenced by rating pain at 3 or less on a 0-to-10 scale 80% of the time (N)
• comply with medication plan (N)
• use nonpharmacologic methods of pain control. (N, HCA)

Skilled nursing services

Care measures

• Perform an initial full assessment of all body systems with emphasis on the respiratory and cardiovascular systems, nutritional status, and cognitive level.
• Obtain a patient history relevant to respiratory and oxygenation status, including oxygen saturation levels.
• Assess breath sounds, breathing patterns, chest movements, secretions, and skin and mucous membrane color.
• Assess for signs of cerebral anoxia, activity intolerance, and chest pain.
• Assess the patient's need for suctioning, such as coarse adventitious breath sounds, coughing, respiratory distress and inability to clear secre-

tions, and characteristics of tracheal secretions.

• Monitor oxygen therapy use, if ordered; obtain or arrange for ABG analysis as ordered.

• Evaluate swallowing ability.

• Assess for anxiety and depression.

• Assess the level of care and compliance of the patient and caregiver with tracheostomy care, including dressing changes, inner cannula changes, and suctioning.

• Assess medication compliance, and monitor for signs and symptoms of adverse effects.

Patient and family teaching

• Teach the patient and family about the disease process, including the purpose and ramifications of laryngetomy and tracheostomy.

• Review suctioning procedure, including signs and symptoms that indicate the need for suctioning.

• Review tracheostomy care, including assessing for dislodgement of cannula; inflating and deflating cuff (if appropriate); suctioning; and changing the dressing, inner cannula, and tracheostomy ties.

• Discuss cleaning and storing of reusable equipment as well as how and where to obtain necessary equipment and supplies.

• Review peritracheal skin inspection and care measures.

• Identify signs and symptoms of respiratory infection.

• Review oxygen use and safety precautions, if indicated, including how to troubleshoot malfunctioning oxygen equipment and replace the tank.

• Teach aspiration and swallowing precautions.

• Provide information on nutritional therapy and fluid intake, breathing exercises and chest physiotherapy, and tracheostomy precautions (such as avoiding aerosol sprays and smoke, preventing aspiration while bathing and shaving, and avoiding smoke from barbecue grills and fires when outside).

• Discuss alternative methods for communication, such as a paper and pen, magic slate, and communication board.

• Cover energy conservation measures.

• Urge the use of a medical alert bracelet that identifies the patient as a neck breather.

• Instruct on medication therapy, including drug, dose, frequency, adverse effects, and signs and symptoms to report.

• Discuss signs and symptoms to report to the physician.

• Remind about follow-up immunizations.

Interdisciplinary actions

Dietitian

• Nutritional evaluation for calorie needs

• Recommendations for support with enteral nutrition and supplements as necessary

• Review foods and liquids for prescribed consistency

Home care aide

• Personal care

• Assistance with ADLs

• Assistance with nutrition and feeding

Speech pathologist
- Speech training and alternate modes of communication (such as voice synthesizer)
- Evaluation of swallowing skills and swallowing training

Occupational therapist
- Energy conservation
- ADL training
- Use of adaptive equipment

Physical therapist
- Home exercise program
- Pulmonary physical therapy — breathing exercises and chest physiotherapy as indicated
- Endurance training

Respiratory therapist
- Use of respiratory equipment, such as nebulizer, oxygen, and tracheostomy supplies
- Breathing exercises and chest physiotherapy

Social worker
- Community resources
- Support groups
- Counseling and referrals

Discharge plan
- Safe management of laryngectomy in the home with physician and community follow-up services
- Independence with all aspects of laryngectomy care
- Return to optimal level of functioning with ability to make needs known
- Referral for outpatient speech therapy for continued instruction in alternate communication methods
- Referral to community support groups

- Referral to hospice if diagnosis is terminal

Documentation requirements
- Skilled assessment, including vital signs; respiratory status (breath sounds, ease of respirations, character and amount of secretions, and oxygen use); tracheostomy care and precautions (dressing change, inner cannula change, and suctioning); understanding of and adherence to all aspects of tracheostomy care; results of blood studies (ABG analysis, if ordered, to support oxygen therapy use)
- Patient's or caregiver's independence with care and therapy regimen
- Patient or caregiver progress toward educational goals
- Patient response to care
- Interdisciplinary team communication: physical therapy, occupational therapy, respiratory therapy, dietitian, and social worker evaluation and need for services; plan for home program; changes in the plan of care, including changes in medication dosages based on blood studies; and patient or caregiver understanding of those changes
- Patient's adherence to instructions and therapy regimen

Reimbursement reminders
- For oxygen therapy to be covered, pulse oximetry or ABG analysis results are required to substantiate the patient's medical need for this therapy. A component also includes the need for skilled observation and evaluation of the patient's response to this therapy and patient and family teaching about when and how to use it.

• Patients receiving home oxygen therapy who had an initial partial pressure of oxygen of 56 or higher or an initial arterial oxygen saturation 89% or higher must have repeated laboratory testing within 60 to 90 days after the start of therapy to demonstrate continued need and, therefore continued coverage of the therapy. Additionally, the physician must see the patient and confirm the continued need for this service.

• Medicare won't reimburse for oxygen therapy ordered "p.r.n."

• Document specific teaching instructions related to oxygen therapy, medications, and safety measures.

• Document any variances to expected outcomes, such as peritracheal infection, increased secretions, and changes in characteristics of secretions.

• A physician order is needed for any plan of care change; document this in the patient's record.

• Specific barriers to learning (impaired vision, impaired mental status and cognitive ability, or caregiver deficiencies) must be identified and recorded.

• If no caregiver is available, willing, and able, documentation must reflect a plan for obtaining a caregiver or plan for an alternative care setting.

• Documentation should reveal if the patient had a laryngectomy recently or is new to medications, oxygen use, aerosol therapy, and chest physiotherapy.

• Specific deficits in initial knowledge level must be addressed and recorded and then progress shown as evidenced by specific concepts and procedures verbalized or demonstrated.

• The following supplies and durable medical equipment are covered by Medicare: nebulizer machine (reimbursed under Medicare part B, 80% of allowable charge if the physician indicates that a metered-dose inhaler alone is insufficient to treat the patient's symptoms), oxygen (reimbursed under Medicare part B, 80% of allowable charge, if the patient's oxygen saturation level is 88% or less), and tracheostomy care supplies (reimbursed under Medicare part B).

• Respiratory therapist services are usually provided by the company supplying the durable medical equipment on a routine or as-needed basis.

Insurance hints

• Present specific data on homebound status, such as bedridden or confined to chair, distance patient is able to ambulate (including use of stairs), changes in muscle strength or endurance.

• Present objective patient findings, changes in clinical condition, and changes in care since previous contact, such as a new physician orders or changes in respiratory or nutritional status.

• Present specifics about patient or caregiver education process, including skills mastered related to tracheostomy care, nutritional therapy, and oxygen use.

• Present progress toward established goals; adjustment issues, such as patient's resistance to or acceptance of therapy; and complications, such as medication adverse reactions or increased shortness of breath.

• Stress comorbid conditions (such as diabetes and chronic heart or lung disease) that would affect the patient's ability to provide self-care.

• Emphasize interventions aimed at avoiding inpatient care.

Leukemia

Leukemia, a progressive, malignant disease of the bone marrow and lymph nodes, is characterized by an uncontrolled proliferation of leukocytes. Immature white blood cells (WBCs) are produced, and thrombocytopenia and anemia soon develop as platelets and red blood cells are affected. Because the immature WBCs are ineffective, they lead to immunosuppression and increased susceptibility to infection. The cause of leukemia is unknown.

The primary focus of home care for the patient with leukemia is education. Some patients with leukemia may receive chemotherapy in the home. Additionally, if the patient is considered terminal with a prognosis of 6 months or less, a referral to hospice is made.

Previsit checklist

Physician orders and preparation
• Nutritional consult for development of individualized neutropenic diet
• Medication therapy as indicated
• Chemotherapeutic regimen as indicated
• Activity orders and restrictions
• Laboratory studies, including complete blood count
• Social worker evaluation for community referrals and counseling
• Physical therapy evaluation for home exercise program and endurance training

• Home care aide assistance with personal care and activities of daily living (ADLs)

Equipment and supplies
• Supplies for standard precautions and proper sharps disposal
• Phlebotomy supplies
• Protective gear for the nurse, including nonpermeable protective gown, shoe covers, goggles, latex gloves, mask, and a container designated for chemotherapeutic wastes (if home chemotherapy is to be given)
• Subclavian dressing care kit and Huber needle for implantable port (if patient has a venous access device)

Safety requirements
• System to assist with adherence to a complex medication regimen, including I.V. chemotherapy
• Emergency plan and access to functional phone and list of emergency phone numbers
• Home safety measures to prevent falls and injury
• Strict safety measures, including using protective equipment for the nurse if chemotherapy is to be given
• Strict sterile technique if a venous access device is to be accessed
• Standard precautions for infection control and sharps disposal
• Instructions on signs and symptoms of adverse reactions from medications, particularly chemotherapy, and actions to take
• Use of granulocytopenic precautions
• Signs and symptoms to report to the physician or emergency personnel

Major diagnostic codes

• Leukemia without/with remission 208.90/208.91

Defense of homebound status

• Risk for infection secondary to decreased WBC count
• Risk for bleeding secondary to decreased platelet count
• Unable to ambulate farther than 10′ (3 m) because of severe fatigue and weakness

Selected nursing diagnoses and patient outcomes

Knowledge deficit related to new diagnosis of leukemia

The patent or caregiver will:
• describe the illness, treatment goals, plan of care, and potential risks and benefits   (N, MD)
• identify care measures to manage common adverse effects of the proposed treatment regimen   (N, HCA)
• demonstrate the ability to perform necessary care measures, such as maintenance of venous access device site and medication administration   (N)
• maintain acceptable level of functioning based on energy levels.
                                                    (N, HCA, PT)

Risk for infection related to decreased WBC count

The patient or caregiver will:
• list signs and symptoms of infection for which to be alert   (N)
• participate in performing meticulous personal hygiene   (N, HCA)

• describe measures to prevent infection   (N, HCA)
• remain free from infection throughout treatment.   (N)

Risk for injury (bleeding) related to decreased platelet count

The patient or caregiver will:
• list signs and symptoms for which to be alert   (N)
• identify medications to avoid that affect blood clotting   (N)
• demonstrate adjustments in lifestyle and personal hygiene to minimize risk of bleeding   (N, HCA)
• remain free from bleeding episodes throughout treatment.   (N)

Pain related to leukemic process

The patient or caregiver will:
• monitor pain intensity, duration, and patterns as well as factors that alleviate or exacerbate pain, and communicate this information to the home care team   (N, MD)
• maintain an acceptable level of pain control   (N, PH)
• verbally contract to comply with pain-relief regimen, avoiding constipation as an adverse effect of pain medications   (N, PH)
• explore alternative supportive therapies for pain relief.   (N, SW)

Altered nutrition: Less than body requirements related to the disease process, chemotherapy, and increased metabolic demands

The patient or caregiver will:
• maintain weight within acceptable parameters   (N, D, HCA)
• identify measures to increase calorie and protein content in foods (N, D)
• remain free from signs and symptoms of nutritional deficiencies. (N, D, HCA)

Anticipatory grieving related to diagnosis of terminal illness

The patient or caregiver will:
- verbalize concerns and feelings (N, HCA, SW)
- use appropriate coping strategies to deal with the diagnosis (N, HCA, SW)
- demonstrate actions indicative of progression to acceptance (N, SW)
- identify resources for support (N, HCA, SW)
- verbalize approval for hospice services. (N, MD, SW)

Skilled nursing services

Care measures
- Perform an initial assessment of all body systems with emphasis on the GI, genitourinary, and integumentary systems as well as nutrition and hydration status and cognitive level.
- Assess the level of care, including observations as the patient or caregiver prepares each day's medication according to the regimen and performs maintenance of the venous access device (if applicable).
- Assess the effectiveness of the treatment regimen (monitor vital signs, check laboratory results frequently, assess for signs and symptoms of infection and bleeding, and assess the level of pain on a scale of 0 to 10).
- Administer chemotherapy as ordered.
- Assess activity and energy level, including complaints of increasing fatigue or weakness.
- Evaluate weight trends.
- Obtain or arrange for laboratory studies as indicated.

Patient and family teaching
- Teach the patient and family about the disease process.
- Review dietary recommendations, including purpose of granulocytopenic diet, how it affects the patient, and foods included on the diet.
- Discuss measures to prevent and control infection.
- Describe the medication regimen, including the name of each drug, adverse effects, and interactions.
- Promote positive coping strategies.
- Discuss dangerous signs and symptoms that require immediate intervention.
- Remind about follow-up appointments for laboratory studies and chemotherapy administration.

Interdisciplinary actions

Dietitian
- Dietary calorie and protein recommendations
- Neutropenic diet plan

Home care aide
- Personal care
- Assistance with ADLs
- Assistance with nutrition

Physical therapist
- Home exercise program
- Endurance training

Discharge plan
- Safe management of leukemia and possible complications at home with physician follow-up services
- Referral to community support services

- Maintenance of optimal level of functional ability
- Pain- and symptom-free until death; death with dignity

Documentation requirements

- Skilled assessment, including subjective and objective data with regard to signs and symptoms of infection, findings from nutritional assessment, and vital signs and weight trends
- Patient or caregiver participation in care (care of venous access device and coordination of medication regimen)
- Patient or caregiver progress toward educational goals (knowledge of medications, disease process, and granulocytopenic precautions)
- Patient response to care, including areas of improvement or deterioration and subsequent need for increased services
- Discussion about the need for hospice care as appropriate
- Patient or caregiver instructions
- Changes in the plan of care, including changes based on blood studies; patient or caregiver understanding of changes, and signs and symptoms to be reported

Reimbursement reminders

- Dietitian services aren't reimbursable under the Medicare home care benefit.
- Teaching for prevention of infection isn't reimbursable.
- Hospice benefit under Medicare doesn't require the patient to be homebound or have identified skilled care needs.

Insurance hints

- Describe objective data about homebound status, such as degree of patient's fatigue and presence of infection.
- Present objective patient findings, including new laboratory values, changes since previous contact, and the need for additional services if the patient's condition begins to deteriorate.
- Present specific data about the patient education progress (diet, medication, and follow-up appointments).
- Discuss the patient's eligibility for and availability of hospice care before the patient requires it.

Liver failure

The patient with liver disease needs to manage his care properly at home to slow progression of the disease and lessen the likelihood of complications, such as ascitic fluid buildup, bleeding tendencies, encephalopathy, and hepatic coma. Depending on the stage of disease, the patient has to make these changes or his caregivers need to learn specifics about his care.

Liver disease includes cirrhosis and liver cancer. Liver damage can be due to alcohol abuse, chemicals, medications, or infection. The focus of home care for this patient includes nutrition education, infection prevention, management of and monitoring for complications, and skin care. The element that probably caused the disease (such as alcohol or medications) needs to be avoided to slow disease progression. The home care nurse should also teach methods of avoiding contributing factors.

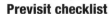

Previsit checklist

Physician orders and preparation

- Diet orders (may include tube feedings or parenteral nutrition)
- Medication orders
- Activity orders and restrictions
- Laboratory studies
- Physical therapy evaluation for therapeutic exercise, transfer techniques, and gait training
- Occupational therapy assistance with activities of daily living (ADLs), muscle reeducation, perceptual motor training, and adaptive equipment
- Nutritional evaluation for diet plan and recommendations
- Speech therapy evaluation for dysphagia and nonoral communications related to esophageal varices, if indicated
- Social worker evaluation for community support and counseling
- Home care aide assistance with personal care and ADLs

Equipment and supplies

- Supplies for standard precautions and proper sharps disposal
- Tape measure
- Fecal occult blood test
- Phlebotomy supplies
- Syringes, dressing, tube feeding bag, and irrigation kit for gastrostomy tube, if needed

Safety requirements

- Standard precautions for infection control and sharps disposal
- System to assist with adherence to a complex medication regimen, including I.V. therapy
- Emergency plan and access to functional phone and list of emergency phone numbers
- Home safety measures to prevent falls and injury, including handrails, grab bars, a shower seat, and a nonskid bathmat for bathroom safety as well as shoes with nonskid soles
- Aspiration precautions
- Use of proper technique in ambulating and transferring patient
- Available support person

Major diagnostic codes

- Cirrhosis:
  - alcoholic 571.2
  - due to Wilson's disease 275.1
  - fatty 571.8
  - liver 571.5
- Liver, metastatic cancer of 197.7
- Liver cancer 155.2

Defense of homebound status

- Unable to ambulate farther than 10′ (3 m) because of shortness of breath from ascites
- Bedridden because of severe weakness
- Unable to safely ambulate outside the home because of confusion or disorientation to time, place, person, and situation due to ammonia buildup
- Unable to leave home secondary to passage of frequent stools as medication effect
- Unable to leave home because of need for continuous parenteral nutrition
- High risk for infection from compromised immune status or high risk for hemorrhage due to esophageal

varices and bleeding tendencies interfering with ability to leave home
• Unable to ambulate without assistance
• Unable to transfer without assistance

Selected nursing diagnoses and patient outcomes

Altered nutrition: Less than body requirements related to altered hepatic function
The patient or caregiver will:
• verbalize the importance of certain nutrients and describe how these nutrients (fats, alcohol, and vitamin K) are metabolized (N, D)
• verbalize knowledge of nutrients and menu selections appropriate to optimize nutrition without contributing to disease progression (N, D)
• demonstrate ability to administer enteral or parenteral feedings, if indicated (N, D)
• verbalize the ability to identify complications of oral, enteral, or parenteral feedings (N, D)
• maintain body weight within acceptable parameters (N, D, HCA)
• demonstrate appropriate measures to combat dysphagia. (N, SP)

Risk for injury (bleeding) related to impaired blood coagulation or bleeding from portal hypertension
The patient or caregiver will:
• provide a safe environment to prevent the patient from falling (N, HCA, OT, PT)
• verbalize measures to prevent bleeding episodes (use of safety razors, fall prevention, use of soft toothbrush, and avoidance of injections and needle sticks) (N)

• verbalize reasons why liver disease may predispose the patient to bleeding episodes (N, MD)
• verbalize signs and symptoms of bleeding (dark stools, coffee-ground emesis, petechiae, and bleeding from the nose or other orifices) (N, MD)
• verbalize emergency measures to control bleeding and emergency plan for obtaining immediate medical attention. (N, MD)

Altered thought processes related to elevated serum ammonia levels and hepatic coma
The patient or caregiver will:
• provide reminders for reality orientation, such as large clock and calendar and current events (N, HCA)
• provide a safe home environment to keep the patient from falling (N, HCA, OT, PT)
• verbalize resources to help with patient supervision. (N, SW)

Diarrhea related to medication therapy for liver failure
The patient or caregiver will:
• verbalize proper medication administration to promote bowel routine by titrating medication to __ bowel movements per day, if ordered (N, MD, PH)
• verbalize measures to reduce episodes of incontinence by offering the bedpan or taking the patient to the bathroom every 2 hours (N, HCA)
• demonstrate proper method of cleaning patient and changing bed linens, if the patient is bedridden. (N, HCA)

Ineffective breathing pattern secondary to ascites
The patient or caregiver will:

- verbalize measures to reduce shortness of breath, such as pacing activities (N, PT)
- demonstrate proper positioning to facilitate optimal breathing (N, PT)
- verbalize emergency plan in case of extreme shortness of breath. (N)

Fluid volume excess related to ascites and portal hypertension
The patient or caregiver will:
- demonstrate how to monitor for fluid buildup (measuring abdominal girth, daily weight, intake and output; checking for edema) (N, HCA)
- verbalize fluid restriction and encouragement, if ordered, and demonstrate how to measure fluids (N, D, HCA)
- state actions, adverse effects, and precautions of diuretics, if ordered (N)
- verbalize knowledge and management of a low-sodium diet. (N, D)

Impaired skin integrity secondary to itching and skin irritation
The patient or caregiver will:
- demonstrate proper skin care to prevent pressure ulcers and maintain skin integrity (N, HCA, PT)
- use topical medications as prescribed to reduce itching. (N, MD, PH)

Knowledge deficit related to (specify disease process, normal liver functioning, nutrition, medications, or complications)
The patient or caregiver will:
- verbalize signs and symptoms of complications, such as mental status changes, signs and symptoms of bleeding, and lethargy (N)
- state components of diet (low sodium, high calorie; advanced stages may require low protein as well) (N, D)

- verbalize causes and manifestations of liver disease (N)
- demonstrate proper technique for administering medications, tube feeding, or parenteral nutrition if indicated (N, D, PH)
- verbalize an emergency plan in case of bleeding or episode of confusion (N)
- demonstrate logging of daily weight, abdominal girth, and intake and output measurements (N, HCA)
- verbalize knowledge of avoidance of alcohol, chemicals, and nonprescription medications (N)
- state an understanding of activity limitations (N, HCA, OT, PT)
- verbalize frequency and importance of follow-up physician visits and laboratory tests. (N)

Ineffective coping (specify Individual or Family) related to disease process
The patient or caregiver will:
- identify coping mechanisms that have worked in the past (N, SW)
- identify resources to assist in caring for patient (N, SW)
- verbalize new coping mechanisms (N, SW)
- use appropriate sources for support. (N, HCA, SW)

Activity intolerance related to fatigue, anemia, and ascites
The patient or caregiver will:
- perform prescribed exercises safely (N, HCA, OT, PT)
- slowly increase activity to build tolerance (N, HCA, OT, PT)
- verbalize limitations and ways to achieve optimal independence with ADLs. (N, OT, PT)

Skilled nursing services

Care measures
● Perform initial assessment of all body systems with emphasis on the mental and nutritional status and neurologic, GI, and cardiovascular systems.
● Assess fluid balance, skin condition, signs and symptoms of bleeding, and patient and family knowledge of infection prevention.
● Obtain and arrange for laboratory studies as ordered.
● Administer I.V. or subcutaneous medications as ordered.
● Administer tube feeding or parenteral nutrition, if newly ordered.
● Assess level of self-care of patient or ability of caregiver to care for patient.
● Assess the effectiveness of the treatment regimen and identify possible complications (tolerance of feedings, signs and symptoms of bleeding, infection, weight gain, changes in mental status).
● Evaluate weight and vital sign changes; measure abdominal girth.
● Assess the need for hospice care.

Patient and family teaching
● Teach about tube feedings or parenteral nutrition.
● Describe medication administration, actions, and adverse effects. Also review administration of subcutaneous injections such as vitamin K.
● Discuss signs and symptoms of complications, such as bleeding, infection, and fluid buildup.
● Instruct on care of the bedridden patient, if applicable.
● Urge the patient to follow the prescribed diet.
● Emphasize proper skin care to prevent irritation and pressure ulcers.

● Demonstrate how to monitor fluid balance (weight, fluid intake and output, and abdominal girth measurement).
● Provide reality orientation and safety measures for the confused patient.

Interdisciplinary actions

Dietitian
● Nutritional evaluation for caloric needs
● Recommendations for nutritional therapy, including enteral or parenteral therapy

Home care aide
● Personal care
● Assistance with ADLs
● Assistance with nutrition

Occupational therapist
● Assistance with ADLs
● Muscle reeducation
● Sensory treatment and perceptual motor training
● Adaptive equipment, if indicated

Physical therapist
● Transfer and gait training
● Therapeutic exercise

Social worker
● Community resources and referrals
● Counseling and coping strategies
● Short-term adjustment to terminal illness
● Referral for hospice care or long-term planning

Speech pathologist
● Evaluation and treatment of dysphagia related to esophageal varices, if indicated

- Nonoral communications due to esophageal varices, if indicated

Discharge plan
- Safe management of liver failure in the home with physician follow-up services
- Ability to demonstrate how to prevent and manage complications
- Referral to community support groups
- Maintenance of optimal level of functional ability
- Referral to hospice if diagnosis is terminal
- Pain- and symptom-free until death; death with dignity

Documentation requirements
- Skilled assessment, including subjective and objective data with regard to signs and symptoms of infection; findings from nutritional assessment; and vital signs, abdominal girth, and weight trends
- Patient or caregiver participation in care (coordination of medication regimen, nutritional therapy, and exercise program)
- Patient or caregiver progress toward educational goals (knowledge of medications, disease process, and bleeding and safety precautions)
- Patient response to care, including areas of improvement or deterioration and subsequent need for increased services; discussion about the need for hospice care as appropriate; the patient's or caregiver's ability to participate in ADLs; medication administration; patient or caregiver understanding of nutritional and fluid requirements and limitations; patient's activity level; and

signs or symptoms of complications (bleeding, fluid buildup, and infection)
- Patient and caregiver instructions

Reimbursement reminders
- Medicare won't pay for maintenance care of the patient with chronic liver disease. Document the need for skilled nursing visits, including new diagnoses, changes in the patient's condition, recent admissions to hospital, and the need for teaching about new treatments.
- Identify how the patient or caregiver is moving toward an attainable and measurable goal. Be specific, for example, "Caregiver is able to demonstrate measurement of tube feeding, flush gastrostomy tube, check for residual. Instructed caregiver on infection control, such as hand washing, storage of tube feeding, and wearing gloves."
- If you are administering injections, document the reason why injections are needed and why the patient or caregiver can't give the injections (for example, lacks manual dexterity and can't hold syringe in hand).
- Dietitian services aren't reimbursable by Medicare.

Insurance hints
- Describe objective data about homebound status, such as degree of patient's fatigue and presence of infection or bleeding.
- Present objective patient findings, including new laboratory values, changes since previous contact, and the need for additional services if the patient's condition begins to deteriorate.
- Present specific data about the patient education progress, including diet, medication, and follow-up appointments.

- Discuss the patient's eligibility for and availability of hospice care before the patient requires it.

Lyme disease

Lyme disease is a complex illness caused by *Borrelia* spirochetes transmitted to humans by way of tick bites. A warm, red lesion forms in the bite area accompanied by headache, neck stiffness, fever, chills, myalgia, arthralgia, malaise, and fatigue. Arthritis of the large joints may develop. Systemic involvement may consist of hepatitis, cardiomegaly, meningeal irritation, and erosion of cartilage. Recognized in at least 32 states, the disease is preventable to some extent with patient education. Early intervention is a necessity to avoid fatality from atrioventricular blocks or left-sided heart failure.

Previsit checklist

Physician orders and preparation
- Oral medication orders as indicated
- Activity orders
- Occupational therapy evaluation for energy conservation and assistance with activities of daily living (ADLs) as patient recovers
- Physical therapy evaluation for individualized exercise program based on extent of musculoskeletal involvement
- Home care aide assistance with personal care and ADLs

Equipment and supplies
- Supplies for standard precautions and proper sharps disposal

- Urine specimen collection container
- Phlebotomy supplies

Safety requirements
- Standard precautions for infection control and sharps disposal
- Information on medication, including dosage, adverse effects, interactions, and safe storage
- Instructions on signs and symptoms of a life-threatening medical emergency and actions to take
- Emergency plan and access to functional phone and list of emergency phone numbers
- Avoidance of exercise that would accelerate joint stress

Major diagnostic code
- Lyme disease 088.81

Defense of homebound status
- Homebound related to joint pain secondary to Lyme disease
- Unable to ambulate unassisted related to meningeal symptoms secondary to Lyme disease
- Bedridden related to heart block and ventricular dysfunction secondary to Lyme disease
- Severe arthritis of the large joints, requiring assistance of another person to ambulate

Selected nursing diagnoses and patient outcomes

Impaired physical mobility related to severe joint inflammation

The patient or caregiver will:
- maintain current level of range of motion of each joint without loss of joint function (N, OT, PT)
- report a manageable level of discomfort, such as rating pain at 3 or less on a 0-to-10 scale (N, PT)
- verbally contract to participate freely in an exercise and therapeutic program (N, OT, PT)
- maintain a calendar with physician and physical and occupational therapy appointments noted.
(N, HCA, OT, PT)

Knowledge deficit related to medication therapy regimen
The patient or caregiver will:
- state the correct dosage for each anti-inflammatory drug in the medication regimen (N, PH)
- identify at least three significant expected adverse effects of medications.
(N, PH)

Pain related to severe joint inflammation
The patient or caregiver will:
- maintain a pain diary, noting episodes of remission and exacerbation
(N, HCA, PT)
- note daily levels of discomfort, verbally contracting to contact the primary care provider when level of discomfort is greater than 5 on a 0-to-10 scale (N)
- use appropriate pain-relief strategies. (N, HCA, PH, PT)

Skilled nursing services

Care measures
- Perform initial assessment of all body systems with emphasis on the neuro-logic, musculoskeletal, cardiovascular, and integumentary systems.
- Assess vital signs and heart rate and rhythm for changes.
- Evaluate patient's neurologic status for changes.
- Assess the effectiveness of the treatment regimen; monitor joint swelling, migratory joint and bone pain, meningeal irritation, hepatitis, and development of atrioventricular blocks, ventricular dysfunction, or cardiomegaly.

Patient and family teaching
- Teach about the medication therapy, including interactions, adverse reactions, dosage, and route for each drug.
- Review signs and symptoms of complications to report to the physician.
- Discuss ways to prevent recurrence of Lyme disease.

Interdisciplinary actions

Home care aide
- Personal care
- Assistance with ADLs

Occupational therapist
- Energy conservation
- ADL assistance and necessary adaptations

Physical therapist
- Home exercise program
- Range-of-motion exercises

Discharge plan
- Safe management of the recovery and rehabilitation phase of Lyme disease in the home with physician follow-up services

- Return to pre-illness level of function
- Referral for outpatient physical therapy if indicated

Documentation requirements

- Skilled assessment, including vital signs and heart rate and rhythm; joint involvement and degree of movement restriction; level of pain and relief measures used, including findings from patient's daily pain log, such as factors exacerbating and relieving pain and periods of remission and exacerbation; extent of fatigue and malaise; results of monitoring progression of potentially life-threatening complications
- Patient or caregiver participation in care, including participation in exercise program and strict adherence to the medication regimen
- Patient response to care
- Patient and caregiver instructions: signs and symptoms of complications, including meningeal irritation, cardiovascular changes, hepatitis, and joint erosion; pain-relief measures; medication therapy regimen; and measures to prevent recurrence of Lyme disease

Reimbursement reminders

- Blue Cross and Blue Shield won't reimburse for occupational therapy as a lone skilled service.
- Registered physical therapist services are reimbursable under the Medicare home care benefit; under Blue Cross and Blue Shield, a registered physical therapist must follow the patient throughout the course of therapy, and the patient can't be followed by a licensed physical therapy assistant for services to be reimbursable.
- Interdisciplinary care coordination must be documented.
- Teaching for prevention of complications secondary to Lyme disease isn't considered a reimbursable skilled nursing service.
- Specific barriers to learning and variance to expected outcomes, such as the development of complications, must be recorded.
- Initial knowledge deficits (regarding medication in particular) should be recorded, followed by details about the patient's progress as evidenced by specific concepts and information demonstrated or verbalized.
- Measures that help achieve patient goals and the steps being taken to decrease frequency of visits as goals are met are keys to reimbursement.
- Changes in the patient's condition that require continual skilled care or physician contact must be documented.

Insurance hints

- Describe objective data about homebound status (joint inflammation, neurologic symptoms, and cardiac symptoms).
- Present objective patient findings and changes since previous contact, such as results of laboratory studies and diagnostic tests (most recent erythrocyte sedimentation rate, multiple gated acquisition scan, EEG, magnetic resonance imaging scan, and electrocardiography scan as appropriate).
- Report specific data about the patient education progress (such as knowledge gained in relation to medications and the exercise program).

Mastectomy care

Treatment of breast cancer by local management requires breast surgery. The size, type, and stage of the tumor, as well as the woman's age, physical condition, and personal preference, determine the type of surgery. Modified radical mastectomy is the excision of a breast tumor, the entire breast, and the axillary lymph nodes. A partial (or segmental) mastectomy is the removal of a tumor and a small wedge of normal surrounding tissue. A total mastectomy is removal of the breast. A radical mastectomy (removal of the breast, pectoral muscles, and axillary nodes) is rarely done. Mammaplasty is reconstruction of the breast. Mastectomy care provided by the home care nurse must focus on wound care, pain, body image, fear of dying, coping skills, and disease management (from self-breast examinations to chemotherapy).

Previsit checklist

Physician orders and preparation
- Medications, including chemotherapy and hormonal agents
- Restrictions on use of affected side for phlebotomy, blood pressure, and activity
- Comfort and pain control measures
- Wound care
- Prosthesis (as indicated)
- Evaluation by physical therapist for therapeutic exercises, and range of motion (ROM) of affected arm
- Evaluation by occupational therapist for prosthesis and device application and use of adaptive equipment

- Visit by social worker for referral to community resources and financial assistance
- Home care aide assistance with personal care and activities of daily living (ADLs)

Equipment and supplies
- Supplies for standard precautions and proper medical waste disposal
- Dressing and wound care supplies: sterile dressings, sterile gauze and toppers, rolls of conforming gauze bandages (such as Kling and Kerlix rolls), nonadherent pads, sterile solutions, ointments, sterile applicators, sterile gloves
- Device for measuring wound
- Wound culturing supplies
- Scale

Safety requirements
- Standard precautions for infection control and medical waste disposal
- Instructions on symptoms of complications or medical emergency, particularly signs of infection or an embolus, and actions to take
- Adaptation of lifestyle and ADLs to conserve energy and minimize strain on affected arm
- Preoperative patient teaching, if indicated
- Information on medications, including dosage, adverse effects, interactions, and safe storage of multiple medications
- Allergies verified and documented
- Occupational Health and Safety Administration–approved clean-up (spill) kit for in-home chemotherapy

• Emergency plan and access to functional phone and list of emergency phone numbers

• Identification and correction of environmental hazards and patient-specific concerns (for example, inability to open cans, handrails on the unaffected side, and night-lights)

• Medical identification bracelet stating no venipuncture or compression to affected arm

Major diagnostic codes

• Cancer of the breast, unspecified 174.9

• Fibrocystic disease 610.1

• Lumpectomy, partial mastectomy 85.43

• Metastases, general/bone 199.1/198.5

• Radiation, enteritis/myelitis 558.1/990

• Radical mastectomy 85.45

• Secondary malignant breast neoplasm 198.81

• Simple mastectomy 85.41

• Wound dehiscence 998.3

• Wound infection 998.51

Defense of homebound status

• Bedridden or confined to chair; out of bed less than twice daily

• Immunosuppressed patient requiring open wound dressing care

• Weakness and pain due to surgery, chemotherapy, or radiation therapy; unable to ambulate without assistance

• Prescribed activity restriction due to extensive reconstructive surgery following mastectomy

Selected nursing diagnoses and patient outcomes

Pain

The patient or caregiver will:

• articulate factors that intensify pain and modify behavior accordingly (N)

• rate pain at 3 or less on a 0-to-10 scale 80% of the time (N)

• carry out appropriate pharmacologic and nonpharmacologic interventions for pain relief. (N, MD)

Risk for infection related to surgical wound

The patient or caregiver will:

• remain infection-free and afebrile (N)

• verbalize or demonstrate an understanding of correct postoperative wound and hemovac care (N)

• exhibit wound healing without complications (N)

• adhere to medical regimen (N, HCA, OT, PT)

• experience decrease in complications from chemotherapy or radiation therapy. (N)

Dressing and grooming self-care deficit

The patient or caregiver will:

• meet personal care needs (N, HCA, OT, PT)

• apply information related to disease process and possible complications to ADLs (N, HCA, OT, PT, SW)

• have an increase in strength, mobility, and endurance (N, HCA, OT, PT)

• implement and maintain home exercise schedule (N, HCA, OT, PT)

• return to self-care with presurgery independence levels. (N, HCA, OT, PT)

Body image disturbance related to changes in appearance secondary to mastectomy and adverse effects of radiation and chemotherapy

The patient or caregiver will:
• verbalize knowledge regarding prosthetic devices and items available
(N, OT, PT)
• demonstrate understanding of need for alteration in ADLs (N, OT, PT)
• verbalize understanding of change in body image (N)
• contact and use identified community support systems and resources, including breast cancer support groups such as Y-Me (N, OT, PT, SW)
• verbalize knowledge of complications or changes warranting notification of a nurse or physician (N)
• be comfortable with physical reconstruction. (N, HCA, OT, PT, SW)

Skilled nursing services

Care measures
• Conduct an initial full assessment of all systems, focusing on skin integrity, nutrition, coping skills, signs of depression, signs of infection, and ROM of the affected arm.
• Assess the surgical site, including wound location, dimensions, condition of surrounding tissue, granulation, drainage, edema, and odor.
• Assess and measure wound and hemovac drainage.
• Instruct the patient and caregiver in postoperative wound care as indicated and ordered.
• Monitor response to care and medications.
• Assess the affected arm, hand, and fingers for color, edema, and circulatory problems.

• Assess emotional response to illness and effectiveness of coping mechanisms.
• Implement bowel regimen, and monitor for constipation related to pain medications or diarrhea related to antibiotics.
• Assess the patient's response to the plan of care, and contact the physician for needed changes in the plan of care.
• Culture wound and track results, communicating results to other health team members.

Patient and family teaching
• Teach about procedures for wound care, signs of healing, and infection.
• Discuss increased risk of infection related to lymphedema and an open wound.
• Review chemotherapy and radiation regimen and schedule.
• Explain the need to keep the affected arm protected and elevated to minimize lymphedema.
• Discuss activity limitations related to the use of the affected arm. Reinforce the importance of ROM exercises prescribed for the affected arm to prevent edema and atrophy at each visit.
• Emphasize the importance of preventing use of the affected arm use for venipuncture, blood pressure, or other procedures. Instruct the patient not to wear constrictive clothing or jewelry on the affected arm.
• Demonstrate the use of antiembolism sleeves to decrease edema and the risk of clot formation.
• Make the patient aware of potential complications as a result of immunocompromised state and the need for preventive health care, such as pneumonia and influenza vaccinations and

avoiding of people with infectious conditions, such as colds and chickenpox.
• Review skin care needs and methods of preventing breakdown.
• Identify coping mechanisms and relaxation methods.
• Teach about medication use, including contraindications and adverse effects.
• Explain the importance of nutrition and hydration for tissue healing.
• Stress the need to perform regular breast self-examinations.
• Identify signs and symptoms to report to the physician.
• Discuss when to call emergency medical personnel.

Interdisciplinary actions

Home care aide
• Assistance with personal care and ADLs
• Participation in home exercise program

Occupational therapist
• Evaluation
• Teaching about safe performance of ADLs
• Breast prosthesis introduction

Physical therapist
• Evaluation and development of home exercise program for active and resistive exercises to prevent "frozen shoulder"
• Instruction and supervision of home exercise program

Social worker
• Evaluation and identification of problems

• Eligibility for additional services or resources
• Referrals to appropriate community resources
• Psychosocial counseling related to altered body image, discussing feelings with husband or significant other, and grieving process over the loss of her breast
• Assistance to the patient in obtaining prosthesis (Reach to Recovery)

Discharge plan
• Safe management of recovery from mastectomy in home with physician follow-up
• Follow-up appointments scheduled with physician
• Pain- and symptom-free until death; death with dignity
• Discharged to care of hospice and physician

Documentation requirements
• Skilled assessment, including subjective and objective signs and symptoms related to wound status and care, pain management, and presence or absence of postoperative complications
• Skilled assessment of surgical site, including wound location, dimensions, condition of surrounding tissue (macerated, erythematous, indurated), condition of wound base (color, presence of eschar), color of surrounding tissue, granulation, drainage, edema, odor, culture obtained, and drainage from hemovac
• Specific care, treatments, and medications administered
• Instructions given, demonstrated, and provided in writing

- Patient and caregiver response to care and instructions as well as progress toward educational goals, including ability to look at wound, change dressing, perform breast self-examination, and record of initial versus current weight
- Coordination of patient care with other members of the health care team and communication of changes in the plan of care
- Assessment of progress toward goals as well as prevention of complications usually associated with patients receiving radiation, chemotherapy, or surgical interventions

Reimbursement reminders

- Make sure that schedule changes or additional services or treatments by any discipline have an accompanying order from the physician.
- Monitor the patient's response to changes in the plan of care.
- Identify any barriers to learning resulting in the need for ongoing visits, such as no willing or available caregiver, and dysfunctional coping skills such as denial.
- Report comorbid conditions or specific factors that affect the patient or wound healing, such as diabetes, osteoporosis, smoking, or no available caregiver.
- Check for an authorized laboratory because many insurance companies have contracts with specific laboratories for processing specimens.
- Dressing and wound care supplies aren't considered routine and therefore are billable when specifically identified in the plan of care as ordered by the physician and entered into Loca

tor 14 (Supplies) of Health Care Finance Administration Form 485 or ordered by the physician within the specific order for treatment requiring the use of certain supplies and entered into Locator 21 (Orders for Treatment).

- When billing for medical supplies, always include the name of supply item, date supply was used, number of units used, and charge per unit.
- Ensure that if daily care is ordered (for postoperative wound care or as the patient's condition declines), there must be a beginning and ending date for the expected time that daily visits will be necessary.

Insurance hints

- Determine initially how often to report clinical conditions, and always notify the insurance company immediately if patient changes affect the frequency or duration of initial care planning.
- Present subjective and objective data specific to established goals, including wound healing, pain level on a 0-to-10 scale, use of the affected arm, and weight changes.
- Provide updates on homebound status, including specifics, such as the inability to get out of bed more than twice daily and ambulating with assistance less than 10′ (3 m).
- Provide alerts to possible barriers to care and learning, including lack of an available caregiver, poor vision, comorbid conditions, advanced age, depression, and weakness.
- Provide updates on progress toward specific goals and prevention of complications.

Ménière's disease

Ménière's disease is a disorder of the inner ear that causes vertigo, tinnitus, a feeling of fullness or pressure in the ear, and fluctuating hearing loss. Even though the underlying cause is unknown, the disease is believed to result from fluctuating fluid pressure within the inner ear. An attack begins with a fullness or aching in one or both ears accompanied by hearing changes or tinnitus. Shortly thereafter, severe vertigo, imbalance, nausea, and vomiting occur. The average attack lasts 2 to 4 hours but may appear in clusters. Weeks, months, or years may pass between episodes. Most of the physical problems in the patient with Ménière's disease are focused on manifestations associated with the vertigo and imbalance, tinnitus, and long-term hearing loss. For these issues, teaching is needed for the families of patients with this health condition and should focus on support of the patient during an acute episode, recognition of the onset of an episode, patient safety, and fluid and electrolyte balance caused by the nausea and vomiting.

Previsit checklist

Physician orders and preparation
• Medications, including antiemetics and antivertigo agents
• Comfort and nausea control measures
• Social worker evaluation for community resources and financial assistance
• Dietitian for menu planning and alternatives to meet dietary needs

• Orders for nutritional supplements and restrictions (sodium, caffeine, alcohol, monosodium glutamate)
• Home care aide for assistance with personal care and activities of daily living (ADLs)

Equipment and supplies
• Supplies for standard precautions
• Sample nutritional supplements
• Scale
• Suction supplies

Safety requirements
• Standard precautions for infection control
• Identification and correction of environmental hazards and patient-specific concerns (for example, placement of grab bars and supportive devices in the bathroom, removal of throw rugs and carpeting, night-lights, indirect lighting)
• Aspiration precautions
• Safe use of suction equipment
• Skin care and protection, including frequent position changes
• Emergency plan and access to functional phone and list of emergency phone numbers

Major diagnostic codes
• Audible and objective 388.32
• Auditory vertigo 386.19
• Central deafness 389.14
• Chronic hypotension 458.1
• Cochlear 386.02
• Cochleovestibular 386.01
• Combined deafness 389.08
• Dizziness 780.4
• Electrolyte and fluid disorders 276.9
• Functional deafness 300.11
• Ménière's disease, unspecified 386.00

- Ménière's disease, vestibular 386.03
- Middle ear deafness 389.03
- Nausea 787.02
- Nausea with vomiting 787.01
- Orthostatic hypotension 458.0
- Sensory deafness 389.11
- Subjective 388.31
- Tinnitus, unspecified 388.30
- Transient ischemic deafness 388.02
- Vestibular neuronitis 386.12
- Volume depletion 276.5

Defense of homebound status

- Unable to leave home environment because of unpredictable periods of vertigo
- Potential for hypotensive episodes because of fluid imbalance caused by nausea and vomiting
- Ongoing episodes of tinnitus with unpredictable pattern of residual deafness

Selected nursing diagnoses and patient outcomes

Risk for trauma
   The patient or caregiver will:
- recognize the onset of an acute attack of vertigo   (N)
- demonstrate moving the patient to a reclining position   (N)
- demonstrate how to keep a safe home environment because of the unpredictability of the onset of symptoms
                                        (N, HCA)
- demonstrate comfort measures during the acute phase of vertigo   (N)
- recognize the potential for social isolation because of the unpredictability of the disease process   (N, SW)

- plan to obtain a medical identification bracelet as a precautionary measure.   (N)

Sleep pattern disturbance
   The patient or caregiver will:
- recognize that tinnitus can be disturbing to the normal sleep pattern (N)
- demonstrate alternatives to mask the tinnitus, such as playing a radio softly, using a white-noise system, wearing a hearing aid with a low tone to "cover up" the tinnitus, or wearing a hearing aid that amplifies ambient sound   (N)
- demonstrate safe use of medications to treat tinnitus and promote rest and sleep, such as meclizine or diazepam.
                                        (N, MD)

Altered nutrition: Less than body requirements
   The patient or caregiver will:
- demonstrate alternatives to regular eating patterns, such as finger foods and frequent small amounts of fluid during the acute phase of an attack
                                        (N, D)
- consume at least ___ calories daily.
                                        (N, D)

Sensory-perceptual alteration (auditory)
   The patient or caregiver will:
- realize that chronic hearing loss can lead to progressive deafness   (N)
- verbalize adaptations to work environment or other accommodations to cope with hearing impairment or tinnitus   (N)
- recognize that impaired verbal communication doesn't reduce the value of the individual   (N, SP)

- recognize that hearing loss may cause speech impairment and use techniques obtained by speech therapy to maximize speech recovery   (N, SP)
- recognize that having a speech impairment doesn't mean that the patient can't hear, so yelling is unnecessary; speak clearly and face the patient when conversing   (N, SP)
- demonstrate waiting an adequate time for a response from the patient when communicating   (N, SP)
- demonstrate facing the patient when communicating and speaking slowly   (N, SP)
- demonstrate the use of short, simple statements and questions to permit the processing of information   (N, SP)
- recognize frustration and anger as a normal response to the loss of functioning   (N, SP)
- determine alternative methods to enhance communication, including writing tablets and flash cards. (N, SP)

Ineffective individual coping
The patient or caregiver will:
- identify signs and symptoms of depression and low self-esteem that stem from having a chronic, disabling disorder   (N, SW)
- demonstrate methods to aid in coping with the unpredictability of Ménière's disease and acute attacks.   (N)

Anticipatory grieving
The patient or caregiver will:
- recognize the loss of hearing as a significant change in normal functioning   (N)
- plan time to evaluate life goals and the impact of the hearing loss on those goals   (N, SW)

- demonstrate effective coping with hearing impairment.   (N)

Impaired physical mobility related to vertigo
The patient or caregiver will:
- realize that sudden attacks of vertigo will affect balance and ambulation   (N)
- recognize the onset of an attack and seek a safe environment to reduce the chance of injury   (N)
- demonstrate alternative approaches to routine activities of daily living to support the sudden onset of vertigo.   (N)

Skilled nursing services

Care measures
- Perform a skilled nursing assessment, focusing on cardiovascular, neurologic, and fluid status; mobility; and balance.
- Assess medication compliance and evaluate whether the patient has all medications as ordered, knows how to take them, and understands common adverse effects.
- Observe response to prescribed medication.
- Assess home safety.

Patient and family teaching
- Review home safety measures.
- Explain that during an acute episode the patient should lie down on a firm surface, stay as motionless as possible, and keep the eyes open and fixed on a stationary object; then when the severe vertigo (spinning) passes, get up slowly.

- Emphasize that the patient shouldn't sip or drink water during an acute episode because it may induce vomiting.
- Discuss the hydrops diet regimen with an overall goal of providing stable body fluid and blood levels and avoid secondary fluctuations in inner ear fluid. Food and fluid intake should be distributed evenly throughout the day and from day to day.
- Emphasize the need to eat approximately the same amount of food at each meal, not to skip meals and, if snacks are eaten, to have them at regular times.
- Explain that foods or fluids with a high salt or sugar content should be avoided because they can cause fluctuations in the inner ear fluid pressure and may increase symptoms.
- Encourage a diet high in fresh fruits, vegetables, and whole grains and low in canned, frozen, or processed foods.
- Discuss drinking adequate amounts of fluid daily, including water, milk, and low-sugar fruit juices (for example, cranberry).
- Teach about anticipating fluid loss that occurs with exercise or heat, and replacing these fluids before they are lost.
- Explain that caffeine-containing fluids and foods — such as coffee, tea, soft drinks, and chocolate — should be avoided because they are diuretics and also have stimulant properties that may make symptoms worse.
- Discuss the need to limit or eliminate alcohol intake. Alcohol can affect the inner ear directly, changing the volume and concentration of the inner ear fluid and increasing symptoms.

- Explain that foods containing monosodium glutamate (often present in prepackaged and Chinese foods) may increase symptoms in some patients and should be avoided.
- Identify triggers that can bring on or increase symptoms, including stress, allergies, menstruation, pregnancy, visual stimuli, and changes in barometric pressure.

Interdisciplinary actions

Home care aide
- Assistance with routine ADLs until patient is able to resume normal activity
- Instructions for caregiver on routine basic care to assist the patient during acute periods of the disease

Social worker
- Referral to community resources and support groups for people with Ménière's disease
- Counseling and referral for stress management and reduction
- Financial evaluation and referral for assistance in meeting home maintenance needs
- Resources to assist with disability issues related to incapacitation and deafness

Speech pathologist
- Recognition of the cause of the speech impairment and use of techniques obtained by speech therapy to maximize speech recovery

Discharge plan

- Safe management of acute phases of the disease by the patient and caregivers
- Understanding by the patient and caregivers of ways to minimize symptoms while maintaining a safe environment
- Minimization of hearing loss as a complication of this disease
- Management of the disease process in the home by the patient and caregivers with physician and community support system follow-ups
- Scheduling a follow-up appointment with the physician

Documentation requirements

- Assessment of all body systems, focusing on neurologic symptoms, nutrition (weight), hydration status (adequate intake, urination), skin integrity, and mental status
- Patient's and caregiver's responses to instruction
- Observation of the patient and caregiver's ability to perform basic care, use oropharyngeal suctioning for aspiration precautions, and practice safety with mobility
- Changes in hearing and balance

Reimbursement reminders

- Ensure that there is a predictable and realistic date for discharging the patient from home care.
- Teaching for prevention (for example, long-term complications and prevention of acute attacks) *alone* isn't considered a reimbursable skilled nursing service.

- Registered dietitian services aren't reimbursable under the Medicare home benefit.

Insurance hints

- Provide review of hospitalization (if appropriate) or the latest visit to see the primary care physician and current condition of the patient, home environment, and availability of caregivers. Review alternatives, such as acute care or skilled nursing facilities, that are being considered.
- Provide objective review of systems, including physical abilities, ambulation, use or need for assistive devices.
- Document the number of episodes of nausea and vomiting. Include what foods and fluids the patient can tolerate.
- Record current laboratory values.
- Provide objective evaluation of respiratory and nutritional status, including initial and current weight. If the patient is able to be supported by oral nutrition, objectively evaluate the patient and caregiver's ability to maintain a patent airway.

Multiple sclerosis

Classified as a disorder of the central nervous system, multiple sclerosis (MS) is characterized by loss of the myelin sheath (the conductive covering of nerve cells) in multiple areas, leaving scar tissue, also called sclerosis. The sclerosis slows or blocks the transmission of nerve impulses in that area of the nervous system. Symptoms of the disease depend upon the nerve cell area that is inflamed and include weakness, paralysis, tremor, muscle spasticity, muscle atrophy, progressive dysfunctional movements, numbness, tingling, facial pain, extremity pain, muscle spasms, vertigo, and changes in vision, coordination, balance, urinary elimination, speech, and cognition. Care of the patient with MS focuses on maximization of mobility and independence, management of pain, communication, bladder retraining, and respiratory muscle dysfunction. For these issues, teaching is needed for the patients with this health condition and their families and should focus on promoting independence, preventing complications, maximizing respiratory functioning, and providing care for basic needs.

Previsit checklist

Physician orders and preparation

- Indwelling urinary catheter
- Physical therapy to strengthen weakened or uncoordinated muscles with range-of-motion (ROM) and stretching exercises
- Speech therapy to improve communication or swallowing related to weakness or poor coordination, which includes exercises, voice training, and the use of special devices
- Occupational therapy to teach energy conservation techniques for completing activities of daily living (ADLs), making best use of assistive devices, and adapting the environment for safety and efficiency
- Specialty bed, wheelchair, and other assistive devices
- Social worker assistance with financial counseling needs and information about provisions in the Americans with Disabilities Act to help the patient get back to work

- Nutritional requirements
- Home suctioning equipment and oxygen

Equipment and supplies

- Supplies for standard precautions and proper sharps disposal
- Indwelling catheter or intermittent catheter kits
- Wound and skin care supplies
- Suctioning kits (oropharyngeal)
- Scale

Safety requirements

- Leg bag or urinary bag attachment device
- Aspiration precautions
- Standard precautions for infection control and sharps disposal
- Information on medications, including dosage, adverse effects, interactions, and safe storage of multiple medications
- Allergies verified and documented
- Emergency plan and access to functional phone and list of emergency phone numbers
- Identification and correction of environmental hazards and patient-specific concerns (for example, placement of grab bars and supportive devices in the bathroom and kitchen and removal of throw rugs and carpeting)
- Oxygen precautions, safe handling and placement of home oxygen equipment, and notification of local fire and police departments of oxygen use in the home
- Safe use of suction equipment
- Skin care and protection, including frequent position changes
- Avoidance of extremes in temperature to the skin (ice and heat)

- Extremity supports to keep limbs in normal anatomic alignment

Major diagnostic codes
- Abnormal involuntary movements 781.0
- Abnormality of gait 781.2
- Atony of bladder 596.4
- Demyelinating diseases of the central nervous system 341.8
- Disturbance of skin sensation 782.0
- Incontinence of urine 788.3
- Incontinence without sensory awareness 788.34
- Lack of coordination 781.3
- Mixed incontinence 788.33
- Multiple sclerosis 340
- Neurogenic bladder 596.54
- Other functional disorder of the bladder 596.59
- Paralysis of bladder 596.53
- Stress incontinence 625.6
- Urge incontinence 788.31

Defense of homebound status
- Unable to ambulate farther than 10′ (3 m) because of imbalance and lack of coordination
- Unable to perform self-care activities unattended
- Unable to control bladder functioning
- Questionable cognitive status due to interrupted transmission of neural impulses
- Unable to leave home safely without assistance

Selected nursing diagnoses and patient outcomes

Impaired physical mobility related to neurologic dysfunction
    The patient or caregiver will:
- recognize that the degree of physical debilitation will change after every exacerbation of the disease
                    (N, HCA, OT, PT, SW)
- demonstrate the use of assistive devices to support independence with physical mobility.   (N, OT, PT)

Total incontinence related to loss of sensation
    The patient or caregiver will:
- recognize incontinence as being an uncontrollable element to the disease process   (N)
- demonstrate methods to support routine elimination patterns through the use of a bowel and bladder regimen.
                    (N)

Urinary retention related to neurogenic bladder
    The patient or caregiver will:
- recognize urinary retention as an uncontrollable element to the disease process   (N)
- demonstrate methods to expel urine, including manual stimulation, bladder manipulation, and intermittent catheterization.   (N)

Fatigue related to disease process
    The patient or caregiver will:
- recognize fatigue as an uncontrollable element of the disease process
                    (N, OT)

• state ways to incorporate frequent rest periods into ADLs   (N, OT)
• demonstrate energy-saving techniques and the use of adaptive equipment to reduce fatigue caused by routine ADLs.   (N, OT)

Feeding, bathing-hygiene, dressing-grooming, and toileting self-care deficits related to loss of strength and sensation

The patient or caregiver will:
• recognize limitations in abilities to perform self-care activities, including hygiene, dressing, toileting, and eating   (N, OT)
• demonstrate maximum participation in self-care activities while conserving energy.   (N, OT)

Ineffective airway clearance related to respiratory compromise and decreased mobility

The patient or caregiver will:
• recognize signs and symptoms that indicate respiratory compromise (N)
• use home suction apparatus to support effective airway clearance   (N)
• demonstrate methods to reduce the likelihood of respiratory compromise.   (N)

Altered nutrition: Less than body requirements

The patient or caregiver will:
• recognize the need for adequate food and fluid intake to support physiologic functioning   (N, D)
• demonstrate adequate food and fluid intake by maintaining body weight and fluid status.   (N, D)

Altered sexuality patterns related to loss of sensation, lubrication, and erection as well as to psychosocial effects of partner as caregiver

The patient or caregiver will:
• recognize the effects of the disease on normal sexual functioning   (N)
• state ways to support sexual functioning needs, including honest communication with the partner and alternative forms of sexual expression.   (N)

Impaired verbal communication

The patient or caregiver will:
• recognize the effects of the disease on verbal communication and perform exercises to strengthen and coordinate muscles associated with speech   (N, SP)
• state alternative methods to communicate, including picture boards, charts, and hand or eye signals (N, SP)
• demonstrate alternative methods of communication.   (N, SP)

Ineffective individual coping or *Ineffective family coping: Compromised*

The patient or caregiver will:
• recognize the effects of the disease on the family unit   (N, SW)
• state activities and resources to support the family's ability to cope with the illness, such as respite care, flexibility with home maintenance schedule.   (N, SW)

Impaired home maintenance management

The patient or caregiver will:
• recognize the impact of the disease on the patient's ability to perform routine home maintenance   (N, SW)

- state alternatives to help the patient complete necessary home chores

  (N, SW)
- demonstrate ways to complete necessary home chores. (N, OT, SW)

Powerlessness

The patient or caregiver will:

- recognize that although the disease has no cure, it can be managed with adherence to prescribed medication and rehabilitation therapy

  (N, MD, OT, PT, SW)
- demonstrate effective coping mechanisms to reduce feelings of powerlessness (N)
- state ways to encourage the patient to participate and function to his maximum level. (N, OT, PT, SW)

Skilled nursing services

Care measures

- Perform a skilled assessment with emphasis on neurologic status, skin integrity, swallowing, bowel and bladder function, speech, and motor function. Include signs of aspiration, pneumonia, and urinary tract infection from urinary retention, which are the primary causes of death in patients with MS.
- Assess the home for assistive device needs.
- Assess nutritional status.
- Assess management of complex or new medication regimen as well as compliance, need, and knowledge of medications.
- Evaluate whether the patient has all prescribed medications, knows how to take them, and understands common adverse effects and any special instructions if part of a clinical trial.

- Evaluate social and emotional functioning of the patient and caregivers, including depression.

Patient and family teaching

- Provide dietary instruction, including the need for a high-fiber and high-fluid diet to stimulate bowel movement and decrease the risk of urinary tract infection; offer the use of supplemental feedings if indicated.
- Emphasize the need to report worsening or new symptoms to the physician.
- Review safety measures.
- Describe activity limitations, exercise regimen, and ways to minimize fatigue.
- Discuss bowel and bladder training programs.
- Identify strategies to cope with MS and measures to minimize symptoms and exacerbations, such as avoiding heat, bathing in warm or tepid water, keeping cool, and using air conditioning or ice packs.
- Encourage the patient to maintain relationships and activities to reduce feelings of isolation and powerlessness.
- Teach about oropharyngeal suctioning.
- Review enteral feeding procedures and gastrostomy tube care (if applicable).
- Demonstrate application of splints.
- Discuss skin care as well as frequent turning and repositioning.
- Explain preventive care, including infection-control measures and the need for influenza and pneumonia vaccinations because illnesses such as influenza are associated with exacerbations of MS. Remember, vaccination is *not* recommended while the patient is taking immunosuppressants.

Interdisciplinary actions

Physical therapist
• Rehabilitation program, including splint application, transferring, standing, and walking
• Assessment of equipment needs, functional features, and safety factors at home
• Continuation of the rehabilitation program as prescribed to increase strength, function, ROM, and coordination

Occupational therapist
• Assessment of ADLs
• Provision of adaptive devices as indicated
• Provision of therapies addressing fine motor skills
• Instruction in energy conservation techniques

Speech pathologist
• Assessment of swallowing
• Evaluation of airway while ingesting foods and fluids
• Instruction to caregivers on aspiration precautions

Social worker
• Assessment of need for community resources
• Provision of emotional support and counseling
• Referral to support group

Home care aide
• Encouragement of the patient and caregiver to provide care
• Reduction of frequency of home care aide interventions as the patient and caregiver gain confidence in providing care as directed

• Assistance with ADLs
• Assistance with personal care
• Participation in home exercise program

Discharge plan
• Patient ambulatory and independent with ADLs with moderate assistance
• Improvement in mobility level, with demonstration of self-care activities appropriate to the level of physiologic functioning
• No development of integumentary, respiratory, GI, or genitourinary complications

Documentation requirements
• Patient's and caregiver's responses to instruction
• Observation of the patient's and caregiver's ability to perform oropharyngeal suctioning, gastrostomy tube feedings (if applicable), use of assistive devices, repositioning, and transfers
• Changes in integumentary, respiratory, GI, genitourinary, or neurologic functioning
• Ability of caregiver to care for the patient

Reimbursement reminders
• An air conditioner may significantly reduce symptoms and may be tax-deductible if recommended by the physician.
• Ensure that wound care is done *exactly* as prescribed (to be reimbursable).

• All nonroutine supplies must be specifically ordered by the physician and entered into Locator 14 (Supplies) of Health Care Finance Administration Form 485 or ordered by the physician within the specific order for treatment requiring the use of certain supplies and entered into Locator 21 (Orders for Treatment).

• When billing for medical supplies, always include the name of supply item, date supply was used, number of units used, and charge per unit.

Insurance hints

• Report current condition of the patient, home environment, availability of caregivers, and alternative care situations being considered such as a skilled nursing facility.

• Provide objective review of systems, including physical abilities, ambulation, use or need for assistive devices.

• Provide thorough skin assessment, and report objective findings. In the event of open or reddened areas, provide accurate wound dimensions, color, granulation, prescribed dressing, and capabilities of caregivers to perform wound care.

• Provide objective evaluation of respiratory and nutritional status. If the patient is receiving gastrostomy tube feedings, provide patient tolerance to feedings, patency of gastrostomy tube, and condition of skin surrounding the tube. If the patient is able to be supported by oral nutrition, objectively evaluate the patient's and caregiver's ability to maintain a patent airway. Report initial and current weight.

• Provide objective review of communication pattern, cognitive level, and ability to comprehend instructions.

Myocardial infarction

Myocardial infarction (MI) results from prolonged ischemia of the heart muscle. Decreased blood flow to the heart may be caused by coronary artery spasm, thrombus formation, or atherosclerosis. Heart failure may result because the dying tissue is unable to contract. Care focuses on lifestyle modification and management of weakness, fear of dying, and subsequent infarctions.

Previsit checklist

Physician orders and preparations

• Order for medications
• Parameters for acceptable vital signs
• Activity restrictions
• Nutritional consultation for instruction on low-fat, low-cholesterol, low-sodium diet
• Oxygen
• Occupational therapy evaluation for energy conservation and assistance with functional ability, including adaptive devices as necessary
• Social worker evaluation for community referrals, financial assistance, and counseling
• Home care aide assistance with personal care and activities of daily living (ADLs)
• Physical therapy for strengthening, endurance, and development of a home exercise program

Equipment and supplies

• Scale
• Phlebotomy supplies
• Oxygen

Safety requirements
- Information on medications, including dosage, adverse effects, interactions, and safe storage of multiple medications
- Allergies verified and documented
- Emergency plan and access to functional phone and list of emergency phone numbers
- Identification and correction of environmental hazards and patient-specific concerns (for example, nightlights and smoke detectors)
- Oxygen precautions, safe handling and placement of home oxygen equipment, and notification of the local fire and police departments of oxygen use in the home
- Medical identification bracelet
- Signs and symptoms to report to the physician

Major diagnostic codes
- Angina 413.9
- Atrial fibrillation 427.31
- Atrial flutter 427.32
- Congestive heart failure 428.0
- Heart block 426.9
- Hypertension 401.9
- Myocardial infarction, acute, unspecified 410.9

(To assign a fifth digit, see appendix A, page 638.)

Defense of homebound status
- Prescribed activity limitation
- Poor endurance; out of bed to chair with assistance only twice per day
- Unable to ambulate farther than 10′ (3 m) because of dyspnea, dizziness, or angina
- Assistance required for transfer or ambulation
- Unable to climb stairs; unable to leave home without assistance

Selected nursing diagnoses and patient outcomes

Fatigue related to decreased cardiac output, secondary to mechanical or electrophysiologic heart problems
The patient or caregiver will:
- comply with the medication regimen (as evidenced by pulse rate and blood pressure within parameters)   (N)
- report no dizziness or chest pain (N)
- have clear breath sounds upon auscultation   (N)
- report a stable weight.   (N)

Risk for injury related to difficulty ambulating, shortness of breath, or anginal episodes
The patient or caregiver will:
- remain injury-free (N, HCA, PT, OT)
- verbalize the importance of avoiding obstacles, such as climbing stairs, wearing shoes without nonskid soles, and attempting to extricate self from a bathtub without assistance.
(N, HCA, PT, OT)

Knowledge deficit related to heart-healthy lifestyle
The patient or caregiver will:
- verbalize the importance of a heart-healthy lifestyle, including low-fat, low-cholesterol, low-sodium diet; cardiac rehabilitation and exercise program; smoking cessation; and adherence to medication regimen   (N, D, OT, PT)
- verbalize food choices in accordance with prescribed diet   (N, D)

• demonstrate physical activities in accordance with cardiac rehabilitation and prescribed exercise regimen.
(N, OT, PT)

Skilled nursing services

Care measures
• Conduct a complete physical assessment, including evaluating vital signs, weighing the patient, listening to the apical pulse for irregularities, S_3 heart sounds, and murmurs.
• Check skin color and temperature.
• Auscultate for breath sounds.
• Assess for chest pain and peripheral edema.
• Assess for nausea, vomiting, or constant cough caused by medications.
• Assess patient's activity level.
• Evaluate patient's response to the plan of care and medications.

Patient and family teaching
• Provide information about medications, including actions, interactions, therapeutic and adverse effects, and safe storage.
• Demonstrate procedure for assessing of blood pressure and pulse, and encourage caregivers to learn cardiopulmonary resuscitation.
• Teach energy conservation measures.
• Reinforce dietary restrictions and alternative selections.
• Identify signs and symptoms to report, such as weight gain greater than 5 lb (2.2 kg) in 1 week or greater than 2 lb (1 kg) in 1 day, decreased exercise tolerance, or confusion.
• Review oxygen therapy use and safety precautions.
• Teach stress-reduction techniques.

• Encourage smoking cessation and moderation of alcohol use (less than two drinks per day).

Interdisciplinary actions

Dietitian
• Consultation for development of individualized low-sodium, low-fat, low-cholesterol diet and complete nutritional assessment

Physical therapist
• Referral as part of the cardiac rehabilitation program

Occupational therapist
• Energy conservation techniques
• Best use of adaptive devices

Social worker
• Financial support and support groups

Home care aide
• Assistance with personal care and ADLs

Discharge plan
• Safe management of recovery from MI in the home by the patient and caregiver with physician follow-up
• Scheduling of appointment for follow-up with the physician
• Referral to outpatient services
• Minimization of complications and death with dignity

Documentation requirements
• Physical assessment findings, including vital signs, weight, presence of

chest pain, shortness of breath, or edema. Note site, severity, reaction, and physician contact for any episode of chest pain, actions taken, and outcome.
● Medication regimen compliance and adverse reactions
● Patient and family teaching and progress toward educational goals
● Factors keeping the patient homebound such as inability to climb stairs
● Patient's response to treatment, including activity tolerance, weight loss, improved vital signs

Reimbursement reminders
● Medicare won't cover oxygen ordered "as needed." Oxygen is covered under Medicare part B (80% of allowable charge) if the patient's oxygen saturation level is 88% or less; re-evaluation is required every 3 weeks and repeated laboratory testing is required within 90 days after therapy initiation to demonstrate continued need. Additionally, the physician must see the patient and confirm the continued need for oxygen.
● Identify complications or noncompliance, subsequent changes to the plan of care, and communication with team members.
● Identify progress toward goals.

Insurance hints
● Present objective patient findings and changes since last update, including weight changes, calf circumference, vital signs within parameters for ___ days.
● Direct interventions toward palliation and avoidance of inpatient hospitalization if complete recovery isn't an option.

● Report on continuing homebound status of the patient.

Osteoarthritis

Classified as a degenerative joint disease of the articular cartilage in synovial joints, osteoarthritis isn't caused by a systemic inflammatory process. Seen primarily in older adults, osteoarthritis occurs when collagen fibers in the cartilage of major weight-bearing joints break down. As more areas of cartilage are lost, underlying bone is exposed at the margins and subchondral areas of the joints, leading to pain.

Osteoarthritis is primarily seen in the hips and knees but is also found in the fingers, wrists, first joint in the big toe, and the spine. Pain is typically localized to the affected joints and described as a deep ache. Motion or use of the affected joint aggravates the pain, and rest reduces it. Over time, the person with osteoarthritis can develop enlarged joints that are typically bony-hard and cool to the touch. This disorder leads to pain and crepitus with movement, muscle spasms, stiffness, limited joint range of motion (ROM), referred pain, joint instability, and deformity with advanced disease.

Most of the care for the patient with osteoarthritis focuses on maximizing mobility and joint ROM, managing self-care, reducing pain or discomfort, and preventing complications of immobility. For these issues, teaching is needed for the families of patients with this health condition and should focus on maximizing physical functioning to achieve independence, pain management, and prevention of complications.

Previsit checklist

Physician orders and preparation
- Medication and administration regimen
- Laboratory orders, including prothrombin time, international normalized ratio, and complete blood count
- Wound care
- Physical therapist evaluation to increase strength and endurance, ROM, transfer abilities, and for gait training
- Occupational therapist evaluation for use of adaptive equipment and energy conservation
- Social worker evaluation for community resources and financial assistance
- Durable medical equipment order for specialty bed, wheelchair, high hip chair, and other assistive devices
- Activity orders and restrictions, including weight-bearing status, maximal flexion, and ROM per the physician order

Equipment and supplies
- Supplies for standard precautions and proper sharps disposal
- Pain scale evaluation form
- Phlebotomy supplies
- Wound care supplies
- Scale, if weight loss is recommended

Safety requirements
- Standard precautions for infection control and sharps disposal
- Correct and safe use of adaptive devices (for example, high hip chair, grab bars, walker)
- Identification and correction of environmental hazards and patient-specific concerns (for example, secure placement of grab bars, supportive devices, and nonskid mat in the bathroom; removal of throw rugs and carpeting; keeping walkways clutter-free; keeping stairways well lit and in good repair)
- Skin care and protection, including frequent position changes
- Safe use of ice or heat to the affected joints for pain relief
- Extremity supports to keep limbs in normal anatomic alignment as indicated
- List of signs and symptoms to report to the physician
- Information on medications, including dosage, adverse effects, interactions, and safe storage of multiple medications
- Allergies verified and documented
- Bleeding precautions
- Emergency plan and access to functional phone and list of emergency phone numbers

Major diagnostic codes
- Ankylosis of joint 718.5
- Contracture of joint 718.4
- Difficulty walking 719.7
- Effusion of joint 719.0
- Internal derangement of knee 717.0
- Joint crepitus 719.6
- Osteoarthrosis, generalized 715.0
- Osteoarthrosis, localized:
  – ankle and foot 715.07
  – forearm 715.03
  – hand 715.04
  – lower leg 715.06
  – pelvis region and thigh 715.05
  – shoulder 715.01
  – upper arm 715.02
- Other derangement of joint 718.0
- Pain in joint 719.4

- Pathological joint dislocation 718.2
- Stiffness of joint 719.5

Defense of homebound status

- Progressive inability to ambulate farther than 10′ (3 m) because of pain in weight-bearing joints
- Progressive inability to perform self-care activities without maximal assistance
- Unable to leave home without assistance
- Need to have leg elevated most of the day

Selected nursing diagnoses and patient outcomes

Chronic pain related to physical agents
The patient or caregiver will:
- recognize that pain is subjective and can be evaluated according to a pain scale (N)
- determine nonpharmacologic pain-reduction measures, such as distraction, meditation, guided imagery, and relaxation techniques (N)
- recognize the need for pain medication and take it appropriately (N, MD)
- demonstrate methods to promote joint rest (N, PT)
- demonstrate good body mechanics and posture to reduce stress on affected joints (N, OT, PT)
- demonstrate the application of splints or other assistive devices to support affected joints. (N, OT, PT)

Impaired physical mobility related to pain
The patient or caregiver will:

- state ways to facilitate movement from sitting to standing, lying to sitting, and lying to standing (N, OT, PT)
- demonstrate methods to facilitate normal ADLs, such as stair climbing and moving into and out of a bathtub or shower (N, OT, PT)
- demonstrate passive and active ROM exercises (N, OT, PT)
- demonstrate isometric, progressive resistance, and low-impact aerobic exercises (N, PT)
- demonstrate the use of ambulatory aids, such as a cane or walker, to facilitate independence with ambulation and mobility. (N, OT, PT)

Feeding, bathing-hygiene, dressing-grooming, and toileting self-care deficits related to musculoskeletal impairment
The patient or caregiver will:
- recognize the impact of upper extremity osteoarthritis on the ability to perform toileting, bathing, dressing, eating, and grooming (N, HCA, OT)
- demonstrate alternative methods to achieve self-care needs (N, HCA, OT)
- use assistive devices to maximize independence with self-care needs. (N, OT)

Risk for disuse syndrome related to prolonged inactivity
The patient or caregiver will:
- recognize the impact of "guarding" a joint as further reducing the joint's functioning (N, OT, PT)
- demonstrate effort to use the affected joints to their maximum ability (N, OT, PT)
- maintain muscle strength, tone, and joint ROM without evidence of contractures (N, OT, PT)

• show no evidence of decreased chest movement, cough stimulus, or depth of ventilation; also show no pooling of secretions or signs or symptoms of infection. (N)

Impaired home maintenance management due to pain on movement
The patient or caregiver will:
• recognize limitations with performance of home maintenance activities (N, OT)
• demonstrate methods to achieve home management needs with the use of assistive devices. (N, OT)

Risk of injury
The patient or caregiver will:
• recognize potential home hazards that could jeopardize safe ambulation (N, HCA, OT, PT)
• recognize potential for complications due to misuse or nonuse of affected joints (N, OT, PT)
• demonstrate safety in the home. (N, HCA, OT, PT)

Skilled nursing services

Care measures
• Perform a skilled nursing assessment, including physical capabilities and cardiovascular, respiratory, neurologic, and musculoskeletal functioning.
• Assess nutritional status and progress toward weight-loss goals as indicated.
• Assess medication compliance, need, and knowledge of medications.
• Evaluate whether the patient has all prescribed medications, knows how to take them, and understands common adverse effects.

• Assess social and emotional functioning of the patient and home, including recognizing depression.

Patient and family teaching
• Review safety measures, including bleeding precautions if on warfarin and fall precautions if ataxic.
• Teach about activity limitations and exercise regimen; explain how increased muscle strength decreases joint stress.
• Review the use of assistive devices and orthotics.
• Demonstrate skin and wound care.
• Teach how to turn and reposition.

Interdisciplinary actions

Physical therapist
• Initiation of rehabilitation program to include transferring, standing, walking, and ROM, isometric, and aerobic exercises
• Assessment of equipment needs, functional features, and safety factors at home
• Continuation of rehabilitation program as prescribed

Occupational therapist
• Assessment of ADLs
• Provision of adaptive devices as indicated
• Provision of therapies addressing fine motor skills
• Instruction in energy conservation techniques

Social worker
• Assessment of need for community resources
• Provision of emotional support and counseling

Home care aide

- Encouragement of the patient and caregiver to provide care and assist as needed
- Reduction of frequency of home care aide interventions as the patient and caregiver gain confidence in providing care as directed
- Assistance with ADLs

Discharge plan

- Patient ambulatory with the use of assistive devices
- Maximal mobility level with demonstration of self-care activities appropriate to the level of joint mobility
- No development of integumentary, respiratory, GI, or genitourinary complications despite risk due to immobility

Documentation requirements

- Instructions given; patient's and caregiver's responses to instruction
- Observation of the patient's and caregiver's ability to perform passive ROM exercises, use assistive devices, maintain normal anatomical alignment, achieve repositioning, and perform transfers
- Changes in integumentary, respiratory, GI, genitourinary, or neurologic functioning
- Ability of caregivers to care for the patient

Reimbursement reminders

- Durable medical equipment is covered under Medicare part B.
- Emergency telephone response systems aren't covered by Medicare or most insurance plans. Though expensive, they may be particularly helpful for patients without available support persons.
- Five or more visits per week are considered "daily" and must have a specified and predictable end.
- Medicare covers phlebotomy supplies.
- Check for an authorized laboratory because many insurance companies have contracts with specific laboratories for processing specimens.
- All nonroutine supplies must be specifically ordered by the physician and entered into Locator 14 (Supplies) of HCFA Form 485 or ordered by the physician within the specific order for treatment requiring the use of certain supplies and entered into Locator 21 (Orders for Treatment).
- When billing for medical supplies, always include the name of the supply item, date the supply was used, number of units used, and charge per unit.

Insurance hints

- Include a brief summary of hospitalization (if appropriate) and current condition of the patient, home environment, and availability of caregivers.
- Provide objective review of systems, including physical abilities, ambulation, use or need for assistive devices.
- Provide thorough skin assessment, and report objective findings. In the event of open or reddened areas, provide accurate wound dimensions, color, granulation, prescribed dressing, and capabilities of caregivers to perform wound care.
- Provide initial and current laboratory values, including prothombin time, international normalized ratio, and complete blood count, as indicated.

• Provide objective evaluation of respiratory and nutritional status, including weight change, pulse oximetry, and activity tolerance due to dyspnea (measured in feet).

• Provide objective review of cognitive level and ability to comprehend instructions. Report progress toward educational goals, including independence with wound care, ambulation, and pain management.

• Report risk of falls, including injuries, physical findings, safety hazards in the home. Describe "near falls," including instructions given to the patient and caregiver and the patient's and caregiver's response.

Osteomyelitis

Osteomyelitis is an infection of the bone. Because of the likelihood of complications, osteomyelitis must be treated immediately. When microorganisms enter the bone, the body's natural defenses can't react quickly enough, permitting the invading organism to multiply unhindered. The growing infection stimulates osteoclastic activity (breakdown), leading to a weakened bone structure, which impedes bone microcirculation and finally causes bone necrosis and death. The primary cause of osteomyelitis is the bacteria *Staphylococcus aureus;* however, fungi, parasites, and viruses can also cause bone infection. Pathogenic organisms reach the bone through open wounds (as seen in some fractures), from within the body (as seen with urinary tract infections), or from an infected wound (such as in stasis ulcers).

Care of the patient who has osteomyelitis is focused on prevention of the transmission of infection, pain control, and problems related to immobility. For these issues, teaching is needed for the families of patients with this health condition and focuses on maximizing physical functioning to achieve maximal independence, pain management, and prevention of complications.

Previsit checklist

Physician orders and preparation

• Order for wound care to include dressing type and frequency

• Order for I.V. antimicrobial therapy

• Acceptable temperature parameters

• Physical therapist evaluation for therapeutic exercises, range of motion (ROM) of the affected extremity

• Occupational therapist evaluation for prosthesis and device application and use of adaptive equipment

• Social worker evaluation for community resources and financial assistance

• Order for durable medical equipment, including specialty bed, wheelchair, and other assistive devices

• Activity orders and restrictions

Equipment and supplies

• Supplies for standard precautions and proper sharps disposal

• Phlebotomy supplies

• Pain scale evaluation form

• Wound care supplies

• Wound culture container

• I.V. access supplies

• I.V. medication

Safety requirements

• Standard precautions for infection control and sharps disposal

- Home assessment for placement of grab bars and supportive devices in the bathroom; removal of throw rugs and carpeting
- Skin care and protection, including frequent position changes
- Observation of dressing changes to reduce continued wound infection or contamination
- Extremity support to keep limb in normal anatomic alignment, if applicable
- Information on medications, including dosage, interactions, adverse effects, allergies, and safe storage
- Emergency plan and access to functional phone and list of emergency phone numbers

Major diagnostic codes

- Acute osteomyelitis 730.0
- Bone infection 730.9
- Chronic osteomyelitis 730.1
- Difficulty walking 719.7
- Electrolyte and fluid disorders 276.9
- Fever 780.6
- Infection, bacterial 041.9
- Malaise and fatigue 780.7
- Osteomyelitis, periostitis, and other infections involving bone 730
- Skin ulcer 707.9
- Unspecified osteomyelitis 730.2
- Volume depletion 276.5

Defense of homebound status

- Prescribed activity restriction and need to have extremity elevated 75% of each day
- Unable to ambulate farther than 10′ (3 m) because of painful bone infection or frequent falls
- Unable to perform self-care activities because of painful bone infection
- Unable to leave home because of pain or adverse effects of pain medication
- Morbid obesity and inability to maintain nonweight-bearing status

Selected nursing diagnoses and patient outcomes

Risk for infection
    The patient or caregiver will:
- recognize the need for long-term antimicrobial therapy to cure osteomyelitis   (N, MD)
- understand that long-term antimicrobial therapy will place the patient at risk for developing a superinfection   (N, MD)
- demonstrate infection-control techniques in the home environment by proper disposal of wound dressings and body fluids   (N)
- recognize the need for adequate nutritional intake for wound healing. (N)

Hyperthermia related to infection
    The patient or caregiver will:
- evaluate the patient's temperature as prescribed   (N)
- record temperature, alerting health care personnel with readings outside acceptable parameters   (N, HCA)
- support the patient with warm clothing in the event of chills associated with a fever   (N)
- support the patient with one layer of dry clothing and a cool environment in the event of diaphoresis associated with a fever   (N)
- recognize the need for adequate fluid intake to combat potential dehydration   (N)

- demonstrate providing antimicrobial therapy as prescribed to ensure a consistent blood level to combat the microorganism causing the infection. (N)

Impaired physical mobility related to musculoskeletal infection

The patient or caregiver will:
- monitor the degree of pain associated with the infection and provide adequate pain management   (N, MD)
- use alternative methods to support pain management, such as distraction, guided imagery, and stress management techniques   (N)
- support the affected extremity with splints or pillows   (N, OT, PT)
- avoid subjecting the affected limb to stress or unnecessary movements
                                        (N, OT, PT)
- recognize the need for some activity to the affected extremity to prevent contractures   (N, OT, PT)
- demonstrate passive ROM to the affected extremity to prevent joint immobility.   (N, OT, PT)

Pain related to bone infection

The patient or caregiver will:
- recognize the source of pain as swelling, inflammation, and by-products of tissue destruction   (N)
- use splints to prevent injury and contracture   (N, OT)
- use prescribed pain medication up to 30 minutes before anticipated activity to the affected extremity
                                        (N, OT, PT)
- use assistive devices when appropriate to aid in activities while minimizing unnecessary exacerbation of pain   (N, OT, PT)
- avoid excessive manipulation or movement of the affected extremity to

prevent unnecessary pain exacerbation.   (N, OT)

Anxiety and *Powerlessness related to chronic illness and immobility*

The patient or caregiver will:
- recognize feelings of helplessness
                                        (N, SW)
- demonstrate compassion when providing care to the patient   (N)
- encourage patient participation in care to aid in feelings of control over the situation.   (N)

Fear related to loss of limb, loss of independence, and death

The patient or caregiver will:
- encourage verbalization of feelings regarding the outcome of the infective process   (N)
- demonstrate methods to help alleviate the fears.   (N)

Ineffective individual coping related to diagnosis, immobility, loss of independence

The patient or caregiver will:
- discuss recent stressful events and describe related emotions   (N)
- cooperate with nurse to plan care
                                        (N)
- identify problems, make plans, and take action   (N)
- request assistance and support from family, friends, and community resources as needed   (N, SW)
- identify and use at least two healthy coping behaviors such as relaxation techniques.   (N)

Ineffective family coping: Compromised

The patient or caregiver will:
- recognize the signs and symptoms of stress   (N, SW)

- recognize that the chronic nature of the illness can lead to feelings of depression and despair (N, SW)
- establish a routine beneficial to both the patient and family (N)
- help the family identify and use available support systems. (N)

Skilled nursing services

Care measures
- Conduct a skilled nursing assessment, focusing on physical capabilities and cardiovascular, respiratory, neurologic, and musculoskeletal functioning.
- Assess nutritional and fluid status.
- Assess vital signs.
- Assess medication compliance, need, and knowledge of medications.
- Evaluate whether the patient has all prescribed medications, knows how to take them, and understands common adverse effects.
- Provide I.V. antibiotic therapy.
- Obtain prescribed wound cultures.
- Assess the social and emotional functioning of the patient and caregivers, including recognizing depression.

Patient and family teaching
- Discus precautions to maintain safety with ambulation and reduce the risk of infection recurrence.
- Identify signs and symptoms that should be immediately reported the physician, including nagging bone pain, local tenderness and inflammation, and fever and chills.
- Review activity limitations and exercise regimen.
- Teach about the use of assistive devices.

- Demonstrate the application of splints for maintenance of anatomic alignment.
- Teach about skin care.
- Emphasize the need for regular turning and repositioning.
- Review I.V. antimicrobial therapy.

Interdisciplinary actions

Physical therapist
- Initiation of rehabilitation program, including transferring, standing, walking, and ROM, isometric, and aerobic exercises
- Assessment of equipment needs, functional features, and safety factors at home
- Continuation of rehabilitation program as prescribed

Occupational therapist
- Assessment of ADLs
- Provision of adaptive devices as indicated
- Instruction in energy conservation techniques

Social worker
- Assessment of need for community resources
- Provision of emotional support and counseling

Home care aide
- Encouragement of the patient and caregiver to provide care
- Reduction of frequency of home care aide interventions as the patient and caregiver gain confidence in providing care as directed
- Assistance with ADLs

Discharge plan

• Patient ambulatory with the use of assistive devices

• Attainment of maximal mobility level with demonstration of self-care activities appropriate to the level of capabilities

• Verbalization and demonstration of preventive measures to counteract risks associated with immobility that cause integumentary, respiratory, GI, or genitourinary complications

• Progressive reduction in the signs and symptoms associated with osteomyelitis, including fever, pain, and swelling of the affected extremity

Documentation requirements

• Patient's and caregiver's responses to instruction

• Observation of the patient and caregiver's ability to perform home I.V. antimicrobial therapy, passive ROM exercises, use of assistive devices, and maintenance of normal anatomic alignment, repositioning, and transfers

• Culture results and subsequent physician notification and change to plan of care

• Changes in integumentary, respiratory, GI, genitourinary, or neurologic functioning

• Ability of caregivers to care for the patient

Reimbursement reminders

• Medicare covers phlebotomy supplies.

• Check for an authorized laboratory because many insurance companies have contracts with specific laboratories for processing specimens.

• All nonroutine supplies must be specifically ordered by the physician and entered into Locator 14 (Supplies) of HCFA Form 485 or ordered by the physician within the specific order for treatment requiring the use of certain supplies and entered into Locator 21 (Orders for Treatment).

• When billing for medical supplies, always include the name of supply item, date supply was used, number of units used, and charge per unit.

• Identify progress toward educational and clinical goals and plan for cessation of services. Five or more visits in a week are considered daily visits and must have a foreseeable and planned end.

Insurance hints

• Provide a review of hospitalization (if appropriate) and current condition of the patient, home environment, and availability of caregivers.

• Provide objective review of systems, including physical abilities, ambulation, use or need for assistive devices.

• Provide thorough skin assessment, and report objective findings. In the event of open or reddened areas, provide accurate wound dimensions, prescribed dressing, and capabilities of caregivers to perform wound care.

• Provide initial and current laboratory values for comparison.

• Provide objective evaluation of ambulatory and nutritional status.

• Provide objective review of cognitive level and ability to comprehend instructions.

• Provide the patient's and caregiver's response to the caregiver's provision of I.V. antimicrobial therapy.

- Arrange for home delivery of medication and supplies needed for antimicrobial therapy.

Osteoporosis

Osteoporosis is the pathologic process by which bones become porous, causing them to weaken. This weakening leads to increases in fractures, most commonly affecting the spine and hip. Women represent 89% of those affected by osteoporosis. Home care nurses don't generally care for patients who have osteoporosis as their primary diagnosis; however, patients recovering from hip fractures account for a large number of home care patients who have osteoporosis. Fractures of the vertebral spine account for the next most common group of patients seen in home care with osteoporosis.

Previsit checklist

Physician orders and preparation
- Medications, including hormones (such as estrogen), antiosteoporotic agents (such as alendronate), calcium, and vitamin D
- Activity restrictions and exercise regimen
- Comfort and pain control measures for compression fractures or hip fractures
- Durable medical equipment, including splints and ambulation devices, such as a cane or walker (as indicated)
- Physical therapist evaluation for therapeutic exercises and range of motion (ROM)

- Occupational therapist evaluation for use of adaptive equipment for activities of daily living (ADLs) and home safety evaluation for patient at risk for falls
- Dietitian evaluation for menu planning and alternatives to meet dietary needs of increased calcium
- Social worker evaluation for community resources and financial assistance

Equipment and supplies
- Supplies for standard precautions and proper sharps disposal
- Scale
- Educational literature related to osteoporosis and prevention of complications

Safety requirements
- Standard precautions for infection control and sharps disposal
- Information on medications, including dosage, adverse effects, interactions, and safe storage of multiple medications
- Allergies verified and documented
- Emergency plan and access to functional phone and list of emergency phone numbers
- Identification and correction of environmental hazards and patient-specific concerns (for example, clear walkways, night-lights, and removal of some furniture to accommodate adaptive equipment)

Major diagnostic codes
- Closed fractures:
  - femur 821.0
  - femur open reduction internal fixation 79.35

– vertebral, cervical 806.0
– vertebral, thoracic 805.2
• Osteoporosis, generalized/idiopathic 733/733.02
• Pain, thoracic spine 724.1
• Pain with radicular and visceral spine 724.4

Defense of homebound status

(Home care nurses should be aware of the need to clarify the patient's primary diagnosis for each episode of home care. The diagnosis on reimbursement forms should reflect the care being given to the patient. For osteoporosis, the primary diagnosis will probably focus on the patient's fractures or other disabilities unless the patient has had numerous recent admissions to the emergency department or hospital and qualifies for skilled management and evaluation.)
• Unable to ambulate farther than 10′ (3 m) without increase in symptoms of pain and exhaustion due to fatigue
• Unable to ambulate or unsafe without assistance because of recent or severe fracture
• Unable to transfer from bed to chair without significant change in symptoms, including pain and fatigue

---

Selected nursing diagnoses and patient outcomes

Knowledge deficit related to use of adaptive equipment (walker or wheelchair)
    The patient or caregiver will:
• verbalize knowledge of how to use a walker or wheelchair   (N, OT, PT)

• demonstrate proper use of walker or wheelchair   (N, OT, PT)
• demonstrate proper posture and distribution of weight while using a walker   (N, OT, PT)
• explain and use methods to bathe using a walker and other assistive devices to get in and out of the shower or bathtub   (N, OT, PT)
• be free from injury.   (N, OT, PT)

Chronic pain related to decrease in intervertebral disk mass and fractures
    The patient or caregiver will:
• verbalize proper analgesia use and rate pain as 3 or less on a 0-to-10 scale 80% of the time   (N)
• have optimal movement related to proper pain control   (N)
• use adjuvant pain therapy for bone pain properly, including anti-inflammatory medication   (N)
• verbalize methods of preventing constipating adverse effects of analgesic use   (N)
• report satisfaction with sleep pattern   (N)
• be able to participate in home exercise program.   (N, PT, OT)

Impaired physical mobility related to pain and limited motion from inflamed joints
    The patient or caregiver will:
• demonstrate measures to prevent contractures   (N, PT)
• demonstrate measures to minimize or prevent muscle spasms   (N, PT)
• perform at expected level of independent self-care   (N, OT, PT)
• maintain functional mobility and ROM   (N, OT, PT)
• maintain optimal functional independence   (N, OT, PT)

- complete home exercise program
(N, PT, OT)
- maintain activity within prescribed
limitations (N, PT, OT)
- demonstrate proper posture while
using a walker, wheelchair, or other
adaptive equipment. (N, PT, OT)

*Impaired walking related to pain and
fear of falling*
The patient or caregiver will:
- express satisfaction with gait pattern, endurance, and coordination
(N, OT, PT)
- express feelings of increased strength
(N, OT, PT)
- verbalize need to increase activity
gradually (N, OT, PT)
- demonstrate progressive tolerance
to activity. (N, OT, PT)

*Dressing-grooming self-care deficit re-
lated to limited mobility*
The patient or caregiver will:
- be clean, properly groomed, and free
from body odor (N, HCA, OT, PT)
- be free from injury
(N, HCA, OT, PT)
- verbalize knowledge of home safety
plan to prevent falls
(N, HCA, OT, PT, OT)
- rearrange home for use of a walker
or wheelchair (N, HCA, OT, PT)
- demonstrate proper walker or wheelchair storage (N, HCA, OT, PT)
- modify home to increase walkway,
lighting, and space for adaptive equipment. (N, OT, HCA)

Skilled nursing services

Care measures
- Recognize that the patient may need
rehabilitation services only.

Patient and family teaching
- Teach how to prevent injury by by
maintaining clear walkways, night-
lights, and grab bars; increasing calcium intake and progressive weight-
bearing exercises; and adhering to medication regimen, including special
orders (such as taking alendronate after rising for the day, on an empty stomach, and then withholding food and all
beverages except tap water for at least
30 minutes after administration).

Interdisciplinary actions

Physical therapist
- Home exercise program
- Safety planning
- Transfer training
- Strength and endurance training

Occupational therapist
- Assistance with management of
ADLs
- Energy conservation
- Best use of assistive devices and
adaptation of home environment

Home care aide
- Hygiene, grooming, and dressing
- Energy conservation measures

Social worker
- Assistance in obtaining community
resources, such as transportation and
home support services

Discharge plan
- Ability to return to normal routine
following recovery from fractures
- Attainment of maximal mobility level with demonstration of appropriate
self-care activities

• Safe management of disease process in the home with physician, outpatient, and community support system follow-up services
• Pain-, injury-, and symptom-free until death

Documentation requirements

• Description of functional losses or gains in clear terms: distance walked with walker or wheelchair and self-care ability
• Evaluation of effectiveness of pain control regimen
• Description of plan to improve patient function whenever progress stalls
• Appropriateness of the patient's home environment
• Long-term needs of the patient, suitability of residence, and presence of caregiver

Reimbursement reminders

• Recognize that the need for a walker or wheelchair doesn't make a patient homebound. Be clear about functional limitations; the patient's ability to use a walker or wheelchair, especially upper body strength; and the presence of other injuries such as paresis.
• Demonstrate coordination of care with rehabilitation services.
• Occupational therapy can be ordered if the patient needs energy conservation and to work with home care aide in transfers in the bathroom.
• Medicare doesn't cover conditions that are essentially "debilitation"; the patient must show continued progress toward goals. When progress has plateaued, the patient is custodial and should be discharged. If osteoporosis

is the primary diagnosis, duration of care should be brief.

Insurance hints

• Describe progressive levels of self-care (dressing, toileting, bathing, grooming, dressing) and abilities, including use of adaptive equipment. Emphasize rehabilitation potential.
• Describe progress toward rehabilitation goals, such as safe use of stairs, transfers from sitting to standing.
• List the collaborative plan of care for all team members providing services.
• Compare and contrast the roles of each rehabilitation team member.
• Explain what long-term care will be needed and explore placement issues.
• Describe any other conditions such as chronic lung disease and how it affects the patient's use of a walker or wheelchair.

Ostomy care

An ostomy is a surgically created opening of the abdominal wall and the bowel or bladder for drainage of stool or urine. Tumors of the urinary tract and lower GI tract, ulcerative colitis, Crohn's disease, trauma to the GI tract, and bowel obstructions may force a patient to have an ostomy. Coverage for supplies is limited, but each insurance company varies. Patients with ostomies require individualized attention and support while adjustment of the elimination process is completed. Patient teaching for self-care of the ostomy is the goal. Careful nutritional management, physical activity tolerance, coping, and lifestyle adjustments are the basis for the return to health for patients with ostomies.

Previsit checklist

Physician orders and preparation
- Dietary restrictions and fluid encouragement
- Irrigation (frequency, irrigant solution)
- Medications
- Activity orders and restrictions
- Order for enterostomal therapist consult for assistance with designing an individualized skin care and ostomy maintenance regimen
- Dietitian evaluation for menu planning and alternatives for a low-residue diet
- Social worker evaluation for community resources and financial assistance

Equipment and supplies
- Supplies for standard precautions and proper waste disposal
- Ostomy supplies (bags, wafers, skin protectant, secure devices, deodorizers)
- Irrigation (device, solution)

Safety requirements
- Standard precautions for infection control and waste disposal
- Avoidance of foods high in fiber, impaction prevention plan
- Abdominal care for pouch and stoma
- Adequate rest periods
- Signs and symptoms (including abdominal pain, fever, progressive inflammation and skin breakdown of ostomy site) to be reported to the physician or nurse
- Information on medications, including dosage, adverse effects, interactions, and safe storage of multiple medications
- Allergies verified and documented
- Emergency plan and access to functional phone and list of emergency phone numbers
- Identification and correction of environmental hazards and patient-specific concerns (for example, no running water, no electricity, no support person in home)

Major diagnostic codes
- Colostomy and enterostomy complications 569.9
- Impaction of intestine 560.3
- Irritable colon 564.1
- Peptic ulcer 533
- Urinary obstruction 599.6

Defense of homebound status
- Unable to ambulate farther than 10′ (3 m) because of fatigue
- Unable to ambulate farther than 10′ because of ostomy leakage or soiling
- Unable to leave home because of draining ostomy

Selected nursing diagnoses and patient outcomes

Risk for impaired skin integrity related to ostomy appliance

The patient or caregiver will:
- verbalize or demonstrate skin care treatment of peristomal area (N, ET)
- report stomal cuts or tears, narrowing of stomal lumen, and separation of the stoma away from the abdominal wall or bulging around the stoma.

(N, ET, MD)

Fluid volume deficit related to dehydration

The patient or caregiver will:
- maintain adequate fluid intake (N, D)
- report signs and symptoms of dehydration, such as dry skin and oral mucus membranes, extreme thirst, decreased urine output, feeling faint when changing positions, and weakness or fatigue. (N)

Altered nutrition: More (or Less) than body requirements related to change in stool elimination

The patient or caregiver will:
- follow the recommended diet (N, D)
- describe an appropriate meal plan for elimination concerns and target weight (N, D)
- verbalize or demonstrate knowledge of care of ostomy (N, ET)
- verbalize a plan for obtaining ostomy supply equipment after discharge (N, ET, SW)
- verbalize knowledge and management of a low-residue diet (N, D)
- verbalize understanding of activity endurance (N, HCA, PT)
- demonstrate the ability to cope with changes of fecal elimination through an ostomy. (N, ET)

Body image disturbance related to effect of ostomy on activities of daily living (ADLs)

The patient or caregiver will:
- participate in care of the ostomy (N, ET)
- participate in odor-control strategies, diet modifications, and acceptance of ostomy. (N, ET, SC)

Activity intolerance related to fatigue

The patient or caregiver will:
- increase activity endurance (N, HCA, PT)
- participate in ADLs. (N, HCA)

Skilled nursing services

Care measures
- Conduct a skilled assessment focusing on mental and cognitive status, nutrition, hydration, and integumentary (mucus membranes), GI, and genitourinary systems.
- Assess level of care of the patient and caregiver with ostomy changing, skin care, and emptying of appliance.
- Assess effectiveness of treatment regimen by dietary intake, weight gain or loss, dehydration signs and symptoms.

Patient and family teaching
- Demonstrate the use of ostomy equipment: appliance, securing device, skin care treatment, and irrigation.
- Describe dehydration prevention measures: drinking 8 to 10 glasses of water or other fluids per day, applying lip ointments for dry lips, maintaining cool temperature of the environment, and seeking attention for signs and symptoms of dehydration.
- Explain how to prevent stoma complications or peristomal skin alterations by using prescribed skin care treatments, adhering to appliance fit, and reporting stoma changes or changes in output.
- Review measures to prevent food blockage by limiting high-fiber foods; taking a warm shower to relax abdominal muscles; drinking warm fluids; massaging the peristomal area to stimulate peristalsis; reporting signs and

symptoms, including high-volume fluid output, abdominal cramps, nausea, and vomiting; and irrigating as prescribed.

Interdisciplinary actions

Dietitian
• Consultation for nutritional needs, a low-fiber diet, and foods that produce gas or excessive odor

Enterostomal therapist
• Consultation for management of ostomy

Social worker
• Referral to community resource programs and support groups

Discharge plan
• Management of ostomy care in the home by the patient and caregiver with physician and community support system follow-ups
• Continuation of home care visits for a homebound patient with skilled care needs
• Ensuring that the patient is pain- and symptom-free until death; death with dignity

Documentation requirements
• Subjective and objective data in regard to ostomy care, hydration, elimination factors, dietary intake, weight gain or loss, abdominal feelings, peristomal skin site, and appliance concerns
• Ostomy care, including type, time, and frequency of irrigation, and appliance change

• Patient and caregiver participation in care
• Patient and caregiver progress toward educational goals
• Patient response to care
• Variances to expected outcomes
• Barriers to learning (physical deformities, visual impairment, and availability of support person)
• Initial level of knowledge and progress toward educational goals

Reimbursement reminders
• Ostomy supplies are covered by Medicare and private insurance companies.
• Remember that appliances, irrigation sets, and skin care ointments are based on the type of system used.
• When billing for medical supplies, always include the name of supply item, date supply was used, number of units used, and charge per unit.
• Registered dietitian services aren't reimbursable under Medicare benefits except under certain conditions.
• Obtain a telephone order for any plan of care change, and document it in the chart.
• Identify patient instructions given and progress toward educational goals.

Insurance hints
• Present objective data about homebound status, including frequency of soiling when standing and walking or that the patient was out of bed no more than twice daily.
• Report any new laboratory findings that change the plan of care.
• Report specifics about patient learning progress.

Pain management

Persistent, chronic pain can decrease quality of life; uncontrolled pain can stop a successful career or make responsibilities of daily living impossible to manage. There are three basic types of pain that require treatment. Acute or subacute pain is recent-onset pain (3 months or less) related to a specific condition other than cancer (for example, fractures or shingles). Chronic pain is pain from a long-term condition (for example, lower back pain, leg pain, and phantom limb pain). The third category is cancer pain — pain caused by a malignant condition or by the treatment of cancer.

For years, pain was largely undertreated because of fears of narcotics addiction and inadequate education of patients and health care professionals. Poor assessment techniques and documentation often resulted in undermedication. In the last 5 years, pain management has become a recognized medical specialty that concentrates on diagnosis, treatment, and management of all three types of pain. The goal of pain management is to identify the cause of pain and to cure it. If this isn't possible, pain management is used to reduce the impact of pain and restore as much quality of life as possible.

Numerous centers for pain management have been started all across the country. There have been significant advances in pain management techniques. There are new medications available, such as local anesthetics, nerve blocks, and intraspinal and epidural medications. Other pain treatments include transcutaneous and intraspinal electrical stimulation, ayurvedic medicine (treatment using plants and drugs indiginous to India), acupuncture, yoga, and meditation. The World Health Organization now recognizes a three-step analgesic ladder to treat pain. The first step is mild pain that is treated with over-the-counter (OTC) medications. The second step is mild to moderate pain that is treated with weak opioids, with or without OTC medications and adjunctive therapies. Finally, step three is moderate to severe pain, treated with strong opioids, either alone or with adjunctive therapy to provide optimum control. This stepped approach to pain control is primarily being used to treat cancer-related pain.

Because pain, whether acute or subacute, chronic or cancer-related, reduces function and the quality of life, patients with pain have some very specific needs. One of their main needs is to have their pain taken seriously — not only by their health care team but by family and caregivers. It's important to educate those who interact with the patient on a regular basis as to the origin and severity of pain. Instruction needs to be given to alleviate misconceptions regarding narcotics addictions and exaggerations of pain. Pain needs to be assessed with each visit and the patient and caregiver need to be instructed in the use of a pain journal that will rate pain on a scale of 0-to-10 at onset and after medication. After this, the major focus is pain control and the prevention or minimization of complications of therapy.

Previsit checklist

Physician orders and preparation

- Dose, route, type, and frequency of pain medication or treatment (a physician may use a combination of drugs intended to work together to alleviate pain; for example, when drugs such as some anticonvulsants, antihypertensives, and antidepressants are added to opioids, the dose of opioid required is much less and pain control is better)
- Medications ordered in addition to analgesics (steroids, antidepressants, anticonvulsants, stool softeners and laxatives, antiemetics, and stimulants)
- Activity level and restrictions
- Order for support services as indicated (physical therapy, occupational therapy, home care aide assistance)
- Oxygen as indicated

Equipment and supplies

- Supplies for standard precautions and proper sharps disposal
- Pain assessment tool
- Pain journal or notebook with written instructions on how to use it effectively
- Medication information and interaction sheets
- Injection or I.V. supplies
- Oxygen supplies

Safety requirements

- List of signs and symptoms to report to the physician, including signs of overdose
- Standard precautions for infection control and sharps disposal
- Information on medications, including dosage, adverse effects, interactions, and safe storage of multiple medications
- Allergies verified and documented
- Emergency plan and access to functional phone and list of emergency phone numbers
- Oxygen precautions, safe handling and placement of home oxygen equipment, and notification of local fire and police departments of oxygen use in the home
- Identification and correction of environmental hazards and patient-specific concerns (for example, night-lights and smoke detectors)
- Restrictions regarding operating a vehicle or machinery while medicated

Major diagnostic codes

- Pain management, generalized 780.9

Defense of homebound status

- Unable to ambulate farther than 10′ (3 m) because of severe pain on movement
- Poor endurance related to pain and shortness of breath
- Use of patient-controlled analgesia pump for pain relief; unable to leave home without assistance because of adverse effects of pain medication
- Maximum assistance needed for all activities
- Severe pain with movement

Selected nursing diagnoses and patient outcomes

Pain related to cancer, fractures, spasms, shingles, surgery, or burns
  The patient or caregiver will:

- rate pain before and after pain medication on a 0-to-10 scale, maintaining a rating of 3 or less 80% of the time (N)
- identify factors that aggravate or relieve pain and modify behavior accordingly (N, OT)
- carry out alternative pain control measures such as heat or cold applications (N)
- report more than 4 hours of sleep nightly (N)
- decrease amount and frequency of pain medication within 72 hours (N)
- verbalize that others validate that the pain exists (N, SW)
- practice selected noninvasive pain-relief measures to manage the pain (N)
- verbalize improvement of pain and increase in daily activities as evidenced by (specify). (N, OT)
- describe comfort from others during the pain experience. (N)

Altered nutrition: Less than body requirements related to inability to ingest foods

The patient or caregiver will:
- verbalize understanding of special dietary needs and plan an appropriate diet (N, D)
- name foods and beverages that don't increase nausea (N)
- report decreased nausea (N)
- increase oral intake as evidenced by (specify) (N, D)
- describe a meal plan for weight gain (N, D)
- initiate a flexible meal time to increase oral intake during pain reduction or pain-free time. (N)

Activity intolerance related to uncontrolled pain

The patient or caregiver will:

- identify factors that reduce activity tolerance (N)
- schedule activity during pain-free or reduced pain periods (for example, during peak of pain medication) (N)
- demonstrate energy conservation measures (N, HCA, OT)
- identify types of activities that can be tolerated. (N, OT)

Skilled nursing services

Care measures
- Perform skilled nursing assessment, including psychosocial, nutritional, integumentary, cardiovascular, genitourinary, respiratory, and hydration status.
- Incorporate bowel regimen into patient's lifestyle.
- Obtain a complete medical and pain history. Facilitate the expression of fears, anxieties, and physical discomfort. Assess pain belief (kinds of things the patient and family have done in the past to relieve painful situations) and pain history to help identify problems and related factors that describe and contribute to the painful situation. Identify the factors that precipitate or hasten the occurrence of the pain. Identify the factors that affect the pain and quality of life. Identify the sites of discomfort, character and description, duration, intensity, and frequency.
- Assess level of pain using a 0-to-10 scale at each visit.
- Assess effectiveness of pain regimen.
- Demonstrate a belief in the patient's report of pain intensity, be supportive (pain is subjective, and one of the patient's greatest needs is for validation).
- Assess ability to perform activities of daily living (ADLs).

- Assess for medication adverse effects and interactions.
- Instruct the patient in possible medication adverse effects and plan of action (overmedication, constipation, dizziness, nausea).
- Assess nutrition and hydration, and monitor for weight loss and gain.
- Assess the impact pain has on the family and environment.
- Assess coping mechanisms and support systems that are in place.
- Encourage and instruct the patient in the use of nonpharmacologic techniques to assist with pain management (diversion, guided imagery, music, comedy, and laughter).
- Assess the need for and make a referral to and conference with other support services.

Patient and family teaching
- Review care of the bedridden patient.
- Describe how to check for and remove impaction as needed.
- Explain how to recognize medication effects, adverse effects, and interactions; review safe storage.
- Identify home safety needs.
- Emphasize the need for energy conservation and pacing.
- Discuss oxygen use and safety precautions.

Interdisciplinary actions

Dietitian
- Consultation for nutritional needs

Home care aide
- Assistance with bathing and personal care and, when indicated, light housekeeping, meal preparation, and laundry

Social worker
- Assessment of coping mechanisms, short-term counseling
- Referral to community agencies and support services

Physical therapist
- Development and instruction in individualized home exercise program (pain patients can quickly become weak and lose muscle mass secondary to inactivity related to pain; a home exercise program will enable them to improve their strength and stay as active as possible)
- Evaluation for and instruction in use of nonpharmacologic pain control measures, such as biofeedback, heat or cold application, and transcutaneous electrical nerve stimulation

Occupational therapist
- Assessment and instruction on adaptive aids and performance of ADLs

Discharge plan
- Verbalization and demonstration by the patient that pain is either resolved or minimized (pain should be rated at 3 or less on a 0-to-10 scale 80% of the time)
- Verbalization of an accurate comprehension of causes
- Demonstration of an understanding of pain management plan of care
- Identification of activities that increase and decrease pain
- Independence with ADLs
- Management of the disease process by the patient and caregiver in the home with physician and community support system follow-ups

- Patient remains homebound; continues to need skilled intermittent care
- Patient condition declines — discharged to hospice
- Patient requires 24-hour skilled care — discharged to a skilled nursing facility
- Pain- and symptom-free until death; death with dignity

Documentation requirements

- Assessment of all systems
- Pain assessment (subjective) with each visit using same method of evaluation (0-to-10 scale)
- All objective signs and symptoms of pain
- Effectiveness of pain management plan of care using same evaluating device (0-to-10 scale)
- Effect of pain on quality of life and care environment
- Ability to perform ADLs
- All signs and symptoms of medication adverse effects and any relieving interventions used
- Referrals to and conferences with other support services
- Nutrition and hydration status
- Caregiver and family reaction to pain (validation or nonvalidation)
- Patient and caregiver instruction and progress toward educational goals (such as pain medication administration via patient-controlled analgesia or subcutaneous injection)

Reimbursement reminders

- Medicare will reimburse for subcutaneous injections that are medically necessary for chronic intractable pain if the patient can't administer the injections or the caregiver is unable or unwilling to do so.
- Ensure that when daily care and visits have been ordered, goals need to be specific; be sure to indicate when daily visits are expected to end.
- Each service needs a corresponding diagnosis.
- All medication and treatment changes need corresponding physician orders.
- Obtain telephone orders for any change in the plan of care, and document it in the chart.
- Identify specific barriers to learning (impairments, handicaps, unavailability or inability of caregiver, and unwillingness of caregiver).
- Identify specific deficits in initial knowledge level, progress as evidenced by specific concepts, and information that was demonstrated and verbalized.
- Registered dietitian services aren't reimbursable under current Medicare home care benefits.
- Document pain accurately and consistently using the same method of measurement.
- Acupuncture is covered by some reimbursement plans if done by a physical therapist or physician but not by an acupuncturist.
- Skilled nursing visits won't be reimbursed if the patient is already dead before the nurse arrives unless the patient is in hospice.

Insurance hints

- Present objective data with regard to homebound status, including the patient's inability to ambulate farther than 10′ (3 m) because of nausea, weakness, and breathlessness.
- Know and report all objective signs and symptoms of pain (even though

pain is subjective), including guarding, diaphoresis, vital sign changes, and weakness.

● Give specifics about patient progress toward education goals and education needs.

● State how interventions provide palliative relief; mention all options considered, including inpatient care, if applicable.

Pancreatitis

Pancreatitis can be described as an acute or chronic inflammation of the pancreas. It results from changes in the structure or function of the pancreas, typically resulting from chronic alcohol abuse. Autodigestion occurs as pancreatic enzymes digest pancreatic tissues. Common signs and symptoms include an increased white blood cell count, fever, nausea, and vomiting. Because chronic pancreatitis primarily results from chronic alcohol abuse, it's the responsibility of the home care nurse to intervene to the extent possible to provide counseling for the alcoholic and his family members.

Previsit checklist

Physician orders and preparation
● Order for medications
● Order for I.V. antibiotics and fluids as needed
● Order for tube feedings as needed
● Order for social worker to provide link to alcoholic rehabilitation
● Nutritional consultation for comprehensive nutritional assessment

Equipment and supplies
● Supplies for standard precautions and proper sharps disposal
● I.V. supplies
● Tube feeding supplies

Safety requirements
● List of signs and symptoms to report to the physician
● Standard precautions for infection control and sharps disposal
● Information on medications, including dosage adverse effects, interactions, and safe storage of multiple medications
● Allergies verified and documented
● Emergency plan and access to functional phone and list of emergency phone numbers
● Identification and correction of environmental hazards and patient-specific concerns (for example, clear walkways, grab bars, and night-lights)
● Fall precautions
● Aspiration precautions and action plan in the event of aspiration

Major diagnostic codes
● Pancreatitis:
    – acute (annular, apoplectic, clacerous, edematous, hemorrhagic, recurrent) 577.0
    – chronic, recurrent 577.1
    – cystic 577.2
    – syphilitic 095.8

Defense of homebound status
● Bedridden; out of bed less than twice daily because of severe weakness or dizziness
● Random acute attacks of severe pain

- Physician orders for bathroom privileges only
- Unable to leave home unattended
- Unable to ambulate without assistance because of weakness or unsteady gait

Selected nursing diagnoses and patient outcomes

Pain related to autodigestion of pancreatic tissues

The patient or caregiver will:
- report a level of discomfort that is no greater than 3 on a 0-to-10 scale
(N, MD)
- relate signs and symptoms of complications, such as hypotension, tachycardia, and tachypnea, and action plan if they occur (N)
- verbalize nonpharmacologic measures to combat pain, including distraction and meditation. (N)

Powerlessness related to illness-related regimen

The patient or caregiver will:
- express feelings of lack of control
(N)
- contract to enter an alcoholic rehabilitation program (N, SW)
- verbalize understanding of the threat to physical health that continued use of alcohol poses (N)
- verbalize at least three alternative coping methods that may be used other than use of alcohol (N)
- identify specific factors in the illness-related regimen over which control can be maintained, and plan appropriate action. (N)

Risk for poisoning related to external factors

The patient or caregiver will:
- state method for safekeeping of dangerous or potentially dangerous products (removal of all alcohol from premises) (N)
- verbalize signs and symptoms related to ingestion of alcohol (N)
- verbalize understanding of physical harm alcohol will cause the patient.
(N)

Skilled nursing services

Care measures
- Perform a skilled assessment focusing on mental and cognitive status, nutrition, hydration, and the GI system.
- Make certain that the patient is being managed with a nasogastric tube during acute attack of pancreatitis because oral intake may further precipitate an attack.
- Administer meperidine for pain relief as prescribed.
- Administer I.V. antibiotics if ordered for replacement of lost fluid volume and to avoid infection from the autodigestion process.
- Monitor closely for signs of complications, such as hypotension, tachycardia, and tachypnea.

Patient and family teaching
- Teach about medications, including dosage, adverse effects, interactions, and medication schedule.
- Emphasize the importance of avoiding alcohol, proper rest, weight management, and optimal nutrition.
- Emphasize the importance of compliance to the regimen.
- Emphasize the importance of medical follow-up.

• Identify signs and symptoms to report to the physician.

Interdisciplinary actions

Dietitian
• Comprehensive nutritional consultation and design of individualized dietary plan

Social worker
• Consultation for access to alcoholic rehabilitation program

Discharge plan
• Safe management of recovery from pancreatitis in the home by the patient and caregiver with physician follow-up and outpatient services
• Demonstration of understanding and willingness to comply with the plan of care for prevention of further complications of alcoholism
• Continuation of home care visits for a homebound patient with skilled care needs

Documentation requirements
• Variances to expected outcomes, including noncompliance to the treatment regimen
• Specific care that was provided as well as teaching instructions, and progress toward educational and clinical goals
• Laboratory values and findings that necessitate a change in the plan of care

Reimbursement reminders
• Identify all episodes of acute pain and the interventions provided for assistance.
• Note all attempts to encourage the patient to access alcoholic rehabilitation services.
• Identify abnormal laboratory values, compare with previous results, report to the physician, communicate changes in the plan of care to health team members, and document.
• Identify specific learning barriers to teaching that was provided.
• Medicare covers phlebotomy supplies.
• Check for an authorized laboratory because many insurance companies have contracts with specific laboratories for processing specimens.

Insurance hints
• Present objective patient findings and changes since last update.
• Present interventions directed toward avoiding inpatient hospitalization.
• Report symptoms and changes since last communication.
• Present other information and measurable changes that communicate the status of the patient and the need for skilled home care services.

Parkinson's disease

Parkinson's disease — a progressive, degenerative, neurologic disease — is characterized by tremors, bradykinesia, and muscle rigidity. It most commonly affects older adult men with symptoms first appearing around age 50. In Parkinson's disease, there is an atrophy of the neurons that produce dopamine, a neurotransmitter. This chemical helps regulate nerve impulses to control motor functioning. The levels of dopamine decrease, leading to a concurrent increase in acetylcholine. It's this increase in acetylcholine that causes the clinical manifestations of the disease, including fatigue, tremors, uncoordinated movements, and unsteady gait. The most pronounced symptoms of Parkinson's disease are bradykinesia, nonintention tremors, and muscle rigidity. Care for the patient focuses on maximizing mobility and self-care, controlling medication adverse effects, nutritional support, and airway protection. For these issues, teaching is needed for the families of patients with this health condition and should focus on maximizing physical functioning to achieve maximal independence, preventing medication complications, and reducing the feelings of social isolation.

Previsit checklist

Physician orders and preparation
- Order for bladder regimen
- Order for bowel regimen
- Order for physical and occupational therapy
- Order for speech therapy to maximize recovery of speech and minimize aspiration risk
- Order for durable medical equipment, including specialty bed, wheelchair, and other assistive devices
- Activity orders and restrictions
- Order for nutritional supplements and tube feedings as indicated
- Order for home suctioning equipment

- Orders for as-needed skilled nursing visits to evaluate and manage tube problems

Equipment and supplies
- Supplies for standard precautions and proper sharps disposal
- Intermittent urinary catheter kit as per the physician order for urinary retention
- Dressing supplies to change dressing around gastrostomy feeding tube, if indicated
- Irrigation kit for gastrostomy tube
- Sterile water
- Suctioning kits (nasotracheal and oropharyngeal)

Safety requirements
- List of signs and symptoms to report to physician
- Standard precautions for infection control and sharps disposal
- Information on medications, including dosage, adverse effects, interactions, and safe storage of multiple medications
- Allergies verified and documented
- Emergency plan and access to functional phone and list of emergency phone numbers
- Identification and correction of environmental hazards and patient-specific concerns (for example, placement of grab bars and supportive devices in the bathroom, removal of throw rugs and carpeting, and placement of three-pronged grounded outlets for medical equipment)
- Aspiration precautions
- Fall precautions, including supportive, well-fitting, nonslip footwear
- Safe use of suction equipment

- Skin care and protection to include frequent position changes
- Safe disposal of incontinence pads

Major diagnostic codes

- Abnormal involuntary movements 781.0
- Abnormality of gait 781.2
- Associated with orthostatic hypotension 333.0
- Dysphasia 438.12
- Lack of coordination 781.3
- Parkinsonism 332.0
- Tremor 781.0

Defense of homebound status

- Unable to ambulate farther than 10′ (3 m) because of bradykinesia, nonintentional tremors, and muscle rigidity
- Unable to maintain patent airway
- Unsafe to leave unattended

Selected nursing diagnoses and patient outcomes

Impaired physical mobility
    The patient or caregiver will:
- recognize limitations with ambulation   (N, OT, PT)
- recognize that tremors, gait, and balance can lead to unsafe independent activities   (N, OT, PT)
- demonstrate passive range of motion to extremities stiffened by the disease   (N, OT, PT)
- demonstrate ability to ambulate at least four times per day to maintain muscle tone and joint flexibility
(N, OT, PT)

- demonstrate the use of assistive devices to promote ambulation and self-care independence   (N, OT, PT)
- recognize home assistive devices that can be used to maximize independence, such as a raised toilet seat, grab bars, and improved lighting in and around the home environment.
(N, OT, PT)

Impaired verbal communication due to decreased voice amplitude and muscle control
    The patient or caregiver will:
- demonstrate adaptations to work environment or other accommodations to cope with difficult verbalization
(N, SP)
- recognize that impaired verbal communication doesn't reduce the value of the individual   (N, SP)
- recognize the cause of the speech impairment and use techniques obtained by speech therapy to maximize speech recovery   (N, SP)
- recognize that having a speech impairment doesn't mean the patient can't hear   (N, SP)
- demonstrate waiting an adequate time for a response from the patient when communicating   (N, SP)
- demonstrate facing the patient when communicating and speaking slowly, without yelling   (N, SP)
- demonstrate the use of short, simple statements and questions to permit processing of information (N, SP)
- recognize frustration and anger as a normal response to the loss of functioning   (N, SP)
- recognize that the disease affects the patient's vocal amplitude and muscle control   (N, SP)

- demonstrate alternative methods of communication (N, SP)
- encourage the patient to speak as loudly as possible to facilitate speech recognition. (N, SP)

Altered nutrition: Less than body requirements

The patient or caregiver will:
- recognize that tremors, gait, impaired chewing, and impaired swallowing can lead to nutritional problems with the patient (N, D)
- recognize alternative nutritional approaches to ensure an adequate intake of calories and fluids (N, D)
- demonstrate assessment of the swallowing reflex prior to meals (N, SP)
- demonstrate the patient's ability to feed himself independently, with the use of assistive devices (N, OT)
- recognize different food consistencies that will facilitate adequate nutrition based upon the patient's chewing and swallowing limitations (N, SP)
- demonstrate an adequate nutritional intake by a stable weight evaluated weekly (N)
- demonstrate methods to decrease tremors by incorporating purposeful activities (purposeful activities decrease nonintention tremors) (N, OT, PT)
- recognize foods high in bulk and fiber to ensure a routine bowel elimination pattern. (N, D)

Sleep pattern disturbance

The patient or caregiver will:
- recognize that rigidity and weakness reduce the ability to move and change positions while sleeping, leading to periods of wakefulness (N)

- recognize that several medications can interfere with the normal rapid-eye-movement sleep cycle, leading to vivid dreams with periods of wakefulness (N, MD)
- recognize the need to incorporate frequent periods of rest and sleep throughout the day to support the body's need for rest and sleep (N)
- demonstrate limiting stimulants, such as caffeine and chocolate, around the hour of sleep (N)
- recognize that warm milk before bedtime, which produces a sedative effect, can aid in falling asleep (N)
- demonstrate reducing noise and other environmental stimulation to aid in falling asleep. (N)

Risk for aspiration

The patient or caregiver will:
- recognize that changes in swallowing can affect the patient's ability to maintain a patent airway (N, SP)
- demonstrate the use of home suction equipment in the event of an airway obstruction. (N)

Feeding, bathing-hygiene, dressing-grooming, and toileting self-care deficits

The patient or caregiver will:
- recognize physical limitations with self-care activities, such as toileting, grooming, bathing, dressing, and feeding (N, HCA)
- demonstrate alternative approaches and the use of assistive devices to maintain independence with self-care activities. (N, HCA)

Sexual dysfunction

The patient or caregiver will:

- recognize there is an altered self-concept with the disease because of muscle rigidity and loss of flexibility (N)
- express recognition of alternative approaches to ensure sexual functioning. (N)

Ineffective individual coping

The patient or caregiver will:
- recognize the sense of hopelessness and powerlessness due to the progression and prognosis of the disease (N)
- demonstrate a positive outlook and praise for performing routine activities to maintain optimal independence. (N)

Ineffective family coping: Compromised

The patient or caregiver will:
- recognize the degree of stress the disease process can place on the family unit (N, SW)
- demonstrate patience and understand the need for family members to want a break in caring for the patient. (N, SW)

Risk for impaired skin integrity

The patient or caregiver will:
- recognize the need to help the patient with position changes because of muscle rigidity (N)
- demonstrate frequent position changes to reduce pressure on bony prominences (N)
- demonstrate an intact integumentary status. (N)

Skilled nursing services

Care measures

- Perform a skilled assessment with emphasis on neurologic status, skin integrity, swallowing function, bowel and bladder function, speech, mobility, and balance.
- Assess the home for assistive device needs.
- Assess nutritional status.
- Provide dietary instruction, and offer the use of supplemental feedings, if indicated.
- Assess medication compliance, need, and knowledge of medications.
- Evaluate whether the patient has all prescribed medications, knows how to take them, and understands common adverse effects.
- Evaluate social and emotional functioning of the patient and caregivers, including recognizing depression.

Patient and family teaching

- Review safety tips, including how to maintain safety in the bathroom (typically the most dangerous room); for example, install grab bars near the commode and in the shower, attach suction cups to the soap dish, use a long-handled sponge or brush, an electric razor, and a shower mat or strips to minimize the risk of slipping on wet surfaces.
- Explain activity limitations and exercise regimen.
- Discuss bowel and bladder training programs.
- Identify strategies for coping with Parkinson's disease.
- Discuss the maintenance of relationships and activities to reduce feelings of isolation and powerlessness.
- Demonstrate oropharyngeal suctioning.
- Teach about enteral feedings and gastrostomy tube care (if applicable).
- Demonstrate application of splints.
- Review skin care.

- Identify the best methods for turning and repositioning.

Interdisciplinary actions

Physical therapist
- Initiation of rehabilitation program, including splint application, transferring, standing, walking, gait, and balance
- Assessment of equipment needs, functional features, and safety factors at home
- Continuation of rehabilitation program as prescribed

Occupational therapist
- Assessment of activities of daily living (ADLs)
- Provision of adaptive devices as indicated
- Provision of therapies addressing fine motor skills and to control nonintention tremors
- Instruction in energy conservation techniques

Speech pathologist
- Assessment of swallowing
- Evaluation of airway while ingesting foods and fluids
- Instruction to caregivers on aspiration precautions

Social worker
- Assessment of need for community resources
- Provision of emotional support and counseling

Home care aide
- Encouragement to the patient and caregiver to provide care
- Reduction of frequency of home care aide interventions as the patient and caregiver gain confidence in providing care as directed
- Assistance with ADLs

Discharge plan
- Stability with ambulation and gait
- Achievement of maximum independence with ADLs with moderate assistance
- Improved mobility level with demonstration of self-care activities appropriate to the level of physiological functioning
- Implementation of measures to prevent or minimize integumentary, respiratory, GI, or genitourinary complications

Documentation requirements
- Patient and caregiver's responses to instruction
- Observations of the patient and caregiver's ability to perform oropharyngeal suctioning, gastrostomy tube feedings (if applicable), use of assistive devices, repositioning, and transfers
- Tube types, sizes, and prescribed feeding and changing schedules
- Changes in integumentary, respiratory, GI, genitourinary, or neurologic status
- Ability of caregivers to care for the patient

Reimbursement reminders
- Emergency telephone response systems aren't covered by Medicare even though they're usually warranted for

those in the advanced stages of Parkinson's, especially those living alone.

● Documentation must reflect the patient's condition; all interventions and instructions provided to the patient; the patient and family's response and understanding of interventions, instructions, or notifications; care coordination among the disciplines providing patient care through the agency; and the plan for follow-up care or discharge from the agency. Medicare doesn't pay for ongoing debilitation; progress toward goals must be demonstrated.

● Use exacerbation of a chronic illness or document changes, such as new medication regimen or dramatic change in functional level, causing the patient to require care for a chronic condition.

● Reflect the patient's continuing need for care.

● Document specific skilled care provided and how it relates to the diagnosis and plan of care.

● Justify the need to repeat instructions or reinstruct.

● Refer to the plan of care and the patient's progress toward outcomes identified in the plan.

Insurance hints

● Provide review of hospitalization (if appropriate) and current condition of the patient, home environment, and availability of caregivers.

● Present objective data about homebound status and patient findings; use quantifiable terms, such as distance patient is able to ambulate, pain rating scale or muscle strength measurements, or specific safety hazards; specify how care is skilled.

● Provide objective review of systems to include physical abilities, ambulation, use or need for assistive devices.

● Provide thorough skin assessment, and report objective findings. In the event of open or reddened areas, provide accurate wound dimensions, prescribed dressing, and capabilities of caregivers to perform wound care.

● Provide current laboratory values, and compare them to recent and initial values.

● Provide objective evaluation of swallowing, respiratory, and nutritional status. If the patient is receiving gastrostomy tube feedings, describe the patient's tolerance of feedings, patency of gastrostomy tube, and condition of skin surrounding the tube. If the patient can be supported by oral nutrition, objectively evaluate the patient's and caregiver's ability to maintain a patent airway.

● Provide objective review of communication abilities, cognitive level, and ability to comprehend instructions.

Peripheral vascular disease

Peripheral vascular disease can affect veins or arteries and can be acute or chronic. Because it alters blood flow to the extremities, it may lead to acute arterial occlusion. As an artery progressively narrows, it may lead to chronic arterial occlusion and intermittent pain. In the veins, an exacerbation or complication of peripheral vascular disease can be a thrombus in a blood vessel of the leg that causes pain, redness, warmth, and tenderness, leading to easy palpation of the vein. When this condition develops, precautions are necessary to ensure that the clot doesn't break free and move into the systemic circulation into the lungs.

Previsit checklist

Physician orders and preparation
- Order for medications
- Activity restrictions

Equipment and supplies
- Measuring tape
- Scale
- Supplies for standard precautions and proper sharps disposal

Safety requirements
- List of signs and symptoms to report to the physician
- Standard precautions for infection control and sharps disposal
- Information on medications, including dosage, adverse effects, interactions, and safe storage of multiple medications
- Allergies verified and documented
- Emergency plan and access to functional phone and list of emergency phone numbers
- Identification and correction of environmental hazards and patient-specific concerns, such as sharp-cornered cabinets, throw rugs, and kerosene heaters
- Safety precautions related to decreased sensation and protection from heat and cold, including supportive, well-fitting footwear

Major diagnostic codes
- Amputation, infected right or left (below knee or above knee) 997.62

- Amputation, transmetatarsal (right or left) 84.12
- Arterial insufficiency 447.1
- Arterial occlusive disease 447.1
- Congestive heart failure 428.0
- Coronary artery disease 414.00
- Diabetes mellitus, with complications, adult 250.90
- Gangrene of toe 785.4
- Pain in limb 729.5
- Peripheral vascular disease 443.9
- Varicose leg ulcer 454.9
- Vascular insufficiency 459.9
- Venous insufficiency 459.81

Defense of homebound status
- Weakness and decreased ability to bear weight
- Limited activity due to leg wound
- Restricted activity (leg to be elevated most of the day)
- Assistance required to ambulate
- Confined to chair or bedridden, out of bed no more than twice daily
- Open, infected wound

Selected nursing diagnoses and patient outcomes

Altered tissue perfusion (peripheral) related to interruption of arterial or venous flow
The patient or caregiver will:
- indicate feelings of comfort, either verbally or through behavior   (N)
- demonstrate palpable peripheral pulses   (N)
- report no numbness, tingling, pallor or rubor, edema, or loss of motor function of affected extremity   (N)
- verbalize the rationale for keeping feet warm, dry, and clean   (N)

- decrease weight by the established amount weekly (N)
- achieve therapeutic anticoagulant blood values (N, MD)
- state precautions and symptoms associated with anticoagulant therapy (N)
- demonstrate skills needed to follow self-care regimen, including bleeding precautions. (N)

Pain related to peripheral ischemia and inflammatory process
The patient or caregiver will:
- verbalize actions that aggravate or alleviate pain and modify behavior accordingly (N)
- demonstrate techniques and body positions to alleviate or avoid pain (N)
- apply warm, moist compresses to prevent venous occlusion (N)
- demonstrate proper use of elastic hose to prevent venous occlusion in unaffected limb (N)
- measure limb circumference daily and notify the nurse of any increase (venous occlusion). (N)

Skilled nursing services

Care measures
- Perform a skilled assessment, focusing on nutrition and hydration status as well as the integumentary and cardiovascular systems.
- Perform dressing changes as ordered.
- Assess redness, temperature, amount of swelling at site.
- Evaluate healing process.
- Perform a nutritional assessment related to diabetes, weight, constipation, and immobility.
- Check pedal pulses for equality, rate, and strength.

Patient and family teaching
- Review home safety information: bleeding precautions, fall precautions, and signs and symptoms that should be reported to the physician.
- Discuss the antibiotic regimen as indicated.
- Explain how to observe for skin and wound site changes.
- Instruct the patient to keep the leg elevated at all times.
- Demonstrate the procedure for application of antiembolism stockings.
- Describe the additional risk of infection from swelling and decreased perfusion.
- Emphasize the importance of medical follow-up and adherence to medication regimen.
- Review the dietary regimen and activity restrictions.

Interdisciplinary actions

Physical therapist
- Consultation for patient's ability to walk, chair-bound versus bed-bound, status, and use of assistive or prosthetic devices

Discharge plan
- Ability of the patient and caregiver to manage peripheral vascular disease and safety needs in the home with physician and community support system follow-ups
- Referral to outpatient services for physical therapy, laboratory specimens
- Continuation of home care visits for homebound patient with skilled care needs

Documentation requirements

• Physical assessment findings, including weight and peripheral circumference measurements
• Skin status, including wound healing, condition, and location of new ulcers
• Changes in neuromuscular functioning
• Results and complications of anticoagulant therapy
• Physical status, including endurance and ability to walk
• Compliance with medication therapy, diet changes, and any adverse reactions

Reimbursement reminders

• Document variances to expected outcomes.
• Document specific teaching instructions and progress toward educational goals.
• Medicare covers phlebotomy supplies.
• Check for an authorized laboratory because many insurance companies have contracts with specific laboratories for processing specimens.
• All nonroutine supplies must be specifically ordered by the physician and entered into Locator 14 (Supplies) of Health Care Finance Administration Form 485 or ordered by the physician within the specific order for treatment requiring the use of certain supplies and entered into Locator 21 (Orders for Treatment).
• When billing for medical supplies, always include the name of supply item, date supply was used, number of units used, and charge per unit.

• Document wound status, indicating stage, drainage, color, amount; document progress or deterioration in wound healing; and measure at least once weekly.

Insurance hints

• Present objective patient findings and changes since last update.
• Report symptoms and changes in the skin and evidence toward healing since last communications.
• Keep in mind that documentation must reflect the patient's condition; all interventions and instructions provided to the patient; the patient's and family's response and understanding of interventions, instructions, or notifications; care coordination among the disciplines providing patient care through the agency; plan for follow-up care or discharge from the agency. Medicare doesn't pay for ongoing debilitation; progress toward goals must be demonstrated.
• Detail exacerbation of a chronic illness or new developments, such as new medication regimen or a dramatic change in functional level, which cause the patient to require care for a chronic condition.
• Reflect the patient's continuing need for care.
• Document specific skilled care that was provided and how it relates to the diagnosis and plan of care.
• Justify the need to repeat instructions or reinstruct.
• Refer to the plan of care and the patient's progress toward outcomes identified in the plan.

Pernicious anemia

Pernicious anemia is caused by a lack of intrinsic factor, a substance needed to absorb vitamin B_{12} from the ileum. The resulting deficiency of vitamin B_{12} causes serious neurologic, gastric, and intestinal abnormalities. The lack of B_{12} results in inhibition of cell growth, particularly of red blood cells, leading to insufficient and large, pale red blood cells with poor oxygen-carrying capacity. Untreated pernicious anemia may lead to permanent neurologic disability.

There is a genetic predisposition toward this disease and a significantly higher incidence in patients with autoimmune diseases, such as thyroiditis, myxedema, and Graves' disease. In addition, dietary intake and vitamin B_{12} absorption may diminish with age, resulting in reduced erythrocyte mass and decreased hemoglobin levels and hematocrit. Homebound patients may require visits to ensure that adequate vitamin B_{12} levels are maintained, focusing on education regarding diet, treatment, and blood study follow-up.

Previsit checklist

Physician orders and preparation
- Oral medications, including vitamin B_{12}
- Injectable vitamin B_{12}
- Dietitian evaluation of nutritional status and design individualized diet to compensate for inadequacies
- Oxygen administration, including arterial blood gases and pulse oximetry
- Complete blood count or hematocrit and hemoglobin level

Equipment and supplies
- Supplies for standard precautions and proper sharps disposal
- Phlebotomy supplies
- Injectable vitamin B_{12}
- Syringes and alcohol wipes
- Pulse oximeter if decreased oxygenation possible
- Oxygen, if ordered

Safety requirements
- Standard precautions for infection control and sharps disposal
- System to assist with adherence to a complex medication regimen
- Information on medications, including dosage, adverse effects, interactions, allergies, and safe storage
- Emergency plan and access to functional phone and list of emergency phone numbers
- Identification and correction of environmental hazards and patient-specific concerns (for example, adequate lighting, nonslip rugs, and bathroom handrails)
- Signs and symptoms requiring notification of the physician

Major diagnostic codes
- Alcoholic neuropathy 357.5
- B_{12} deficiency (dietary) 281.1
- Epistaxis 784.7
- Iron-deficiency anemia 280.9
- Malaise and fatigue, other 780.79
- Pernicious anemia 281.0

Defense of homebound status
- Unable to ambulate farther than 10′ (3 m) because of severe shortness of breath upon activity

- Maximal assistance for ambulation required
- Use of assistive device because of weakness, ataxia, and dizziness
- Unable to leave home without assistance of another
- Bedridden or confined to chair; not out of bed more than twice daily

Selected nursing diagnoses and patient outcomes

Fatigue related to nutritional deficit
The patient or caregiver will:
- demonstrate energy conservation measures   (N, HCA)
- use oxygen therapy as necessary and ordered to enhance functional ability   (N)
- report a decrease in fatigue   (N)
- demonstrate a decrease in episodes of ataxic gait   (N)
- demonstrate independence in performing ADLs.   (N, HCA)

Altered nutrition: Less than the body requirements related to inability to ingest or digest food or absorb nutrients due to biological, psychological, or economic factors
The patient or caregiver will:
- verbalize an understanding of pernicious anemia   (N)
- consume a diet of at least 1,200 calories daily   (N, D)
- verbalize menu planning consistent with dietary needs.   (N, D)

Knowledge deficit of disease process and treatment related to lack of exposure
The patient or caregiver will:
- verbalize an understanding of the disease process   (N)

- verbalize an understanding of the need for treatment   (N)
- demonstrate proper technique for administering vitamin B_{12} injections.   (N)

Skilled nursing services

Care measures
- Perform a skilled assessment with emphasis on nutrition and hydration, integumentary integrity, and mental and cognitive status. Also focus on assessing vital signs, weight, and any complaints of shortness of breath, dyspnea, and chest pain at each visit.
- Monitor oxygen therapy use if ordered; obtain or arrange for blood gases as ordered.
- Administer vitamin B_{12} injections monthly.
- Observe I.M. site for adverse reactions.
- Perform medication management.
- Perform blood specimen collection.

Patient and family teaching
- Teach about medication therapy, including dosage, frequency, adverse effects, and symptoms to report such as symptoms of infection at injection site.
- Emphasize the importance of adhering to a high-protein, high-iron diet.
- Review safety precautions, including oxygen safety measures.
- Discuss energy conservation measures.
- Emphasize the importance of compliance with the medical regimen and follow-ups.
- Identify signs and symptoms to be reported to the physician, such as increased shortness of breath, dizziness, or a fall.

Interdisciplinary actions

Dietitian
• Consultation for assessment of nutritional status and development of individualized dietary plan

Home care aide
• Assistance with ADLs
• Energy conservation measures

Discharge plan
• Safe management of pernicious anemia in the home by the patient and caregiver with physician and community support system follow-ups
• Follow-up appointments with physician at recommended intervals
• Follow-up appointments for blood studies in the authorized laboratory
• Patient and caregiver understanding and control of pernicious anemia; knowledge of preventive measures and signs and symptoms of recurrence

Documentation requirements
• Patient response to care and any variance to expected outcomes
• Results of baseline hematology report as indicated, including action taken and changes in the plan of care
• Assessment of findings of all body systems, such as pallor, dyspnea, glossitis, or peripheral neuropathies
• Any equipment used, such as oxygen and phlebotomy supplies
• Patient and caregiver instructions and progress toward educational goals such as independence in giving vitamin B_{12} injections

• Safety precautions
• Signs and symptoms to be reported
• Proper sharps disposal
• Objective evidence of continuing homebound status

Reimbursement reminders
• Note specific rationale for continuing homebound status.
• Refer to Medicare's Home Health Agency Manual, Chapter II, section 205.1, if the patient receives Medicare, for specific information related to anemias.
• Medicare covers phlebotomy supplies.
• Check for an authorized laboratory because many insurance companies have contracts with specific laboratory for processing specimens.
• All nonroutine supplies must be specifically ordered by the physician and entered into Locator 14 (Supplies) of Health Care Finance Administration Form 485 or ordered by the physician within the specific order for treatment requiring the use of certain supplies and entered into Locator 21 (Orders for Treatment).
• When billing for medical supplies, always include the name of supply item, date supply was used, number of units used, and charge per unit.
• Medicare won't reimburse for oxygen therapy orders "as needed."

Insurance hints
• Present objective patient findings and changes since last update, including progress toward goals, such as independent I.M. injection and current versus pretreatment hematocrit.

- Update regarding communications with physicians and caregivers and changes to the plan of care.
- Report changes in mental status, particularly deterioration.
- Report laboratory changes, weight loss, and problematic adverse effects caused by multiple medications.
- Present specific data on homebound status such as inability to walk farther than 10′ (3 m) because of dizziness.

Pneumonia

Pneumonia is an inflammation of the lung caused by an infectious agent (virus, bacteria, fungi) or by inhalation of foreign substances (such as food) into the lungs. Bacteria are responsible for most cases of pneumonia. Common risk factors for the development of pneumonia include chronic illness, viral respiratory infections, chronic lung disease, influenza, cancer, abdominal or thoracic surgery, general anesthesia, smoking, malnutrition, alcoholism, immunosuppression, advanced age, immobility, and an artificial airway. Symptoms include cough, sputum production (green, yellow, or rust color), chills, fever, pleuritic chest pain, shortness of breath, malaise, and poor appetite. Auscultation of the lungs may reveal diminished breath sounds in a particular area, crackles, rhonchi, or wheezing.

Treatment of pneumonia may include any or all of the following: antibiotics, oxygen if hypoxia is present, bronchodilators, expectorants, chest physiotherapy, and pain medication. Care of the homebound patient with pneumonia should focus on the need to perform deep breathing exercises, maintenance of adequate nutrition and hydration, the need for frequent position changes, and interventions that can help to prevent pneumonia.

Steps should be taken to minimize the spread of infection. Instruct high-risk individuals to avoid exposure to infectious disease whenever possible. Teach about good hand-washing techniques to help prevent transmission of infection and about avoidance of respiratory irritants.

Previsit checklist

Physician orders and preparation
- Specific initial and ongoing physician orders
- Care and teaching orders for each discipline
- Medication regimen
- Aerosol therapy as indicated
- Oxygen therapy as indicated
- Chest physiotherapy as indicated
- Activity orders and restrictions

Equipment and supplies
- Supplies for standard precautions and proper sharps disposal
- Phlebotomy supplies
- Pulse oximeter
- Metered-dose inhaler as indicated
- Nebulizer with prescribed medication as indicated
- Oxygen as indicated
- Incentive spirometer

Safety requirements
- Standard precautions for infection control and sharps disposal
- Emergency plan and access to functional phone and list of emergency phone numbers

- Identification and correction of environmental hazards and patient-specific concerns (for example, night-light, smoke detectors, and fire evacuation plan)
- Oxygen precautions if indicated
- Equipment care and storage instructions
- Allergies verified and documented
- Information on medications, including dosage, adverse effects, interactions, and safe storage
- Proper disposal of expired drugs
- Instruction on signs and symptoms of medical emergency and actions to take

Major diagnostic codes
- Bacterial pneumonia 482.9
- Bronchopneumonia 485
- Chest physiotherapy 93.99
- Nebulizer therapy 93.94
- Pneumococcal pneumonia 481
- Pneumonia, organism unspecified 486
- Pneumonia, specified organisms not elsewhere classified 483.8
- Viral pneumonia 480.9

Defense of homebound status
- Unable to ambulate farther than 10′ (3 m) because of dyspnea with minimal exertion
- Unable to ambulate farther than 10′ because of fatigue and poor endurance related to infectious process
- Unable to negotiate stairs due to profound shortness of breath
- Unable to leave home without assistance
- Dependence on oxygen therapy
- Unable to transfer independently

- Severe weakness or dyspnea with any activity

Selected nursing diagnoses and patient outcomes

Ineffective breathing pattern related to pneumonia and respiratory muscle fatigue
The patient or caregiver will:
- demonstrate achievement and maintenance of adequate respiratory functioning.   (N, PT)

Ineffective airway clearance related to bronchospasm and increased pulmonary secretions
The patient or caregiver will:
- demonstrate effective coughing and increased air exchange in the lungs
(N, PT, RT)
- demonstrate clear breath sounds
(N, PT)
- maintain pulse oximetry oxygen saturation levels at greater than 90%.
(N, RT)

Risk for infection
The patient or caregiver will:
- demonstrate meticulous proper handwashing technique and measures to control transmission of infection by discharge   (N)
- demonstrate knowledge of risk factors associated with infection and practice appropriate precautions to prevent infection   (N)
- demonstrate pulmonary status free from signs and symptoms of acute infection.   (N)

Ineffective management of therapeutic regimen: Individual related to complexity of therapeutic regimen

The patient or caregiver will:
• describe disease process, causes, and factors contributing to symptoms and the regimen for disease management (N, PT, OT)
• demonstrate improved management of therapeutic regimen as evidenced by improved pneumonia management practices (specify medications, oxygen use, incentive spirometer use, breathing exercises, and activity restrictions). (N, OT, PH, PT, SW)

Activity intolerance related to shortness of breath

The patient or caregiver will:
• identify factors that reduce activity tolerance (N, OT, PT)
• exhibit a decrease in hypoxic signs associated with increased activity (for example, pulse, blood pressure, and respirations) (N, OT, PT)
• progress to the highest level of mobility possible (N, OT, PT)
• identify measures to conserve energy. (N, OT, PT)

Knowledge deficit related to pneumonia management, including oral medications, aerosol therapy, oxygen therapy, breathing exercises, chest physiotherapy, and incentive spirometry

The patient or caregiver will:
• state correct dose and time for each medication prescribed and adverse effects and precautions for each (N, PH)
• demonstrate correct technique for administration of aerosol therapy (metered-dose inhaler, nebulizer treatment) (N, PH, RT)

• verbalize understanding of parameters for use of "as needed" oral and inhaled medication (N, PH)
• demonstrate correct use of oxygen and understanding of oxygen safety precautions (N, RT)
• demonstrate ability to perform breathing exercises (N, PT, RT)
• demonstrate ability to perform chest physiotherapy (N, PT, RT)
• demonstrate ability to use incentive spirometer (N)
• verbalize understanding of infection control measures. (N)

Skilled nursing services

Care measures
• Perform a skilled assessment of the respiratory system, including patient history relevant to respiratory and oxygenation status.
• Perform a skilled assessment of cardiovascular functioning, mental and cognitive status, and nutrition and hydration.
• Assess energy and fatigue level.
• Assess ability to mobilize and remove secretions by coughing.
• Assess for the presence of chills and diaphoresis with temperature elevation.
• Evaluate knowledge of disease process.
• Assess level of care and compliance of the patient and caregiver with the use of a metered-dose inhaler, oral medications, oxygen, incentive spirometer as ordered.
• Assess adherence to chest physiotherapy and postural drainage regimen as ordered.
• Assess signs and symptoms of hypoxia and respiratory distress.

- Administer medications as ordered.
- Supervise home oxygen therapy.

Patient and family teaching

- Explain the disease process, including appropriate infection control measures.
- Review the oral and aerosol medication regimen including dosage, frequency, purpose, potential adverse effects, and interactions.
- Describe body positioning to enhance upper airway availability (generally semi-Fowler's or sitting upright or leaning over bed table).
- Discuss the use of oxygen and safety precautions if ordered.
- Review abdominal deep breathing and coughing exercises.
- Explain how to use incentive spirometry to mobilize secretions.
- Teach about chest physiotherapy if ordered.
- Discuss the importance of adequate nutrition and hydration to meet the patient's metabolic needs.
- Emphasize the need to consult the physician regarding receiving influenza vaccine (annually) and pneumonia vaccine. (See *Pneumonia vaccine.*)

Interdisciplinary actions

Physical therapist

- Development and instruction of an individualized home exercise program
- Performance and instruction of pulmonary physical therapy — breathing exercises and chest physiotherapy as indicated

Occupational therapist

- Instruction in energy conservation techniques

Pneumonia vaccine

When educating your patient about the pneumonia vaccine, be sure to include the following facts:

- The vaccine protects against most bacteria that cause pneumococcal pneumonia.
- One vaccination lasts most people a lifetime.
- The vaccine is especially important for people age 65 or older; those with chronic illness, such as heart or lung disease and diabetes; and those with a compromised immune system from cancer, human immunodeficiency virus, or organ transplant medication.
- Adverse effects (such as fever, muscle pain, and swelling and soreness at injection site) are generally mild and last a short time.
- The vaccine is covered by Medicare and some insurance companies.

- Provision of training for activities of daily living
- Assessment of the need for and instruction in the use of adaptive equipment

Home care aide

- Assistance with personal care and hygiene needs

Social worker

- Referral to community resources and support groups
- Counseling and referral for stress management and reduction

Discharge plan

- Effective management of pneumonia care in the home by the patient and caregiver with physician follow-up
- Follow-up appointments with physician at recommended intervals
- Follow-up appointment for blood studies in the authorized laboratory
- Referral to community resources for assistance

Documentation requirements

- Subjective and objective data related to respiratory assessment, including breath sounds; dyspnea; energy level; temperature; pulse oximetry measurements; response to care, such as with inhalers, nebulizers, and oxygen therapy; and other systems assessment, particularly cardiac and nutrition
- Instructions given related to pneumonia management, including increased fluid intake, energy conservation, pneumonia vaccination, and prevention of recurrence such as with smoking cessation
- Skilled procedures performed, such as nebulizer treatment, chest physiotherapy
- Understanding of and adherence to medication regimen
- Understanding of and adherence to oxygen use, including rate, mode of delivery, and when used
- Patient and caregiver progress toward educational goals
- Patient response to care
- Instruction in signs and symptoms to be reported
- Laboratory results, such as results of sputum culture and chest X-ray; physician notification; and changes in the plan of care
- Interdisciplinary communication
- The patient's activity restriction, such as an inability to ambulate farther than 10′ (3 m) because of dyspnea on exertion
- Availability, willingness, and ability of caregiver
- Unfamiliarity of patient with medications, aerosol therapy, oxygen use, chest physiotherapy
- Specific deficits in initial knowledge level, then progress as evidenced by verbalization or demonstration of specific concepts and procedures

Reimbursement reminders

- Indicate expected endpoint of daily visits when daily visits have been ordered.
- Obtain a physician order for any change in the plan of care, and document this in the patient's record.
- The following supplies and durable medical equipment are covered by Medicare: nebulizer machine (Medicare part B, 80% of allowable charge; physician must indicate that metered-dose inhaler alone is insufficient to treat patient's symptoms), oxygen (Medicare part B, 80% of allowable; patient's oxygen saturation level must be 88% or less).
- Respiratory therapist services are usually provided by the company supplying the durable medical equipment, on a routine or as needed basis.
- Medicare covers phlebotomy supplies.
- Check for an authorized laboratory because many insurance companies have contracts with specific laboratories for processing specimens.

• All nonroutine supplies must be specifically ordered by the physician and entered into Locator 14 (Supplies) of Health Care Finance Administration Form 485 or ordered by the physician within the specific order for treatment requiring the use of certain supplies and entered into Locator 21 (Orders for Treatment).

• Identify specific barriers to learning (for example, impaired vision or impaired mental status and cognitive ability).

• When billing for medical supplies, always include the name of supply item, date supply was used, number of units used, and charge per unit.

Insurance hints

• Present objective data about homebound status, such as inability to ambulate farther than 10′ because of dyspnea or weakness, inability to leave home without assistance because of oxygen therapy and weakness.

• Present objective patient findings, changes in clinical condition, and changes in care since last contact (for example, physician increased oxygen delivery in response to decreased pulse oximetry).

• Present progress toward established clinical and educational goals.

Postmortem care

Postmortem care involves caring for the patient's body after death and preparing it for removal from the home. This may include removing or capping of any tubes or equipment attached to the patient, bathing the patient, and dressing the patient and the bed in clean clothes or linens.

Giving support to family members and seeing that their spiritual, physical, and emotional needs are met is a large part of postmortem care. Sensitivity, calmness, and control will reassure and support the family members during this difficult time. You should be aware of the patient's preferences, cultural traditions, or religious practices involving death and postmortem care. For instance, people of the following faiths may oppose autopsy: Islam, Judaism, and Russian Orthodox. If you don't know, ask the family. Attending the patient's funeral and conducting bereavement follow-up with family members are vital parts of supporting family members during their grieving process.

The home care nurse needs to be aware of the agency policy and state and local regulations regarding postmortem care, whom to notify, and the nurse's responsibilities. In many states the attending nurse pronounces the patient dead. This isn't the case in every state, and you should have a clear knowledge of your legal limits, mandates, and agency policy. If you have a question regarding your legal limits, your state licensing board will have up-to-date information on federal, state, and local laws and mandates.

Previsit checklist

Physician orders and preparation

• Do-not-resuscitate orders, advance directives, and knowledge of any premade funeral arrangements, such as cremation society or funeral home of choice (this information should be in the home as well as in the patient's chart)

Equipment and supplies
- Supplies for standard precautions
- Bath supplies
- Clean gown or clothing of the family's choice
- Clean bed linen
- Death certificate (if mandated)
- Accurate list of whom to contact and in what order (this list will vary according to state and local mandates and agency policy; if it appears that death isn't related to the disease for which you are seeing the patient [fall or accidental death], the notification procedure will probably be different and may involve the medical examiner and autopsy)

Safety requirements
- Standard precautions for infection control and treatment of soiled linen
- Safety precautions for in-home durable medical equipment

Major diagnostic codes
- Postmortem examination 89.8

Defense of homebound status
- Homebound status defense already established

Selected nursing diagnoses and patient outcomes

Spiritual distress related to loss of family member

The family or caregiver will:
- express grief   (N, SC, SW)
- describe the meaning of the death or loss   (N, SC)
- share grief with significant others.   (N, SC)

Decisional conflict related to inexperience with decision making or disagreement within support systems

The family or caregiver will:
- relate the advantages and disadvantages of choices   (N)
- share fears and concerns regarding choices and responses to others   (N)
- make informed choices.   (N)

Skilled nursing services

Care measures
- Perform a skilled assessment for absence of vital signs: listen for apical pulse, feel for carotid pulse for 1 minute. (Brachial pulse is taken for 1 minute in infants and children up to age 8.)
- Assess for spontaneous respirations.
- Check for fixed and dilated pupils.
- Establish time of death.
- Close the patient's eyes if possible.
- Cover the body with a sheet only if this isn't upsetting to the family.
- Notify the physician, coroner, or local authorities according to regulations and agency policy.
- Remove or cap any tubes or support devices attached to the patient, if regulations and agency policy allow.
- Check with family members regarding religious rituals related to care of the body after death (for example, leaving the window open to allow the patient's spirit to depart), and adapt your care as possible to accomodate the family's wishes.
- Bathe the body, and redress it in a clean gown or clothing of the family's choice. The body should be in good

alignment on a clean bed. The family may wish to assist with bathing and dressing of the body. Family members should be supported in performing these duties.

• Place an incontinence pad securely under the buttocks and between the legs.

• Raise the head of the bed slightly to prevent pooling of fluids in the head and face.

• Place dentures in the mouth if possible.

• Provide emotional support to the family.

• Assist with notification of clergy, family members, and other support persons if the family desires.

• Remain with the family and caregiver until the body is removed and support systems are in place and functioning.

• Conduct bereavement follow-up with the family and caregivers.

Family teaching

• Inform the family of routine procedures regarding postmortem care.

• Familiarize the family with the proper procedures to follow to arrange a funeral.

Interdisciplinary actions

Social worker

• Counseling, referral to community resources and support groups

• Assistance with bereavement counseling and follow-up

Discharge plan

• Patient discharged at time of death

Documentation requirements

• Physical assessment (lack of apical, carotid, and or brachial pulses for 1 minute, no spontaneous respirations, and pupils fixed and dilated)

• Time of death

• Time that the physician and appropriate authorities were notified

• Time last seen by the patient's primary care physician

• Care and disposition of the body

• All communication and care measures and the time they occurred

• Family members' reaction to death and care given

• Referrals or conferences with other disciplines

• Instructions to family members, their responses, and arrival of any support services

Reimbursement reminders

• The postmortem care skilled nurse visit is reimbursable under current Medicare home care benefits.

• When billing for medical supplies, always include the name of supply item, date supply was used, number of units used, and charge per unit.

Insurance hints

• Notify the insurance company of the date and time of the patient's death.

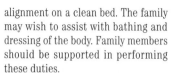

Pressure ulcer care

A pressure ulcer is an observable pressure-related alteration of intact skin. Pressure ulcers can be due to a combination of factors and situations. On a cellular level, ischemia occurs to the tissue when too much pressure is applied for a prolonged period. This pressure is normally from a bony prominence on one side and a hard surface on the other side. The resulting ischemia leads to necrosis of the soft tissue between the surfaces. Skin discoloration or redness may actually indicate necrosis of underlying adipose or muscular tissue. Friction and shearing forces can also cause tissue necrosis. Factors such as the patient's general health, nutritional status, skin texture and turgor, body weight, and mobility are key in the development of pressure ulcers. Not only do these factors need to be assessed during treatment of pressure ulcers, but good assessment of these factors can be helpful in prevention.

Treatment of pressure ulcers depends on the depth of the ulcer; however, the initial assessment procedure is the same. The home care nurse is responsible for a thorough assessment of the wound, including its stage, location, size, and appearance (amount and type of drainage, amount of necrotic tissue or granulation, wound color, and presence or absence of odor); presence of any tunneling, pockets, sinus tracts, or undermining; and appearance of tissue surrounding the wound for maceration, induration, rash, tape burns, or tenderness. (See *Wound and skin assessment tool,* pages 368 and 369.) The home care nurse is also responsible for monitoring for infection as well as nutritional and hydration status. Focus in the home should also be given to patient and caregiver teaching needs in regard to wound care and wound prevention.

Previsit checklist

Physician orders and preparation

- Wound care, with actual end date specified (updated as wound heals)
- Cleaning method
- Type of dressing
- Frequency of dressing changes, with actual end date specified
- Pressure-relieving or support devices
- Dietary restrictions, calorie allowance
- Oral, I.V., or topical medications
- Activity orders and restrictions
- Physical therapy evaluation for home exercise program, transfer training, and endurance training
- Occupational therapy evaluation for energy conservation and assistance with functional ability, including adaptive devices as necessary
- Nutritionist evaluation for prescribed dietary needs
- Social worker evaluation for community referrals, financial assistance, and counseling
- Home care aide for assistance with personal care and activities of daily living

Equipment and supplies

- Supplies for standard precautions
- Wound care supplies (dressing materials, cleaning solutions)
- Gloves
- Nutritional intake and weight log
- Wound and skin assessment tool
- Wound measuring device
- Plastic bags for disposal of used dressing materials
- Camera, film, and consent form for photographing wound

Safety requirements

- Standard precautions for infection control
- Signs and symptoms of infection and plan of action
- Emergency plan and access to functional phone and list of emergency phone numbers
- Identification and correction of environmental hazards and patient-specific concerns (for example, smoke detectors, night-light, water heater thermostat set at 120° F (48.8° C) or less for patients with decreased sensation to prevent burns)
- Information on antibiotics, including dosage, adverse effects, and interactions
- Allergies verified and documented

Major diagnostic codes

- Debridement 86.22
- Decubitus ulcer 707.0
- Diabetes mellitus, with complications 250.9
- Peripheral vascular disease, unspecified 443.9
- Ulcer, ischemic 707.9
- Ulcer, lower extremity 707.1
- Ulcer, skin chronic, unspecified 707.9 (To assign a fifth digit, see appendix A, page 638.)

Defense of homebound status

- Bedridden or out of bed less than twice daily; prescribed activity includes elevating extremity most of the day
- Open, draining, or infected wound
- Prescribed non-weight-bearing status secondary to foot ulcer

- Unable to ambulate farther than 10′ (3 m) because of lower extremity ulcer
- Maximum assistance needed to ambulate or transfer

Selected nursing diagnoses and patient outcomes

Impaired skin integrity related to mechanical factors, physical immobilization, extremes in age, moisture, altered fluid status, altered metabolic state, skeletal prominence, immunological deficit, altered nutritional state, altered skin turgor, or altered circulation

The patient or caregiver will:
- identify causative factors for pressure ulcers   (N)
- identify a causative rationale for prevention and treatment   (N)
- participate in the prescribed treatment plan to promote wound healing
                                            (N, PT)
- demonstrate progressive healing of dermal ulcer.   (N)

Altered nutrition: Less than body requirements related to actual or potential metabolic needs in excess of intake

The patient or caregiver will:
- increase oral intake as evidenced by (specify)   (N, D)
- describe causative factors when known   (N)
- describe the rationale and procedure for treatment.   (N, D)

(Text continues on page 370.)

Wound and skin assessment tool

Primary diagnosis _Left CVA_

Secondary diagnosis _Diabetes_

Pertinent medical history _Right-side weakness, depression, IDDM_

WOUND LOCATION:

Site _Right heel_   Date of outset   _8/25/00_

(circle affected area)

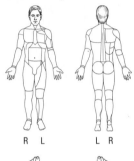

R L   L R   L   R

         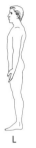 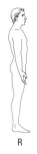

L   R   ·L   R

DATE (M/D/Y)	TERM	TYPE #	LENGTH, WIDTH (cm)	DEPTH (cm)	TUNNELING (cm, o'clock)	COLOR (R/Y/B/M)	DRAINAGE (amount and type)	ODOR & TYPE (Y/N)
8/25/00	ST 2	2	4 x 3	< 0.1	∅	14	Scant, serous	N

Wound and skin assessment tool *(continued)*

CLASSIFICATION	TERMS	TYPE
Pressure ulcers	**ST1** — nonblanchable erythema of intact skin; heralding lesion of skin ulceration	**1.** Stage 1
	ST2 — partial-thickness skin loss involving epidermis or dermis; ulcer is superficial; presents as an abrasion, blister, or shallow crater	**2.** Stage 2
	ST3 — full-thickness skin loss involving damage or necrosis of subcutaneous tissue that may extend down to, but not through, underlying fascia; ulcer presents as a deep crater with or without tunneling of adjacent tissue	**3.** Stage 3
	ST4 — full-thickness skin loss with extensive destruction, tissue necrosis, or damage to muscle, bone, or support structures	**4.** Stage 4
	ST3 or ST4 (?) — wound completely covered with necrotic tissue; cannot be staged until wound base is visible	**5.** Stages 3 – 4 (?)
Wound	**PTW** (partial-thickness wound) — loss of epidermis and partial loss of dermis	**6.** Skin tear
	FTW (full-thickness wound) — tissue destruction, extending through the dermis and involving the subcutaneous layer; may involve muscle or bone	**7.** Surgical
		8. Vascular ulcer
		9. Other
Color	**R** — clean, healthy, granulating tissue	**10.** Red
	Y — presence of slough or fibrotic tissue	**11.** Yellow
	B — presence of eschar	**12.** Black
	M — two or more colors present in wound (specify color by letters)	**13.** Mixed
Skin condition	**SC** (skin condition) — an abnormal finding on the surface of the skin	**14.** Rash
		15. Incontinence-related
		16. Bruises
		17. Other

PAIN (Y*/N)	PHOTO (Y/N)	ADJUNCTIVE THERAPIES OR PRODUCTS AND ADDITIONAL COMMENTS	SIGNATURE, TITLE
N	Y	☒Support Surface ☒Nutritional Intervention ☐New Orders Obtained T & P 2 hours, heel protectors, heels elevated	J. Hughes, RN, BSN

Patient's Name (Last, Middle, First)	Attending Physician	Room Number	ID Number
Stevens, Arlene	Dr. T. Elliot	123-2	01726

Source: Cathy Thomas Hess, RN, BSN, CWOCN, President, Wound Care Strategies, Inc., © 1998.

Body image disturbance related to changes in appearance secondary to open draining wound

The patient or caregiver will:

- implement new coping methods
(N, SW)
- verbalize and demonstrate acceptance of appearance (N, SW)
- demonstrate a willingness and ability to resume care and other responsibilities (if possible) (N)
- initiate new or re-establish existing support systems. (N, SW)

Skilled nursing services

Care measures

- Perform skilled assessment of mental and cognitive status; and cardiovascular, GI, genitourinary, integumentary systems (particularly noting high-risk areas: sacral, bony prominence, feet); and nutrition and hydration.
- Assess wound per agency protocol.
- Assess level of self-care of patient and capabilities of caregivers.
- Perform dressing changes.
- Assess level of pain and effectiveness of pain medication.
- Assess for signs and symptoms of infection.
- Assess wound healing and effectiveness of treatment.
- Assess environment and contributing factors for development of pressure ulcer.
- Assess vital signs.
- Perform wound cultures as ordered.
- Administer medications as ordered.

Patient and family teaching

- Demonstrate wound care and observe return demonstration.

- Identify signs and symptoms of infection.
- Discuss methods of pain management, including use of antiembolism stockings.
- Describe nutritional practices that promote healing and explain how to keep a dietary intake log.
- Emphasize the need for range-of-motion exercises, 2-hour turning, frequent shift of position while sitting, prevention of heels and bony prominence from resting on mattress and other hard surfaces, and elevation of affected extremity when sitting or resting.
- Teach about antibiotic use and adverse effects where applicable.
- Identify signs and symptoms that need to be reported to the physician.
- Emphasize the need to administer pain medication 30 minutes prior to painful dressing changes.
- Review infection control measures.

Interdisciplinary actions

Home care aide

- Personal care and, when indicated, light housekeeping, meal preparation, and laundry

Social worker

- Counseling and referral to community agencies and support groups

Dietitian

- Consultation for nutritional needs (increased protein and caloric intake to promote healing)

Physical therapist

- Development and instruction in individualized home exercise program

Discharge plan

- Wound healing without signs or symptoms of infection
- Any infection resolved
- Patient and caregiver independent with wound care
- Verbalization by the patient and caregiver of comprehension of risk factors; prevention methods in place and functioning
- Follow-up appointments with physician at recommended intervals

Documentation requirements

- Skilled assessment of body systems
- Skilled assessment of wound, including wound sizing (for accurate tracking of healing, measure the wound at each visit and document its size, using the same evaluation tool each time)
- Staging a wound is required by most third-party payers. The Pressure Ulcer Scale for Healing (PUSH) tool gives a precise measurement of healing. Developed by the National Pressure Ulcer Advisory Panel (NPUAP) as a quick, reliable tool for monitoring the changes in pressure ulcer status over time, it combines measurements of the ulcer's length and width and the amount of exudate and the tissue type present. A copy of the PUSH tool is available at www.npuap.org/pushins.htm, and more information can be obtained by contacting the NPUAP at (314) 909-6815.
- Photograph of wound on initial visit and every 3 weeks thereafter (or per agency policy)
- Wound drainage, odor, and amount
- The patient's activity level
- Vital signs

- Subjective and objective data related to signs and symptoms of infection and pain management
- Wound care carefully recorded, including the patient's response to care (level of pain)
- Notation of changes or stressors in the patient or environment
- Notation of factors contributing to skin breakdown; measures established to promote healing and prevent future pressure ulcers
- Patient and caregiver participation in care
- Any patient or caregiver teaching conducted and response
- Nutritional and hydration status, recommended dietary changes, intake flowchart
- Referrals to and conferences with other disciplines
- Patient and caregiver progress toward established goals
- Any laboratory results
- Safety precautions
- Infection control measures
- Signs and symptoms that need to be reported to the physician

Reimbursement reminders

- Document wound healing, measuring wound with each visit. Most reimbursement agencies and Medicare require staging for reimbursement.
- Be aware of the following constraints and the best use of them: While some reimbursement agencies will allow skilled home health involvement until wound is healed, many private plans only grant a limited number of visits to be divided between skilled services. Independence with wound care by either the patient or caregiver should be established as soon as possible.

• The Interim Payment System pays for patients covered by Medicare part A. Payments should cover nursing visits as well as routine and nonroutine supplies (including surgical dressings). The patient doesn't have any copayments for visits or supplies. However, because of some unclear language in the regulations, some home care agencies may choose not to provide nonroutine supplies. In such a case, the patient is forced to acquire needed dressings from a supplier. If the patient has Medicare part B coverage, the surgical dressing policy governs payment to the supplier. The patient must pay the supplier 20% of the Medicare allowable charge. If the patient doesn't have part B coverage and the home care agency doesn't supply the dressings, the patient must purchase the products himself.

• Document any barriers or limitations to learning (such as deformities, visual impairment, and no available, able, and willing caregiver).

• Registered dietitian services aren't reimbursable under current Medicare home care benefits.

• Home care aide services are covered by current Medicare home care benefits (as long as a skilled service is present) but aren't covered by many other reimbursement plans.

• Check for an authorized laboratory because many insurance companies have contracts with specific laboratories for processing specimens.

• All nonroutine supplies must be specifically ordered by the physician and entered into Locator 14 (Supplies) of Health Care Finance Administration Form 485 or ordered by the physician within the specific order for treatment requiring the use of certain supplies

and entered into Locator 21 (Orders for Treatment).

• When billing for medical supplies, always include the name of supply item, date supply was used, number of units used, and charge per unit.

Insurance hints

• Have most recent wound measurements and dressing type available, and know any changes that have occurred.

• Be able to support need for skills; demonstrate need for continued teaching or skilled care (change in wound care, no available caregiver, or patient and caregiver unable to change dressing).

• Notify case manager of signs of resolution and interventions that minimize or prevent recurrences and inpatient care.

Prostate cancer

The prostate gland is the most common site of cancer in men in America. Prostate cancer rarely occurs before age 40, and the incidence increases sharply with age. Hormonal changes, viral infections, and environmental influences may all affect development of this virulent form of cancer. Because nonurinary symptoms tend to be vague to such an extent that the disease often isn't diagnosed until it's far advanced, prevention through comprehensive community education is essential. No true primary prevention for prostate cancer exists; therefore, secondary prevention in terms of regular screening for prostate cancer in men over age 40 is extremely important. The home care nurse's focus in caring for the patient with prostate cancer is usually catheter care and pain control.

Previsit checklist

Physician orders and preparation
- Oral medications as indicated
- Chemotherapeutic regimen
- Activity orders and restrictions
- Laboratory work, including prostate-specific antigen
- Enterostomal consultation for treatment of urinary incontinence
- Psychiatric nurse consult for counseling regarding emotional issues related to diagnosis of cancer and possibility of sterility and sexual dysfunction
- Urinary catheter insertions

Equipment and supplies
- Phlebotomy supplies
- Supplies for standard precautions and proper sharps disposal
- Urinary catheters
- Drainage bags
- Disposal equipment appropriate for chemotherapeutic agents
- Scale

Safety requirements
- Standard precautions for infection control and sharps disposal
- System to assist with adherence to a complex medication regimen
- Information on medications, including dosage; adverse effects, particularly estrogenic hormones; interactions; and safe storage
- Allergies verified and documented
- Emergency plan and access to functional phone and list of emergency phone numbers
- Identification and correction of environmental hazards and patient-specific concerns (for example, a nightlight, grab bars in the bathroom, and fall precautions)
- Instructions on signs and symptoms to report to the physician

Major diagnostic codes
- Bone metastasis 198.5
- Prostate cancer:
  - cancer in situ 233.4
  - primary 185
  - secondary 198.82
  - uncertain behavior 236.5
  - unspecified 239.5
- Prostatectomey (transurethral resection of the prostate) 60.2
- Prostatitis 601.9
- Urine incontinence, male 788.3
- Urine retention 788.20

Defense of homebound status
- Fatigue secondary to radiation therapy; unable to ambulate farther than 20′ (6 m)
- Recovering from recent surgery (radical resection of the prostate)
- Bowel and bladder incontinence
- Confined to chair
- Bedridden
- Need for maximal assistance to ambulate or transfer
- Severe pain
- Imminent death

Selected nursing diagnoses and patient outcomes

Knowledge deficit related to surgical experience
The patient or caregiver will:
• describe the nature of surgery and postoperative care (N)
• reinforce discharge restrictions.(N)

Knowledge deficit related to new diagnosis of prostate cancer
The patient or caregiver will:
• describe the illness, treatment goals, plan of care, and potential risks and benefits of treatment (N)
• describe care measures to manage common adverse effects of the proposed treatment regimen (N)
• demonstrate ability to perform recovery care measures such as maintenance. (N)

Risk for infection related to decreased white blood cell count secondary to radiation
The patient or caregiver will:
• list signs and symptoms of infection to watch for (N)
• perform excellent personal hygiene (N)
• identify proper infection control measures (N)
• remain infection-free throughout treatment. (N)

Pain related to cancer progression and surgery
The patient or caregiver will:
• monitor pain intensity, duration, patterns, and factors that alleviate or exacerbate pain and communicate this information to the health care team (N)

• achieve and maintain pain at a level of 3 on a 0-to-10 scale at least 80% of the time. (N)

Functional urinary incontinence and *Bowel incontinence related to adverse effects of prostate surgery*
The patient or caregiver will:
• alter clothing and environment to promote continence (N, ET)
• contract verbally to participate in bowel and bladder retraining programs. (N, ET)

Altered urinary elimination related to prostate cancer and surgical alteration
The patient or caregiver will:
• demonstrate an understanding of causative factors of altered urinary elimination (N)
• identify appropriate measures to minimize symptoms. (N)

Skilled nursing services

Care measures
• Perform a skilled assessment of the genitourinary, GI, and reproductive systems; assess mental and cognitive status.
• Assess level of care of the patient and caregiver (restoration of urinary and bowel continence, preparation of each day's medication regimen).
• Assess the effectiveness of the treatment regimen.
• Assess laboratory work frequently, especially the complete blood count.
• Assess for signs and symptoms of infection.
• Assess pain on a 0-to-10 scale.
• Assess bowel and bladder control.
• Implement bowel and bladder control regimen.

- Assess nutritional and hydration status.
- Assess catheter care.
- Change urinary catheter as directed.
- Perform venipuncture as ordered.
- Assess urinary output.
- Administer medications as ordered.
- Assess for adverse effects of medications, chemotherapy, and radiation therapy.
- Collect urine cultures.

Patient and family teaching

- Emphasize the need for infection control when the patient is immunosuppressed.
- Identify symptoms of a urinary tract infection or obstruction.
- Identify symptoms of cancer metastasis (low back pain, aching in legs, and hip pain).
- Review pain control measures — both comfort and pharmacologic.
- Describe the medication regimen, including dose, frequency, purpose, and adverse effects.
- Explain disease process and management.

Interdisciplinary measures

Enterostomal therapist

- Consultation for treatment of urinary incontinence

Psychiatric nurse

- Counseling regarding emotional issues related to diagnosis of cancer and possibility of sterility and sexual dysfunction

Discharge plan

- Safe management of prostate cancer and its various complications by the patient and caregiver in the home with physician follow-up
- Follow-up appointments for blood studies in the authorized laboratory
- Follow-up appointments with physician at recommended intervals
- Referral to community resources for assistance

Documentation requirements

- Complete physical assessment findings, including incontinence, skin integrity, weight, wound drainage, and activity tolerance
- Subjective and objective data with regard to signs and symptoms of infection and bowel and bladder incontinence
- Findings from psychiatric consultation and action plan to address needs
- Findings from enterostomal therapist evaluation
- Laboratory results
- Safety precautions, including signs and symptoms to be reported
- Patient and caregiver response to and participation in care (coordination of medication regimen and management of incontinence)
- Patient and caregiver progress toward educational goals (knowledge of medication, disease process, radiation therapy, and prognosis)

Reimbursement reminders

- Indicate when daily visits are expected to end if daily care has been ordered.

- Teaching for prevention of infection isn't reimbursable.
- Document specific deficits in initial knowledge level, then progress as evidenced by demonstration or verbalization of specific concepts and information.
- Document care coordination among the disciplines.
- Document any changes in patient condition.
- Medicare covers phlebotomy supplies.
- Check for an authorized laboratory because many insurance companies have contracts with specific laboratories for processing specimens.
- All nonroutine supplies must be specifically ordered by the physician and entered into Locator 14 (Supplies) of Health Care Finance Administration Form 485 or ordered by the physician within the specific order for treatment requiring the use of certain supplies and entered into Locator 21 (Orders for Treatment).
- When billing for medical supplies, always include the name of supply item, date supply was used, number of units used, and charge per unit.

Insurance hints

- Present objective data about homebound status.
- Present objective patient findings and changes since last contact, including weight changes, skin integrity compromise, activity tolerance, and bowel and bladder incontinence.
- Report new laboratory values and any change in clinical condition since last contact.
- Present specifics about patient education progress.

Renal failure

Renal failure is the progressive deterioration of the filtering ability of the kidneys to clear the blood of waste products. The patient is asymptomatic until approximately three-quarters of the renal function is lost. Kidney failure can result from various causes, including congenital disorders, infection, endocrine-related problems such as diabetic nephropathy, or vascular problems. The disease can progress slowly or rapidly. The trajectory of illness generally includes the following phases: reduced renal reserve, renal insufficiency, renal failure, and end-stage renal disease.

The treatment for renal failure is dialysis and kidney transplantation. Medicare doesn't cover home care services for care related to kidney failure. However, home care agencies may care for patients with other conditions who are also receiving dialysis. Care is often provided for skin ulcers, rehabilitation following a stroke, fracture, or other conditions not associated with renal failure.

Previsit checklist

Physician orders and preparation

- Medications
- Activity orders and restrictions
- Comfort measures and pain control orders
- Dialysis schedule
- Wound care orders
- Specific diet
- Venipuncture

Equipment and supplies
- Supplies for standard precautions and proper sharps disposal
- Wound care
- Tape
- Gauze
- Biological dressings
- Wound creams and gels
- Biohazard bag for discarding dressings
- Wound cleanser or normal saline
- Camera, film, and consent form for photographing wound per agency policy
- Biohazard bag for specimen tube while in transport
- Venipuncture supplies

Safety requirements
- Standard precautions for infection control and sharps disposal
- System to assist with adherence to a complex medication regimen
- Information on medications, including dosage, adverse effects, interactions, and safe storage
- Allergies verified and documented
- Emergency plan and access to functional phone and list of emergency phone numbers
- Identification and correction of environmental hazards and patient-specific concerns (for example, night-light, grab bars in bathroom, and other fall precautions)
- Reportable signs and symptoms

Major diagnostic codes
- Diabetic nephropathy 250.4
- Kidney, cystic 753.10
- Nephropathy 583.9
- Nephrosclerosis 403.9
- Renal failure, acute tubular necrosis 584.5
- Renal failure, chronic 585

(To assign a fifth digit, see appendix A, page 638.)

Note: Kidney disease *can't* be the primary diagnosis in patients who are receiving home care; they can only receive care for related conditions other than dialysis. These most commonly include:
- Decubitus ulcer 707.0
- Stroke 436.

Defense of homebound status
- Bedridden
- Unable to ambulate farther than 10′ (3 m) because of fatigue due to anemia
- Unable to ambulate because of prescribed physical restrictions or lower extremity edema
- Dyspnea or dizziness with activity
- Unable to ambulate or transfer without maximal assistance

Selected nursing diagnoses and patient outcomes

Fluid volume excess related to renal disease with minimal or zero output

The patient or caregiver will:
- verbalize understanding of the need to regulate fluid intake   (N)
- maintain weight chart and report weight gains greater than 2 lb (1 kg) in 24 hours to physician   (N)
- be free from fluid volume excess (N)
- demonstrate ability to adhere to fluid and sodium restrictions.   (N)

Powerlessness related to treatment regimen and complications

The patient or caregiver will:

- identify two things that can be controlled (N, SW)
- express a sense of optimism for the future (N, SW)
- use community resources and support systems. (N, SW)

Impaired skin integrity related to skin ulcer

The patient or caregiver will:

- demonstrate or verbalize correct dressing change technique (N)
- verbalize signs and symptoms of infection to report to the physician (N)
- exhibit wound healing without complications (N)
- verbalize or demonstrate proper skin hygiene (N)
- demonstrate how to prevent further skin breakdown. (N)

Altered nutrition: Less than body requirements

The patient or caregiver will:

- maintain weight within normal limits (N, D)
- remain free from signs and symptoms of malnutrition (N, D)
- increase calorie intake. (N, D)

Risk for injury related to chronic pathologic changes of all organ systems

The patient or caregiver will:

- verbalize signs and symptoms to report to the physician (N)
- modify home to clear walkways and increase lighting (N)
- ask for assistance with transfers when fatigued. (N)

Impaired physical mobility related to hemiparesis (for patients with a stroke)

The patient or caregiver will:

- demonstrate correct limitation of activity and use of bedside commode (N, PT)
- demonstrate deep breathing and range-of-motion (ROM) exercises to maintain functional capacity (N, PT)
- demonstrate proper use of assistive devices (N, OT, PT)
- follow exercise and ROM regimen. (N, PT)

Pain related to ischemia

The patient or caregiver will:

- verbalize understanding of pain control regimen (N)
- verbalize one nonpharmacologic method of pain relief such as relaxation (N)
- achieve pain relief (N)
- express an understanding of how ischemia causes pain. (N)

Diversional activity deficit related to poor endurance and inability to maintain social contacts

The patient or caregiver will:

- describe appropriate recreational activities within mobility restrictions (N, SW)
- participate in chosen activities (N, SW)
- use community support groups such as visiting pet therapy, church outreach, and programs for shut-ins.

Sleep pattern disturbance related to prolonged time in bed

The patient or caregiver will:

- remain awake during the day (N)
- express satisfaction with sleep pattern (N)

- demonstrate one relaxation technique to aid in sleeping (N)
- limit stimulants such as caffeine in the evening. (N)

Death anxiety related to chronic life-threatening illness and increasing disability

The patient or caregiver will:
- express fears of death (N, SW)
- seek spiritual support to explore the meaning of life and illness (N, SW)
- make a preliminary plan for advance directives at the end of life, including decisions about termination of dialysis. (N, SW)

Skilled nursing services

Care measures
- Perform skilled assessment of the cardiovascular, pulmonary, integumentary, and musculoskeletal systems; assess nutrition, hydration, and elimination.
- Assess self-care or caregiver ability and compliance.
- Assess the effectiveness of the treatment regimens.
- Follow laboratory results, and communicate with team members.
- Examine wound care as indicated.
- Administer medication and assess for adverse effects and interactions.
- Assess for signs and symptoms of infections.
- Assess dialysis access device.
- Weigh the patient, and monitor intake and output.
- Ascertain need for medical identification bracelet

Patient and family teaching
- Identify signs and symptoms of infections and complications, and review preventive measures.
- Explain how to monitor and record the patient's daily weight and to report a gain of ___ lb daily
- Review pain control methods, including oral, I.M., and subcutaneous options.
- Explain how to maintain ROM.
- Discuss methods to prevent constipation.
- Review medication regimen, including dose, frequency, purpose, interactions, and adverse effects.
- Discuss wound care regimen and shunt care as indicated.
- Describe proper skin care techniques.
- Explain dietary restrictions.

Interdisciplinary actions

Occupational therapist
- Energy conservation techniques
- Bathing and self-care
- Use of adaptive equipment

Physical therapist
- Instruction and monitoring of home exercise program
- Transfer training

Home care aide
- Hygiene assistance and assistance with activities of daily living

Social worker
- Community referrals for independence
- Psychosocial support and coping

Dietitian
- Nutritional support

Discharge plan

- Return of the patient to independent status after wound healing
- Completion of rehabilitation program and return to optimal function
- Follow-up appointments made by patient for blood studies in the authorized laboratory
- Follow-up appointments made by patient with dialysis clinic and physician at recommended intervals
- Referral to community resources for assistance

Documentation requirements

- Skilled assessment, including weight, skin turgor, intake and output, vital signs, edema, shortness of breath, dyspnea, skin integrity and dryness, nausea and vomiting, energy level, and activity tolerance
- Skilled assessment of patient's response to care
- Effectiveness of pain control with rating on a 0-to-10 scale
- Assessment of wound and healing progress with wound measurements and staging
- Notation of any dressing changes performed
- Patient and caregiver instruction, specifically in regard to nutritional intake, wound care, medications, and activity restrictions
- Patient's response to instructions
- Interdisciplinary team communication
- Patient's ability to transfer safely within limited activity
- Laboratory results
- Assessment of dialysis access device
- Vital signs

- Safety precautions
- Signs and symptoms to be reported
- Patient's compliance with instructions and therapy regimen

Reimbursement reminders

- All dialysis-related needs should be performed at the dialysis center. Note Section 230 E of the Health Care Financing Administration's (HCFA's) "Home Health Agency Manual" (HCFA Pub. 11): "Services that are covered under the ESRD [end-stage renal disease] program and are contained in the composite rate reimbursement methodology, including any service furnished to an ESRD beneficiary that is directly related to that individual's dialysis, are excluded from coverage under the Medicare home health benefit. However, to the extent that a service is not directly related to a beneficiary's dialysis, for example, a nursing visit to furnish wound care for an abandoned shunt site, and other requirements for coverage are met, the visit would be covered."
- Skilled nursing visits for epoetin administration are usually covered by Medicare; epoetin is covered if certain conditions are met, such as an average hematocrit of less than 36 preceding administration.
- Wound care supplies are covered by Medicare but require detailed documentation of what, how many, and cost per unit of items used.
- Check for an authorized provider before ordering wound care products because many insurance companies have contracts with specific providers.
- End-stage renal disease can't be the primary diagnosis as the reason for home care; instead, list the reason that

skilled nursing care is needed in the home (such as wound care).

● Home care visits for the administration of epoetin therapy may be covered depending on the frequency and duration. However, the actual drug isn't covered by Medicare home care.

● Document any interdisciplinary coordination and change to the plan of care.

Insurance hints

● Document progress to goals.

● Document size and stage of wound healing.

● Evaluate progress in rehabilitation program.

● Describe adjustment issues such as the patient's resistance or acceptance of imposed activity restrictions.

● Document complications, such as constipation or infection.

● Evaluate pain control.

● Describe gains in knowledge.

● Document skills and concepts mastered in relaxation and prevention of wound recurrence.

● Present specific data on homebound status, such as dizziness, weakness, not out of bed more than twice daily.

● Emphasize the next step in care; show that there is a progressive plan for independence.

● Note any comorbid conditions, such as diabetes or chronic lung or heart disease, that would affect the patient's ability to provide self-care.

Safety assessment of the home

Upon entering the home of a patient, assessment of the environment is an essential responsibility of the home care nurse. Beyond necessary shelter and comfort, the patient's surroundings are observed for existing and potential hazards that might affect the safety and well-being of the patient. Hazards can be structural, such as unsafe stair railings and inadequate lighting; environmental, as in inadequate disposal of infectious materials; or organizational, as in the lack of an emergency plan in case of fire, dangerous weather, or a medical emergency. The patient's ability to function safely within the home should be documented, including the safe use of assistive devices, household appliances and equipment, ambulation, storage and administration of medications, and activities of daily living. Outside the patient's home, the neighborhood and community should be assessed for the presence of threats to physical safety, for example, a high-crime, urban area or a rural location remote from public assistance services. Patient and caregiver education is the focus of the home care team when addressing safety needs in the home.

Previsit checklist

Physician orders and preparation

● Orders specific to patient safety

● Activity limitations

● Medication orders

Equipment and supplies

● Patient education materials on home safety, infection control, and safe use of home medical equipment

● Supplies for standard precautions

Safety requirements

- Standard precautions for infection control
- Information on medications, including dosage, adverse effects, interactions, and safe storage
- Allergies verified and documented
- Correct and safe use of adaptive devices (for example, cane, walker, and wheelchair)
- Correct and safe use of household appliances (for example, microwave and stove)
- Adequate and safe food storage
- Correct and safe use of medical equipment (for example, oxygen and humidifiers)
- Emergency lighting source (flashlight) available and in working order
- Adequate lighting in the home, including night-lights in the bedroom and bathroom
- Electrical cords in good repair and out of the way, no overloaded electrical outlets, and grounded outlets available as needed
- Safe flooring (for example, no waxed or slippery floors, throw rugs, or loose tiles)
- Walkways free from clutter with items put up and out of the way
- Secure handrails and grab bars
- Nonskid mat or adhesive strips in the bathtub
- Stairways well lit and in good repair
- Furniture arranged to allow ease of movement in the home
- Chairs in good repair
- Chemical hazards (for example, cleaning fluids, bleach, poisons) clearly marked and properly stored
- Adequate means for disposal of infectious materials
- Medications clearly labeled and properly stored
- Correct and safe medication administration
- Emergency plan and access to functional phone and list of emergency phone numbers
- Contact person (for example, friend, neighbor, or pastor) to visit the patient at regular intervals for well-being checks
- Patient and caregivers aware of signs and symptoms that need to be reported to the physician

Major diagnostic codes

- Abuse, adult 995.80
- Injury 959.9 (use code to specify cause, for example, Falls from slipping or tripping E885)
- Trauma, complication (early), other specified 958.8
- Walking difficulty related to a joint disorder 719.7
- Weakness, generalized 780.7
- Poisoning, unspecified 977.9 (use code to specify agent, for example, Corrosives and caustics E864)

(To assign a fifth digit, see appendix A, page 638.)

Defense of homebound status

- Activity limitations
- Unable to ambulate farther than 10′ (3 m) because of extreme fatigue
- Unsafe for ambulation without maximal assistance
- Activity restricted by pain
- Assistance required with activities of daily living (ADLs)
- Weakness

- Severe shortness of breath with activity
- Bedridden or confined to chair

Selected nursing diagnoses and patient outcomes

Knowledge deficit related to lack of home safety information (home environment, home medical equipment, medication, emergency situations)

The patient or caregiver will:
- remain safe in home environment (N, HCA)
- demonstrate safe use of medical equipment in home (N)
- demonstrate safe storage of medications (N)
- state measures to take in case of emergency. (N, HCA)

Impaired home maintenance management related to altered health status, insufficient support systems or persons, impaired cognitive or emotional functioning, and inadequate resources

The patient or caregiver will:
- arrange for assistance in managing home maintenance (N, SW)
- use community and family support systems (N, SW)
- have no deficiencies or needs identified in home maintenance. (N)

Risk for injury related to hazards within the home environment

The patient or caregiver will:
- have no injury while in his home environment. (N, HCA, OT, PT)

Skilled nursing services

Care measures
- Assess the patient's and caregiver's functional abilities and willingness to comply with safety measures for the home environment.
- Assess the home environment for safety hazards.

Patient and family teaching
- Teach safety precautions related to impaired mobility or decreased functional ability.

Interdisciplinary actions

Home care aide
- Observation for adherence to safety precautions and reporting of any incident of noncompliance or any concerns related to patient safety

Physical therapist
- Instruction on safe performance of home exercise program and safe use of adaptive equipment

Occupational therapist
- Instruction on safety in performing ADLs and safe use of adaptive devices

Pharmacist
- Answers to community's medication safety questions

Social worker
- Referrals to community resources
- Counseling to the patient and caregiver for coping strategies

Discharge plan

• Patient remains safe in home environment
• Patient returns to optimal levels of self-care and activity
• Follow-up appointments for blood studies in the authorized laboratory
• Follow-up appointments with the physician at recommended intervals

Documentation requirements

• Assessment of the home and surrounding environment for safety hazards
• Patient's and caregiver's functional abilities to maintain safe home environment
• Patient and caregiver compliance with home safety precautions
• Stressors impacting patient and caregiver adherence to safety precautions
• Instructions given in regard to maintaining a safe environment and the patient and caregiver's response
• Implementation of safety measures
• Identification of signs and symptoms to be reported
• Patient and caregiver ability to safely perform care
• Institution of infection control measures and standard precautions

Reimbursement reminders

• Durable medical equipment is covered under Medicare part B but, if equipment is approved, the patient will be responsible for 20% of the allowable charge.
• Five or more visits per week are considered daily visits and must have a finite and predictable end.

• Remember that reimbursement requires the documentation of homebound status, any variance to expected outcomes, any change to the plan of care, any change in the patient's condition, patient education provided and the patient's response, all treatments and procedures covered by physician order.

Insurance hints

• Present objective data regarding risk of injuries, physical assessment findings, coping ability, and safety hazards in the home.
• Present objective data regarding limitations in mobility or activity as related to homebound status.
• Present details of patient education needs and goals.
• Present physician orders and the patient's requests; however, remember that neither will guarantee coverage.

Seizure disorder

A seizure is caused by an excessive and abnormal discharge of electrical activity within the brain. This electrical activity causes a cerebral malfunction, which leads to abnormality in skeletal muscle function, sensation, the autonomic nervous system, behavior, or level of consciousness. A seizure can occur as a single isolated event in an otherwise healthy individual in response to an abnormal condition, such as a high fever, head injury, infection, endocrine disorder, or toxic poisoning. Chronic seizure activity is epilepsy. Typically, electrical activity within the brain isn't synchronized. When something affects this electrical activity, the neurons can start to discharge in a synchronous manner, leading to a seizure. Most of the physical problems in the patient with a seizure disorder focus on providing care during and immediately after a seizure. For these issues, teaching is needed for the families of patients with this health condition and should focus on supporting the patient during and after a seizure, helping with physical comfort, and reducing anxiety about the unpredictability of episodes.

Previsit checklist

Physician orders and preparation
- Order for skilled nursing assessment
- Order for home suction equipment
- Activity orders and restrictions
- Medication
- Venipuncture as needed

Equipment and supplies
- Vital signs equipment
- Supplies for standard precautions and proper sharps disposal
- Sterile water
- Suctioning kits, if indicated, for aspiration precautions

Safety requirements
- Action plan for postseizure care
- Standard precautions for infection control and sharps disposal
- Home assessment for placement of grab bars and supportive devices in the bathroom and removal of throw rugs and loose carpeting
- Seizure and aspiration precautions
- Safe use of suction equipment
- Emergency plan and access to functional phone and list of emergency phone numbers

- Adequate lighting
- Information on medications, including dosage, adverse effects, interactions, and safe storage
- Allergies verified and documented

Major diagnostic codes
- Abnormal involuntary movements 781.0
- Alteration of consciousness 780.09
- Alteration of consciousness, transient 780.02
- Cerebrovascular accident 436
- Convulsions, idiopathic/febrile 780.39/780.31
- Epilepsy, generalized convulsive 345.1
- Epilepsy, generalized nonconvulsive 345.0
- Grand mal status 345.1
- Partial epilepsy, focalized 345.5
- Partial epilepsy with impairment of consciousness 345.4
- Petit mal status 345.0
- Transient ischemic attacks 435.9

(To assign a fifth digit, see appendix A, page 638.)

Defense of homebound status
- Unable to leave home environment because of recent and severe seizure activity
- Risk for aspiration because of the unpredictable seizure activity
- Neurologic impairment
- Paralysis secondary to a cerebrovascular accident
- Unable to safely leave home without assistance
- Bedridden
- Maximal assistance required to ambulate

Selected nursing diagnoses and patient outcomes

Ineffective airway clearance
The patient or caregiver will:
• recognize that during a seizure the patient airway may become obstructed (N)
• recognize signs and symptoms of an obstructed airway (N)
• demonstrate supporting the patient during a seizure, including loosening clothing around the neck, turning the patient on his side, and avoid placing anything in the patient's mouth. (N)

Risk for injury
The patient or caregiver will:
• recognize that uncontrollable extremity movements can cause injury to the patient (N)
• demonstrate helping the patient to a lying position in the event of a seizure (N)
• recognize safety hazards in the home that can contribute to an injury in the event of a seizure, such as smoking alone in bed and locking bedroom doors. (N)

Anxiety related to threatened change in health status secondary to seizures
The patient or caregiver will:
• recognize the causes of anxiety (N, SW)
• demonstrate open communication about seizure disorder with family, friends, and colleagues (N, SW)
• demonstrate proper techniques to help alleviate anxiety. (N, SW)

Risk for aspiration
The patient or caregiver will:
• recognize the potential for aspiration during and immediately after a seizure (N)
• demonstrate the use of the home suction equipment to ensure a patent airway after a seizure (N)
• demonstrate proper techniques for prevention of aspiration. (N)

Ineffective individual coping related to high degree of threat and inadequate opportunity to prepare for stressor
The patient or caregiver will:
• recognize feelings of low self-esteem and depression (N, SW)
• demonstrate patience and understanding while helping the patient resume normal activities and remain seizure-free (N, SW)
• demonstrate healthy coping mechanisms. (N, SW)

Powerlessness related to illness-related regimen
The patient or caregiver will:
• recognize how seizure activity is unpredictable and affects the person's entire life and activities (N)
• demonstrate understanding and support as the patient tries to take control over the seizure activity and frequency. (N)

Skilled nursing services

Care measures
• Conduct a skilled nursing evaluation, including assessment of the patient's neurologic, respiratory, cognitive, and cardiovascular functioning.
• Obtain requested laboratory samples to include blood for medication levels.

- Inform the physician of any changes in condition.
- Monitor medication administration and the patient's response to them.
- Assess signs and symptoms of seizure activity, including onset signals such as an aura.
- Assess vital signs.
- Implement safety measures.

Patient and family teaching
- Review home safety measures.
- Identify signs and symptoms that need to be reported to the physician.
- Emphasize the importance of wearing a medical identification bracelet and adhering to the medication regimen.
- Discuss medication purposes, dosages, frequency, and adverse effects.
- Review seizure precautions.

Interdisciplinary actions

Physical therapist
- Gait training
- Home safety evaluation

Social worker
- Referrals to support services and community services as needed

Discharge plan
- Patient seizure-free or seizures controlled with medication regimen
- Anxiety level decreased or managed
- Ability of the patient and family to institute proper safety measures during the occurrence of a seizure
- Follow-up appointments for blood studies in the authorized laboratory
- Follow-up appointments with the physician at recommended intervals

- Referral to community resources for assistance
- Patient ambulatory and independent with activities of daily living with moderate assistance
- Improved mobility level with demonstration of self-care activities appropriate to the level of physiologic functioning
- No development of integumentary, respiratory, GI, or genitourinary complications

Documentation requirements
- Patient's and caregiver's responses to instruction
- Observation of the patient's and caregiver's ability to perform oropharyngeal suctioning, prevent injury during a seizure, and protect the airway during a seizure
- Changes in neurologic or respiratory functioning
- Ability of caregiver to care for the patient
- Assessment findings
- Safety measures
- Signs and symptoms to be reported
- Instruction in proper seizure precautions to be taken
- Laboratory results
- Seizure activity
- Interdisciplinary communication
- Teaching performed and the patient's and family's response to it

Reimbursement reminders
- Document homebound status.
- Physical therapy services may be indicated for patients with hemiplegia or paralysis.
- Specify any barriers to learning.

Insurance hints

- Provide review of hospitalization (if appropriate) and current condition of the patient, home environment, and availability of caregiver.
- Provide objective review of systems, including type of seizure, aura, postictal response, and airway management.
- Provide current laboratory values.
- Provide objective review of communication pattern, cognitive level, and ability to comprehend instructions.

Spinal cord injury

A spinal cord injury is typically caused by trauma. Although it can occur in any age-group, these injuries are typically seen in adolescent and young adult men who engage in high-risk activities. Spinal cord injuries are classified as being complete or incomplete by the cause of the injury and the level of residual disability. The initial spinal cord injury causes microscopic hemorrhages in the gray matter of the spinal cord and edema in the white matter. As the hemorrhages extend, the size of injury increases. Circulation to the cord is impaired, reducing vascular perfusion and oxygen to the cord tissue. This eventually leads to spinal cord cell ischemia and death.

Most of the physical problems in the patient with a spinal cord injury are focused on maximizing mobility, reducing the complications of immobility, accepting altered body functioning, and promoting self-care. For these issues, teaching is needed for the families of patients with this health condition and should focus on preventing complications, maximizing mobility, and providing care for basic needs.

Previsit checklist

Physician orders and preparation

- Order for an indwelling urinary catheter
- Order for physical, speech, and occupational therapy
- Order for specialty bed, wheelchair, and other assistive devices
- Activity orders and restrictions
- Order for nutritional requirements
- Order for home oxygen therapy
- Medications
- Venipuncture and laboratory studies
- Order for home suctioning equipment

Equipment and supplies

- Indwelling catheter as ordered
- Supplies for standard precautions
- Supplies to change dressing around gastrostomy feeding tube, if indicated
- Irrigation kit for gastrostomy tube
- Sterile water
- Suctioning kits (nasotracheal and oropharyngeal)
- Oxygen equipment
- Wound care supplies (if needed)
- Vital signs equipment
- Leg bag or urinary bag attachment device

Safety requirements

- Standard precautions for infection control
- Home assessment for placement of grab bars, supportive devices in bathroom, removal of loose rugs and carpeting, and wheelchair accessibility
- Aspiration precautions
- Oxygen precautions, safe handling and placement of home oxygen equipment, and notification of local fire and

police departments of oxygen use in the home
- Safe use of suction equipment
- Skin care and protection to include frequent position changes
- Extremity supports to keep limbs in normal anatomic alignment
- Emergency plan and access to functional phone and list of emergency phone numbers
- Night-light
- Proper urinary catheter care

Major diagnostic codes
- Anorexia 783.0
- Aspiration, mucus 933.1 (if due to trauma, use trauma codes)
- Bladder retention 788.20
- Cervical compression 723.4 (if due to trauma, use trauma codes)
- Constipation 564.0
- Contraction, flaccid, paralytic muscle 728.85
- Coordination disturbance 781.3
- Fecal impaction 560.39
- Gait abnormality 781.2
- Hemiplegia 342.9
- Incontinence 788.30
- Lumbar compression 724.4 (if due to trauma, use trauma codes)
- Lumbosacral compression 724.4 (if due to trauma, use trauma codes)
- Muscle spasms 728.85
- Nerve pain not elsewhere classified 729.2
- Neurogenic bowel 564.81
- Paraplegia 344.1
- Spinal cord injury 952.9
- Spinal cord injury:
  – cervical 952.00
  – lumbar 952.2
  – multiple sites 952.8
  – sacral 952.3
  – thoracic 952.1

- Spinal root pain 729.2
- Stasis pneumonia 514 or 426
- Thoracic compression 724.4 (if due to trauma, use trauma codes)

Defense of homebound status
- Unable to ambulate without assistance
- Not independent with self-care needs
- Unable to maintain patent respiratory functioning
- Unable to feed self
- Unable to maintain airway with food and fluids
- Bedridden or confined to wheelchair
- Indwelling urinary catheter

Selected nursing diagnoses and patient outcomes

Impaired physical mobility related to neuromuscular impairment
    The patient or caregiver will:
- recognize the need to perform passive range of motion (ROM) to paralyzed limbs   (N, PT)
- demonstrate ROM exercises to affected limbs   (N, PT)
- identify complications of immobility and demonstrate techniques to reduce complications.   (N, PT)

Impaired gas exchange related to ventilation and perfusion imbalance
    The patient or caregiver will:
- recognize an alteration in respiratory functioning   (N)
- demonstrate aspiration precautions with meals and medications   (N)
- demonstrate turning, repositioning, and coughing to maximize gas exchange.   (N, RT)

Ineffective breathing pattern related to neuromuscular dysfunction

The patient or caregiver will:

• recognize a normal respiratory rate for the patient with a spinal cord injury (N)

• demonstrate proper turning, deep breathing, and coughing techniques with the patient (N, RT)

• maintain adequate oxygenation (N, RT)

• identify proper measures for maintaining adequate oxygenation. (N, PT)

Risk for autonomic dysreflexia

The patient or caregiver will:

• verbalize an understanding of the complication of autonomic dysreflexia (N)

• state signs and symptoms of pending autonomic dysreflexia (N)

• demonstrate knowledge of proper interventions in case the patient exhibits signs and symptoms of autonomic dysreflexia. (N)

Altered urinary elimination related to sensory motor impairment

The patient or caregiver will:

• recognize when the patient has a full bladder (N)

• demonstrate trigger voiding techniques to initiate spontaneous voiding (stroking the inner thigh, pulling pubic hair, tapping on the abdomen over the bladder, and pouring warm water over the perineum for women) (N)

• demonstrate proper urinary self-catheterization (N)

• demonstrate use of self-catheterization to evaluate for residual urine. (N)

Constipation related to decreased motility of the GI tract

The patient or caregiver will:

• demonstrate an understanding of the parts of a comprehensive bowel retraining program (N)

• recognize the role of a high-fluid, high-fiber diet, stool softeners, and digital stimulation and manual removal in a comprehensive bowel retraining program (N)

• have regular bowel movements. (N)

Sexual dysfunction related to altered body structure or function

The patient or caregiver will:

• recognize how the spinal cord injury will affect sexual functioning (N)

• recognize alternatives to ensure adequate sexual functioning to maintain as positive a self-concept as possible. (N, SW)

Self-esteem disturbance

The patient or caregiver will:

• verbalize feelings (N, SW)

• encourage the patient to participate in as much self-care as possible to maximize independence. (N)

Feeding, bathing and hygiene, dressing and grooming, and toileting self-care deficits related to neuromuscular impairment

The patient or caregiver will:

• recognize the patient's limited ability to perform self-care activities (N)

• demonstrate supporting the patient in performing as many self-care activities as physically able. (N, OT)

Anxiety related to threat to change in role function and self-concept

The patient or caregiver will:

- recognize anxiety as being a normal part of the recovery and rehabilitation process (N)
- demonstrate anxiety-reduction techniques. (N)

Risk for disuse syndrome

The patient or caregiver will:

- recognize potential complications from not using extremities and body parts because of the spinal cord injury and demonstrate proper techniques to reduce complications. (N, PT)

Risk for injury

The patient or caregiver will:

- recognize various ways the body can be injured while attempting to perform activities or exercises (N, PT)
- demonstrate safe techniques when performing activities, exercises, and routine care. (N, PT)

Risk for impaired skin integrity

The patient or caregiver will:

- recognize the impact of immobility on the integumentary status (N)
- demonstrate proper turning and repositioning to prevent skin breakdown (N)
- demonstrate proper skin care to prevent skin breakdown. (N)

Skilled nursing services

Care measures

- Conduct a skilled nursing assessment, including evaluation of the neurologic, cardiovascular, respiratory, GI, genitourinary, and integumentary systems as well as nutritional status.
- Assess bowel and bladder function.
- Assess passive and active ROM capabilities.
- Evaluate for the onset of autonomic dysreflexia.
- Assess medication compliance, need, and knowledge.
- Assess the home situation and need for assistive devices or durable medical equipment.
- Evaluate for all prescribed medications, whether the family knows how to provide them to the patient, and whether common adverse effects are understood; provide ongoing assessment for patient and family adherence to the prescribed medication regimen.
- Assess social and emotional functioning of the patient and family.
- Measure vital signs.
- Perform tracheal suctioning as indicated.
- Collect laboratory specimens.
- Provide urinary catheter care.
- Provide wound care and skin care as needed.
- Administer enteral feeding.
- Recognize depression.

Patient and family teaching

- Teach about medication administration, including dosages, purposes, and adverse effects.
- Review home safety measures.
- Demonstrate maintenance of an airway and emergency airway procedures as well as nasotracheal and oropharyngeal suctioning.
- Discuss home oxygen therapy.
- Emphasize the need to establish a respiratory care program, including frequent position changes, turning, chest physiotherapy, postural drainage, use of incentive spirometer, and cough resistance.

- Review gastrostomy tube care.
- Demonstrate proper application of splints.
- Review skin care.
- Detail activity limitations.
- Explain indwelling catheter care.
- Review bowel elimination care.
- Identify signs and symptoms to be reported to the physician.
- Review infection control measures.

Interdisciplinary actions

Physical therapist
- Initiation of prescribed rehabilitation program, including transferring and active and passive ROM exercises
- Assessment of equipment needs, function features, and home safety

Occupational therapist
- Assessment of activities of daily living (ADLs) and education in the use of assistive devices as indicated
- Provision of therapies to address fine motor skills
- Education in energy conservation techniques

Social worker
- Assessment of the need for community services
- Provision of emotional support and counseling

Home care aide
- Assistance with hygiene and ADLs
- Gradual withdrawal of home care aide and homemaker support as the family and other caregivers gain confidence with patient care as directed

Discharge plan
- Care program established
- Bowel and bladder program established and functioning
- Respiratory program to remove excess secretions
- Skin program to prevent skin breakdown
- Performance of regular active and passive ROM exercises
- Participation in an outpatient rehabilitation program
- Follow-up appointment for blood studies in the authorized laboratory
- Follow-up appointments with the physician at recommended intervals

Documentation requirements
- Patient's and caregiver's responses to instruction
- Observation of the patient's and caregiver's ability to perform basic care, bowel and bladder retraining program, turning and repositioning, respiratory function care, gastrostomy tube feedings (if applicable), use of assistive devices, maintenance of normal anatomic alignment, repositioning, and transfers
- Changes in integumentary, respiratory, GI, genitourinary, or neurologic functioning
- Ability of caregiver to care for the patient
- Complete physical assessment
- Laboratory results
- Patient's response to care
- Safety precautions
- Signs and symptoms to be reported
- Patient and caregiver compliance with instruction and therapy regimen

Reimbursement reminders

- Medicare covers phlebotomy supplies.
- Check for an authorized laboratory because many insurance companies have contracts with specific laboratories for processing specimens.
- Note that all nonroutine supplies must be specifically ordered by the physician and entered into Locator 14 (Supplies) of Health Care Finance Administration Form 485 or ordered by the physician within the specific order for treatment requiring the use of certain supplies and entered into Locator 21 (Orders for Treatment).
- When billing for medical supplies, always include the name of supply item, date supply was used, number of units used, and charge per unit.

Insurance hints

- Review hospitalization (if appropriate) and current condition of the patient, home environment, and availability of caregivers.
- Provide objective review of systems to include physical abilities, use or need for assistive devices, need for passive or active ROM exercises.
- Provide thorough skin assessment, and report objective findings. In the event of open or reddened areas, provide accurate wound dimensions, prescribed dressing, and capabilities of caregiver to perform wound care.
- Provide current laboratory values.
- Provide objective evaluation of respiratory and nutritional status. If the patient is receiving gastrostomy tube feedings, provide patient tolerance to feedings, patency of gastrostomy tube, and condition of skin surrounding the tube. If the patient is able to be sup-

ported by oral nutrition, objectively evaluate the patient and caregiver's ability to maintain a patent airway.

Spinal stenosis

Spinal stenosis is defined as any narrowing of the spinal canal or associated structures. Narrowing of the spinal canal occurs as a result of degenerative changes or movement of anatomic structures through injury or the shape of the canal. Almost all incidents of spinal stenosis are secondary to degenerative changes in the spine. Treatment includes decompression laminectomy or spinal fusion for severe cases.

Previsit checklist

Physician orders and preparation

- Medications, dosages, frequencies, routes
- Activity restrictions
- Wound care orders

Equipment and supplies

- Postsurgical wound care
- Skin cleaner
- Dressing supplies
- Tape
- Suture removal kit as ordered
- Biohazard bag for disposal of old dressings
- Supplies for standard precautions
- Vital signs equipment

Safety requirements

- Clear walkways
- Night-light
- Removal of some furniture to accommodate adaptive equipment

- Standard precautions for infection control
- Emergency plan and access to functional phone and list of emergency phone numbers
- Proper body mechanics

Major diagnostic codes

- Backache, unspecified 724.5
- Cervical stenosis 723.0
- Lumbar stenosis 724.02
- Pain, thoracic spine 724.1
- Pain with radicular and visceral spine 724.4
- Stenosis specified region not elsewhere classified 724.09
- Thoracic stenosis 724.01

Defense of homebound status

- Unable to transfer from bed to chair without significant change in symptoms (pain and fatigue)
- Unable to ambulate farther than 10' (3 m) because of musculoskeletal weakness and pain
- Unable to ambulate because of imposed physical restriction

Selected nursing diagnoses and patient outcomes

Knowledge deficit related to use of adaptive equipment (walke or wheelchair)

The patient or caregiver will:

- verbalize knowledge of how to use a walker or wheelchair   (N, OT, PT)
- demonstrate proper walker or wheelchair use   (N, OT, PT)

- demonstrate proper posture when using a walker   (N, PT)
- explain and use safe methods using a walker and other assistive devices to get in and out of the shower and bathtub or on and off the toilet
(N, OT, PT)
- remain free from injury. (N, OT, PT)

Chronic pain related to narrowing of the spinal canal

The patient or caregiver will:

- verbalize proper analgesia use (N)
- demonstrate optimal movement related to proper pain control   (N)
- use adjuvant pain therapy for bone pain, including anti-inflammatory medication   (N)
- verbalize methods of preventing constipating adverse effects of analgesic use   (N)
- report satisfaction with sleep pattern   (N)
- demonstrate ability to participate in home exercise program.   (N)

Pain related to surgical intervention

The patient or caregiver will:

- express satisfaction with the pain-control regimen   (N)
- verbalize dietary and pharmacologic methods to prevent constipation (N)
- demonstrate ability to participate in a home exercise program.   (N, PT)

Impaired physical mobility related to pain and limited motion from pathological or surgical changes in spinal canal

The patient or caregiver will:

- demonstrate an ability to walk with appropriate posture   (N, PT)

- remain free from muscle spasms (N)
- perform at expected level of independent self-care   (N, OT, PT)
- maintain functional mobility and range of motion   (N, OT, PT)
- demonstrate proper home exercise techniques.   (N, OT, PT)

Impaired walking related to pain and weakness

The patient or caregiver will:
- participate in a home exercise program   (N, PT)
- demonstrate normal posture when walking, sitting, and lying down   (N, PT)
- express feelings of increased strength.   (N, OT, PT)

Activity intolerance related to prolonged periods of immobility

The patient or caregiver will:
- participate in a prescribed activity program   (N, OT, PT)
- verbalize need to increase activity gradually   (N, OT, PT)
- demonstrate progressive tolerance to activity.   (N, OT, PT)

Dressing and grooming self-care deficit related to limited mobility and imposed physical restrictions

The patient or caregiver will:
- demonstrate correct adaptive methods for self-care   (N, OT)
- have self-care needs met.   (N)

Risk for injury related to unsteady gait

The patient or caregiver will:
- be free from injury   (N, OT, PT)
- verbalize knowledge of home safety plan to prevent falls   (N, OT, PT)

- rearrange home for use of a walker or wheelchair   (N, HCA, OT, PT)
- demonstrate proper walker or wheelchair storage   (N, OT, PT)
- modify home to increase walkway, lighting, and space for adaptive equipment.   (N, OT)

Impaired skin integrity related to surgical procedure

The patient or caregiver will:
- have surgical incision that will heal without complications   (N)
- demonstrate proper wound care techniques   (N)
- verbalize methods for maintaining skin cleanliness   (N)
- verbalize appropriate dietary intake to aid in wound healing   (N, D)
- demonstrate proper infection control procedures for the home.   (N)

Skilled nursing services

Care measures

- Conduct a complete physical assessment of body systems.
- Demonstrate and evaluate home exercise program.
- Evaluate the patient's response to care.
- Measure vital signs.
- Perform venipuncture and specimen collection as indicated.
- Evaluate incision and care.
- Perform pain medication titration as ordered.
- Evaluate pain management.

Patient and family teaching

- Teach about injury prevention.
- Demonstrate proper wound and incision care.

- Review proper body mechanics.
- Identify methods of pain relief and control.
- Teach about medication administration, including dosages, purposes, frequency, and adverse effects.

Interdisciplinary actions

Physical therapist
- Instruction and evaluation of home exercise program
- Safety planning
- Transfer training
- Strength training
- Instruction in use of assistive devices
- Instruction in signs and symptoms that need to be reported to the physician

Occupational therapist
- Assistance with management of activities of daily living (ADLs)
- Instruction in energy conservation techniques

Home care aide
- Assistance in hygiene and ADLs

Social worker
- Assistance in obtaining community resources, such as transportation and in-home support services

Discharge plan
- Return of the patient to normal routine following recovery from surgery
- Return of the patient to optimal functional level following exacerbation of an acute episode of pain

- Follow-up appointments for blood studies in the authorized laboratory
- Follow-up appointments with the physician at recommended intervals
- Patient functions safely at home

Documentation requirements
- Physical assessment of body systems and any changes noted
- Patient's response to care
- Teaching performed and the patient's and family's response
- Any laboratory results
- Description of functional losses or gains in clear terms: walked with walker or wheelchair; self-care ability in dressing, feeding, bathing, toileting, grooming
- Evaluation of effectiveness of pain-control regimen
- Description of plan to improve patient function whenever progress stalls
- Appropriateness of the patient's home environment
- Healing of surgical wound, signs and symptoms of infection
- Any barriers to learning or physical progress
- Any adaptive devices used
- Coordination with rehabilitative services
- Safety precautions
- Reportable signs and symptoms
- The patient's ability to function safely at home

Reimbursement reminders
- Be aware of the need to clarify the patient's primary diagnosis for each episode of home care. The diagnosis on

the medical treatment plan should reflect the care being given to the patient. For spinal stenosis, if the care is restorative after surgery, the plan of care should reflect an emphasis on restorative care postoperatively. If the patient hasn't had surgery yet, the plan of care should reflect a clear rehabilitative goal. It's important to document continuous progress because rehabilitative services that focus on "debilitative" aren't covered by Medicare. When progress has reached a plateau, the patient is custodial and should be discharged.

• Because these patients are severely disabled, it's essential to clearly describe the expected benefits, collaborative plan of care, and progress toward goals with each visit note, team conference note, and other team communication.

• Demonstrate coordination of care with rehabilitation services.

• Order occupational therapy if the patient needs energy conservation, and work with home care aide in transfers in the bathroom.

• If the patient is initially very weak from surgery, physical therapy and other rehabilitative care can be offered after the patient regains strength and has the ability to benefit from an exercise program.

• Medicare covers phlebotomy supplies.

• Check for an authorized laboratory because many insurance companies have contracts with specific laboratories for processing specimens.

• All nonroutine supplies must be specifically ordered by the physician and entered into Locator 14 (Supplies) of Health Care Finance Administration Form 485 or ordered by the physician within the specific order for treatment requiring the use of certain supplies and entered into Locator 21 (Orders for Treatment).

• When billing for medical supplies, always include the name of supply item, date supply was used, number of units used, and charge per unit.

Insurance hints

• Describe progressive levels of self-care (dressing, toileting, bathing, grooming, dressing) and abilities, including the use of adaptive equipment; emphasize rehabilitation potential.

• Describe progress toward rehabilitation goals, such as safe use of stairs and proper transfers from a reclining to a sitting position and from a sitting to a standing position.

• List the collaborative plan of care for all team members providing services.

• Compare and contrast the roles of each rehabilitation team member.

• Describe how the home care program complements the therapy given prior to discharge from the skilled nursing facility because many of these patients will have come from a skilled nursing facility.

• Describe any other conditions such as chronic lung disease and how it affects the patient's use of a walker or wheelchair.

Suprapubic catheter care

Patients with spinal cord injury or urinary or reproductive tumors may need a suprapubic catheter. This urinary diversion requires skin care attention and monitoring of urine output. The catheter should be changed by sterile technique every 3 months or as needed. Patient and caregiver education, support, and acceptance of urinary elimination are the main components of care of the catheter. Coverage for medical supplies is limited to patients who meet specific criteria. Hydration, altered patterns of urinary elimination, self-image, and activity tolerance are issues that patients with suprapubic catheters may have to confront daily.

Previsit checklist

Physician orders and preparation
- Catheter care, including irrigation and frequency of changes
- Skin care
- Diet restrictions
- Medications
- Activity orders and restrictions

Equipment and supplies
- Urinary catheter
- Urinary drainage bag
- Secure device
- Dressings
- Irrigation or instillation needs
- Urinary specimen cup
- Vital signs equipment
- Supplies for standard precautions

Safety requirements
- Standard precautions for infection control and disposal of supplies
- Skin protection
- Awareness of dangerous signs and symptoms and action plan
- Identification of resource person
- Emergency plan and access to functional phone and list of emergency phone numbers
- Night-light
- Allergies verified and documented

Major diagnostic codes
- Attention to other artificial opening of urinary tract V55.4
- Fitting and adjustment of urinary devices V53.6
- Malignant neoplasm genital organs or tract, female not elsewhere classified (NEC)/male NEC 184.9/187.9
- Malignant neoplasm of bladder, primary, unspecified 188.9
- Malignant neoplasm of kidney, primary/secondary 189.0/198.0
- Malignant neoplasm of prostate, primary 185
- Malignant neoplasm of a urinary organ 189.9
- Neurogenic bladder 596.54
- Rupture of bladder or sphincter 596.6
- Suprapubic tube 596.5
- Unspecified disorder of urethra and urinary tract 599.9
- Urinary abnormality NEC 788.69
- Urinary infection (tract) NEC 599.0
- Urinary retention 788.20

Defense of homebound status
- Unable to ambulate farther than 10′ (3 m) because of fatigue

* Unable to ambulate farther than 10' (3 m) because of draining catheter
* Unable to leave home because of catheter
* Maximum assistance required for ambulation or transfers
* Paralysis

Selected nursing diagnoses and patient outcomes

Knowledge deficit related to suprapubic catheter management, including site care, catheter, and activity
The patient or caregiver will:
* verbalize or demonstrate correct technique for washing the catheter insertion site   (N)
* verbalize techniques to keep the insertion site clean and free from infection   (N)
* verbalize or demonstrate correct techniques to maintain flow of urine and to empty catheter bag.
                    (N, HCA)

Altered urinary elimination related to suprapubic catheter
The patient or caregiver will:
* record urinary output and characteristics of urine   (N, HCA)
* drink 8 to 10 glasses (2,400 to 3,000 ml) of water or juice daily.   (N)

Risk for infection related to invasive suprapubic catheter
The patient or caregiver will:
* use clean techniques while washing around the catheter insertion site and emptying the drainage bag   (N, HCA)
* report temperature elevation, drainage, presence of swelling, pain or redness at the insertion site.   (N)

Body image disturbance related to changed urinary elimination patterns
The patient or caregiver will:
* verbalize positive self-worth (N, SC)
* accept the suprapubic catheter as a part of daily routine.   (N, HCA, SC)

Altered sexuality patterns related to suprapubic catheter
The patient or caregiver will:
* accept the suprapubic catheter and continue with sexual activity   (N)
* verbalize feelings in regard to the suprapubic catheter.   (N)

Skilled nursing services

Care measures
* Perform skilled assessment of mental and cognitive status, hydration, and integumentary, reproductive, genitourinary systems.
* Assess level of care of the patient and caregiver; observe how they perform catheter management techniques, skin care, and emptying of urinary bag.
* Assess amount of urinary drainage, color, odor, and intake of fluids.
* Change the catheter (as ordered).
* Irrigate catheter as indicated per physician order.
* Perform proper skin care at the catheter insertion site.
* Collect urine specimens as ordered.
* Evaluate the patient's response to treatments and care.
* Measure vital signs.
* Assess for signs and symptoms of infection.

Patient and family teaching
* Discuss catheter supplies needed and purposes.

- Review methods to prevent hydration.
- Identify signs and symptoms of dehydration and infection and when the physician needs to be notified.
- Review methods to prevent skin breakdown and infection of the catheter site.
- Demonstrate proper skin care at the insertion site and catheter care.
- Explain how to change the drainage bag.

Interdisciplinary actions

Physical therapist
- Development and education in an increased exercise and activity endurance program

Home care aide
- Hygiene and grooming needs

Discharge plan
- Safe management of suprapubic catheter care in the home by the patient and caregiver with physician follow-up
- Follow-up appointments for urine specimens in the authorized laboratory
- Follow-up appointments with the physician at recommended intervals

Documentation requirements
- Subjective and objective data with regard to suprapubic catheter care — hydration, urinary elimination factors, catheter insertion site, and sexuality concerns

- Assessment of suprapubic catheter care, type, time and frequency of changing
- Patient and caregiver participation in care
- Patient and caregiver progress toward educational goals
- Patient response to care
- Safety precautions
- Signs and symptoms to report to the physician
- Infection control
- Teaching performed and the patient's or family's response
- Any change in patient condition

Reimbursement reminders
- The following suprapubic catheter supplies are covered by Medi-care and many private insurance companies: catheters, irrigation sets, drainage bags, skin care ointment, dressings, and secure devices based on type of system used.
- Registered dietician services aren't reimbursable under Medicare benefits pending certain conditions.
- Document any variances to expected outcomes.
- Document any barriers to learning (physical deformities, visual impairment, and availability of support person).
- Obtain an order for any change in the plan of care and document it in the chart.
- Document initial level of knowledge and progress to educational goals.
- Check for an authorized laboratory because many insurance companies have contracts with specific laboratories for processing specimens.
- All nonroutine supplies must be specifically ordered by the physician

and entered into Locator 14 (Supplies) of HCFA Form 485 or ordered by the physician within the specific order for treatment requiring the use of certain supplies and entered into Locator 21 (Orders for Treatment).

• When billing for medical supplies, always include the name of supply item, date supply was used, number of units used, and charge per unit.

Insurance hints

• Present objective data about home-bound status.
• Report any new laboratory findings that change the plan of care.
• Report specifics about the patient's learning progress.

Surgical patient care

Patients who have undergone surgical procedures require varied and specialized home care. Beyond the care of the surgical wound, physiologic, psychosocial, and role function concerns must be addressed. Surgery can affect multiple body systems, mental and emotional status, and functional abilities. With many types of surgery being performed in the outpatient setting, patient education regarding postoperative care and expectations is vital to the well-being of the home care patient. Please refer to the sections related to specific disorders and treatments for more information.

Previsit checklist

Physician orders and preparation

• Wound care frequency and instructions

• Activity limitations
• Medication orders
• Laboratory test orders

Equipment and supplies

• Dressing supplies
• Wound measurement device
• Consent form and camera to photograph wound
• Supplies for standard precaution
• Vital signs monitoring equipment
• Laboratory draw equipment
• List of medications, administration regimen, allergies, storage, potential adverse effects, and interactions

Safety requirements

• Correct and safe use of adaptive devices (for example, walker or wheelchair)
• Adequate lighting in the home
• Clear, uncluttered floors
• Safe flooring (for example, no throw rugs or loose tiles)
• Secure handrails and grab bars
• Emergency plan and access to functional phone and list of emergency phone numbers
• Standard precautions for infection control
• Education in regard to reportable signs and symptoms

Major diagnostic codes

• Acute inflammation 614.3
• Amputation, arm/hand/leg 887.4/ 887.0/897.4
• Aneurysm, aortic 441.9
• Appendicitis, acute 540.9
• Bowel obstruction 560.9
• Cholecystectomy 51.22
• Coronary artery bypass graft, complication 996.61

- Deep vein thrombosis 451.19
- Fistula, anal 565.1
- Gastrojejunostomy V45.3
- Generalized purulent infection 038.1
- GI bleed, unspecified 578.9
- Hickman catheter insertion 39.98
- Hysterectomy (abdominal) 68.4
- I & D of abscess 86.04
- Ileus, postoperative 997.4
- Other aftercare following surgery V58.4
- Pancreatitis, acute 577.0
- Peritonitis, postoperative infection 998.7
- Pneumonia, postoperative 997.3
- Spleen, traumatic injury 865.0
- Tracheostomy, complication 519.0
- Urinary tract infection, not elsewhere classified 599.0
- Uterine bleeding, abnormal 626.9
- Wound, open/surgical nonhealing 879.8/998.83
- Wound dehiscence 998.3
- Wound infection, postoperative 998.59

Defense of homebound status

- Postoperative weakness or pain
- Postoperative fatigue or dyspnea
- Presence of open wound, drains
- Activity restrictions
- Maximal assistance required with transfers and ambulation
- Unsteady gait
- Activity limited by pain
- Assistance required with activities of daily living (ADLs)

Selected nursing diagnoses and patient outcomes

Knowledge deficit related to postoperative care, including pain medications and antibiotics; activity restrictions; prescribed antiembolism stockings or abdominal binder; wound or drain care, signs and symptoms of complications, and prescribed exercise regimen

The patient or caregiver will:
- state the correct dose and time for prescribed pain medications or antibiotics and the adverse effects and precautions for each   (N, PH)
- adhere to prescribed activity restrictions, such as limitations on exercise, driving, sexual activity, weight bearing, lifting, or range of motion
                                      (N, OT, PT)
- wear antiembolism stockings or abdominal binders as ordered   (N)
- demonstrate ability to care for surgical wound using correct technique
                                      (N)
- demonstrate ability to empty drains and accurately record drainage and to perform drain site care using correct technique   (N)
- state signs and symptoms of wound complications (pain, increased redness and drainage, change in type of drainage, and fever) and report them to the physician   (N)
- demonstrate correct technique in performing prescribed postoperative exercises, including coughing and deep breathing exercises and incentive spirometry.   (N, PT)

Pain related to surgical procedure
The patient or caregiver will:
• report decreased need for pain medications (N)
• return to optimal activity levels.
(N, PT, OT)

Risk for infection related to surgical procedure
The patient or caregiver will:
• have no wound infection. (N)

Impaired skin integrity related to surgical incision
The patient or caregiver will:
• have incision well-approximated (N)
• report no redness, swelling, or drainage from the incision (N)
• report no pain the at the incision site.
(N)

Impaired gas exchange related to surgical procedure
The patient or caregiver will:
• make clear breath sounds (N)
• have an effective cough (N)
• show no purulent sputum (N)
• have no complaints of dyspnea (N)
• have a pulse oximetry level greater than 90% on room air. (N)

Risk of constipation related to immobility and pain medications
The patient or caregiver will:
• return to normal bowel pattern
(N, PH, PT)
• experience no pain with defecation.
(N, PH, PT)

Impaired physical mobility related to surgical procedure
The patient or caregiver will:
• exhibit increased ambulation, activity, and range of motion (N, OT, PT)

• show ability to perform ADLs safely and without complications.
(N, OT, PT)

Ineffective individual coping related to postoperative stressors
The patient or caregiver will:
• verbalize feelings related to emotional state (N, SW)
• identify actions resulting in effective coping (N, SW)
• identify strengths and factors to enhance coping and weaknesses and factors that inhibit effective coping.
(N, SW)

Caregiver role strain related to demands of care
The caregiver will:
• exhibit no signs and symptoms of strain (for example, crying, short temper, depression) (N, SW)
• identify and continue activities that are important for self (N, SW)
• accept outside help. (N, SW)

Skilled nursing services

Care measures
• Perform a skilled assessment of the musculoskeletal, integumentary, genitourinary, and cardiopulmonary systems; assess nutrition, hydration, and mental and cognitive status.
• Assess level of care of the patient and caregiver, including ability to perform wound care, drain care, medication compliance, adherence to activity limitations, and adherence to pulmonary hygiene measures.
• Assess effectiveness of treatment regimen, including wound healing, pain management, and activity level.

- Obtain laboratory specimens (for example, prothrombin time, wound culture, complete blood count, and urinalysis and culture) as ordered.
- Administer medications.
- Provide wound care, skin care, and dressing changes.
- Perform venipuncture as ordered.
- Evaluate and manage pain.
- Assess for signs and symptoms of infection.
- Assess vital signs.

Patient and family teaching

- Discuss the types of supplies needed and where to obtain them.
- Describe techniques (clean or sterile) for wound care and provide step-by-step procedures and instructions.
- Explain how to properly dispose of infectious materials.
- Identify signs and symptoms of wound complications to report to the physician.
- Demonstrate how to empty surgical drains and record drainage.
- Identify signs and symptoms of complications related to drain sites and drainage.
- Discuss wearing supportive apparel, such as abdominal binders and antiembolism stockings and orthopedic appliances, such as braces or slings.
- Explain the use of incentive spirometry and emphasize the importance of frequent coughing and deep breathing exercises.
- Teach about medication management, including indications, dosages, times, and adverse effects for all medications.
- Review home safety instructions, including adequate lighting, uncluttered floors, easy access to telephone, having emergency numbers on hand.

- Discuss pain management.
- Review infection control measures.

Interdisciplinary actions

Home care aide

- Assistance with personal hygiene and ADLs

Physical therapist

- Instruction on home exercise program and safe use of ambulation equipment

Occupational therapist

- Instruction on adaptive techniques and devices for increased self-care in ADLs

Pharmacist

- Answers to community's medication regimen questions

Social worker

- Assistance obtaining necessary supplies and equipment
- Referrals to community resources
- Counseling the patient and caregiver in coping strategies

Dietitian

- Nutritional support to promote wound healing
- Counseling and instruction on specific dietary requirements related to surgery or the disease process

Discharge plan

- Safe management of wound care in the home by the patient and caregiver
- Return of the patient to optimal levels of self-care and activity

- Follow-up appointments for blood studies in the authorized laboratory
- Follow-up appointments with the physician at recommended intervals

Documentation requirements

- Patient and caregiver education, including instruction on wound care, safety, activity, diet, and medications
- Skilled assessment of the wound site, including measurements, description, photographs, and specific signs and symptoms of complications (the patient must sign a consent form for the wound to be photographed)
- Patient and caregiver participation in wound care
- Activity level and safe use of adaptive equipment
- Pertinent body systems
- Medication management
- Patient response to treatment and progress toward goals
- Stressors affecting patient adherence to the therapeutic regimen
- Safety precautions
- Signs and symptoms to report to the physician
- Infection control measures
- Laboratory results

Reimbursement reminders

- Durable medical equipment is covered under Medicare part B (dressing supplies are only covered if there is a physician order). The patient will be responsible for paying 20% of the allowable charge if the equipment is approved; if it's not approved, the patient is responsible for the entire charge. The charge for dressings may be ab-

sorbed into the agency's costs, depending on policy.

- Five or more visits per week are considered to be daily visits and must have a finite and predictable end.
- Reimbursement requires the documentation of homebound status, variances to expected outcomes, changes to the plan of care, change in patient condition, and patient education provided and the patient's response to it.
- Document all treatments and procedures covered by a physician order.
- Medicare covers phlebotomy supplies.
- Check for an authorized laboratory because many insurance companies have contracts with specific laboratories for processing specimens.
- When billing for medical supplies, always include the name of supply item, date supply was used, number of units used, and charge per unit.

Insurance hints

- Present all data related to wound care, including wound assessment, care, and patient and caregiver education.
- Present objective data regarding wound condition, including pertinent laboratories, measurements, and any changes.
- Present objective data regarding limitations in mobility or activity as related to homebound status.
- Present details of patient education needs and goals.
- Present physician orders and the patient's requests; however, remember that neither will guarantee coverage.

Tracheostomy care

A tracheostomy is the stoma, or opening, made by a surgical incision into the trachea (tracheotomy) for the purpose of establishing an airway. Indications for placement of a tracheostomy tube are relief of upper airway obstruction (for example, tumor, upper airway edema, infection), management of secretions, prevention of aspiration, and long-term mechanical ventilation.

Some tracheostomy tubes have an inner and an outer cannula. The outer cannula stays in place; the inner cannula can be removed for cleaning. The tracheostomy tube is held in place by twill tapes or Velcro straps. A replacement tracheostomy tube should be kept near the patient in the event that the patient's tracheostomy tube is accidentally dislodged.

The presence of a tracheostomy tube makes effective coughing difficult and reduces the patient's ability to raise tracheobronchial secretions. Suctioning is used to remove these secretions and help maintain a patent airway.

Tracheostomy tubes are either cuffed or noncuffed. Cuffed tubes aren't required for all patients but should be used if the patient is at risk for aspiration. Noncuffed tubes are primarily used in long-term situations where there is minimal risk for aspiration and minimal secretions. A fenestrated tracheostomy tube is often used for patients who can swallow without risk of aspiration but still require suctioning. The fenestrated tracheostomy tube has one or more openings on the outer cannula that permit air from the lungs to flow over the vocal cords.

Tracheostomy care is required for patients in the home setting who don't have a caregiver able to provide this care. Able caregivers receive tracheostomy care training in the home.

Previsit checklist

Physician orders and preparation
- Care and teaching orders for each discipline
- Oral medication as indicated
- Aerosol therapy as indicated
- Chest physiotherapy as indicated
- Oxygen orders as indicated
- Activity orders and restrictions
- Orders for blood gas monitoring

Equipment and supplies
- Supplies for standard precautions and sharps disposal
- Oxygen as indicated
- Tracheostomy care supplies, including tracheostomy care kit containing two soaking trays, plastic forceps, sterile gauze pads, sterile precut tracheostomy dressing, cleaning brush, pipe cleaners, sterile applicators (cotton-tipped swabs), sterile drape, and twill tape or Velcro tracheostomy ties; disposable inner cannula or spare nondisposable inner cannula of same size as that currently in use; hydrogen peroxide; sterile and nonsterile gloves; extra tracheostomy tube of same size and type as one currently in place; obturator
- Suction kit containing sterile gloves, container for sterile water or normal saline solution, and sterile suction catheter
- Suction machine with connecting tubing
- Sterile water or normal saline solution

- Manual resuscitation bag connected to oxygen source if indicated

Safety requirements
- Standard precautions for infection control and sharps disposal
- Emergency plan and access to functional phone and list of emergency phone numbers
- Fire evacuation plan, functional smoke detectors, and access to functional fire extinguisher
- Oxygen precautions, safe handling and placement of home oxygen equipment, and notification of local fire and police departments of oxygen use in the home
- Power outage plan (local power companies need to know if a patient in the home requires electrical power for life-support equipment)
- Night-light
- Information on medications, including dosage, adverse effects, interactions, and safe storage
- Proper disposal of expired drugs
- Instructions on signs and symptoms of medical emergency and actions to take

Major diagnostic codes
- Acute laryngotracheitis with obstruction 464.21
- Attention to tracheostomy V55.0
- Cancer
  - of esophagus 150.9
  - head, face, and neck 195.0
  - of larynx 161.9
  - of trachea 162.0
- Foreign body 934
  - in bronchioles or lung 934.8
  - in main bronchus 934.1
  - in trachea 934.0
- Permanent tracheostomy 31.29
- Pneumonia 486
- Revision of tracheostomy 31.74
- Temporary tracheostomy 31.1
- Tracheitis, acute without/with obstruction 464.10/464.11

Defense of homebound status
- Bedridden; requires total care
- Unable to ambulate; requires maximum assistance to transfer from bed to chair
- Unable to ambulate farther than 10' (3 m) due to dyspnea with minimal exertion

Selected nursing diagnoses and patient outcomes

Ineffective airway clearance related to increased pulmonary secretions and difficulty clearing secretions
The patient or caregiver will:
- demonstrate effective coughing and increased air exchange in the lungs (N, PT, RT)
- demonstrate stable physiological status as well as signs and symptoms of improved respiratory status (optimal breathing). (N)

Risk for infection related to tracheostomy
The patient or caregiver will:
- demonstrate an understanding of signs and symptoms of infection (N, RT)
- remain free from signs and symptoms of acute respiratory infection (N)
- demonstrate intact peritracheal skin that is free from signs and symptoms of infection. (N)

Knowledge deficit related to tracheostomy care and disease process

The patient or caregiver will:

• verbalize understanding of disease process related to tracheostomy and purpose of tracheostomy (N)

• demonstrate ability to perform all aspects of tracheostomy care, including suctioning and care of equipment. (N, RT)

Impaired verbal communication related to tracheostomy

The patient or caregiver will:

• demonstrate ability to communicate using alternate forms of communication. (N, SP)

Body image disturbance related to alteration in structure, function, and appearance

The patient or caregiver will:

• demonstrate at least two coping mechanisms, such as participation in a support group and engaging in a hobby or activity (N, OT, SW)

• demonstrate appropriate measures for managing changes in body image and lifestyle, such as not going out on a boat and avoiding situations that increase risk (N, OT, SW)

• verbalize fear of rejection or reactions of others (N, SW)

• demonstrate knowledge of appropriate community resources. (N, SW)

Altered nutrition: Less than body requirements, related to decreased oral intake, altered taste sensation, and difficulty swallowing

The patient or caregiver will:

• demonstrate adequate nutrition and hydration status (N, D)

• maintain weight within planned parameters. (N, D)

Skilled nursing services

Care measures

• Assess for abnormal breathing patterns, sounds, chest movements, secretions, and skin and mucous membrane color.

• Assess for signs of cerebral anoxia, activity intolerance, and chest pain.

• Assess need for suctioning, ability to clear secretions, characteristics of tracheal secretions, peritracheal skin integrity, and swallowing ability.

• Assess for anxiety and depression.

• Assess level of self-care and compliance of patient and caregiver with tracheostomy care, including dressing changes, inner cannula changes, and suctioning.

• Perform a complete systems assessment.

Patient and family teaching

• Explain disease process as well as purpose and ramifications of tracheostomy.

• Provide instruction on all aspects of tracheostomy care, including suctioning; changing dressing, inner cannula, and tracheostomy ties; cleaning reusable equipment with soap and water, then rinsing, air-drying, and storing it in a clean plastic bag; assessing for tracheostomy tube dislodgment and securing or replacing tube; deflating and inflating tracheostomy; inspecting peritracheal skin; and recognizing signs and symptoms of infection.

• Review how and where to obtain necessary equipment and supplies, oxygen use and safety precautions, actions to take for malfunctioning oxygen equipment, and use of backup tank replacements.

• Discuss tracheostomy precautions; for example, avoiding aerosol sprays, preventing aspiration while bathing, and taking precautions while outside.
• Explain how to perform cardiopulmonary resuscitation with a tracheostomy.
• Emphasize need for adequate nutrition and fluid intake of 2 to 3 L daily, unless contraindicated, to liquefy secretions and upright feeding position to prevent aspiration.
• Discuss good oral hygiene.
• Teach deep-breathing exercises.
• Explain alternate means of communication, such as paper and pen, magic slate, communication board, or voice prosthesis.
• Describe energy conservation measures.

Interdisciplinary actions

Dietitian
• Assessment of nutritional status and hydration
• Assessment of the patient's calorie needs and development of a plan to meet those needs
• Instruction in caloric and nutritional needs and goals

Home care aide
• Assistance with personal care and hygiene needs

Occupational therapist
• Instruction in energy conservation techniques and performance of activities of daily living
• Assessment of need for and instruction in use of adaptive equipment

Physical therapist
• Development of and instruction about individualized home exercise program
• Performance of and instruction in pulmonary physical therapy (breathing exercises and chest physiotherapy as indicated)

Respiratory therapist
• Instruction in use of respiratory equipment (nebulizer, oxygen, tracheostomy supplies)
• Instruction in breathing exercises, chest physiotherapy

Social worker
• Referral to community resources (especially those that may assist with expenses of home tracheostomy care) and support groups
• Counseling and referral for stress management and reduction

Speech pathologist
• Recommendation for safe and effective swallowing and communication

Discharge plan
• Effective management of all tracheostomy care by patient and caregiver in the home with physician follow-up services
• Signs and symptoms minimized; death with dignity
• Referral to hospice

Documentation requirements
• Subjective and objective data related to respiratory assessment and assessment of other systems

- Instructions given related to tracheostomy care and precautions
- Skilled procedures performed, including tracheostomy dressing change, inner cannula change, and suctioning
- Understanding of and compliance with all aspects of tracheostomy care
- Progress of patient and caregiver toward educational goals
- Patient response to care
- Specific barriers to learning (for example, impaired vision, and impaired mental status and cognitive ability)
- Absence of available, willing, and able caregiver
- Patient newly diagnosed with tracheostomy
- Patient new to medications, oxygen use, aerosol therapy, or chest physiotherapy
- Specific deficits in initial knowledge level, then progress as evidenced by specific concepts and procedures verbalized and demonstrated

Reimbursement reminders

- When daily visits have been ordered, indicate expected end point of daily visits.
- Obtain a physician order for any plan of care change, and document this in the patient's record.
- Supplies and durable medical equipment covered by Medicare: nebulizer machine (Medicare part B, 80% of allowable charge; physician must indicate that metered-dose inhaler alone is insufficient to treat the patient's symptoms), oxygen (Medicare part B, 80% of allowable charge; patient's oxygen saturation level must be 88% or lower), tracheostomy care supplies (Medicare part B, check with supply company for specific information, such as coverage and quantity).

- Respiratory therapist services are usually provided on a routine or as-needed basis by the company supplying the durable medical equipment.

Insurance hints

- Present objective data about homebound status.
- Present objective patient findings, changes in clinical condition, and changes in care since last contact (for example, new physician orders).
- Present specifics about patient and caregiver education process and progress toward established goals.

Tuberculosis

Tuberculosis (TB) is a preventable and mostly curable disease that requires constant public surveillance. Primarily thought of as a pulmonary disease, it may affect other body parts or body systems, such as the larynx, GI tract, lymph nodes, skin, skeletal system, nervous system, urinary tract, and reproductive system. Extrapulmonary forms of TB may accompany the acquired immunodeficiency syndrome virus. Because of the increasing prevalence of multidrug-resistant TB, initial therapy now consists of treating the disease with at least four different drugs and increased support to encourage adherence to the medical regimen and follow-up care. Transmission of the organism from one person to another must be prevented by strict adherence to respiratory isolation, particularly for persons within the household.

Previsit checklist

Physician orders and preparation
- Use of respiratory isolation
- Initial medication regimen of four drugs
- Nutritional consult to assess current dietary intake
- Social work to assess need for alternative housing and need for contact screening

Equipment and supplies
- Supplies for standard precautions and proper sharps disposal
- Gloves
- Particulate respirator masks
- Alcohol wipes
- Sterile container for sputum for culture and sensitivity testing
- Vacutainers; needles for blood-drawing for culture and sensitivity testing

Safety requirements
- Standard precautions for infection control and sharps disposal
- Chart listing how to apply respiratory isolation precautions to prevent infection of other people in household
- Compliance with local health department codes for reporting active TB cases
- Information on multiple medications, including dosage, adverse effects, interactions, and safe storage

Major diagnostic codes
- Tuberculosis, unspecified (NOS) 011.90

Defense of homebound status
- Severe weakness; out of bed no more than twice daily
- Gait disturbance; unsafe, unsteady gait
- Unable to ambulate farther than 10′ (3 m) unassisted related to extreme fatigue
- Non-weight-bearing status due to infectious disease process of the bones

Selected nursing diagnoses and patient outcomes

Ineffective airway clearance related to increased sputum and fatigue level
Patient or caregiver will:
- increase fluids to 68 oz (2,000 ml) per day to thin secretions so they may be more easily cleared from airway (N)
- arrange for scheduled rest periods at regular intervals throughout the day to prevent overwhelming fatigue. (N)

Knowledge deficit regarding infectious disease process (spread and treatment) related to lack of exposure to information
Patient or caregiver will:
- verbalize method by which TB is spread and measures necessary to prevent transmission of TB (for example, remain on medication regimen, cover mouth and nose when coughing or sneezing, wear a mask as indicated to prevent inadvertent aerosolizing) (N)
- identify basic food groups and explain how nutritionally adequate diet will be achieved (N, D)

- state name, dose, actions, interactions, and adverse effects of prescribed medications (N)
- verbalize knowledge of medication regimen and need for certain drugs to be administered simultaneously (N)
- verbally contract to notify health care provider if, for any reason, medication can't be taken (N)
- state knowledge of scheduled physician's appointments and tests (sputum test or X-ray) (N)
- demonstrate knowledge of signs and symptoms that indicate need for immediate medical care (increased cough, hemoptysis, unexplained weight loss, fever, night sweats). (N)

Skilled nursing services

Care measures
- Perform skilled assessment of mental and cognitive function as well as of respiratory, skeletal, integumentary, GI, nervous, urinary, and reproductive systems.
- Assess the level of care performed by patient and caregiver and adherence to the medication regimen.
- Assess the effectiveness of the treatment regimen: check results of monthly sputum sample, assess for signs and symptoms of complications developing, assess nutritional status.

Patient and family teaching
- Explain about drugs used to treat TB, including name, dose, actions, and adverse effects of prescribed medications, as well as rationale for combining certain drugs.
- Emphasize the importance of thorough follow-up and communication with the physician to improve outcome

(for example, drug interactions, such as the impaired effectiveness of protease inhibitors and nonnucleoside reverse transcriptase inhibitors [used to treat human immunodeficiency virus] when combined with rifampin [used to treat TB] may be avoided).
- Provide a basic understanding of how TB is spread, measures to prevent transmission, symptoms indicating further deterioration, and when to notify nurse or physician.
- Provide basic understanding of foods included in nutritionally sound diet.
- Explain schedule of future physician's appointments.

Interdisciplinary services

Dietitian
- Consultation to determine nutritional needs and meal planning to provide a nutritionally adequate diet

Home care aide
- Assistance with personal care and activities of daily living (ADLs)

Occupational therapist
- Energy conservation techniques to improve ability to perform ADLs
- Need for assistive or adaptive devices (including positioning devices) and teaching

Physical therapist
- Assessment of safety related to transfers and gait
- Assessment of body strength to maintain function, mobility, and range of motion and perform ADLs
- Establishment of home exercise program

Social worker

• Identification of community resources or support services available

• Financial counseling related to loss of job or income due to illness

• Evaluation of patient coping mechanisms and adjustment to chronic illness

Discharge plan

• Safe management of recovery from TB by patient and caregiver with physician follow-up services and community services as needed and without development of long-term complications

Documentation requirements

• Skilled assessment, including subjective and objective data with regard to signs and symptoms of TB and development of systemic involvement

• Results of monthly sputum culture

• Care coordination among multiple disciplines case conferences, team meetings, or phone conferences regarding the patient and findings from social work evaluation

• Patient and caregiver participation in self-care (medication compliance)

• Patient response to care

• Specific deficits in initial knowledge level and progress toward educational goals as evidenced by specific concepts and information demonstrated and verbalized

• Care coordination among the disciplines

• Changes in patient's condition that require continued skilled care or physician contact

• Specific instructions given to patient and family regarding respiratory isolation techniques, infection control precautions, communicable waste disposal, medication regimen and compliance, disease process, home safety, and emergency measures

Reimbursement reminders

• If daily care has been ordered, goals should indicate specific date when daily visits are expected to end.

• Teaching for prevention of complications isn't considered reimbursable under Medicare's home health care benefit.

• Registered dietitian services aren't reimbursable under Medicare.

Insurance hints

• Present objective data about homebound status.

• Present objective patient findings and changes since last contact.

• Report new laboratory values and any change in clinical condition since last contact.

• Present specifics about patient education progress.

Ulcer care, diabetic foot

The development of most diabetic foot ulcers can be linked to distal peripheral neuropathy. Frequently, the ulcer results following minor trauma to a foot that lacks protective sensation. When unnoticed trauma occurs in the presence of impaired peripheral circulation, healing is substantially delayed. Impaired host defenses in the person with diabetes can further complicate

Identifying diabetic foot ulcers

This pie graph illustrates the primary etiology of diabetic foot wounds. The accompanying chart shows characteristics of diabetic foot wounds by etiology.

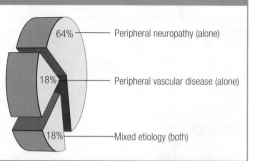

- 64% — Peripheral neuropathy (alone)
- 18% — Peripheral vascular disease (alone)
- 18% — Mixed etiology (both)

ETIOLOGY	TYPICAL PRESENTATION	COMMON MECHANISM OF INJURY	UNDERLYING PATHOLOGY
Peripheral neuropathy	• Plantar surface of foot • Round shape with even borders • Low to moderate drainage	• Minor trauma • Repetitive pressure to plantar bony prominences	• Loss of sensation in lower extremities impairs protective responses • Foot deformities cause abnormal pressure at bony prominences
Peripheral vascular disease	• Gangrenous or necrotic lesions on toes • Decreased temperature of affected extremity	• Trauma	• Impaired circulation delays healing and promotes infection

this sequence by greatly increasing the risk for infection.

Patients with diabetic foot ulcers that don't heal well are prevalent in the home health care setting. (See *Identifying diabetic foot ulcers*.) A variety of wound care regimens, from the simple to the advanced, are available for home treatment. Protocols, guidelines, and wound care teams are frequently used by home care agencies to guide the selection of a wound care regimen.

Because skilled home nursing visits are generally periodic and intermittent, patients and their caregivers must play an active role in the management and treatment of these chronic wounds. They require instruction on the prevention of future ulcer development and also on the development of osteomyelitis. Wound care is dynamic; therefore, treatments and visit frequency require regular evaluation and adjustment. In cases where osteomyelitis has been diagnosed, the patient may begin a regimen of I.V. antibiotics in the home.

Previsit checklist

Physician orders and preparation

- Wound care and treatment orders (cleaning method, type of dressing, and frequency of change)
- Medication orders (oral agents or insulin)
- Diet orders
- Treatment of infection (if applicable), including antibiotic agents and blood cultures
- Blood glucose monitoring, including frequency and timing, target ranges, sliding scale insulin, and parameters for notifying physician of blood glucose results
- Laboratory blood studies, including glycosylated hemoglobin
- Activity orders and restrictions
- Enterostomal therapy evaluation for wound care
- Podiatrist consultation for foot, nail, and wound care
- Dietitian evaluation for diet and teaching about possible increased needs due to ulcer
- Physical therapy evaluation for modified exercise and activity program
- Occupational therapy evaluation for assistance and adaptations secondary to functional limitations imposed by ulcer
- Social work evaluation for community resources and financial assistance for equipment and supplies

Equipment and supplies

- Supplies for standard precautions and proper sharps disposal
- Wound treatment and dressing supplies, including irrigating solutions, dressings, packing, and topical debridement agents
- Blood glucose monitoring supplies, including glucose meter, test strips, lancing device and lancets, and patient blood glucose logbook or diary
- Phlebotomy equipment
- Camera, photography consent form, and supplies to document wound appearance (be sure to follow agency protocol for frequency of photographing wound)

Safety requirements

- Standard precautions for wound care, infection control, and sharps disposal
- System to enable adherence to complex medication regimen, including insulin injections (sliding scale) as appropriate
- Emergency plan and access to functional phone and list of emergency phone numbers
- Signs and symptoms of infection, circulatory impairment, and impaired wound healing
- Emergency treatment measures for hyperglycemia and hypoglycemia
- Foot care and sick day measures
- Allergies

Major diagnostic codes

- Diabetes type 1, uncontrolled 250.03
- Diabetes type 2, uncontrolled 250.02
- Diabetes with peripheral circulatory disorders 250.7

Defense of homebound status

- Non-weight-bearing status on lower extremity due to diabetic foot ulcer or prescribed activity restrictions

• Visual impairment requiring assistance of another person to leave home
• Inability to ambulate farther than 10′ (3 m) due to chronic open lower extremity wound or ulcer

Selected nursing diagnoses and patient outcomes

Impaired skin integrity related to development of diabetic ulcer
The patient or caregiver will:
• exhibit signs of ulcer healing in _____ visits or weeks   (N, ET, PT)
• demonstrate measures to maintain skin integrity of other extremity
  (N, ET, HCA, PO, PT)
• identify nutritional needs related to ulcer   (N, D)
• remain free from signs and symptoms of infection and circulatory impairment on each visit   (N, ET, PT)
• demonstrate procedure for independent wound care by discharge.
  (N, ET, PT)

Risk for injury related to loss of sensation to lower extremities
The patient or caregiver will:
• demonstrate measures to prevent further injury to lower extremities by discharge   (N, OT, PT)
• demonstrate ability to perform self-examination on feet and identify reportable problems.   (N, PO, PT)

Risk for infection related to ulcer development and complications associated with diabetes mellitus
The patient or caregiver will:
• remain free from signs and symptoms of infection throughout duration of care   (N, ET, HCA, PT)

• exhibit vital signs within acceptable parameters   (N, HCA)
• demonstrate appropriate measures to prevent infection   (N, ET, PT)
• identify early signs and symptoms of infection requiring notification of the physician.   (N, ET, PT)

Knowledge deficit related to diabetes self-management and ulcer care
The patient or caregiver will:
• verbalize understanding of diabetic self-management   (N, D)
• demonstrate measures to control blood glucose levels   (N, D)
• perform ulcer care treatment independently by discharge   (N, ET, PT)
• identify danger signs and symptoms to notify physician   (N, ET, PT)
• demonstrate adherence to plan of care and follow-up.
  (N, ET, HCA, MD, OT, PT)

Skilled nursing services

Care measures
• Perform initial skilled assessment of the wound, including information on location; size; depth; presence of necrosis, sinus tracts, and odor; presence and type of exudates; condition and color of wound base; condition of surrounding tissue (warmth, erythema, crepitus, and induration); and signs and symptoms of localized infection.
• Perform skilled assessment of neurovascular status of lower extremities, including extent and amount of edema, circumference measurements, and degree of pitting; skin color and temperature; capillary refill; complaints of pain, including type, onset, duration, frequency, and relief measures; presence of pulses; complaints of numb-

ness or tingling or evidence of paralysis.

- Assess for signs and symptoms of systemic infection, such as fever, chills, and generalized malaise.
- Assess blood glucose control, including patient techniques (blood glucose monitoring and insulin injection), effectiveness of treatment regimen (check patient's blood glucose, refer to patient's logbook, or use memory function of patient's meter), signs and symptoms of hypoglycemia and hyperglycemia, complaints, and measures taken.
- Obtain or arrange for blood studies, including glycosylated hemoglobin.
- Assess effectiveness of treatment regimen.
- Perform wound care as ordered, including cleaning with normal saline solution or other nontoxic agents and applying dressing to protect the wound. Keep ulcer tissue moist, keep surrounding tissue dry, fill wound cavities, and alleviate pressure on wound bed.
- Observe patient's and caregiver's ability to perform prescribed wound care.

Patient and family teaching

- Explain need for complete rest for the injured part as necessary component for healing.
- Describe signs and symptoms of infection to report promptly if they occur.
- Explain that management of blood glucose is essential for wound healing.
- Provide diabetic education to assist in meeting blood glucose target ranges.
- Emphasize importance of adequate nutrition and hydration in wound healing.

- Review wound care and treatment if applicable.
- Detail infection control measures, including safe disposal of soiled dressings.
- Teach how to observe and report wound characteristics.
- Outline measures to prevent future ulceration, including daily care and self-examination of feet with prompt attention to problems, selection of proper footwear, special attention to scar tissue from healed ulcer as it may be prone to breakdown, and regular and ongoing care from a podiatrist.

Interdisciplinary actions

Dietitian

- Evaluation for appropriate dietary plan
- Consultation for complex nutritional needs and optimal diet for wound healing (may include increased fluid, protein, and calorie intake)

Enterostomal therapist

- Evaluation of wound
- Consultation for wound care regimen, including specialized products and equipment

Home care aide

- Assistance with personal care, hygiene, and nutrition
- Infection control measures
- Assistance with ambulation

Occupational therapist

- Evaluation for assistive devices
- Instruction in use of adaptive aids for diabetes self-care (including foot care and wound care) as indicated

• Instruction and assistance for activities of daily living with non-weight-bearing status

Physical therapist
• Mobility assessment
• Exercise program to maintain physical condition while preventing weight bearing to affected area

Podiatrist
• Evaluation for foot deformities that could predispose the patient to future ulceration
• Preventive care in the patient with loss of protective sensation
• Prescription for therapeutic footwear
• Referral to footwear specialist for construction of custom-fit shoes when prescribed

Social worker
• Referral to community resources and support groups for people with diabetes
• Counseling and referral for stress management and reduction
• Financial evaluation and referral for assistance with securing supplies and equipment
• Identification of resources to assist with disability issues related to injury

Discharge plan
• Self-management of disease process in home with physician and community support systems follow-up
• Demonstration of independence in wound care and evidence of healing wound
• Maintenance on antidiabetic medication therapy with blood glucose levels within targeted parameters

• Understanding of measures to prevent recurrence of ulcers and further injury
• Follow-up appointments planned for blood studies and with physician at recommended intervals
• Referral to outpatient physical therapy if indicated

Documentation requirements
• Skilled assessment, including wound care diagnosis and any supporting diagnosis
• Wound assessment, including location (using proper anatomical terms, such as plantar or flexor, distal or proximal, medial or lateral); dimensions (in centimeters); condition of surrounding tissue (for example, macerated, erythematous, and indurated); condition of wound base (for example, color, presence of slough, and eschar); presence or absence of signs and symptoms of infection; and healing progress
• Successive photographs (patient must sign a consent form for the wound to be photographed.)
• Current treatment
• Patient and caregiver ability or inability to perform the procedures
• Recent blood glucose results and adherence to diabetic regimen
• Patient and caregiver instructions, including procedure for wound care, signs and symptoms of healing, danger signs and symptoms (indicating infection or circulatory impairment) to report to physician, dietary plan, home exercise program, infection control and safety measures, measures to reduce risk of complications, signs and symptoms of complications, and use of assistive or adaptive devices

Prescription footwear

Patients who have had a diabetic foot ulcer can reduce their risk for future ulceration by wearing prescription footwear. Special footwear can prevent foot injury by redistributing pressure, controlling extraneous motion, and cushioning the foot. Medicare part B covers 80% of the reasonable cost for special shoes and orthoses for patients who meet certain criteria. Secondary insurance or the patient is responsible for the other 20%.

Who's covered?

Patients with one or more of the following conditions are eligible for Medicare part B coverage of prescription footwear:

- history of partial or complete foot amputation
- history of previous foot ulcer
- history of preulcerative callus
- peripheral neuropathy with callus formation
- foot deformity
- peripheral vascular impairment.

How is coverage obtained?

- Physician certifies that patient has one or more of the above conditions and is being treated for diabetes.
- Physician or podiatrist writes footwear prescription.
- Qualified dispenser (podiatrist or orthotist) constructs and fits the prescribed footwear and files the appropriate claim forms.

Reimbursement reminders

- Long-term wound care is reimbursable under Medicare if the following criteria are documented: the wound is complex and requires skills of a nurse; there is regular contact with physician regarding treatment, orders, and wound progress; and attempts to try new procedures have been made if wound isn't responsive to current treatment.
- Daily wound care is reimbursable under Medicare if the following criteria are documented: daily services are medically necessary, daily care can't be performed less frequently without jeopardizing medical outcome, and there is a predictable and realistic date for ending daily services.
- Medicare reimburses the home care agency for most, but not all, wound care

supplies. Gloves are *not* reimbursable. Check with agency billing department for coverage benefits of specific supplies.

- Medicare will reimburse for some in-home podiatry services and prescription footwear. (See *Prescription footwear.*)
- For coverage of special footwear, the physician certifies that the patient has one or more of the above conditions and is being treated for diabetes. The physician or podiatrist writes the footwear prescription and a qualified dispenser (podiatrist or orthotist) constructs and fits the prescribed footwear and files the appropriate claim forms.

Insurance hints

- Present objective findings and changes in wound status since previous contact, including dimensions. Describe color of wound base and amount of exudate being produced; this will dictate choice of treatment. Note if eschar or signs of infection are present.

• Report recent blood glucose results and patient's adherence to diabetic regimen.

• Describe patient adherence to mobility restrictions and non-weight-bearing status.

• Report patient's and caregiver's level of participation in wound care and treatment.

• Discuss eligibility for prescription footwear and plan for obtaining it after wound has healed.

Ulcerative colitis

Ulcerative colitis is a chronic inflammation of the mucosa and submucosa of the distal colon. Chronic ulceration leads to GI bleeding with remissions and exacerbations of the inflammation. Patients with ulcerative colitis are rarely homebound for long periods of time. As with other chronic illnesses, patients develop a high degree of self-care ability. Patients are more likely to be referred to home care after corrective surgery, which removes portions of the colon, rather than during acute inflammatory episodes. The primary focus for the home care nurse is patient and caregiver education, wound care, and ostomy care.

Previsit checklist

Physician orders and preparation
• Dietary orders and consult
• Activity orders

• Comfort measures and pain control orders
• Wound care if postoperative
• Enterostomal therapy consult
• Order to photograph wound

Equipment and supplies
• Supplies for standard precautions
• Wound care supplies if postoperative from colon surgery, including skin cleaner, dressing supplies, tape, and suture removal kit when ordered
• Camera, film, and a consent form
• Ostomy supplies, including irrigation bag, tubing, and solutions; stoma measurement device; ostomy bags and devices (same size as devices currently in use); odor repellent drops; and stoma paste

Safety requirements
• Standard precautions for infection control
• Emergency plan and access to functional phone and list of emergency phone numbers
• Plan for signs of infection, dehydration, and dehiscence
• Fire evacuation plan, functional smoke detectors, and access to functional fire extinguisher

Major diagnostic codes
• Colitis, membranous 564.1
• Colitis, ulcerative 556.9
• Colitis due to radiation 558.1
• Colostomy, temporary and permanent 46.11 and 46.13
• Ileostomy 46.2

Defense of homebound status

• Unable to ambulate farther than 10′ (3 m) due to fatigue, poor endurance
• Uncontrolled wound or ostomy drainage causing leakage or soiling of clothes
• Pain with movement, out of bed less than twice daily

Selected nursing diagnoses and patient outcomes

Knowledge deficit related to disease process

The patient or caregiver will:
• verbalize medications, actions, and adverse effects for treatment of ulcerative colitis   (N)
• state dietary modifications necessary to control symptoms   (N, D)
• verbalize understanding of disease process and treatment modalities (N)
• state importance of adhering to plan of care as ordered by physician for prevention and control of symptoms (N)
• demonstrate knowledge of wound and ostomy care   (N, ET)
• verbalize knowledge of signs and symptoms of infection, GI bleeding, intestinal obstruction, and dehydration and when to report symptoms to physician.   (N)

Powerlessness related to treatment regimen and complications

The patient or caregiver will:
• identify two things that can be controlled in his or her life   (N, SW)
• express a positive outlook about the future.   (N, SW)

Diarrhea related to GI changes

The patient or caregiver will:
• have normal pattern of elimination and formed stools   (N)
• identify dietary modifications necessary to control gas and diarrhea
                                                            (N, D)
• comply with medication schedule to control diarrhea and pain   (N)
• demonstrate skill in titrating medication to control diarrhea through episodes of remission and exacerbation of inflammation.   (N)

Ineffective individual coping related to negative effects of chronic illness and disability

The patient or caregiver will:
• discuss feelings about illness
                                                         (N, SW)
• participate in treatment planning
                                                         (N, SW)
• identify community support groups and agencies available.   (N, SW)

Altered nutrition: Less than body requirements

The patient or caregiver will:
• maintain weight within limits established by the physician   (N, D)
• be free from signs and symptoms of malnutrition   (N)
• express satisfaction with oral intake.
                                                          (N, D)

Risk for fluid volume deficit related to GI upset

The patient or caregiver will:
• provide mouth care four times a day to maintain intact oral mucous membranes   (N)
• monitor intake and maintain fluid balance   (N, D)
• maintain electrolyte levels within normal limits   (N, D)

• be free from symptoms of dehydration. (N)

Impaired physical mobility related to weakness

The patient or caregiver will:
• demonstrate measurably increased strength and endurance in activities of daily living (ADLs), ambulation, and transfers (N, OT, PT)
• demonstrate deep-breathing and range-of-motion exercises to maintain functional capacity. (N, OT, PT)

Knowledge deficit related to GI alterations and surgical procedure

The patient or caregiver will:
• verbalize one nonpharmacologic method of pain relief, such as relaxation (N)
• express understanding and purpose of ostomy in relation to ulcerative colitis (N, ET)
• demonstrate understanding of all aspects of wound and ostomy care, including emptying bags, cleaning site, irrigation, danger signs, and symptoms to recognize. (N, ET)

Sleep pattern disturbance related to GI discomfort

The patient or caregiver will:
• express satisfaction with sleep patterns (N)
• demonstrate one relaxation technique to aid in sleeping (N)
• limit stimulants, such as caffeine, in the evening. (N)

Skilled nursing services

Care measures
• Perform initial full assessment, including GI function, nutrition and hydration, elimination, skin and mucous membrane appearance; also assess for signs of infection, obstruction, or increased pain levels.
• Perform skilled assessment of surgical site, including wound location, dimensions, condition of surrounding tissue (for example, macerated, erythematous, indurated); condition of wound base (for example, color, presence of eschar); color of surrounding tissue, granulation, drainage, edema, and odor; also assess and measure wound or Hemovac drainage.
• Provide postoperative wound care, as indicated and ordered; culture wound and track results. Communicate results to other health team members.
• Monitor patient's response to care and medications; assess patient's response to plan of care and contact physician for needed changes in plan; and assess effectiveness of treatment.
• Assess emotional response to illness and effectiveness of coping mechanisms.
• Implement ordered bowel regimen and monitor for constipation related to pain medications or diarrhea related to antibiotics.
• Assess self-care for patient and family related to poor endurance.

Patient and family teaching
• Describe signs and symptoms of infections and possible complications.
• Review pain control (pharmacologic and nonpharmacologic).
• Emphasize maintenance of oral intake (adequate fluids and fiber).
• Teach about prevention of diarrhea (foods to avoid, medication effects, and adverse effects).
• Discuss surgical wound care or ostomy care, including ostomy irrigation;

appliance changes; bag changes; skin care and preparation before applying devices; cleaning reusable equipment with soap and water before rinsing, air-drying, and storing in clean plastic bags; obtaining equipment and supplies; assessing for appliance fit, skin breakdown, and infection; customizing appliance fit; and protecting skin.

Interdisciplinary actions

Dietitian
• Instructions on modifications of diet to control symptoms of disease

Enterostomal therapist
• Consultation for ostomy care

Occupational therapist
• Instruction in energy conservation with ADLs and increased endurance

Physical therapist
• Assessment for safety in ADLs, ambulation, and transfers
• Instruction in home exercise program

Social worker
• Information and referrals for community services and psychosocial support and coping, especially those that may assist with expenses of ostomy care

Discharge plan
• Return to independent status after recovery from acute GI inflammation or surgery
• Effective wound care and ostomy care by patient in home with physician follow-up

• Discharge to care of physician for follow-up of medication regimen

Documentation requirements
• Skilled assessment, including the patient's response to care, effectiveness of pain control, effectiveness of dietary modifications, elimination pattern, and appearance of stoma
• Patient and caregiver instruction, including dietary modifications, diarrhea prevention and control, activity restrictions, fluid and hydration status, wound care, and ostomy care
• Interdisciplinary team communication and changes to plan of care
• Homebound status as needed for coverage of Medicare and other insurance

Reimbursement reminders
• Identify factors causing homebound status, action plan, and target date for discharging from home care.
• Identify factors affecting the patient's ability to be independent in care, such as denial or decreased attention span due to pain and fatigue.
• Describe the stages of wound healing for incision and progression toward intact skin and mucous membranes.
• All nonroutine supplies must be specifically ordered by the physician and entered into Locator 14 (Supplies) of Health Care Financing Administration Form 485, or ordered by the physician within specific order for treatment requiring use of certain supplies and entered into Locator 21 (Orders for Treatment).
• When billing for medical supplies, include the following information: name of supply item, date item was

used, number of units used, and charge per unit.

Insurance hints
- Identify progress toward goals.
- Describe healing of surgical wound incision.
- Describe gains in knowledge, such as skills and concepts mastered in relaxation, prevention of reoccurrence of inflammation, and independence with ostomy care.
- Present specific data on homebound status.
- Emphasize the next step in care; show that there is a progressive plan for independence.
- Note any comorbid conditions, such as diabetes or chronic lung or heart disease, that would affect the patient's ability to provide self-care.

Unna's boot therapy

Unna's boot therapy, first described in the 1890s, is one of the most common forms of compression dressings for chronic leg ulcers. Success is often limited, however, and treatment generally involves many weeks of therapy. The patient may not meet Medicare eligibility criteria for the entire duration of care as he often isn't homebound. Varicose ulcers resulting from venous insufficiency achieve the best result from Unna's boot therapy; it generally isn't considered effective for ulcers resulting from arterial disease. The treatment involves wrapping the affected extremity with a bandage that has a mixture of glycerin, zinc, and a gelatin in it. Unna's boots can be changed from once per day to weekly; they can be open- or close-heeled. Home care focuses on assessment of the wound, educating the patient or caregiver, and maximizing independence.

Previsit checklist

Physician orders and preparation
- Wound care orders
- Activity and transfer orders
- Diet orders to encourage wound healing
- Comfort measures and pain control
- Review notes of other team members to coordinate care
- Consent for photographing wound if planning to take pictures

Equipment and supplies
- Supplies for standard precautions
- Wound care supplies, including tape; elastic bandage; biologic dressings impregnated with gelatin, zinc, and glycerin; biohazard bag for discarding dressings; and wound cleaner or normal saline
- Camera for photographing wound per agency policy, film for camera, and a consent form

Safety requirements
- Standard precautions for infection control
- List of danger signs and symptoms to report to physician, including those that indicate hemorrhage, infection, and contracture
- Identification and correction of environmental hazards and patient-specific concerns, such as night-lights and clear pathways for wheelchair or other assistive devices
- Avoidance of sitting for long periods of time; elevation of leg

Major diagnostic codes

- Coronary atherosclerosis, unspecified 414.00
- Decubitus ulcer 707.0
- Heredity and familial telangestasis resulting in ulcers 448.0
- Peripheral vascular insufficiency, unspecified 443.9
- Varicose vein of lower extremities with ulcer/with inflammation/with ulcer and inflammation 454.0/454.1/454.2

Defense of homebound status

- Non-weight-bearing status related to leg ulcers
- Unable to ambulate due to prescribed activity restrictions
- Unable to transfer from wheelchair to car without assistance

Selected nursing diagnoses and patient outcomes

Knowledge deficit related to diagnosis and use of Unna's boot

The patient or caregiver will:
- demonstrate knowledge of nutritional requirements for wound healing and any specific diet orders (such as a diabetic diet)   (N, D)
- verbalize knowledge of community agencies who are able to provide food in home if no caregiver is available and patient isn't able to purchase and prepare food due to non-weight-bearing status

(N, SW)
- demonstrate standard precautions for infection control with dressing technique, activity, and transfer

(N, OT, PT)

- demonstrate knowledge of proper use of Unna's boot, including safe use of equipment, and name and number of durable medical equipment company to be contacted if repair or replacement is necessary   (N)
- demonstrate and verbalize infection control principles   (N)
- identify signs and symptoms of infection and hemorrhage to report to the physician   (N)
- verbalize and demonstrate proper skin hygiene   (N)
- demonstrate and verbalize correct dressing change technique of Unna's boot.   (N)

Altered physical mobility related to venous ulcer

The patient or caregiver will:
- demonstrate elevation of leg as ordered and compliance with activity restrictions as ordered   (N, OT, PT)
- demonstrate increased levels of strength and endurance in performing activities of daily living   (N, OT, PT)
- perform range-of-motion exercises or home exercise program as prescribed by physician and therapist

(N, OT, PT)
- maintain activity within prescribed limitations.   (N, OT, PT)

Pain related to venous insufficiency

The patient or caregiver will:
- verbalize knowledge of use, actions, and adverse effects of medications for pain control   (N, PH)
- identify at least one nonpharmacologic method of pain relief, such as deep breathing or relaxation techniques (N)
- achieve pain relief   (N)
- express understanding of factors precipitating pain   (N)

• perform activities to minimize pain, for example, progressive ambulation. (N, OT, PT)

Body image disturbance related to chronic leg ulcer
The patient or caregiver will:
• verbalize understanding of change in body. (N)

Skilled nursing services

Care measures
• Perform skilled assessment of cardiovascular and integumentary systems and nutrition and hydration status
• Assess self-care for patient and family related to safe transfer, wound care; and observe as they perform dressing change.

Patient and family teaching
• Detail signs and symptoms of infection.
• Emphasize need for elevation of affected leg.

Interdisciplinary actions

Occupational therapist
• Use of adaptive equipment and energy conservation measures

Physical therapist
• Strength and endurance training of muscles
• Development of home exercise program

Social worker
• Referrals for community services (such as Meals On Wheels)

Discharge plan
• Safe management by patient and caregiver of Unna's boot therapy, disease process, and transfers in the home with physician follow-up

Documentation requirements
• Skilled assessment, including patient's response to care, adjustment to body image, and effectiveness of pain control
• Wound care assessment, including changes in the size and character of ulcer (dimensions, color, drainage, odor, and wound edge appearance) and patient or caregiver's ability to provide care related to dressing change
• Patient and caregiver progress toward educational goals
• Interdisciplinary team communication and changes to plan of care

Reimbursement reminders
• Dressing supplies are covered by Medicare; managed care plans may require that dressings be obtained from a specific provider.

Insurance hints
• Record progress toward goals; for example: "Wound care was q.d. now is q.o.d, will go to twice a week beginning ___[date]; wound healing: ulcer size has decreased by ___%."
• Describe adjustment to such issues as patient's resistance or acceptance to providing self-care, dressing changes, and activity; progress toward goals in self-care for hygiene and dressings.
• Describe gains in knowledge (skills and concepts mastered).

- Present specific data on homebound status (such as prescribed leg elevation most of day and inability to transfer without assistance).
- Emphasize the next step in care; show that there is a progressive plan for patient to assume wound care.
- Note any comorbid conditions, such as diabetes and chronic lung or heart disease, that would affect the patient's ability to provide self-care and delay wound healing.

Urinary catheter care, indwelling

Patients may have an indwelling urinary (Foley) catheter following a surgical procedure or for other reasons, such as obstruction from tumors or scarring and strictures of the urethra. An indwelling catheter can be easily managed at home with the use of a few guidelines for positioning of the drainage bag, keeping the system closed, emptying the drainage bag, and proper perineal cleaning. Patient and caregiver education is the key to successful management of the indwelling urinary catheter system. Education about prevention of infections and complications and symptoms to report to the nurse or physician is of primary importance. An indwelling urinary catheter doesn't qualify a patient for homebound status; therefore, a primary diagnosis that resulted in the need for the catheter would have to be the focus of the plan of care.

Previsit checklist

Physician orders and preparation
- Irrigation or instillation frequency
- Catheter insertion date
- Catheter care
- Hydration status
- Activity orders and restrictions
- Oral medications

Equipment and supplies
- Supplies for standard precautions
- Catheter (size)
- Urinary drainage bag
- Device for securing urinary catheter tube (Velcro or rubber)
- Irrigation or instillation needs

Safety requirements
- Standard precautions for infection control and disposal of supplies
- Preventive skin care
- Instructions about signs and symptoms of medical emergency and actions to take
- Specific warning about ambulation and increased risk of falls from tripping on tubing
- Resource person

Major diagnostic codes
- Digestive-genital tract fistula, female 619
- Hyperplasia of prostate 600
- Neurogenic bladder 596.54
- Other specified disorders of the urinary tract 599.8
- Prolapse of vaginal wall 618.0
- Stricture of ureter 593.3
- Urinary incontinence, unspecified 788.30
- Urinary obstruction 599.6

- Urinary tract infection, unspecified 599.0

Defense of homebound status

- Unable to ambulate farther than 10′ (3 m) due to pain secondary to surgery
- Bedridden
- Unable to ambulate farther than 10′ secondary to disease process (such as multiple sclerosis, spinal cord injury, or head trauma resulting in neurogenic bladder)

Selected nursing diagnoses and patient outcomes

Knowledge deficit related to indwelling urinary catheter
    The patient or caregiver will:
- verbalize knowledge of signs and symptoms of urinary tract infections and preventive measures   (N)
- demonstrate proper techniques for change of drainage and leg bag by return demonstration   (N)
- identify prevention techniques for keeping urinary meatus clean and free from infection   (N)
- demonstrate and verbalize correct techniques for maintenance of flow of urine and emptying catheter bag. (N)

Altered urinary elimination related to indwelling catheter
    The patient or caregiver will:
- record adequate urine output and characteristics of urine   (N)
- verbalize signs and symptoms of urinary tract infection and when to report to nurse or physician   (N)
- drink 8 to 10 glasses of water or juice daily.   (N)

Body image disturbance related to changed urinary elimination patterns
    The patient or caregiver will:
- verbalize positive self-worth   (N)
- accept indwelling urinary catheter as a part of daily routine.   (N)

Altered sexuality patterns related to indwelling urinary catheter
    The patient or caregiver will:
- adapt lifestyle and identify where to obtain current information on options for incontinence and impotence   (N, SW)
- discuss alternate forms of intimacy.   (N, SW)

Skilled nursing services

Care measures
- Perform skilled assessment of mental and cognitive function, hydration status, and integumentary, reproductive, and genitourinary systems.
- Assess level of care of patient and caregiver; observe how they perform catheter care and emptying of urinary drainage bag.
- Assess amount of urinary drainage, color and odor of drainage, and fluid intake.

Patient and family teaching
- Teach about indwelling urinary catheter care, including where and how to get supplies, changing catheters, changing and cleaning urinary drainage bags, use of tape or security devices (Velcro and rubber devices), and use of irrigation or instillation supplies.
- Describe signs and symptoms of infection and provide an action plan.
- Emphasize role of hydration in keeping urinary tract clean and need to pre-

vent dehydration; encourage drinking 8 to 10 glasses of water or juice per day and seeking attention for signs and symptoms of dehydration.

• Discuss using clean technique with any catheter care to prevent urinary infection.

Interdisciplinary actions

Home care aide
• Assistance with activities of daily living, such as bathing and range-of-motion exercises
• Assistance with nutrition through meal preparation

Physical therapist
• Development of and instruction about an increased exercise and activity endurance program

Social worker
• Counseling for issues relating to chronic illness

Discharge plan
• Safe management of indwelling urinary catheter care by the patient and caregiver in the home with physician follow-up services

Documentation requirements
• Subjective and objective data regarding indwelling urinary catheter care, including hydration, urinary elimination factors, catheter insertion site, and sexuality concerns; indwelling urinary catheter type; and time and frequency of changing

• Participation of patient and caregiver in care
• Progress of patient and caregiver toward educational goals
• Response of patient and caregiver to care

Reimbursement reminders
• Indwelling urinary catheter supplies are covered by Medicare and most third-party payers.
• Catheters, irrigation sets, drainage bags, skin care ointment, dressings, and security devices are based on type of system utilized.
• Registered dietitian services aren't reimbursable under Medicare benefit pending certain conditions.
• Record patient response to treatment, variances to expected outcomes, barriers to learning (physical deformities, visual impairment), and availability of support person.
• Obtain a telephone order for any plan of care change and record in the patient's chart.
• Identify initial level of knowledge and progress to educational goals.

Insurance hints
• Present objective data about homebound status.
• Report any new laboratory findings that change plan of care.
• Report specifics about client learning progress, such as acceptance or resistance to independent catheter care, leaving home, and handling complications.

Valvular heart disease

Heart disease, as both a primary and a secondary diagnosis, covers a large number of patients receiving home health care. Valvular diseases of the heart can be congenital, but are most often a chronic acquired disease of any of the four cardiac valves. The patient may have a resulting obstruction (stenosis) or insufficient closure (regurgitation) due to valvular degeneration. More than one valve may be involved, and both stenosis and regurgitation may be present. Home health care of these patients depends on the symptoms presented and the severity of the disease. Complications include heart failure due to a decreased cardiac output and arrhythmias.

Previsit checklist

Physician orders and preparation
- Weight parameters
- Dietary limitations
- Fluid restrictions
- Activity limitations
- Medications, including antiarrhythmic drugs and anticoagulant drugs
- Laboratory specimens, including prothrombin time and international normalized ratio
- Oxygen

Equipment and supplies
- Supplies for standard precautions and proper sharps disposal
- Scale
- Venipuncture supplies
- Oxygen tank and tubing

Safety requirements
- Standard precautions for infection control and sharps disposal
- Instructions about signs and symptoms of complications and actions to take
- Functional limitations due to decreased endurance
- Preoperative patient teaching if indicated
- Oxygen precautions, safe handling and placement of home oxygen equipment, and notification of local fire and police departments of oxygen use in the home
- Use of antibiotic prophylactically, such as for dental procedures

Major diagnostic codes
- Aortic insufficiency, congenital 746.3
- Aortic regurgitation, congenital 746.4
- Atrial fibrillation 427.31
- Congestive heart failure 428.0
- Dysrhythmias 427.9
- Endocarditis, acute and subacute 421
- Hypertension, benign/malignant 401.1/401.0
- Mitral insufficiency, congenital 746.6
- Mitral stenosis, congenital 746.5
- Multiple vessel percutaneous transluminal coronary angioplasty 36.05
- Pacemaker V45.0
- Tricuspid stenosis, congenital 746.1
- Valve replacement, unspecified 35.20

Defense of homebound status
- Cardiac restrictions on activity
- Poor endurance related to decreased cardiac output

- Dyspnea on exertion, unable to walk farther than 10′ (3 m) without resting
- Bedridden or confined to chair; out of bed no more than twice daily

Selected nursing diagnoses and patient outcomes

Decreased cardiac output related to mechanical factors

The patient or caregiver will:

- demonstrate stable cardiovascular and respiratory status as defined by _____ (parameters)   (N)
- achieve laboratory values within normal limits by _____(date)   (N)
- demonstrate adherence to plan of care as demonstrated and verbalized by caregiver and patient findings
                                        (N, OT, PT)
- report decrease in shortness of breath and chest pain by _____(date).
                                                        (N)

Risk for injury related to activities of daily living

The patient or caregiver will:

- demonstrate increasing levels of strength and endurance while performing transfers, ambulation, and other activities of daily living (ADLs)
                                        (N, OT, PT)
- demonstrate knowledge of safety factors to be used to prevent falls and injuries   (N, OT, PT)
- demonstrate compliance with range-of-motion exercises and home exercise program   (N, OT, PT)
- demonstrate use of proper techniques for transfers in order to maintain safety.   (N, OT, PT)

Knowledge deficit related to disease process

The patient or caregiver will:

- demonstrate knowledge of use, adverse effects, and interactions of anticoagulant therapy medications   (N)
- demonstrate knowledge of bleeding precautions (anticoagulation therapy)
                                                        (N)
- verbalize understanding of and adhere to medication regimens   (N)
- state importance of monitoring weight and reporting gains or losses outside of parameters to physician
                                                    (N, MD)
- verbalize knowledge of bowel program and report regular bowel movements   (N)
- demonstrate knowledge of disease process and signs and symptoms to report to physician.   (N)

Ineffective individual coping

The patient or caregiver will:

- contact and use identified community support systems and resources
                                                    (N, SW)
- adapt lifestyle to relieve symptoms and improve quality of life (N, OT, SW)
- demonstrate at least two acceptable coping mechanisms, such as seeking assistance and verbalizing feelings.
                                                    (N, SW)

Skilled nursing services

Care measures

- Perform skilled assessment of all body systems, especially cardiopulmonary.
- Monitor vital signs and weight.
- Assess fluid status, intake and output, and presence of edema.
- Observe for jugular vein distention.
- Auscultate for extra heart sounds and murmurs.

- Prepare for surgical intervention as indicated.
- Monitor amount and type of exercise.
- Assess emotional response to illness and effectiveness of coping mechanisms.
- Monitor lifestyle adaptation methods.
- Monitor medication use and adverse effects.
- Implement bowel regimen.
- Assess the patient's response to care plan and report to physician.
- Perform venipuncture per physician orders.

Patient and family teaching

- Demonstrate how to take a radial pulse.
- Emphasize the need to measure intake and output and record daily weights using the same scale.
- Discuss the ordered exercise program or therapy plan.
- Describe coping mechanisms and relaxation methods.
- Teach about medication use, contraindications, and adverse effects.
- Identify diet changes as indicated.
- Explain energy conservation techniques.
- Review safe use and care of home oxygen if indicated.
- Identify signs and symptoms to report to physician and indicate when to call emergency medical personnel.
- Emphasize the importance of compliance to the treatment plan.

Interdisciplinary actions

Dietitian

- Patient teaching regarding hydration and nutrition
- Education regarding specific diet and restrictions

Home care aide

- Assistance with personal care and ADLs

Occupational therapist

- Evaluation of and education in energy conservation techniques

Physical therapist

- Evaluation of and instruction about cardiac exercise program for increased endurance and strength and safe mobility

Social worker

- Evaluation and identification of problems that would benefit by referrals to appropriate community resources
- Psychosocial counseling

Discharge plan

- Patient remains safely at home with a return to self-care and physician follow-up
- Referral to outpatient services when no longer homebound

Documentation requirements

- Skilled assessment, including cardiopulmonary status, progress toward goals, and indicated subjective and objective signs and symptoms: irregular pulse changes, murmurs, arrhythmias;

weight and fluid status; shortness of breath and abnormal breath sounds; and activity tolerance changes

• Specific care, treatments, and medications administered

• Instructions given, demonstrated, and provided in writing

• Patient and caregiver response to care and instructions

• Coordination of patient care with other members of the health care team

Reimbursement reminders

• Identify progress toward goals.

• Indicate level of skilled assessment and evaluation of patient signs and symptoms beyond what the patient could assess (for example, apical pulse rate and rhythm, or heart sounds).

• Ensure that any schedule changes by any team member have an accompanying order from the physician.

• Record laboratory results and notification of the physician with the visit note.

• Record medication changes and specific need to monitor the patient's response to change.

• Identify any barriers to learning, resulting in the need for ongoing visits.

• Continuously document multidisciplinary planning and communication.

• Blood-drawing supplies are considered routine and are nonbillable.

Insurance hints

• Determine how often to report clinical conditions, and always notify the physician immediately if patient changes affect initial care planning frequency or duration.

• Present objective data specific to patient's established goals.

• Identify possible barriers to care and learning.

• Update progress toward specific goals.

Venous leg ulcer

Venous leg ulcers are chronic, commonly recurrent wounds that can take months to heal. Typically irregularly shaped and producing copious drainage, venous ulcers are most likely to develop at the medial malleolus. The ulcers may be painful and cause sensations of aching, stinging, or burning. Patients with a history of thrombophlebitis and lower extremity edema are at highest risk for the development of venous leg ulcers. Effective treatment of this problem addresses two areas — local wound care and the reduction of underlying venous hypertension.

Venous leg ulcers are usually associated with an impairment of valvular function in one or both of the lower extremities. The increased pressure gradient allows blood to pool in the areas of highest gravity, causing fluid leaks from the capillaries. As a result, edema makes the skin vulnerable to injury. These wounds are complicated by impaired healing processes that result from compromised circulatory status.

Compression bandages are the cornerstone of therapy for patients with venous ulcers. Traditionally, the rigid compression dressing using impregnated nonelastic gauze (Unna's boot) has been the gold standard of treatment. Recently, multilayer flexible compression bandages are advocated for their ability to sustain a more effective compression for up to a week while absorbing wound exudates. Aggressive treatment for severe ulcers may include use of mechanical intermittent compression pumps, skin grafting, or the use of growth factors.

Local wound care of the venous ulcer usually consists of a primary dressing to manage drainage. The most important factor in dressing selection is the amount of exudate produced by the wound. Alginates, fiber dressings, and foams are indicated for wounds with moderate to large amounts of drainage. As drainage is absorbed into the dressing, the wound surface moisture should be maintained to promote a moist healing environment. Care for these patients focuses on wound care, skilled assessment of the wound, and education of patient and caregivers regarding dressing change technique, signs of complications such as infection and vascular compromise, and prophylactic measures to minimize the risk of recurrences.

Previsit checklist

Physician orders and preparation
- Local wound treatment orders, including cleaning method, dressing type (for example, alginate, hydrocolloid, foam, or gel) and frequency of change
- Compression dressing orders, including type of dressing (for example, elastic bandage, Unna's boot, or multilayer dressing) and frequency of application
- Activity restrictions or rehabilitation orders as indicated
- Pain control instructions
- Consent to photograph wound

Equipment and supplies
- Wound care supplies, including bandages and dressings
- Supplies for standard precautions and proper sharps disposal
- Blood glucose monitoring supplies
- Camera, film, and consent form

Safety requirements
- List of danger signs and symptoms to report to the physician, including those indicating infection and neurovascular compromise
- Standard precautions for infection control and sharps disposal
- Information on medications, including dosage, adverse effects, interactions, and safe storage
- Allergies documented
- Emergency plan and access to functional phone and list of emergency phone numbers
- Identification and correction of environmental hazards and patient-specific concerns (for example, nightlights, clear paths, and no sharp corners, to prevent falls)

Major diagnostic codes
- Chronic venous insufficiency, without ulceration 459.81
- Ulcer of lower limb, except decubitus 707.1
- Varicose veins of lower extremities with ulcer/with inflammation/with ulcer and inflammation 454.0/454.1/454.2

Defense of homebound status
- Lower extremity rest and elevation required to promote wound healing

- Unable to ambulate farther than 10′ (3 m) due to severe pain of lower extremity wound

Selected nursing diagnoses and patient outcomes

Knowledge deficit related to self-care management

The patient or caregiver will:

- express interest in self-care and desire to understand disease process (N)
- verbalize and demonstrate understanding of wound care, medication regimen, nutrition, fluid intake parameters, prevention of injury, and promotion of health (such as weight reduction and cessation of smoking).
(N, D, ET, PT)

Impaired skin integrity

The patient or caregiver will:

- experience healing of open wound in _____ visits or weeks without signs or symptoms of infection or complications (N, ET)
- verbalize signs and symptoms for which to call physician (N, ET)
- demonstrate proper wound care.
(N, ET)

Fluid volume excess

The patient or caregiver will:

- demonstrate proper lower extremity positioning and exercises to improve venous return in _____ visits or weeks (N, OT, PT)
- verbalize rationale and demonstrate nonpharmacologic measures to decrease edema (N, OT, PT)
- have no more than +1 lower extremity edema in _____ visits or weeks.
(N)

Pain (specify type and location)

The patient or caregiver will:

- rate pain at 3 or less on a 0-to-10 scale 80% of the time (N)
- verbalize adverse effects and interactions of analgesic use and plan of action to minimize or prevent same (including constipation, decreased mental alertness, and lethargy) (N)
- demonstrate nonpharmacologic measures to treat pain, such as distraction, positioning of affected area, and relaxation and visualization exercises.
(N)

Risk for injury related to lower extremity edema

The patient or caregiver will:

- have no further injury to lower extremities at discharge
(N, HCA, OT, PT)
- verbalize knowledge of safety techniques to avoid injury
(N, OT, PT)
- identify potential hazards and state how to adapt the environment to minimize or eliminate hazards.
(N, OT, PT)

Skilled nursing services

Care measures

- Provide skilled assessment of vital signs, skin, cardiopulmonary function, nutritional status, lower extremities (edema and induration, color and temperature, and pulses), and wound (location, size, appearance, and surrounding tissue changes).
- Provide skilled care to local wound (cleaning and dressing) and apply compression measures.

Patient and family teaching

• Emphasize importance of keeping affected extremity elevated and positioned properly as much as possible to decrease edema and promote healing.

• Explain the purpose and importance of diuretic medication if ordered.

• Review fluid intake parameters as ordered by the physician.

• Discuss maintenance of adequate nutrition to promote wound healing.

• Teach how to protect lower extremities from further injury.

• Identify signs and symptoms of infection that should be reported.

• Review use of analgesics as ordered.

• Explain how weight reduction and smoking cessation can lead to improved outcomes and decrease the risk for recurrence (if applicable).

• Teach that the use of topical emollients on lower extremities may cause stasis dermatitis and should be avoided.

• Explain that after healing is achieved, compression hosiery should continue to be worn whenever ambulatory.

• Emphasize that the physician should be notified immediately should severe chest pains begin or if other signs and symptoms of thrombus or embolus occur.

Interdisciplinary actions

Dietitian

• Education regarding diet and hydration

Home care aide

• Assistance with bathing, hygiene, and grooming

• Meal preparation and light household duties

Physical therapist

• Strengthening to aid in position changes

• Mobility exercises to improve venous return

Social worker

• Referral to community resources

• Financial assistance as needed

Discharge plan

• Management of venous ulcer by patient and caregiver in the home with physician and community support systems follow-up services

• Referral to outpatient services

• Continued home care visits for homebound patient with skilled care needs

Documentation requirements

• Correct statement of wound care diagnosis and any supporting diagnosis

• Wound assessment to include location (using proper anatomical terms such as anterior or posterior, medial or lateral); dimensions (in centimeters), including depth and condition of surrounding tissue (for example, macerated or erythematous); condition of wound base (for example, color, presence of slough, and moisture); presence or absence of signs and symptoms of infection; progress of healing; and current treatment

• Patient and caregiver ability or inability to perform the procedures

Reimbursement reminders

• Long-term wound care is reimbursable under Medicare if the following criteria are documented: wound is complex and requires the skills of a nurse; there is regular contact with the physician regarding treatment, orders, and wound progress; and attempts to try new procedures have been made if the wound isn't responsive to current treatment. (Most of these items can be documented by using photos, but patient permission is needed to release the photograph.)

• Daily wound care is reimbursable under Medicare if the following criteria are documented: daily services are medically necessary, daily care can't be performed less frequently without jeopardizing medical outcome, and there is a predictable and realistic date for ending daily services.

• Medicare reimburses the home care agency for most but not all wound care supplies. Gloves are *not* reimbursable. Check with agency billing department for coverage benefits of specific supplies.

• All nonroutine supplies must be specifically ordered by the physician and entered into Locator 14 (Supplies) of Health Care Financing Administration Form 485 or ordered by the physician within the specific order for treatment requiring the use of certain supplies and entered into Locator 21 (Orders for Treatment).

• When billing for medical supplies, include the following information: name of supply item, date supply was used, number of units used, and charge per unit.

Insurance hints

• Present objectives, findings, and changes in wound status since previous contact.

• Describe the amount of exudate being produced because this will dictate choice of treatment.

• Objectively describe the current degree of lower extremity edema.

• Describe patient adherence to use of compression devices, lower extremity elevation, and mobility restrictions.

• Present objective findings regarding level of pain and effectiveness of current treatment.

Walker instruction

Walking with the use of assistive devices helps stabilize the patient's gait and assists in preventing injury from falls. Walkers come in a variety of sizes and styles. A simple aluminum walker with front wheels is most commonly used after hip surgery, strokes, and other injuries. The use of a walker alone won't qualify the patient for home care; however, the primary disease or injury for which the patient is receiving skilled intermittent home care would qualify him or her for home instruction in the use of walkers by a physical or occupational therapist. This important education can maintain safety and prevent falls in patients with conditions or diseases that result in a loss of balance, decreased endurance, shortness of breath, syncope, or neuropathy.

Previsit checklist

Physician orders and preparation
- Review of rehabilitation team notes
- Medical orders and activity restrictions
- Physical therapy evaluation for therapeutic exercises and range of motion of affected leg
- Occupational therapy evaluation for use of adaptive equipment

Equipment and supplies
- Orders for any additional needs, such as wound or pin care supplies
- Orders for splints or other assistive devices as needed
- Elevated toilet seat (after hip fracture or replacement)

Safety requirements
- Clear walkways, with furniture, electrical cords, throw rugs, and so on moved or removed as needed to accommodate walker
- Emergency plan and access to functional phone and list of emergency phone numbers
- Identification and correction of environmental hazards and patient-specific concerns (for example, objects placed on low surfaces for patients with hip or knee disorders)

Major diagnostic codes
- Cerebrovascular accident 436
- Chronic obstructive pulmonary disease, NOS 496
- Closed fracture
  – ankle (right or left), unspecified 824.8

  – femur (right or left), unspecified 821.00
  – hip (right or left), unspecified 820.8
  – pelvis, unspecified 808.8
- Congestive heart failure 428.0
- Degenerative joint disease, hip/lower leg or knee 715.95/715.96
- Hip replacement (total right or left) 81.51
- Neuropathy (unspecified) 357.9
- Parkinsonism, primary/secondary 332.0/332.1
- Syncope 780.2

Defense of homebound status
Because use of walker increases patient's ability to ambulate, nurse will need to clearly document functional limitations. The need for a walker isn't sufficient to justify that the patient is homebound; however, the patient may be so debilitated by primary diagnosis that homebound status is clear from functional limitations.
- Activity intolerance; unable to ambulate farther than 10′ (3 m)
- Decreased endurance; unable to ambulate farther than 10′ without increase in symptoms of pain or shortness of breath
- Unable to transfer safely from the bed to a chair
- Unable to ambulate safely due to diagnoses affecting balance

Selected nursing diagnoses and patient outcomes

Knowledge deficit related to use of walker
The patient or caregiver will:

- demonstrate safe and proper walker use (N, OT, PT)
- demonstrate proper posture when using a walker (N, OT, PT)
- demonstrate proper distribution of weight on hands while using a walker. (N, OT, PT)

Pain related to fracture, surgery, or trauma to soft tissue
The patient or caregiver will:
- verbalize proper analgesia use (N)
- demonstrate optimal movement and rate pain at 3 or less on a 0-to-10 scale 80% of the time (N, OT, PT)
- report satisfaction with sleep patterns. (N)

Impaired physical mobility related to hemiparesis
The patient or caregiver will:
- be free from joint contractures (N, OT, PT)
- be free from muscle spasms (N, OT, PT)
- demonstrate increasing levels of strength and endurance in activities of daily living (ADLs) (N, OT, PT)
- demonstrate independence in ADLs through compensatory techniques involving the unaffected side (N, OT, PT)
- improve or maintain functional mobility and range of motion in affected limb (N, OT, PT)
- achieve functional independence (N, OT, PT)
- perform home exercise program as ordered (N, OT, PT)
- express satisfaction with mobility (N, OT, PT, SW)
- maintain activity within prescribed limitations. (N, OT, PT)

Risk for injury related to unsteady gait

The patient or caregiver will:
- remain free from injury or falls (N, OT, PT)
- demonstrate competency in the use of the walker while performing transfers for ADLs, including bathing and toileting (N, OT, PT)
- demonstrate safety through postural control for sitting balance and balance during transfers (N, OT, PT)
- demonstrate increased strength secondary to home therapy programs (N, OT, PT)
- verbalize knowledge of home safety plan to prevent falls (N, OT, PT, SW)
- demonstrate proper walker storage when not in use (N, OT, PT)
- demonstrate knowledge of the durable medical equipment company to contact for repairs or maintenance of equipment (N, OT, PT)
- maintain clear, well-lit walkways to allow space for safe use of the walker (N, OT, PT)
- have access to emergency services and know who to contact in an emergency, including an emergency fire evacuation plan. (N)

Skilled nursing services

Care measures
- Patient may need rehabilitation services only.

Patient and family teaching
- Emphasize injury prevention.

Interdisciplinary actions

Home care aide
- Assistance with hygiene, dressing, and grooming

Occupational therapist
- Assistance with management of ADLs and energy conservation

Physical therapist
- Home exercise program
- Safety planning
- Transfer training
- Strength training

Social worker
- Assistance in obtaining community resources, such as transportation, in-home support services, and medical emergency call buttons if available in the area

Discharge plan
- Return of patient to normal routine following recovery

Documentation requirements
- Description of functional losses or gains in clear terms (feet walked with walker), self-care ability (dressing, feeding, bathing, toileting, and grooming)
- Evaluation of effectiveness of pain control regimen
- Description of plan to improve patient function whenever progress stalls
- Assessment of appropriateness of patient's home environment
- Assessment of long-term needs of patient, suitability of residence, and presence of caregiver

Reimbursement reminders
- Be clear about functional limitations and patient's ability to use a walker, especially upper body strength, presence

of other injuries, and paresis; the need for a walker doesn't make a patient homebound.
- Demonstrate coordination of care with rehabilitation services.
- Order occupational therapy if patient needs energy conservation and work with home care aide in transfers in bathroom.
- Medicare doesn't cover conditions that are essentially "debilitation"; patient must show continued progress toward goals. When patient's progress reaches a plateau, care is considered custodial and patient should be discharged.

Insurance hints
- Describe progressive levels of self-care (dressing, toileting, bathing, and grooming) and ability, including use of adaptive equipment; and emphasize rehabilitation potential.
- Describe progress toward rehabilitation goals, such as safe use of stairs and transfers sitting to standing.
- Describe increased strength and endurance for ambulation and ADLs.
- List the collaborative plan of care for all team members who are providing services.
- Compare and contrast the roles of each rehabilitation team member.
- Explain what care will be needed in the long term, as well as placement issues.
- Describe any comorbid conditions, such as chronic lung disease, and how it affects the patient's use of a walker.

Wound care

Wound care is a common reason for initiating home health care. Management problems can occur due to a combination of factors and situations. The patient's general health, nutritional status, skin texture and turgor, body weight, and mobility are key players in the progression of healing; in addition, friction and shearing forces can cause trauma to the wound site. All of these factors need to be assessed during wound care; good assessment can be helpful in shortening the duration of healing.

Care for these patients focuses on ongoing evaluation of the wound and patient's risk factors for poor healing. Education of patients or caregivers in wound care skills, mobility enhancement, and pain assessment should be done on admission and periodically thereafter as indicated.

Previsit checklist

Physician orders and preparation
- Wound care orders (updated as the wound heals): cleaning method, type of wound, frequency of dressing changes
- Pressure-relieving or support devices
- Dietary restrictions, calorie allowance
- Oral, I.V., or topical medications
- Activity orders and restrictions

Equipment and supplies
- Supplies for standard precautions and proper disposal of sharps and used dressing materials
- Wound care supplies (will vary according to treatment of choice): dressing materials, gloves, cleaning solutions (such as normal saline solution, peroxide, soap and water)
- Nutritional intake and weight log
- Measuring device

Safety requirements
- Standard precautions for infection control and disposal of sharps and used dressing materials
- List of danger signs and symptoms to report to the physician, including signs of infection
- Information on medications, including dosage, adverse effects, interactions, and safe storage
- Allergies documented
- Emergency plan and access to functional phone and list of emergency phone numbers
- Identification and correction of environmental hazards and patient-specific concerns (for example, smoke detectors, night-light and sharp edges to furniture)

Major diagnostic codes
- Disruption of operation wound 998.3
- Dressing of wound 93.57
- Immobilization, pressure, and attention to wound 93.5
- Open wound of hip and thigh without complications 890.0
- Open wound of other and unspecified/multiple sites 879/879.8
- Wound irrigation 96.59

Defense of homebound status
- Bedridden
- Bed rest
- Open, draining, or infected wound
- Non-weight bearing secondary to foot wound
- Unable to ambulate farther than 10′ (3 m) due to lower extremity wound

Selected nursing diagnoses and patient outcomes

Impaired skin integrity
The patient or caregiver will:
• identify causative rationale for prevention and treatment of complications, such as infection, edema, and pain
(N)
• participate in the prescribed treatment plan to promote wound healing
(N, HCA)
• demonstrate progressive healing of wound through progressive reduction in dimensions and healthy granulation.
(N)

Altered nutrition: Less than body requirements related to actual or potential metabolic needs in excess of intake
The patient or caregiver will:
• increase oral intake of protein and high-calorie foods unless otherwise indicated
(N, D)
• demonstrate compliance with recording fluid and food intake (a weekly weight may be indicated) (N)
• verbalize knowledge of special diet and specific nutritional requirements.
(N, D)

Body image disturbance related to changes in appearance secondary to open draining wound
The patient or caregiver will:
• demonstrate at least two new coping methods, such as verbalizing feelings and humor
(N, SW)
• demonstrate willingness and ability to resume self-care and role responsibilities (where possible)
(N)
• initiate new or reestablish existing support systems.
(N, SW)

Skilled nursing services

Care measures
• Provide skilled assessment of mental and cognitive function, nutrition and hydration, and cardiovascular, GI, genitourinary, and integumentary systems.
• Assess wound and stage.
• Assess patient's level of self-care and capabilities of caregiver.
• Perform dressing changes.
• Assess level of pain and effectiveness of pain medication.
• Assess for signs and symptoms of systemic or local infection each visit (such as fever, increased erythema, induration, tenderness, and increased pain).
• Assess wound healing and effectiveness of treatment.
• Describe the appearance of wound (amount and type of drainage, amount of necrotic tissue and granulation, wound color, and presence or absence of odor); also assess for any tunneling, pockets, sinus tracts, or undermining.
• Assess appearance of tissue surrounding wound for maceration, induration, rash, and tape burns, and assess for tenderness.
• Document all assessment information in medical record.
• Assess the cause of the wound and make reversal or improvements of conditions prophylactically; assess environmental factors (bedridden and limited mobility) and contributing factors (such as nutrition factors [underweight, poor intake, or obesity]) for development of pressure ulcer.
• Make sure wound site is free from pressure at all times.
• Encourage as much mobility as possible.

- Clean patient thoroughly after urination and defecation; use moisture barrier ointments to protect skin.
- Apply moisturizing lotions to intact skin immediately after bathing; never massage stage I areas because this may increase tissue damage.
- Keep skin clean and dry; use urinary and fecal collection devices (for example, catheter) if wound contamination is a problem.

Patient and family teaching

- Describe wound care and signs and symptoms of infection.
- Explain methods of pain management and suggest administering pain medication 30 minutes before painful dressing changes.
- Review nutritional practices that promote healing and explain how to keep an intake log.
- Teach range-of-motion exercises and explain that they should be carried out at least three times per day.
- Discuss turning or changing positions every 2 hours; for patients confined to a wheelchair, weight should be shifted every hour while in the chair, and custom cushions should be used to alleviate pressure.
- Demonstrate prevention of pressure from resting on mattress and other hard surfaces.

Interdisciplinary actions

Dietitian

- Consultation for nutritional needs (increased protein and calorie intake to promote healing)

Home care aide

- Personal care

- When indicated, light housekeeping, meal preparation, and laundry

Physical therapist

- Development of and instruction in individualized home exercise program

Social worker

- Counseling and referral to community agencies and support groups

Discharge plan

- Wound healing without signs and symptoms of infection
- Resolution of any infection
- Independence of patient and caregiver with wound care
- Verbalized comprehension of risk factors by patient and caregiver; placement of functioning prevention methods

Documentation requirements

- Skilled assessment of wound sizing and accurate tracking of wound healing; wound should be measured with each visit
- Subjective and objective data related to signs and symptoms of infection and pain management
- Careful recording of wound care given, including patient's response to care and level of pain
- Notation of any changes or stressors in patient or environment
- Notation of factors contributing to wound and measures put in place to promote healing and prevent future trauma
- Participation of patient and caregiver in care

• Nutritional and hydration status, recommended dietary changes, and food diary
• Referrals to and conferences with other disciplines
• Progress of the patient and caregiver toward established goals

Reimbursement reminders

• Accurately record wound healing and measure wound at each visit; most reimbursement agencies still require staging for reimbursement.
• Although some reimbursement agencies will allow skilled home care involvement until wound is healed, many private plans only grant a limited number of visits to be divided among skilled services. Be aware of those constraints and the best use of them. Establish independence with wound care by either patient or caregiver as soon as possible.
• Accurately document any barriers or limitations to learning (such as deformities, visual impairment, and no available, able, and willing caregiver).
• Registered dietitian services aren't reimbursable under current Medicare home care benefits.
• Home care aide services are covered by current Medicare home care benefits as long as a skilled service is present but they're rarely covered by other reimbursement plans.

Insurance hints

• Always have available the most recent wound measurements and dressing type, and be aware of any changes that have occurred.
• Be able to support the need for skilled care, demonstrate need for continued teaching or skilled care (change in wound care, no available caregiver, or patient and caregiver unable to do dressing change).

Maternal-neonatal disorders and treatments

Breast-feeding

Breast-feeding is the easiest, safest, and least expensive method of infant nutrition. It also promotes bonding between mother and child and carries health benefits to both of them. Infant benefits of breast-feeding include passive immunity against illness, proteins to promote brain development and, some researchers believe, lower incidence of hospital readmission for diarrhea and respiratory infections. Breast-feeding promotes involution of the uterus because of hormone production and helps the new mother lose weight more quickly due to the burning of calories involved in milk production. Additionally, it provides satisfaction to the mother that she is meeting her infant's nutritional needs. Another significant benefit of breast-feeding is the time and effort it saves. Breast-feeding is free, convenient, and always available; however, it's sometimes difficult in the initial stages. The new mother may be tired or recovering from surgery. She may worry that the milk produced isn't enough to provide adequate nutrition for the infant. The new mother may also experience common, self-limiting problems, such as breast engorgement, sore nipples, or difficulty in let-down of milk. All of these problems can be greatly reduced through patient education and with the support of the health care team and family.

Previsit checklist

Physician orders and preparation
• Order indicating the need for the visit
• Delivery information, including route of delivery and medications used during birth
• Infant information, including time of delivery, birth weight, discharge weight, and any concurrent medical problems or nutritional needs

Equipment and supplies
- Infant scale
- Documentation forms
- Educational handouts
- Breast pump, if applicable

Safety requirements
- Standard precautions for infection control
- Newborn safety checklist

Major diagnostic codes
- Disorders relating to high birth weight and long gestation 766
- Extreme immaturity (birth weight less than 1,000 g (2 lb) and gestation less than 28 completed weeks) 765.0
- Feeding problems in the newborn 779.3
- Fetal growth retardation, unspecified 764.9
- Fetal malnutrition without mention of small for gestational age (SGA) 764.2
- Neonatal dehydration 775.5
- Neonatal hypoglycemia 775.6
- Other preterm infants 765.1
- SGA, weight unspecified, malnutrition not mentioned 764.0
- SGA with mention of malnutrition 764.1

(To assign a fifth digit, see appendix A, page 638.)

Defense of homebound status
- Fatigue or weakness postpartum
- Need to elevate legs frequently because of preeclampsia

Selected nursing diagnoses and patient outcomes

Ineffective family coping: Compromised, related to neonatal health problems

The parents will:
- identify and use at least two healthy coping behaviors (N)
- demonstrate ability to meet neonate's special care needs (N)
- identify and use available support systems (N)
- express a feeling of increased control over their lives (N)
- identify how to access professional health care assistance if necessary. (N)

Sleep pattern disturbance related to external factors

The parents will:
- describe factors that prevent or facilitate sleep (N)
- incorporate rest and sleep periods within daily routine (for example, multitasking, sleeping when neonate sleeps, and accepting family support) (N)
- exhibit no physical signs or behaviors that indicate sleep deprivation. (N)

Ineffective breast-feeding related to limited maternal experience or dissatisfaction with breast-feeding process

The mother will:
- demonstrate proper positioning of the neonate during breast-feeding and proper technique to encourage the neonate to latch on to the nipple correctly (N, LC)
- express physical and psychological comfort with breast-feeding techniques (N, LC)

- observe that the neonate feeds successfully on both breasts and appears satisfied for at least 2 hours after feeding (N, LC)
- observe that the neonate's weight remains within an accepted range and his nutritional needs appear to be met (specifically, showing no signs or symptoms of dehydration and normal patterns of elimination) (N)
- state at least one resource for breast-feeding support (N, LC)
- verbalize understanding of breast-feeding techniques and demonstrate measures to minimize discomfort. (N, LC)

Ineffective infant feeding pattern related to neurologic impairment or developmental delay
The neonate will:
- demonstrate adequate breast-feeding ability with an effective sucking reflex as well as a coordinated suck and swallow response (N, LC)
- show no signs or symptoms of dehydration, normal patterns of elimination, urine output of 1 ml/kg/day, good skin turgor, moist mucous membranes, and flat fontanels (N)
- return to birth weight by 10 days after delivery. (N)

Knowledge deficit related to lack of information about neonatal care
The mother will:
- demonstrate understanding of increased calorie intake to meet the nutritional needs of breast-feeding, including adequate hydration for optimal health maintenance and milk supply (N, D, LC)
- demonstrate ability to care for neonate independently or with minimal assistance (N)

- contact community resources when necessary. (N, LC)

Pain related to postpartum physiologic changes (specifically nipple soreness and breast engorgement)
The mother will:
- verbalize understanding of techniques to prevent or treat nipple soreness and breast engorgement (N, LC)
- empty breasts regularly. (N, LC)

Caregiver role strain related to discharge of a family member with significant home care needs
The parents will:
- identify and develop a realistic appraisal of each stressful situation (N)
- demonstrate appropriate coping mechanisms for each stressful situation (N)
- identify and use support systems and resources. (N, LC)

Altered family processes related to inclusion of new member
The parents will:
- identify support systems available in the community (N)
- share feelings about neonate with each other (N)
- assume new or additional responsibilities as needed. (N)

Altered parenting related to inadequate attachment to high-risk neonate
The parents will:
- demonstrate safe and supportive care to neonate (N, LC)
- initiate regular contact with neonate (N)
- stay informed of neonate's condition (N)

- display appropriate attachment behaviors, including providing neonate with appropriate verbal, tactile, and auditory stimulation (N)
- set realistic goals for neonate. (N, LC)

Skilled nursing services

Care measures
- Perform initial full assessment of all systems of patient admitted to home care.
- Perform skilled assessment of mother's basic knowledge, including breast-feeding; infant feeding (latching on, sucking reflex, and swallowing); infant elimination patterns, hydration status, and weight patterns for age; signs and symptoms of let-down reflex; infant breast-feeding positioning; mother and infant communication patterns; and need for community support (such as nursing mothers league, lactation consultant, and LaLeche League).

Patient and family teaching
- Review anatomy of breast structure and infant oral structure.
- Discuss breast-feeding problems, including poor latch-on, ineffective sucking, or nonsupportive significant other.
- Explain how to minimize maternal discomforts, sore nipples, insufficient emptying of breast at feeding, dehydration, and actual or perceived inadequate milk supply.
- Describe normal newborn elimination patterns and normal newborn feeding patterns.
- Identify need for supplementation.
- Identify need for breast pump and instruction in its use.

Interdisciplinary services

Dietitian
- Nutritional recommendations to meet increased nutritional demands

Lactation consultant
- Ongoing support and surveillance of the breast-feeding process

Discharge plan
- Mother's ability to manage breast-feeding with physician and community support system follow-up services
- Follow-up appointments with physician planned for mother and infant at recommended intervals

Documentation requirements
- Mother's level of knowledge and progress toward educational goals
- Problems mother is experiencing (for example, breast engorgement making latch-on difficult, flat nipples, infant regurgitation, and infant exhibiting weak suck and tongue thrusting)
- Areas in which instruction is given (such as use of a breast pump) along with objective outcomes (such as length of time pumped and milk collected)
- Length and frequency of feedings
- Effectiveness of breast-feeding, including breast and nipple comfort, infant satisfaction, and infant elimination patterns
- Variances to expected outcomes
- Measures taken to correct breast-feeding problem, such as involvement of community support and a lactation consultant

Reimbursement reminders

• Most insurers are reluctant to pay for breast-feeding visits unless provided by certified lactation specialists.

• Rental or purchase of breast pumps usually isn't covered.

• Dietitian services aren't reimbursable without extenuating circumstances.

• Specify any barriers to learning, such as physical deformities, visual impairment, and lack of available support persons.

Insurance hints

• Focus on the infant problem or medical condition rather than breast-feeding difficulty.

• Provide ICD-9 codes corresponding to medical condition.

• Describe specifics about patient's learning progress and gains in mastery of concepts and skills.

• Report progress toward goals (for example, infant weight gain, normal elimination patterns, and independence with care).

• Report complications, such as regurgitation, sleep deprivation, and dehydration.

• Report communication with other health team members and changes in the plan of care.

Cesarean section postcare

Postpartum care of the new mother involves caring for both the mother and the neonate. The mother who has delivered her baby by cesarean section poses a problem as a patient recovering from surgery as well as a postpartum patient. Cesarean deliveries are done for a variety of reasons — cephalopelvic disproportion, fetal distress, failure to progress, active herpes, and cases where it isn't advisable to let the mother labor. Today's cesarean section delivery is a relatively common procedure with few surgical risks. Recovery from a cesarean delivery is slightly more difficult than that from a vaginal birth because the new mother must also recover from a surgical incision.

This patient has special needs that may require a home health care nurse to check the incision or remove staples from the incision. The new mother is less mobile during recovery, and positioning the baby for feeding may be a challenge. The new mother is cautioned against lifting; if there are other children in the home, avoidance of activity may be a problem. The home care nurse's function is to see that the surgical incision is healing properly and that the new mother is able to care for the incision. Home health care may be directed toward wound care or other complications of the surgery. The home health care nurse must help the patient function as normally as possible during the postpartum period.

Previsit checklist

Physician orders and preparation

• Orders regarding postoperative care and activity orders and restrictions

• Discharge summary from hospital or physician's office indicating reason for cesarean section delivery and any complications of recovery

Equipment and supplies
- Supplies for standard precautions and proper sharps disposal
- Wound care supplies as prescribed (such as suture removal kit, cleaning solutions, dressings, and adhesive tape)
- Camera, film, and consent form for photographing wound
- Teaching materials

Safety requirements
- Standard precautions for infection control and sharps disposal
- Emergency plan and access to functional phone and list of emergency phone numbers
- Fire evacuation plan, functional smoke detectors, and access to functional fire extinguisher
- Instructions about signs and symptoms of medical emergency and actions to take
- Information on medications, including dosage, adverse effects, interactions, and safe storage

Major diagnostic codes
- Antepartum hemorrhage, unspecified 641.00
- Cesarean section delivery with/without complications 669.39/669.71
- Cesarean section wound dehiscence 674.12
- Chorioamnionitis 762.7
- Complications of obstetrical surgical wounds, such as hematoma and infection 674.34
- Postpartum hemorrhage, unspecified 666.00

Defense of homebound status
- Inability to leave the home without the assistance of another person secondary to severe fatigue
- Postsurgical recovery (open wound site)
- Signs of infection
- Fatigue, weakness, and shortness of breath that limit activity
- Activity restriction prescribed by obstetrician
- Protection of newborn from infection without other available caregivers

Selected nursing diagnoses and patient outcomes

Knowledge deficit regarding self-care, cesarean section delivery, nutritional and hydration needs, and infant care
The mother will:
- demonstrate knowledge of the need for increased hydration and dietary changes to improve or avoid constipation that often accompanies analgesic therapy   (N, D)
- be able to follow physician orders regarding cesarean delivery care as evidenced by return demonstration (N)
- verbalize understanding of incision healing process and any signs or symptoms to report immediately   (N)
- accomplish self-care and infant care.   (N)

Pain secondary to surgical incision
The mother will:
- verbalize knowledge of medication regimen, including analgesics, their use, adverse effects, and interactions   (N)

• demonstrate knowledge of at least two nonpharmacologic pain management strategies, such as relaxation, distraction, guided imagery, positive self-talk, and thought-stopping (N)
• rate pain at 3 or less on a 0-to-10 scale 80% of the time. (N)

Risk for infection
The mother will:
• identify signs and symptoms of an infected incision (redness, elevated temperature, and drainage), a postpartum infection, or a urinary tract infection; verbalize when they should be reported to the physician; and outline follow-up actions (N)
• demonstrate wound care using standard precautions for infection control. (N)

Caregiver role strain
The parents will:
• demonstrate adequate coping strategies (N)
• verbalize stress-management techniques (N)
• demonstrate knowledge of outside support and community resources if necessary. (N, SW)

Fatigue
The parents will:
• demonstrate knowledge regarding the need to allow adequate rest periods (N)
• identify basis of fatigue and individual areas of control (N)
• identify appropriate interventions to promote more sleep and rest, such as napping when infant naps or using social supports. (N)

Altered urinary elimination
The mother will:
• return to normal urinary patterns without signs of infection (N)

Risk for constipation
The mother will:
• regain normal bowel function. (N)

Ineffective breast-feeding
The mother will:
• demonstrate knowledge of the lactation process, correct positioning, and infant feeding cues (N, LC)
• identify procedures to improve or prevent engorgement, soreness of nipples, cracking of nipples, or blisters (N)
• demonstrate alternative positioning of infant for breast-feeding to reduce pain of incision site (N)
• identify community resources available for breast-feeding support (such as LaLeche League). (N, LC)

Skilled nursing services

Care measures
• Perform a full assessment of body systems; evaluate vital signs, involution of uterus, lochial flow, nutrition and hydration, psychosocial status, presence or absence of lactation, and pain level for incision, perineum, and breasts and nipples.
• Assess coping skills.
• Evaluate the home environment for safety concerns.
• Perform or arrange for venipuncture as ordered by the physician.
• Evaluate elimination status and offer suggestions for comfort and measures to return to normal elimination patterns.

• Evaluate mother's knowledge of infant care and level of confidence in providing care.
• Assess infant's feeding patterns.
• Assess newborn's vital signs.
• Determine if neonatal jaundice is present and take appropriate measures.
• Evaluate cesarean section incision for signs and symptoms of healing; remove staples and photograph wound as ordered (the patient must sign a consent form for the wound to be photographed).

Patient and family teaching
• Describe incisional care, including aseptic technique with prescribed regimen.
• Discuss signs of healing and healthy tissue as well as signs and symptoms of infection and dehiscence and actions to take.
• Develop coping skills individualized to the needs of the patient (age extremes, comorbidities, and multiple births).
• Review alternative expressions of intimacy and sexuality for use during immediate postpartum period.
• Emphasize need for follow-up care and immunizations for mother and baby.
• Demonstrate care of the infant.
• Explain family planning options.
• Identify comfort measures for new mother.
• Provide information on community resources available for the new family (particularly high-risk groups, including young mothers and those with multiple births, challenged infants, or lack of familial support).
• Discuss signs and symptoms of newborn illness.

Interdisciplinary actions

Dietitian
• Recommend menu plans to meet nutritional needs within mother's preferences
• Evaluation of mother's goals and development of a realistic plan to attain ideal body weight

Home care aide
• Housekeeping assistance

Lactation consultant
• Review of common lactation problems and options for resolution
• Identification of community resources to assist with breast-feeding

Social worker
• Information on financial assistance
• Counseling for long-range planning
• Contingency emergency care planning
• Psychosocial assessment and evaluation

Discharge plan
• Mother's postpartum course normal and without complications
• Adequate knowledge about self-care following delivery
• Ability of mother to verbalize comfort measures
• Ability of mother to understand physician discharge orders
• Stable vital signs exhibited by mother and neonate
• Mother's success in feeding infant and performing newborn care
• Verbalization of newborn signs and symptoms requiring medical attention

and identification of care provider for infant

• Ability of mother to demonstrate correct technique for taking infant temperature

• Ability of mother to demonstrate adequate bonding with infant

• Ability of mother to verbalize signs and symptoms of postpartum depression and appropriate measures to take

• Ability of mother to perform incision care and verbalize signs and symptoms of impaired healing

Documentation requirements

• Healing of incision and staple removal

• Description of wound length, width, depth; color of drainage; and odor if wound care is performed at every visit

• Record of vital signs with regard to any changes noted since discharge

• Physical assessment findings related to the postpartum course, including any variances from normal

• Physician notification of any changes in condition or variances from normal

• Mother and baby interaction

• Infant feeding method and mother's ability to provide adequate nutrition

• Educational needs of the mother

• Unusual family dynamics

• Educational booklets and materials provided and community resource material discussed

• Variances to expected outcomes, interaction with physician and team members, and orders for any change in the plan of care

• Barriers to learning, such as weakness, fatigue, and lack of familial support and assistance

• Continued needs and follow-up plans

Reimbursement reminders

• Home care services are more likely to be reimbursed when an ICD-9 code is present to indicate the reason for visits beyond newborn care and teaching needs.

• Identify factors that require skilled assessment and teaching.

• Identify factors that prevent patient from leaving home or getting to follow-up appointments for mother and infant.

Insurance hints

• Present patient's ability or inability to learn wound care.

• Provide an estimated end point for services.

• Present objective data.

• Present any variances from normal postpartum course.

• Report laboratory values in relation to previous levels.

• Emphasize factors that indicate potential need for hospitalization if not managed with skilled nursing services (assessment, treatment, and education).

• Notify the case manager when home care is discontinued.

Formula-feeding

Infant nutrition is an area of newborn care where the new mother will exhibit preference for either breast-feeding or formula-feeding; both methods provide adequate nutrition for the newborn. The mother may choose one method over the other for several reasons: personal preference, concern over body image, cultural beliefs, medical necessity, or a conscious effort to enlist the help of an alternate caregiver. Perhaps the most important reason one method is chosen over another is the direct intervention of the delivery room staff. The new mother is most vulnerable during the immediate postpartum period and is open to suggestions made by the professional staff.

Many new mothers elect to formula-feed their newborns. Next to breast-feeding, formula is the best food source for the neonate and can be administered by anyone. The American Academy of Pediatrics recommends commercially prepared formula over animal's milk for the infant's first year. Commercially prepared formulas supply all necessary vitamins and nutrients — manufacturers are constantly striving to duplicate breast milk. Easily obtained, formula is available in several types, such as ready-to-feed or powdered (advance preparation needed). Varieties of formula are also available for infants with specific digestive problems. Because of the uniformity of the manufacturing process, one brand of formula is identical from state to state.

Previsit checklist

Physician orders and preparation
- Order indicating the need for visits
- Delivery information, including route of delivery, time of delivery, birth weight, discharge weight, and any concurrent medical problems or nutritional needs

Equipment and supplies
- Infant scale
- Educational handouts

- Commercial formula
- Bottles and nipples

Safety requirements
- Home assessment for adequate water source, refrigeration, and storage space
- Standard precautions for infection control
- Newborn safety checklist
- Safety requirements specific to formula feeding, such as avoidance of microwaves to heat formula, adequate assessment of formula temperature prior to feeding, and avoidance of bottle propping

Major diagnostic codes
- Disorders relating to high birth weight and long gestation 766
- Disorders relating to short gestation and unspecified low birth weight 765
- Extreme immaturity (birth weight less than 1,000 g (2 lb) and gestation less than 28 completed weeks) 765.0
- Feeding problems in the newborn 779.3
- Fetal growth retardation, unspecified 764.9
- Fetal malnutrition without mention of small for gestational age (SGA) 764.2
- Neonatal dehydration 775.5
- Neonatal hypoglycemia 775.6
- Other preterm infants 765.1
- SGA with/without mention of malnutrition 764.0/764.1
(To assign a fifth digit, see appendix A, page 638.)

Defense of homebound status

• Fatigue, weakness, and shortness of breath limiting activity
• Confined to home because of instability of diabetes mellitus
• Activity restriction prescribed by obstetrician
• Protection of newborn from infection

Selected nursing diagnoses and patient outcomes

Sleep pattern disturbance
The parents will:
• describe factors that prevent or facilitate sleep   (N)
• incorporate rest or sleep periods within daily routine (such as multitasking, sleeping while neonate sleeps, and accepting family support)   (N)
• exhibit no physical signs or behaviors that indicate sleep deprivation.
                                    (N)

Caregiver role strain related to discharge of a family member with significant home care needs
The parents will:
• identify support systems available in the community   (N)
• share feelings about neonate with each other   (N)
• assume new or additional responsibilities as needed.   (N)

Altered family processes
The parents will:
• demonstrate family involvement and support   (N)

Knowledge deficit related to neonatal care
The parents will:
• demonstrate the ability to care for neonate independently or with minimal assistance   (N)
• contact community resources when necessary   (N, SW)
• identify common problems of formula-feeding and demonstrate knowledge of measures to correct problems
                                (N, SP)
• verbalize understanding of formula-feeding techniques.   (N)

Ineffective infant feeding pattern
The neonate will:
• achieve satisfying bottle-feeding regimen with normal growth and development   (N)
• demonstrate weight gain consistent with nutritional intake and appropriate for age   (N)
• demonstrate normal patterns of elimination   (N)
• show no signs of dehydration, maintaining moist mucous membranes and flat fontanels   (N)
• demonstrate adequate formula-feeding ability.   (N)

Skilled nursing services

Care measures
• Perform skilled assessment of basic formula-feeding knowledge and evaluate infant feeding, including latching-on, sucking reflex, and swallowing; infant elimination patterns; infant weight patterns for age; infant formula-feeding positioning; and mother and infant communication patterns.
• Provide support of the mother's choice of feeding method.

Patient and family teaching

• Discuss formula-feeding problems, including spitting or regurgitation, choking on nipple, and using a pillow to position infant.

• Review normal newborn elimination patterns and feeding patterns.

• Describe formula preparation and storage.

• Teach about asepsis in preparation and storage of formula.

• Emphasize the importance of good handwashing, follow-up appointments for preventive care with pediatrician, and immunizations.

• Discuss lactation suppression.

• Demonstrate burping positions.

• Identify signs and symptoms of formula intolerance.

Interdisciplinary actions

Speech pathologist

• Evaluation of sucking and swallowing reflex, if applicable

Social worker

• Identification of and referral to community resources

Discharge plan

• Pattern of normal infant growth and development

• Infant thriving and gaining weight appropriate for age

• No sanitation issues in the home precluding preparation and storage of formula, such as lack of running water and refrigeration

Documentation requirements

• Caregiver's level of knowledge

• Teaching methods used

• Problems caregiver may be experiencing and corrective measures used

• Infant feeding cues and preparation of formula prior to feeding

• Infant weight

• Infant feeding length, amount of formula taken, quality of sucking, and regurgitation or feeding difficulties

• Maternal or caregiver level of satisfaction with feeding

• Areas in which further instruction is needed

• Physician order stating necessity of visits

• Postvisit follow-up care

• Variances to expected outcomes

Reimbursement reminders

• Identify need for visits and outcomes achieved, such as infant crying to be fed, taking formula at rate of 1 oz (30 ml) every 15 minutes, adequate burping, and presence or absence of regurgitation.

• Compare infant's weight at time of visit to discharge weight.

• Note objective findings identified at time of visit, such as weak infant sucking and gagging on nipple.

• Identify adequate preparation and storage of formula.

• Use ICD-9 codes appropriate for problem that necessitated visit; newborn status alone is unacceptable for most insurance plans.

Insurance hints

• Most insurers are reluctant to pay for infant formula feeding assessment unless a concurrent medical problem is present.

- Focus on the infant problem or medical condition rather than breast-feeding difficulty.
- Provide ICD-9 codes that correspond to the medical condition necessitating the visit.
- Report changes noted after visits to case manager with plans for continued follow-up if necessary.

Gestational diabetes mellitus

Diabetes mellitus is a disorder of carbohydrate, protein, and fat metabolism characterized by an increase in fasting blood glucose and abnormal glucose tolerance levels. Pregnant women with diabetes are at risk for complications of pregnancy, as are the infants of diabetic mothers. Complications that may occur in a pregnant diabetic include hyperglycemia, severe infection, neuropathy, pregnancy-induced hypertension, abruptio placentae, polyhydramnios, and injuries associated with the delivery of a macrosomic infant, such as vaginal lacerations and postpartum hemorrhage.

Medical management of the patient with gestational diabetes may include dietary restrictions in mild cases or insulin therapy. Oral hypoglycemics aren't advised because the medications cross the placental barrier. In addition, a number of women with gestational diabetes go on to develop diabetes later in life if dietary modifications and lifestyle changes aren't made. In most cases of gestational diabetes, blood glucose levels fall to normal after delivery. All pregnant women should receive testing for diabetes between the 24th and 26th week of pregnancy. An early delivery may be scheduled if the diabetes is poorly controlled or the infant is growing too large.

Goals for home monitoring of a patient with gestational diabetes include keeping the blood sugar levels within normal levels, assessing the fundal height, checking fetal heart tones, and educating the patient in blood glucose monitoring. If insulin is needed for control, instructions are given with an emphasis on return demonstration. If the physician orders a special diet for control of the diabetes, nutritional counseling is given. In either case, gestational diabetes is a significant, life-changing event and follow-up care is vital. (Also see "Diabetes mellitus," page 209.)

Previsit checklist

Physician orders and preparation
- Orders for parameters of care
- Obstetric history of present pregnancy
- Diet orders

Equipment and supplies
- Supplies for standard precautions and proper sharps disposal
- Insulin and administration supplies
- Vital signs equipment
- Doppler stethoscope for fetal heart tones
- Supplies for blood glucose monitoring, including blood glucose meter, alcohol swabs, lancing device, and log book

Safety requirements

- Standard precautions for infection control and sharps disposal
- Instructions about signs and symptoms of medical emergencies and actions to take
- Emergency plan and access to functional phone and list of emergency phone numbers
- Refrigeration appropriate for storage of insulin

Major diagnostic codes

- Antepartal hyperglycemia 648.83
- Diabetes, type 1, uncontrolled 250.03
- Diabetes, type 2, uncontrolled 250.02
- Diabetes mellitus 648.0
- Diabetes mellitus, gestational 648.8
- Diabetes with complications 250.9
- Obesity (morbid) 278.00 (278.01)
- Polyhydramnios 761.3

Defense of homebound status

- Concurrent medical problem present or unstable diabetes with recent syncopal episodes
- Confined to home by obstetrician
- Protection of newborn from infection

Selected nursing diagnoses and patient outcomes

Risk of constipation related to lactation, fatigue, and decreased activity
   The patient will:
- maintain adequate fluid intake (N)
- increase natural fiber in the diet to prevent constipation and decrease glycemic index of foods to stabilize blood glucose (N)
- follow prescribed diet. (N, D)

Knowledge deficit regarding medical plan of care
   The patient will:
- verbalize accurate knowledge of the disease process and treatment regimen (N)
- perform the necessary procedures correctly and indicate understanding of reasons for actions (N)
- demonstrate plan for necessary life changes (N)
- identify interferences to learning and specific actions to deal with them (N)
- demonstrate knowledge of medication regimen and blood glucose testing with return demonstration (N)
- demonstration of knowledge of nutritional requirements and new diet as ordered by the physician. (N, D)

Fear related to new diagnoses and possible complication of pregnancy
   The patient will:
- acknowledge and discuss fears, recognizing healthy versus unhealthy fears (N)
- verbalize desire to undertake tasks to effect change (N)
- report feelings of self-confidence with progress made. (N)

Altered role performance
   The patient will:
- demonstrate appropriate behaviors regarding parenting role (N)
- participate in the development of a mutually agreeable treatment plan and goals. (N)

Skilled nursing services

Care measures

- Assess current disease process, develop a plan of care, schedule follow-up appointments, and evaluate compliance with the plan of care and lifestyle modifications.
- Assess vital signs.
- Assess fetal well-being and fundal height.
- Assess blood glucose levels, trends, and patient's management of insulin needs.
- Assess patient's understanding of diagnosis and treatment.
- Assess current nutritional status, diet tolerance, and maternal weight gain.
- Assess patient's psychosocial status and home environment.

Patient and family teaching

- Describe signs and symptoms of hypoglycemia and hyperglycemia and actions to take.
- Emphasize the need for activity and rest.
- Explain how to collect specimens and monitor blood glucose levels.
- Teach how to monitor fetal movement and make kick counts.
- Review safety measures regarding medication storage and proper sharps disposal; emphasize the need to keep emergency information nearby.
- Discuss care of the patient.

Interdisciplinary actions

Dietitian

- Consultation for nutritional needs

Home care aide

(If patient is on bed rest for concurrent medical condition)
- Housekeeping duties
- Care of other family members

Social worker

- Information on financial assistance
- Counseling for long-range planning
- Contingency emergency care planning
- Psychosocial assessment and evaluation

Discharge plan

- Term of pregnancy completed
- Patient able to safely monitor own diabetes in home
- Patient independent in self-care and infant care with assistance of significant others, physician, and community support

Documentation requirements

- Results of skilled assessment, including subjective and objective data, fetal heart rate, presence of fetal movement, patient's vital signs and weight, any symptoms patient may be experiencing, patient reflexes, and results of blood glucose monitoring
- Patient compliance with plan of care
- Emotional needs and concerns of patient
- Daily telephone contact with patient
- Medication modifications
- Variances to expected outcomes
- Barriers to learning
- Continued needs and follow-up plans
- If extra visit needed, reason for visit and condition change precipitating need for visit

Reimbursement reminders

- Indicate compliance with physician orders.
- Home care services are reimbursed when an ICD-9 code is present to indicate reason for visit.
- Instruments, such as blood glucose monitoring machines, lancets, and test strips, are *not* covered by the insurance company unless the patient is a prepregnant diabetic. Check the patient's prescription plan to see if these items may be purchased through the pharmacy plan.

Insurance hints

- Emphasize factors requiring skilled nursing services and potential for acute care needs if assessment, early intervention, and education are lacking (including labile blood sugar and asymptomatic hypoglycemia or hyperglycemia).
- Give an estimated end point for services.
- Present objective data.
- Present any variances from normal.
- Explain patient's capacity for learning self-care objectively.
- Try to develop a therapeutic follow-up plan for patient.

Hyperbilirubinemia

Hyperbilirubinemia is characterized by greater-than-normal amounts of bilirubin in the blood, which occurs when bilirubin is produced and travels to the liver in the unconjugated form. In the liver, bilirubin binds to the albumin in plasma and is converted to conjugated bilirubin; then it's excreted through the biliary tree into the duo-denum and kidneys. In the intestine, it's converted back to unconjugated bilirubin, which is absorbed into the intestinal wall and enters the enterohepatic circulation. Because a newborn has a liver with only a limited ability to excrete excess bilirubin, all newborn infants have elevated levels of serum bilirubin.

Physiologic jaundice is the periodic rise and fall in serum bilirubin levels; the average level is 8 to 12 mg/dl by the 4th day of life, which gradually decreases to about 1.5 mg/dl by the 10th day of life. Jaundice occurs from 24 to 48 hours after birth, when the red blood cells begin to break down and the immature liver is unable to handle the extra load. This condition may give a yellow tint to the skin and the infant is said to be jaundiced. This is a normal and transient condition that is usually self-limiting and requires no treatment.

Pathologic jaundice results when the bilirubin levels increase beyond normal levels or excretion of the excess bilirubin is reduced. These excess bilirubin levels can be the result of many factors: hemolytic disease, polycythemia, abnormal liver function, or extravascular bleeding. Decreased excretion can result from decreased hepatic uptake of bilirubin, impaired transport of conjugated bilirubin, or obstructed bile flow. Both increased bilirubin and decreased excretion may occur more often in preterm infants, infants of diabetic mothers, or infants with prenatal sepsis or postnatal infection. Breast-feeding jaundice may occur in the breast-fed baby due to inhibition of certain enzymes and free fatty acids found in breast milk. This type of jaundice occurs by the 7th day of life, with levels rising as high as 15 mg/dl and lasting for 2 to 3 weeks before decreasing. It may necessitate cessation of breast-feeding for 2 to 4 days. Most of the time, bilirubin levels in healthy full-term infants will decrease without complications.

Treatment of pathologic jaundice in the home setting usually involves phototherapy. A phototherapy unit, such as a Wallaby, is a fiber-optic light source that breaks down excess red blood cells near the skin's surface so they can be transported to the GI system and excreted in urine and feces. This treatment works well in the home setting because the family remains intact — mother and baby aren't separated — which promotes bonding. The Wallaby unit is portable, lightweight, and user-friendly; compliance is high using this outpatient treatment and hospital costs are minimized. Infants must meet certain criteria prior to the initiation of treatment. In addition, the caregiver must be able to assume care for the infant receiving phototherapy, to complete required documentation, and to maintain the equipment involved in the treatment. The caregiver must also understand that the infant will have daily blood work to determine the effectiveness of treatment.

Previsit checklist

Physician orders and preparation
- Initiation of phototherapy with parameters for temperature, feeding, elimination, and bilirubin levels

Equipment and supplies
- Consent to treat and other documentation forms
- Wallaby unit
- Thermometer
- Amber blood tubes
- Lancets
- Alcohol swabs
- Clean 2″ × 2″ gauze pads
- Adhesive bandages
- Relevant laboratory paperwork
- Sharps disposal container
- Infant scale

Safety requirements
- Standard precautions for infection control and sharps disposal
- Emergency plan and access to functional phone and list of emergency phone numbers, including number for poison control center
- Identification and correction of environmental hazards and patient-specific concerns (for example, electrical outlet meets safety requirements, and night-lights)
- Power outage plan (local power companies need to know if a patient in the home requires electrical power for life-support equipment)
- Phone number of durable medical equipment company

Major diagnostic codes
- Hemolytic disease due to Rh isoimmunization/ABO isoimmunization/ other and unspecified isoimmunization 773.0/773.1/773.2
- Hydrops fetalis due to isoimmunization 773.3
- Jaundice from breast milk 774.39
- Kernicterus due to isoimmunization 773.4
- Kernicterus not due to isoimmunization 774.7

- Late anemia due to isoimmunization 773.5
- Neonatal jaundice associated with preterm delivery 774.2
- Neonatal jaundice due to delayed conjugation from other causes, unspecified 774.30
- Perinatal jaundice due to hepatocellular damage 774.4
- Unspecified fetal and neonatal jaundice, transient 774.6

Defense of homebound status

- Infant requires phototherapy
- Fatigue, weakness, and shortness of breath that limit mother's activity
- Confined to home because of instability of maternal diabetes mellitus
- Activity restriction prescribed by obstetrician
- Protection of newborn from infection

Selected nursing diagnoses and patient outcomes

Altered nutrition: Less than body requirements, secondary to interrupted breast-feeding
    The mother will:
- verbalize understanding of neonate's dietary needs and need for frequent feedings   (N, D)
- recognize adequate elimination patterns (two to five bowel movements per day).   (N)
    The neonate will:
- exhibit no symptoms of dehydration (sunken fontanels, no tears when crying, cotton-mouth appearance, and fewer than 6 wet diapers in 24 hours).   (N)

Risk for injury secondary to phototherapy
    The neonate will:
- maintain body temperature   (N)
- exhibit decreasing bilirubin levels   (N)
- develop no complications from phototherapy, such as eye damage because eyes were left unprotected   (N)
- have bilirubin levels within acceptable limits by day of discharge.   (N)

Knowledge deficit (parents) related to phototherapy, infant's condition, prognosis, safety, and treatment
    The parents will:
- identify obstructions to learning and specific actions to deal with them (N)
- demonstrate ability to maintain phototherapy equipment   (N)
- demonstrate compliance with plan of care   (N)
- demonstrate understanding of need to wake infant for frequent feedings because phototherapy may cause excessive sleepiness (feeding increases bowel movements, which is how the body excretes bilirubin)   (N)
- demonstrate ability to maintain adequate documentation of temperature, feeding, and elimination   (N)
- verbalize understanding of symptoms needing immediate nursing or medical intervention   (N)
- verbalize understanding that supplemental water doesn't "flush out" bilirubin but may actually increase levels by decreasing formula or breast milk intake, which increases stool formation where bilirubin is eliminated.   (N)

Skilled nursing services

Care measures
- Perform daily physical assessment of the newborn.
- Assess weight daily.
- Draw blood for daily bilirubin level and other laboratory work as ordered by physician.
- Report daily bilirubin results and progress of treatment to physician.
- Inform caregiver of blood test results.
- Provide psychological support of the caregiver.

Patient and family teaching
- Explain phototherapy procedure to caregivers.
- Discuss necessary documentation.
- Teach caregiver how to take infant's temperature.
- Review requirements for adequate infant nutrition and maintenance of hydration.
- Instruct caregiver in documentation of elimination patterns and correction of inadequate elimination by waking infant for frequent feedings and eliminating water supplementation.
- Educate caregiver about feeding difficulties; explain that therapies, such as phototherapy, don't need to be for long, continuous periods, so the infant can be picked up frequently for bonding and feedings.

Interdisciplinary services

Dietitian
- Nutritional recommendations

Discharge plan
- Acceptable levels of infant bilirubin
- Referral of noncompliant caregiver to social worker; follow-up plan development
- No improvement noted in jaundice; hospitalization necessary for further evaluation

Documentation requirements
- Parental consent prior to initiation of treatment
- Daily physical assessment of the infant, including weight, feeding, elimination, vital signs, response to treatment, and activity
- Caregiver's documentation, including amount of time infant is out of phototherapy for bathing and other care
- Results of daily blood tests
- Response from physician regarding laboratory results
- Changes in plan of care
- Variances in expected outcomes
- Communication with caregivers regarding treatment

Reimbursement reminders
- Daily visits to draw blood test are covered by most insurers.
- Communicate laboratory reports to case manager on a daily basis or at end of therapy.
- Provide correct ICD-9 code to ensure payment.
- Indicate need for bilirubin level to case managers at end of phototherapy treatment due to bilirubin rebound effect.

• Obtain a telephone order for any plan of care change and note reason for it in chart.

Insurance hints
• Present objective data regarding patient.
• Present objective patient findings and changes since last contact.
• Report new laboratory values and changes in clinical condition.
• Notify case manager when home care is discontinued.

Neonatal care

Decreased length of hospital stays, due in part to cost containment and the perception of childbirth as a normal process that doesn't require hospitalization, has greatly increased the importance of postdelivery home care. During the short hospital stay, there is very little time to educate the parents about newborn care. In addition, with mothers and newborns being discharged sooner, many postpartum complications may not show up until after they leave the hospital. The role of the home care nurse, therefore, is to educate the new family in the care of the neonate and to provide assessment of any concerns that may have come up since discharge.

The home care nurse is in the best position to assess the neonate and evaluate the caregiver's level of knowledge and comfort in providing care for the baby. The new caregiver usually has many questions; in the familiar home environment, she feels comfortable asking them. The home care nurse can assess the home environment and suggest changes that may help the family accommodate the newborn.

Assessment of the newborn is important to promoting optimal growth and development and preventing complications; however, not all commercial insurers provide a home visit for this assessment. It's imperative that the discharge planner emphasize the medical necessity of the home visit and provide objective data to the case manager after the visit. Educational visits usually aren't covered by insurers unless the education involves an infant with special needs.

Previsit checklist

Physician orders and preparation
• Physicians orders with specific parameters to be assessed

Equipment and supplies
• Supplies for standard precautions
• Vital signs equipment
• Educational materials
• Any specific adaptive material or supplies relative to care
• Infant scale
• Thermometer

Safety requirements
• Standard precautions for infection control
• Assessment of environment to determine suitability of the home for newborn care
• Emergency phone numbers, including the number for the poison control center

Major diagnostic codes
- Birth trauma 767
- Birth trauma, unspecified 767.9
- Cleft palate/lip/both 749.0/749.1/749.2
- Conditions involving the integument and temperature regulation of the newborn 778
- Disorders relating to long gestation and high birth weight 766
- Disorders relating to short gestation and unspecified low birth weight 765
- Facial nerve injury 767.5
- Feeding problems in the newborn 779.3
- Fracture of the clavicle 767.2
- Hemolytic disease of the newborn 773
- Injuries to scalp 767.1
- Other and ill-defined conditions in the perinatal period 779
- Perinatal disorders of the digestive system 777
- Respiratory problems after birth 770.8

Defense of homebound status
- Fatigue or weakness postpartum
- Instability of diabetes mellitus with serious or recent episodes of altered consciousness
- Activity restriction prescribed by obstetrician
- Protection of newborn from infection

Selected nursing diagnoses and patient outcomes

Ineffective infant feeding pattern
  The neonate will:

- feed successfully and appear satisfied for at least two hours after feeding   (N, LC)
- return to birth weight by 10 days after delivery   (N)
- maintain normal patterns of elimination — urine output of 1 ml/kg/day.   (N)
- show signs of normal growth and development.   (N)

Risk for infection
  The parents will:

- demonstrate knowledge of infection control measures, such as handwashing and proper handling of bottle-feeding equipment   (N)
- verbalize knowledge of signs and symptoms of postpartum infection, such as elevated temperature, change in vaginal discharge, and heat or redness around the incision   (N)
- verbalize knowledge of signs and symptoms of infection in newborn around umbilicus or penis in circumcised male.   (N)

Knowledge deficit regarding newborn care
  The parents will:

- demonstrate knowledge of signs and symptoms of dehydration in the infant   (N)
- demonstrate ability to care for newborn independently   (N)
- demonstrate knowledge of signs of infection or other newborn illness with appropriate resources to contact with concerns   (N)
- verbalize readiness to assume caregiving independently   (N)
- recognize infant cues and identify appropriate responses   (N)
- be familiar with developmental milestones   (N)

• recognize community resources to assist with lactation, newborn issues, and postpartum depression. (N, SW)

Skilled nursing services

Care measures

• Assess newborn vital signs and reflexes; observe for normal newborn behavior or behavior appropriate for age.
• Weigh infant to determine if nutritional needs are being met.
• Perform physical assessment of infant; assess for jaundice and presence of birth complications that would interfere with normal growth and development.
• Observe infant feeding to determine if pattern is effective for growth and development.
• Assess developmental age and structural abnormalities.
• Compare birth weight to present weight to determine nutritional needs.
• Note presence of behaviors indicating continued hunger after feeding.
• Assess infant elimination pattern.
• Observe interaction of other family members with newborn.
• Incorporate parent's observations and suggestions into plan of care.
• Assist caregiver in breast-feeding or formula-feeding infant.
• Assess the caregiver's knowledge of asepsis.
• Refer new family to parenting support groups to assist in adjustment to new roles and responsibilities.

Patient and family teaching

• Discuss anticipated growth and development goals for the infant and corresponding calorie needs.

• Describe signs and symptoms of newborn illness.
• Review normal newborn behavior with the patient and family.
• Teach about temperature-taking methods and provide instruction if infant requires thermoregulation.
• Discuss newborn safety, bathing, cord care, circumcision site care, and perineal skin care.
• Emphasize the importance of making and keeping follow-up appointments for well-baby checks, immunizations, and postpartum checks.
• Teach proper hand-washing technique.
• Instruct the patient and family in baby care, including provision of adequate layers of clothing and proper climate control and common reasons and strategies for infant crying.

Interdisciplinary actions

Social worker

• Assessment of social needs, housing, and finances of new family
• Assistance with applications for government aid
• Assistance with integration of other family members in care of newborn

Lactation consultant

• Ongoing support and monitoring of the breast-feeding process

Discharge plan

• Normal newborn weight gain for gestational age
• Normal newborn behavior patterns for gestational age

- No signs and symptoms of infection in infant
- Ability of parents to provide basic newborn care
- Ability of parents to verbalize understanding of adverse signs in newborn
- Identification of routine health care needs of newborn by parents to health care professional
- Ability of parents to meet nutritional needs of infant shown by adequate feeding times and adequate newborn bowel movement and voiding patterns
- Exhibition by parents of emotional stability to care for newborn

Documentation requirements

- Physical findings of newborn
- Vital signs and weight
- Feeding patterns and effectiveness
- Adverse findings and follow-up physician call, noting any new orders
- Unsafe or health hazards in the home, including action taken to correct problem or instruction provided
- Caregiver ability to provide newborn care
- Caregiver's level of understanding of infant care
- Variances to expected outcomes

Reimbursement reminders

- Mother and infant may have one clinical record.
- Number of visits approved is usually very limited, so coordination of services, care, and teaching is imperative.
- Present objective findings.
- Compare findings to discharge parameters.

- Correlate physical assessment to medical condition.
- Follow physician orders regarding assessment.
- Note follow-up of any problems encountered on the home visit.
- Use designated ICD-9 codes for comorbidity and primary cause for home care consult.

Insurance hints

- Report objective patient findings and changes since last contact.
- Indicate in the plan of care if further visits are needed; state goals and time frame for goals to be achieved.
- Provide discharge summary to case manager at end of care.
- When requesting visit for initiation of care, state medical necessity of visit.
- Use diagnostic code number when requesting initial visit.

Postpartum care

The postpartum period begins immediately after delivery of the placenta and lasts for 6 weeks, during which time a number of physical and mental changes occur in the new mother. The uterus shrinks and descends into the pelvis; this process is known as involution and takes up to 6 weeks, even though by the 10th day postdelivery the uterus can no longer be felt. Breasts enlarge and fill with milk whether or not the new mother is breast-feeding. Vaginal discharge is present for up to 6 weeks postdelivery. Uncomfortable physical complaints, such as hemorrhoids, painful episiotomy, or constipation, may leave the new mother feeling that she isn't well enough to cope

Signs of postpartum depression

More than 80% of new mothers experience some form of "baby blues." In most cases, this is a temporary response to the work involved in caring for a new baby. In some cases, however, more severe signs of postpartum depression can occur and may not resolve for several months.

Mild depression

Typically, baby blues begin in the first days after delivery and last about 2 weeks. Symptoms can include crying, irritability, poor sleep, mood changes, and a sense of helplessness. The new mother may have a poor appetite or, conversely, may crave certain foods. She also may state that something "just isn't right." This self-limiting type of depression is thought to result from a reduction in estrogen levels after delivery. No treatment is needed beyond alleviating symptoms. The new mother should ask for help with newborn care, take frequent rest breaks when the baby is sleeping, and eat small, frequent, well-balanced meals.

More serious symptoms

If mild symptoms don't disappear within 2 weeks or if they worsen and begin to include headaches, hyperventilation, or heart palpitations, the new mother may be suffering from postpartum depression. This disorder, an exaggeration of the baby blues, is characterized by a more severe level of despondency. The depressive behavior may progress to extreme agitation, hallucinations, and a feeling of being "out of control." This behavior isn't short-lived. Postpartum depression usually lasts for 3 to 6 months, and medical intervention is required.

Telling the difference

The keys to differentiating the two conditions are time and severity of symptoms. A new mother with baby blues will feel better after getting rest; the depressed mother won't. The baby blues progressively improve; depression requires treatment. Support groups can offer the new mother opportunities to discuss her new feelings and any concerns she has about the daily care of her new baby. Every new mother should have the phone number of a local support group because this is a condition that affects many new mothers. A clinically depressed mother requires more; she *must* have referral to a professional counselor, psychiatrist, or psychologist.

---

with motherhood. Hormonal changes in the postpartum period, plus the responsibilities of caring for the newborn, make the new mother at risk for depression and anxiety. (See *Signs of postpartum depression.*) The family unit changes with the addition of the newborn, which sometimes brings on marital and family strains, especially if the new mother doesn't have an adequate support system.

It's widely agreed that after childbirth the new mother deserves a period of rest; despite this fact, hospital maternity stays are getting shorter with a 24- to 48-hour stay normal after an uncomplicated delivery. Most insurers consider childbirth a natural occurrence, with the bulk of the recovery to be done in the home setting. Therefore, the home care nurse now provides parenting and newborn care education. The hospital staff provides postdelivery health observation of mother and newborn, but many new mothers leave the hospital setting unprepared to manage postpartum changes and assume care of the newborn.

The early-discharged mother needs home care follow-up to answer questions she may have. Taking care of herself and the baby is an overwhelming job, especially for a young mother. The specific home care needs of the postpartum patient are related to education of the mother regarding self-care and relief from postpartum discomfort, as well to ensure that the new mother is able to provide adequate infant care.

Previsit checklist

Physician orders and preparation
- Orders for care
- Discharge recommendations, including analgesics ordered
- Postdelivery summary sheet indicating route of delivery and any complications that may have occurred during the delivery
- Knowledge of baseline patient laboratory values
- Infant information, including birth weight, feeding method, and any complications that may have been noted while in the nursery

Equipment and supplies
- Supplies for standard precautions and proper sharps disposal
- Vital signs equipment
- Blood-drawing equipment
- Educational handouts
- Infant scale

Safety requirements
- Standard precautions for infection control and sharps disposal
- Home observation for appropriateness for patient care
- Emergency plan and access to functional phone and list of emergency phone numbers
- Infant safety precautions related to prevention of infection and availability of infant safety-related equipment, including car seat, crib, and so on
- Instructions on danger signs and symptoms such as those indicating deep vein thrombosis (positive Homans' sign or pain, redness, swelling, lump in posterior calf) or other medical emergency and actions to take

Major diagnostic codes
(Most insurers will allow the postpartum visit only if the mother has had a complicated postpartum course; a few insurers will, however, allow the visit for a normal postpartum course after a shortened length of stay.)
- Deep vein thrombosis, postpartum, unspecified 671.40
- Disruption of perineal wound, unspecified 674.20
- Fourth-degree perineal laceration 664.3
- Infections of the nipple, postpartum 675.04
- Major puerperal infection, unspecified 670.00
- Mastitis, postpartum 675.14
- Newborn feeding problems 779.3
- Normal, uncomplicated vaginal delivery 650

- Pelvic hematoma, postpartum 665.74
- Postpartal complication of surgical wound, unspecified 674.34
- Postpartum hemorrhage, unspecified 666.00
- Varicose veins of legs, unspecified 671.00

Defense of homebound status

- Mother symptomatic due to low hemoglobin posthemorrhage
- Mother with elevated temperature due to infection postdelivery
- Mother on modified bed rest due to complications from vaginal delivery; out of bed no more than two times daily

Selected nursing diagnoses and patient outcomes

Fatigue
    The mother will:
- demonstrate knowledge of the need for multitasking to allow rest periods while infant is sleeping   (N)
- verbalize acceptance of caregiver assistance with housework and care of newborn to allow patient to rest   (N)
- identify basis of fatigue and individual areas of control   (N)
- identify appropriate interventions to promote more sleep and rest   (N)
- show increased level in coping ability by appropriate expression of feelings, identification of options, and use of resources.   (N, SW)

Altered urinary elimination
    The mother will:
- return to normal urinary patterns without signs of infection or neurologic deficit.   (N)

Risk for constipation
    The mother will:
- regain usual bowel function   (N)
- verbalize knowledge of dietary or medical interventions to correct constipation.   (N)

Knowledge deficit related to care of self and newborn
    The mother will:
- demonstrate knowledge of the lactation process, demonstrate correct positioning, identify infant feeding cues, and identify proper positioning for bottle-feeding, including positioning to promote bonding   (N)
- verbalize understanding of comfort measures to relieve pain   (N)
- verbalize understanding of physician orders regarding analgesia   (N)
- verbalize understanding of postpartum process   (N)
- identify signs and symptoms of infection or complications that require medical intervention   (N)
- assume responsibility for continued learning and seek resources. (N, SW)

Altered sexuality patterns
    The mother will:
- verbalize understanding of changing sexual roles, and indicate understanding of normal postpartum sexual changes   (N)
- verbalize understanding of need for contraception with first and any sexual encounter.   (N)

Skilled nursing services

Care measures
- Evaluate postpartum vital signs.
- Evaluate involution of uterus.
- Assess lochial flow.

- Assess new mother's emotional state.
- Evaluate presence or absence of lactation.
- Evaluate home environment for safety concerns.
- Request laboratory work as ordered by physician.
- Evaluate specific medical condition necessitating visit.
- Evaluate elimination status and offer suggestions for comfort measures.
- Evaluate caregiver's knowledge of infant care and level of confidence in providing care.
- Assess infant's feeding pattern.
- Assess newborn vital signs.
- Determine if neonatal jaundice is present and take appropriate measures.

Patient and family teaching

- Instruct new mother in care of infant.
- Teach postpartum patient about contraception.
- Instruct new mother in comfort measures, routine exercise, and nutrition.
- Review community resources available for new family.
- Provide information on signs and symptoms of newborn illness.

Interdisciplinary services

Social worker

- Information on financial assistance
- Counseling for long-range planning
- Contingency emergency care planning
- Psychosocial assessment and evaluation

Discharge plan

- Normal postpartum course without complications
- Mother knowledgeable about self-care following delivery and verbalizes comfort measures
- Mother understands physician's discharge orders
- Stable vital signs exhibited by mother and newborn
- Ability of mother to perform newborn care and feed infant successfully
- Ability of mother to identify newborn signs and symptoms requiring medical attention
- Mother demonstrates correct infant temperature taking
- Mother identifies care provider for infant
- Mother exhibits adequate bonding with infant
- Mother verbalizes signs and symptoms of postpartum depression as well as appropriate measures to seek assistance

Documentation requirements

- Skilled assessment, including documentation of vital signs with regard to any changes noted since discharge
- Physical assessment findings related to the postpartum course
- Variances from the normal postpartum course
- Notification of physician of any deviations from normal
- Mother-baby interaction
- Infant method of feeding and mother's ability to provide adequate nutrition
- Educational needs of mother
- Unusual family dynamics

- Educational booklets offered and community resource material provided
- Variances to expected outcomes
- Barriers to learning
- Continued needs and follow-up plans

Reimbursement reminders

- Home care services are reimbursed when an ICD-9 code is present to indicate reason for visit.

Insurance hints

- Present objective data.
- Present any variances from normal postpartum course.
- Report laboratory values.
- Notify case manager when home care is discontinued.

Pregnancy-induced hypertension

Pregnancy-induced hypertension (PIH), also called preeclampsia, occurs in 6% to 8% of all pregnancies and is the most common medical complication of pregnancy and a major cause of maternal and infant disease and death worldwide. A rise in blood pressure, protein in the urine, and frequently edema characterize the disorder. Because these signs are prevalent in a normal pregnancy, having one or more of them isn't a definitive diagnosis. PIH is defined as either a systolic blood pressure greater than 30 mm Hg or a diastolic blood pressure greater than 15 mm Hg higher than blood pressure readings taken before 20 weeks' gestation, or greater than 140/90. Women with PIH are at risk for complications of pregnancy, including abruptio placentae, renal failure, cerebral edema, disseminated intravascular coagulation, pulmonary edema, seizures, and HELLP syndrome (characterized by *h*emolysis, *e*levated *l*iver function tests, and *l*ow *p*latelets). Chronic hypertension that wasn't evident until the pregnancy may result in low birth weight infants, stillbirth, neonatal death, and other complications. The aim of treatment is to reduce infant mortality, maintaining the maternal blood pressure as close to normal as possible and delivery of a viable infant without complications.

Most patients develop PIH at or about the third trimester. Due to limits on reimbursement for long-term hospitalization, these patients are generally maintained at home under the close supervision of the home care nurse. The primary functions of the home care nurse are blood-pressure monitoring, evaluation of symptoms, and patient education for self-monitoring. The evaluation of blood pressure requires strict attention to technique to prevent erroneous results. The correct method of taking blood pressure is to have the patient in the left lateral position, which will give the major arteries the most vasodilation. Although diagnosis of PIH is made after two blood pressure readings with a rise of greater than 30 mm Hg over the usual readings with the patient in a sitting position, the preferred method of blood pressure monitoring in the home is to have the patient rest as much as possible in the left lateral supine position to provide uterine displacement. In addition, the homebound patient will have daily urine proteins checks for proteinuria, edema evaluated, and reflexes checked. The patient will be instructed in signs and symptoms that need immediate reporting and telephone contact to determine condition. Visit frequency, after initial stabilization in the hospital, is a minimum of two weekly skilled visits for observation and instruction, with telephone contact daily and as needed.

Previsit checklist

Physician orders and preparation
- Physician orders listing specific parameters (urine protein, blood pressure, and edema)
- Obstetric history pertaining to this pregnancy

Equipment and supplies
- Vital signs equipment
- Urine protein dipsticks
- Reflex hammer
- Doppler stethoscope for fetal heart tones
- Scale for weight

Safety requirements
- Standard precautions for infection control
- Emergency plan and access to functional phone and list of emergency phone numbers
- Fire evacuation plan, functional smoke detectors, and access to functional fire extinguisher
- List of symptoms requiring medical attention
- If home infusion required, adequate electrical outlets and notification of power company that resident has critical need for power

Major diagnostic codes
- Benign essential hypertension of pregnancy 642.0
- Eclampsia 642.6
- Hypertension secondary to renal disease complicating pregnancy 642.1
- Hypertensive complications of pregnancy, childbirth 642
- Mild or unspecified preeclampsia 642.4
- Other preexisting hypertension complicating pregnancy 642.2
- Preeclampsia or eclampsia superimposed on preexisting hypertension 642.7
- Severe preeclampsia 642.5
- Transient hypertension of pregnancy 642.3
- Unspecified hypertensive complications of pregnancy 642.9

(To assign a fifth digit, see appendix A, page 638.)

Defense of homebound status
- Out of bed no more than two times daily
- Unable to leave the home without assistance of another
- Fatigue, weakness, shortness of breath limiting activity
- Activity restriction prescribed by obstetrician
- Infusion therapy

Selected nursing diagnoses and patient outcomes

Activity intolerance

The patient or caregiver will:
- demonstrate compliance with activity limitations   (N)

• verbalize knowledge of disease process and potential adverse reactions to increased activity (N)
• demonstrate energy conservation techniques. (N)

Ineffective family coping: compromised with anxiety related to medical condition
The patient or caregiver will:
• identify appropriate coping mechanisms for stressful situations (N)
• demonstrate knowledge of community agencies available to support financial or other needs. (N, SW)

Fluid volume deficit (isotonic)
The patient or caregiver will:
• maintain normal fluid volume levels (N)
• have normal urinary output. (N)

Knowledge deficit related to medical condition
The patient or caregiver will:
• demonstrate compliance with plan of care, maintain bed rest in left lateral position, comply with medication regimen, monitor vital signs and uterine contractions (N)
• verbalize knowledge of disease process (N)
• demonstrate knowledge of importance of maintaining adequate nutrition (N)
• demonstrate adequate recording of symptoms during times of self-care. (N)

Knowledge deficit related to emergency medical management of condition (signs and symptoms to be aware of)
The patient or caregiver will:
• be aware of signs and symptoms for which to seek medical management, such as headache (frontal or occipital) unrelieved by common analgesics; visual disturbances (flashing lights before eyes and seeing "stars"); hyperreflexia; tremors; unusual nervousness; epigastric or right abdominal quadrant pain; altered sensorium; vaginal bleeding; abdominal or uterine tenderness or pain; and significant changes in uterine activity. (N, MD)

Skilled nursing services

Care measures
• Assess weight of patient.
• Assess for presence of edema (location and degree).
• Assess for presence of hyperreflexia.
• Assess for signs and symptoms of worsening condition.
• Assess fetal heart tones.
• Evaluate patient compliance to plan of care (bed rest in left lateral position).
• Evaluate patient knowledge of symptoms requiring medical management.
• Assess for proper nutrition as prescribed (for example, low sodium).
• Assess psychosocial status and home situation.

Patient and family teaching
• Teach about recording daily weight and contacting physician for a gain of more than 2 lb per day or more than 5 lb per week.
• Demonstrate how to record symptoms, amount and site of edema, and uterine activity monitoring.
• Emphasize need for exercise and scheduled rest periods.
• Teach self-care and infusion therapy instructions.
• Review coping skills.

- Instruct patient in collection of urine for dipstick protein measurement and how to record results.
- Instruct caregiver in care of patient.

Interdisciplinary actions

Home care aide
- Housekeeping duties
- Assistance in care of other family members

Social worker
- Information on financial assistance
- Counseling for long-range planning
- Contingency emergency care planning
- Psychosocial assessment and evaluation
- Information regarding care for other children, if any

Discharge plan
- Admitted to hospital for delivery
- Blood pressure stabilized
- Ability of patient to perform own health observation and verbalize danger signs and symptoms with appropriate action plan for potential situations, such as increased blood pressure, weight gain, bleeding, and signs of labor
- Ability of caregiver to perform health monitoring of patient
- Self-care with assistance of significant others, support of physician, and community resources

Documentation requirements
- Skilled assessment, including subjective and objective data

- Fetal heart tones record, presence of fetal movement
- Blood pressure with patient in left lateral recumbent position
- Edema, location, pitting or nonpitting; note facial edema
- Results of urine protein (clean catch method)
- Patient's vital signs, including weight
- Any symptoms patient may be experiencing
- Patient compliance with plan of care and any variances to expected outcomes
- Patient reflexes
- Emotional needs and concerns of patient
- Daily telephone contact with patient
- Barriers to learning
- Continued needs and follow-up plans

Reimbursement reminders
- Indicate compliance with physician orders.
- Home care services are reimbursed when an ICD-9 code is present to indicate reason for visit.
- Most insurers won't pay for supplies, such as dipsticks to check for proteinuria. The patient may have a pharmacy plan that pays for such materials with the physician orders.
- If extra visits are needed, document reason for visit and condition change precipitating need for visit.

Insurance hints
- Give actual date for end point of services and update it according to patient's progress.
- Present objective data.
- Present any variances from normal.
- Explain patient's capacity for learning self-care objectively.

• Try to develop a therapeutic follow-up plan for patient.

Preterm labor

Preterm labor is defined as the onset of labor after the 20th and before the 38th week of pregnancy. Good fetal outcome is achieved when the pregnancy is maintained to the 36th week of gestation; some tertiary facilities are reporting success rates with infants born at 32 weeks. The goal of pregnancy management is to maintain the pregnancy to as close to term as possible without maternal or fetal compromise.

Most cases of preterm labor have an unknown etiology; however, some factors predispose a patient to the development of preterm labor. These factors include multiple gestation, incompetent cervix, preeclampsia or eclampsia, diabetes, injury, uterine anomalies, or a history of preterm labors. Placental disorders, including hemorrhagic disorders of the placenta, also predispose the patient to preterm labor.

The goal of home health care is to maintain the patient in the home environment as long as possible to reduce hospital costs and allow the mother to maintain bonds with other children and family members. Patients are selected for home management and must be agreeable to the treatment plan and compliant with regards to the plan of care. The home must be suitable for care with emergency access for rapid transfer to the hospital if needed. The home care nurse must be prepared to educate the patient and her family regarding signs and symptoms that must be reported immediately because the speed in which the patient receives

medical intervention may affect the outcome of the pregnancy.

At the present time, there is conflict in the medical community regarding home uterine monitoring. Once a promising observation method, it has recently fallen out of favor due to the cost involved and the frequency of false-positive data given regarding the start of contractions. Home health care in terms of preterm labor is at the discretion of the individual physician. Patient self-palpation for contractions and fetal kick count is generally accepted as an initial assessment before the initiation of home uterine monitoring or the use of tocolysis.

Previsit checklist

Physician orders and preparation
• Physician orders listing guidelines for medical notification
• Obstetric history of present pregnancy

Equipment and supplies
• Vital signs equipment
• Doppler stethoscope for fetal heart tones

Safety requirements
• Standard precautions for infection control
• Emergency plan and access to functional phone and list of emergency phone numbers
• List of symptoms requiring immediate medical attention

Major diagnostic codes
• Antepartum hemorrhage 641

- Early onset of delivery 644.21
- Early or threatened labor 644
- Hemorrhage from placenta previa 641.1
- Hemorrhage in early pregnancy delivered, not delivered 640.01, 640.03
- Other specified hemorrhage in early pregnancy 640.8
- Placenta previa without hemorrhage, antepartal 641.03
- Premature separation of placenta 641.2
- Threatened abortion 640.0
- Threatened premature labor, not delivered during care 644.03
- Unspecified hemorrhage in early pregnancy 640.9

(To assign a fifth digit, see appendix A, page 638.)

Defense of homebound status
- On bed rest
- Unable to leave the home without the assistance of another person
- Skilled services required regarding monitoring

Selected nursing diagnoses and patient outcomes

Anxiety related to medical condition
The patient will:
- demonstrate at least two coping techniques   (N)
- be able to provide return demonstration of two relaxation techniques.   (N)

Altered nutrition: Less than body requirements
The patient will:

- demonstrate ability to maintain adequate nutrition.   (N)

Fluid volume deficit (isotonic)
The patient will:
- maintain normal fluid volume levels   (N)
- have normal urine output.   (N)

Knowledge deficit related to premature labor
The patient will:
- demonstrate compliance with plan of care to assist in delay of premature labor   (N)
- identify and report danger signals of premature labor   (N)
- achieve successful prolongation of pregnancy to term.   (N)

Knowledge deficit related to management of complications of pregnancy
The patient or caregiver will:
- be aware of signs and symptoms that necessitate immediate medical attention   (N)
- demonstrate knowledge of behavioral compliance with medications, activity restrictions, bed rest, and diet   (N)
- verbalize knowledge of disease process   (N)
- demonstrate adequate recording of symptoms during times of self-care.   (N)

Skilled nursing services

Care measures
- Assess weight of patient.
- Check fetal heart tones.
- Evaluate fundal height.
- Evaluate signs and symptoms.

- Assess patient knowledge of symptoms requiring medical management.
- Assess for proper nutrition.
- Assess psychosocial status and home situation.
- Evaluate patient's compliance to plan of care.

Patient and family teaching

- Instruct caregiver in care of the patient.
- Teach about uterine self-palpation.

Interdisciplinary actions

Home care aide

- Housekeeping duties
- Care of other family members

Social worker

- Information on financial assistance
- Counseling for long-range planning
- Contingency emergency care planning
- Psychosocial assessment and evaluation

Discharge plan

- Admitted to hospital for delivery
- Ability of patient to perform own health monitoring
- Ability of caregiver to perform health observation of patient

Documentation requirements

- Skilled assessment, including both subjective and objective data
- Fetal heart tones and presence of fetal movement
- Vital signs, including weight

- Symptoms patient may be experiencing
- Patient compliance with plan of care
- Emotional needs and concerns of patient
- Daily telephone contact with patient
- Variances to expected outcomes
- Barriers to learning
- Continued needs and follow-up plans

Reimbursement reminders

- Indicate compliance with physician orders.
- Home care services are reimbursed when an ICD-9 code is present to indicate reason for visit.
- If extra visit is needed, document reason for visit and condition change precipitating need for visit.

Insurance hints

- Give estimated end point for services.
- Present objective data.
- Present any variances from normal.
- Explain patient's capacity for learning self-care objectively.
- Try to develop a therapeutic follow-up plan for patient.

9 Pediatric disorders and treatments

Acquired immunodeficiency syndrome

Acquired immunodeficiency syndrome (AIDS) is a progressive destruction of the patient's immune system by human immunodeficiency virus (HIV). AIDS makes the patient highly susceptible to infections and malignancies. HIV is transmitted to children by contact with infected blood or body fluids, by contact with mucous membranes during birth, through transfusion of blood products, through sexual conduct, through injection of drugs, or during breast-feeding. Home care of children with AIDS focuses on nutritional and antiviral support as well as disease prevention and infection control.

Previsit checklist

Physician orders and preparation
• Frequency and nature of skilled nursing visits

• Serum glucose and electrolyte levels
• Weight monitoring
• Intake and output monitoring
• Type, rate, frequency, and route of nutritional support, such as total parental or enteral nutrition or oral supplementation
• Nutritional formula and solutions and calorie allotments
• Antiviral and antibiotic orders and immune globulin, including route, rates, and times of administration; and flavoring agents to mask unpleasant medications, if required
• Care of vascular access device and parenteral or enteral nutrition device and insertion sites as appropriate
• Activity orders and restriction
• Dietitian evaluation of dietary and fluid intake, including calorie allotment
• Enterostomal therapy evaluation for enteral tube site care if indicated
• Social worker evaluation for resources, financial assistance, and equipment needs
• Home care aide assistance with personal care, nutrition, and ambulation

Equipment and supplies

- Supplies for standard precautions and proper waste and sharps disposal
- Nutritional support equipment including delivery devices, formula, and site care supplies, such as dressings for long-term central venous access device, I.V. infusion, or feeding pump
- Phlebotomy equipment
- Scale
- Supplies for administering medications, including sterile distilled water for preparing medications; mortar and pestle to grind tablets, if needed; syringes and measuring cups for oral or tube medication administration; and syringes to access device, if used
- Sterile gauze and occlusive dressings
- Heparin and normal saline solution for flushing venous access device if indicated
- Stethoscope, thermometer (axillary temperatures preferred), and sphygmomanometer (with cuff properly sized to fit the child's arm)
- Intake and output form; calorie count record

Safety requirements

- Infant and child safety precautions, including car seat, hot water heater thermostat set at 120° F (48.9° C)
- Standard precautions for infection control and waste and sharps disposal
- System to assist adherence to complex medication regimen, including nutrition therapy
- Activity orders and restrictions
- Action plan for intolerance and device or tube dislodgment
- Working electricity with grounded electrical receptacle for feeding pump
- Power outage plan

- Instructions on signs and symptoms of medical emergency and actions to take as well as signs and symptoms to report to physician
- Emergency plan and access to functional phone and list of emergency phone numbers (local emergency medical service providers should have advance directions to the home, particularly if it's in a hard-to-find location)
- Fire evacuation plan, functional smoke detectors, and access to functional fire extinguisher
- Night-light
- Information on medications, including dosage, adverse effects, interactions, and safe storage
- Infection control precautions to protect child from contact with people who have colds and other infections
- Use of prepared boiled and cooled water or distilled water for ingestion by child brushing teeth and for preparing or swallowing medication because of possible contamination of ground- or municipal water

Major diagnostic codes

- Candidiasis, unspecified 112.9
- Cytomegalovirus 078.5
- Failure to thrive 783.4
- Human immunodeficiency virus infection, symptomatic 042
- Immunodeficiency 279.3
- Septicemia, unspecified 038.9
- Tuberculosis, unspecified 011.9

Defense of homebound status

- Confined to bed due to invasive medical equipment and need for nutritional support

- Unable to ambulate farther than 10' (3 m) due to profound fatigue or weakness secondary to illness or treatment protocol effects
- Bedridden or confined to chair, requiring assistance of one or two persons to transfer
- Severity of immune suppression precludes activity outside home

Selected nursing diagnoses and patient outcomes

Altered nutrition: Less than body requirements related to (specify: effects of disease and medications, need for double the recommended dietary allowance, anorexia secondary to oral lesions, fatigue, or malaise)

The patient or caregiver will:
- offer child-size food portions frequently and record amounts eaten (N, D, HCA)
- offer food following naps or rest periods (N, D, HCA)
- provide soft foods during flare-up of oral lesions (N, D, HCA)
- demonstrate adherence to planned nutritional support therapy, including record of intake and calories (N, D)
- describe appropriate technique for delivering nutritional support (N, D)
- demonstrate an absence of signs and symptoms of electrolyte imbalance and hyperglycemia (N)
- maintain nutritional requirements (N, D)
- demonstrate at least maintenance of current weight with gradual achievement of a target weight of _____ . (N, D, HCA)

Altered family processes related to the impact of the child's condition on role responsibilities, siblings, finances, and responses of relatives, friends, and community

The patient or caregiver will:
- verbalize feelings frequently to professional nurse and to family members (N, SW)
- actively participate in care (N, HCA)
- demonstrate measures to facilitate child role change from sick role to well role (N, SW)
- seek appropriate support from external resources when needed (N, SW)
- verbalize understanding of disease as a terminal illness. (N, MD, SC, SW)

Knowledge deficit related to management of therapeutic regimen secondary to insufficient knowledge of (specify: modes of transmission, risks of live virus vaccines, avoidance of infections, school attendance, and community resources, nutritional support, or actions, preparation and administration, adverse effects, precautions, and interactions of all medications given to child)

The patient or caregiver will:
- describe modes of transmission of HIV (N)
- list alternatives to live virus vaccines (for example, Salk-killed injectable inactivated rather than Sabin live attenuated oral poliomyelitis vaccine) and verbalize when the child can't receive live virus vaccines (N, MD)
- institute measures to protect the child from visitors with infections (N, HCA, MD)
- encourage school attendance as the child's endurance permits (N, SW)

- select community resources appropriate for family situation (N, SW)
- demonstrate adequate skills for administering nutritional support and medication therapy. (N, D)

Skilled nursing services

Care measures

- Perform an initial skilled assessment of all body systems; closely observe immune, neurologic, integumentary, and GI systems.
- Assess level of care provided by caregiver, especially in preparation and administration of medications, nutritional support, and infection control.
- Assess effectiveness of treatment regimen, including vital signs, weight trends, calorie count, intake and output, skin turgor, signs and symptoms of opportunistic infection.
- Assess completeness of immunization status — excluding live virus vaccines — appropriate for age. Live attenuated measles-mumps-rubella vaccine (MMR), should be given per normal schedule. Yellow fever vaccine, oral polio vaccine, and bacillus Calmette-Guérin (BCG) are contraindicated.
- Assess insertion site and perform site care to vascular access device or enteral feeding tube.
- Administer infusions via vascular access devices as ordered.
- Monitor for possible adverse effects of medication therapy.
- Evaluate caregiver's ability to administer medications and nutritional support therapy.
- Check placement of enteral feeding tube, if used.

- Observe caregiver in care of venous access device or enteral feeding tube and site as well as preparation and administration of medications and nutritional supplements as appropriate.
- Obtain or arrange for laboratory tests, such as serum glucose and electrolyte levels, as ordered.

Patient and family teaching

- Teach about assessing vital signs and weight and monitoring intake and output.
- Describe energy conservation techniques and safety measures.
- Discuss infection control measures, including standard precautions.
- Identify signs and symptoms to report to the physician, including any episodes of vomiting, diarrhea, abdominal distention, difficulty swallowing or breathing, and changes in mental status.
- Review signs and symptoms of parenteral or enteral feeding problems, including possible fluid overload.
- Discuss nutrition therapy regimen and care.
- Describe measures to maintain weight.
- Teach about medications, including dosage, frequency, route, preparation, administration, and possible adverse effects.
- Demonstrate vascular access site care, including flushing.

Interdisciplinary actions

Dietitian

- Evaluation for nutritional supplementation by oral, GI, or vascular routes
- Calorie needs and allotment

- Age-appropriate guidance for snacks and other oral foods, incorporating patient's preferences into selections
- Guidance in avoiding food and drug interactions

Social worker
- Referral to community resources and support groups
- Counseling and referral for stress management or reduction
- Assistance in coping with terminal illness

Home care aide
- Assistance with personal care and activities of daily living
- Assistance with oral feeding
- Respite care
- Homemaker services

Discharge plan
- Safe management of child with AIDS in the home, with follow-up services of physician and school nurse (if attending school)
- Continued need for skilled nursing for infusion therapy, if ordered, and episodic follow up by dietitian (for nutritional changes related to disease process and growth and development of child)
- Referral to community social service organizations for crisis intervention
- Referral to hospice care of the child and family with end-stage AIDS
- Death with dignity and minimal discomfort.

Documentation requirements
- Skilled assessment of vital signs; skin and mucous membrane integrity; GI function, including bowel sounds and bowel elimination patterns; urine output; weight; results of blood studies; vascular access device or feeding tube site placement, patency, and care measures; activity level, including type of play; signs and symptoms of opportunistic infection; summary of food log and calorie counts
- Nutritional support and feeding administration (type, amount, timing, residuals, and tolerance)
- Patient and caregiver participation in care
- Patient and caregiver progress toward developmental goals, including managing feelings of being overwhelmed, need for repeated instructions
- Patient and caregiver independence with care and therapy regimen
- Response to medication and nutritional supplements, including adverse reactions, if any
- Use of all durable medical equipment (DME), including frequency of use, settings, and care of equipment
- Status, use, and care of any access devices
- Patient and caregiver instructions
- Caregiver teaching and demonstrated responses to teaching
- Communications with physician and other disciplines
- Complications (evidence or lack thereof)
- Safety and infection control precautions
- Signs and symptoms to be reported
- Blood studies obtained and results, including report to physician
- Changes in plan of care, including changes directly related to results of blood studies; patient and caregiver understanding of changes

Reimbursement reminders

• Care of children with AIDS is covered under the Ryan White Act and the Katie Beckett Act, administered in many states by Medicaid. This care includes skilled nursing in the home and school, dietitian and social worker services, and DME rentals.

• Use of a needleless infusion system, while more expensive, is an appropriate safeguard against sharps injuries and HIV exposure in the community.

• Report any variances to expected outcomes, such as fluid overload, high residuals, or changes in the patient's condition.

• Record any barriers to learning, such as physical deformities; visual impairments; language, culture, or literacy barriers; and a lack of or overburdened support person.

• Note which community resources (such as entitlement programs, early intervention, and school programs) are available.

Insurance hints

• Record complete assessment data each visit, including changes in condition since last visit and progress toward goals, such as maintenance of laboratory values or weight. Include changes in weight, skin turgor, mucous membranes, and intake and output; signs of opportunistic infection; and adjustment issues, such as patient's resistance to or acceptance of diagnosis, nutritional support, therapy, and instructions.

• Report complications, such as nausea, vomiting, diarrhea, fluid overload, skin breakdown, and aspiration.

• Describe gains in knowledge, such as skills and concepts mastered in medication administration, nutritional therapy measures, and infection-control precautions.

• Present specific data on homebound status, such as continued inability to ambulate because of severe fatigue from malnutrition or cachexia, the number of persons needed to assist patient out of chair, and continued limitations in ambulation.

• Present objective patient findings and changes since last contact, such as return of serum glucose or electrolytes to within normal parameters, maintenance of or gradual gain in weight, and improved skin turgor.

• Present objective data about homebound status.

• Report any new laboratory findings that change the plan of care.

• Report specifics about the patient caregiver and family learning progress.

• Detail responses of the child and family to care performed at each visit.

• Review presence, use, and care of equipment at each visit, including settings and rates.

• Describe all teaching of child and family and response to teaching performed at each visit.

• Report all communication with physician and other disciplines — including need for hospice.

Asthma

Asthma is a chronic illness characterized by episodes of wheezing that is caused by bronchospasm, excessive mucus production, and airway constriction. Asthma episodes may be triggered by stressors, such as exercise, heat, and cold, and various allergens including some medications. Episodes may occur suddenly or develop gradually.

More than 5 million children in America have asthma. In 1998, approximately 200 children under age 15 died of asthma — twice the death rate of 10 years ago. The Centers for Disease Control and Prevention estimates nearly a threefold increase in asthma prevalence over the past 20 years; a large proportion of the cases can be directly linked to exposure to environmental tobacco smoke (ETS), or secondhand smoke. Home care for children with asthma focuses on prevention of asthma episodes and prompt care during acute exacerbations.

Previsit checklist

Physician orders and preparation

- Routine medications, such as long-acting beta agonists, inhaled corticosteroids, and cromolyn
- Rescue medications, including short-acting bronchodilators, such as albuterol, and inhaled or systemic corticosteroids
- Peak flow meter monitoring, including frequency, target ranges, and instructions for each range of readings
- Pulse oximeter and settings, with instructions for low (specified) readings, and oxygen for acute exacerbations
- Delivery devices for all ordered medications and treatments, including settings, routes, frequency, duration, and dosage
- Injectable epinephrine for anaphylaxis
- Measures to combat allergens found in child's environment, including elimination of ETS and desensitization

- Immunotherapy such as anti-immune globulin E injections and oral glucocorticosteroids
- Chest physiotherapy to loosen and remove mucus, including type and frequency
- Dietary restrictions or supplementation
- Laboratory and diagnostic tests, such as sputum culture or chest X-ray
- Social worker evaluation for community resources
- Physical therapy evaluation for endurance training and chest physiotherapy

Equipment and supplies

- Supplies for standard precautions and proper waste and sharps disposal
- Agents for cleaning equipment, such as household vinegar, and dishwasher (if available) for sterilization of equipment
- Delivery devices for use with medications and treatments, such as nebulizers, air compressor, suction catheters, suction machine, peak flow meter, pulse oximeter, vibrator, chest percussors, and oxygen equipment, such as tank, flowmeter, and tubing
- Safety devices such as OXYGEN IN USE and NO SMOKING signs; securing devices for oxygen tanks
- Fragrance-free soaps, lotions, and cleaning supplies
- Assessment equipment, such as stethoscope, thermometer, and sphygmomanometer (with cuff sized to fit the child's arm)

Safety requirements

- Standard precautions for infection control and waste and sharps disposal

- System to assist compliance with complex medication regimen, including equipment care
- Emergency plan and access to functional phone and list of emergency phone numbers
- Fire evacuation plan, functional smoke detectors, and access to functional fire extinguisher
- Night-light
- Oxygen precautions, safe handling and placement of home oxygen equipment, and notification of local fire and police departments and utility companies of oxygen use in the home
- Measures to avoid multiple chemical sensitivity, for example, not wearing perfume or cologne, knowing child's allergens, using vinyl gloves if anyone (child, family member, or nurse) has sensitivity to latex, using fragrance-free cleaning products, and avoiding strong household cleaners
- Instructions on signs and symptoms of a medical emergency and actions to take

Major diagnostic codes

- Asthma without/with status asthmaticus 493.90/493.91

Defense of homebound status

- Unable to ambulate farther than 10′ (3 m) due to respiratory distress
- Confined to first level of home; unable to climb stairs secondary to shortness of breath
- Shortness of breath when talking or on exertion

Selected nursing diagnoses and patient outcomes

Ineffective airway clearance related to bronchospasm and increased pulmonary secretions
   The patient or caregiver will:
- demonstrate effective cough and increased air exchange in lungs (N, RT)
- report an improvement in ability to breathe   (N, RT)
- exhibit an absence of chest retractions and wheezing on auscultation
                                              (N, RT)
- demonstrate measures to improve air exchange   (N, RT)
- administer inhaled glucocorticosteroids and bronchodilators, and oxygen at onset of asthma episode to open airway   (N)
- perform chest physiotherapy and suctioning to aid in removal of mucous plugs as airway opens.   (N, RT)

Fear related to episodes of breathlessness and recurrences
   The patient or caregiver will:
- verbalize feelings related to asthmatic episodes   (N, SW)
- communicate overall improvement in control of episodes   (N)
- state confidence in ability to manage episodes.   (N)

Knowledge deficit related to (for example, disease process, medication regimen)
   The patient or caregiver will:
- check oxygen saturation daily and be alert to upcoming asthma episode
                                                 (N)
- demonstrate ability to monitor peak flow daily and be alert to upcoming asthma episode
                                                 (N)

- administer preventive medications, such as cromolyn, to avoid episodes
(N, PH)
- identify triggers (N)
- participate in efforts to rid home of allergens (N)
- verbalize early signs and symptoms of impending asthmatic attack (N, MD)
- demonstrate measures to treat impending attack (N, MD)
- verbalize the need for tapering dosage of corticosteroids with physician guidance (N, MD)
- verbalize the need for removal of mucous plugs after use of bronchodilators to avoid fatal rebound bronchospasm.
(N, MD)

Skilled nursing services

Care measures
- Perform an initial skilled assessment of all systems, including respiratory, cardiovascular, and immune systems.
- Assess level of care provided by patient and caregiver, including attention to safety precautions, avoidance of triggers, and administration of medications and treatments.
- Assess effectiveness of treatment regimen, including auscultation of breath sounds, peak flow meter readings, oxygen saturation, ease of breathing, respiratory rate and depth, sputum production and characteristics.
- Observe patient and caregiver use of medication delivery devices and peak flow meter.
- Obtain or arrange for laboratory tests as indicated.

Patient and family teaching
- Discuss medication therapy, for routine and rescue medications including actions, adverse effects, precautions, possible interactions, and methods of administration.
- Describe signs and symptoms of impending attack, including ranges for peak flow meter readings.
- Review measures to treat an impending attack.
- Discuss danger signs and symptoms requiring emergency treatment.
- Explain use of epinephrine for anaphylaxis.
- Emphasize the importance of preventing long-term or concurrent complications (such as chronic bronchitis, pneumonia, or emphysema) by prompt and thorough treatment during episodes and prevention of episodes.

Interdisciplinary actions

Social worker
- Evaluation for referral to community resources
- Counseling and stress reduction
- Advocacy regarding air quality issues
- Assistance with insurance and financial matters

Respiratory therapist
- Pulmonary evaluation
- Chest physiotherapy

Discharge plan
- Safe independent management of the child with asthma in the home with physician follow-up services
- Follow-up appointments for laboratory testing with authorized laboratory

Documentation requirements

• Skilled assessment of subjective and objective data regarding signs and symptoms of respiratory distress (including respiratory rate and depth, retractions, complaints of shortness of breath, breath sounds, and cough and sputum production and characteristics)

• Results of pulse oximetry or peak flow meter use

• Methods used to reduce exposure to allergens and triggers

• Effects of medications, use of oxygen, and chest physical therapy

• Child and caregiver participation in care, including ability to use delivery devices, caregiver progress toward educational goals, and child's response to care, including frequency of asthmatic episodes and changes in occurrence

• Patient and caregiver instruction

• Complications (evidence or lack thereof)

• Safety precautions

• Signs and symptoms to be reported

• Results of any laboratory or diagnostic tests obtained

• Physical therapy evaluation

• Teaching related to chest physiotherapy

Reimbursement reminders

• Keep in mind that many insurance companies will cover the cost of a nebulizer for patients with asthma experiencing severely impaired respiratory status. However, the reimbursement typically covers one nebulizer for a specified period such as 5 years. If the patient requires a new nebulizer within this period of time, the insurance company may not pay for it.

• Know that devices such as spacers (not provided with the medication itself) may require out-of-pocket payment. However, specific equipment such as allergen reduction devices (for example, air filters) may be covered; check with the patient's third-party payer for details.

• Record results of assessment, including vital signs, breath sounds, and oxygen saturation or peak flow rate.

• Describe reports of asthma episodes, including duration, triggers, (if known), effect of oxygen and medications, responses of child and caregiver, and use of emergency medical services.

• Detail the effect of preventive measures, including medications; allergen removal efforts; and use of devices for early warning of susceptibility to asthmatic exacerbations.

• Record responses of caregiver to teaching, including return demonstration of procedures and verbalization of understanding of information taught.

• Describe any environmental situations that may affect the child's susceptibility to asthma episodes. For example, document high pollen counts, code red or orange days (high heat and humidity), or toxic spraying in child's environment such as for insect control. Include child's exposure to ETS in any settings in which he spends any length of time, such as a babysitter's or relative's home.

• Report all communication with physician and other disciplines, including durable medical equipment providers.

Insurance hints

- Present objective assessment data including results of pulse oximetry or peak flow testing and vital signs for each visit.
- Report any change in child's condition since last contact, including progress or deterioration; development of infection; and ability to recognize early warning signals
- Report adjustment issues, such as the patient's resistance to or acceptance of treatment and the disease
- Report any adverse effects of medications.
- Present specifics about caregiver education progress, such as ability to use nebulizer or inhaled medications, improvement in symptoms, and adherence to desensitization program.

Cancer care

Cancer in children is similar in many ways to cancer in adults. While medical treatment and procedures for the disease are similar, there are many factors that need to be considered when treating children. For example, children generally respond to a diagnosis of cancer with a range of emotions that parallel and sometimes mirror those of their parents or other significant adults in their lives. They may be very ill or in a lot of pain, or they may not feel sick at all. They will have gone through numerous, confusing diagnostic tests, hearing the same words as adults with cancer; however, they may not comprehend them. Because children normally fashion their emotional responses after adults', stabilizing their care environment as quickly as possible is crucial. Home care of children with cancer involves assessment and treatment of the child as well as support for his parents, siblings, and extended family, such as grandparents and close family friends. Referrals to community resources for counseling, support groups (for parents and siblings), financial, and respite services should be made as early as possible.

Previsit checklist

Physician's orders and preparation

- Medications including dosage, route, and frequency
- Laboratory testing, such as drug levels, electrolyte levels, and complete blood counts
- Nutritional support, including enteral feeding if appropriate
- Activity orders and restrictions
- Homebound education (if needed) or in-school infection precautions (depending on school district requirements) and any changes in school-day duration
- Excuse from receiving live virus vaccines ordinarily required for all school children (such as measles, mumps, and rubella (MMR), varicella, and oral polio vaccines [current recommendations are that all children should be receiving injectable polio vaccine only])
- Durable medical equipment such as infusion equipment

Equipment and supplies

- Supplies for standard precautions and proper sharps disposal
- Nutritional monitoring tool and scale
- Developmental, social, psychological, and emotional evaluation tool

- Patient information sheets for parents on drug interactions and adverse effects
- Wound care supplies
- Clean-up (spill) kit for in-home chemotherapy approved by the Occupational Safety and Health Administration (OSHA)

Safety requirements

- Information on medications, including dosages, adverse effects, interactions, and safe storage
- Written safety precautions involving medications and equipment around children
- Documentation of allergies
- Emergency plan and access to functional phone and list of emergency phone numbers, including that of Poison Control Center
- Night-light
- Use of standard precautions for prevention of infection
- List of OSHA requirements and precautions for use of in-home chemotherapy drugs

Major diagnostic codes

- Adrenal cancer 194.0
- Brain cancer 191.9
- Esophagus, cancer of 150.9
- Head or neck, cancer of 195.0
- Hickman catheter insertion 38.98
- Leukemia, acute 208.0
- Leukopenia 288.0
- Lung cancer 162.9
- Metastases, general/bone 199.1/198.5
- Multiple myeloma 203.0
- Pancreatic cancer 157.9
- Pleural effusion 197.2
- Spinal cord tumor 239.7

Defense of homebound status

- Most private insurance companies and Medicaid won't require a child to be homebound. Written explanation of any homebound status requirements should be requested from the third-party payer.

Selected nursing diagnoses and patient outcomes

Risk for altered growth and development related to impaired ability to achieve developmental tasks
    The child will:
- demonstrate growth and development in social skills, language, cognition, and motor activities appropriate to age-group (specify).   (N)

Coping, ineffective family: Compromised
    The family will:
- frequently verbalize feelings to nurse and each other   (N, SW)
- participate in care of ill family member   (N, SW)
- facilitate return of ill family member from sick role to well role   (N, SW)
- maintain functional support system for each other   (N, SW)
- seek appropriate external resources when needed.   (N, SW)

Home maintenance management impairment related to inadequate resources, housing, or impaired caregivers
    The family will:
- identify factors that restrict self-care and home management   (N, SW)

- demonstrate ability to perform skills necessary for care of the individual or home   (N)
- express satisfaction with home situation.   (N, SW)

Risk for parental role conflict related to separation secondary to frequent hospitalizations
   The parents will:
- identify source of role conflict   (N, SW)
- define the parental role desired   (N, SW)
- participate in decision-making regarding care of child   (N, SW)
- participate in care of child at level desired.   (N, SW)

Risk for social isolation (child and family) related to altered state of wellness
   The patient and family will:
- express sadness   (N, SW)
- discuss losses periodically (N, SW)
- identify possible sources of social interaction   (N, SW)
- utilize available resources.(N, SW)

Skilled nursing services

Care measures
- Closely monitor for adverse effects of treatment (nausea, vomiting, decreased white blood cell count, electrolyte imbalance, and loss of appetite).
- Monitor developmental, social, emotional, psychological, and educational status. Note abnormalities and focus interventions and evaluation on those areas.
- Assess nutrition and fluid intake.
- Monitor laboratory test results and report abnormalities and evaluation of interventions as needed.

- Assess skin turgor and monitor weight with each visit (in contrast to weekly adult weights, children lose weight and dehydrate very quickly).
- Assess care environment and social interactions (friends, siblings, parents, and grandparents). Families may need to be encouraged to constructively discipline their child who has cancer because he can quickly become out of control and unsettled by changes in behavior standards, which can add to parental stress. Also, the child can often feel that he is sicker than told because of the lapse in discipline and the change in rules, which can also be confusing to siblings.
- Make referrals to and conference with other support services; encourage patient and family participation in available support systems.

Patient and family teaching
- Provide tips on administering medications; for example, for a minimal additional charge, most pharmacies will flavor drugs with child's flavor of choice.
- Teach caregiver to perform wound care or treatments. Discuss incorporating play or story time into procedure routines to help relax and distract a child or using that time to allow an adolescent patient to share his feelings, receive news about friends and family, or exchange jokes or riddles to help remove the intensity and fear that can normally accompany medical procedures and wound care. (Frequent use of the three Hs [humor, hope, and hugs] will make these tasks easier.)
- Instruct family in medication and equipment safety.

• Instruct caregiver to post Poison Control Center and emergency contact numbers by the telephone.

• Instruct family in methods to increase oral intake. For example, children with open mouth lesions will find frozen popsicles and juice popsicles soothing. Also, some drugs can be frozen in juice and administered as a frozen pop (check with pharmacist first).

• Instruct caregiver that if child can't attend school, most public school systems have homebound programs in place to accommodate him. These programs keep children from losing ground educationally and help maintain and promote social and developmental growth. If a child is able to attend school, accommodations can be made to prevent exposure to infection.

Interdisciplinary actions

Social worker

• Assessment of emotional, psychological, developmental, and educational needs
• Assessment of family coping and stressors
• Short-term counseling
• Referral to community resources

Discharge plan

• Safe independent management of child with cancer with follow-up services of physician and school nurse (if attending school)
• Stable care environment with support systems in place and functioning

Documentation requirements

• Developmental, psychological, and emotional levels and any changes
• Formal education needs and referrals made to support services, type of education source to be used (in home, in school, protected environment)
• Results of all conferences with support services
• Sibling reaction to disease and treatment process
• Interactions between parents, patient, siblings, extended family, and friends
• Availability of support system and level of current function; carefully document changes in support systems and need for new instruction
• Methods used to decrease patient anxiety and promote patient cooperation
• Method of medication administration (such as incorporated into frozen popsicles, crushed in foods, or flavor added by pharmacist)
• Patient's favorite comfort toy or blanket and its name
• Skin turgor and weight with each visit (in contrast to weekly weight monitoring in adults)
• Name and type of educational materials given to parents and patient, including reactions to these materials
• Patient activity level and any changes
• All safety instructions and safety measures in place and when established
• Patient, family, and support system progress toward established goals

Reimbursement reminders

• Medicaid and many private insurance companies list cancer as a catastrophic illness and have catastrophic coverage, but many health maintenance organizations do not.

• Frequently, limited visits are available, so it's important to know the allowable number of visits at the beginning of home care and to prioritize visit goals.

• Individuals can contact the American Cancer Society for information on available additional funding for equipment, supplies, emergency housing, and travel. They are also a valuable resource for interacting with insurance companies.

Insurance hints

• Present objective data regarding homebound status.

• Make a list of all objective patient findings and changes since last contact prior to interaction with case manager.

• Know new laboratory values and any new change in clinical condition.

• Give specifics regarding the patient and caregiver education progress.

Cerebral palsy

Cerebral palsy, a complex of chronic neurologic disabilities affecting body movement and coordination, isn't progressive or communicable. It's caused by damage to one or more specific areas of the brain prenatally, perinatally, or during infancy and most often involves lack of oxygen to the brain. Depending on the area of brain damage, the effects may include muscle tightness or spasm, involuntary movement, disturbance in gait and mobility, abnormal sensation and perception, seizures, mental retardation, feeding difficulties, learning disabilities, arthritis, breathing problems caused by postural difficulties, pressure ulcers, or impairment of sight, hearing, or speech.

An estimated 500,000 children and adults have one or more symptoms of cerebral palsy. Each year, about 5,000 infants as well as 1,200 to 1,500 preschool-age children are diagnosed with cerebral palsy. Home health care of children with cerebral palsy focuses on anticipatory guidance, skilled assessments (including developmental assessments), and therapeutic regimens to specifically treat neuromuscular disabilities and associated symptoms.

Previsit checklist

Physician orders and preparation

• Medications, including dosage, route, and frequency (commonly analeptics or antispasmodics)

• Instructions for seizure precautions, including suction

• Activity orders and restrictions

• Nutritional support, including enteral feeding if appropriate

• Braces or orthopedic appliances

• Laboratory tests and testing for serum levels of analeptics, antispasmodics, and other medications

• Physical therapy evaluation for home exercise program, transfer and gait training, and assistive devices

• Speech pathologist evaluation for language training and swallowing program

- Occupational therapy evaluation for activities of daily living (ADLs) training and assistive devices
- Social worker evaluation for financial assistance, referral, and community support
- Dietitian evaluation of nutritional needs and appropriate supportive therapies
- Home care aide assistance with ADLs, personal hygiene, and exercise program

Equipment and supplies
- Supplies for standard precautions and proper waste and sharps disposal
- Supplies for Denver II Developmental Screening test or other developmental assessment tool as appropriate. (Some agencies supply standardized kits; otherwise, bring supplies as specified in the test.)
- Wound care supplies, if pressure ulcers present
- Physical assessment and neurologic testing equipment, including cotton wisps, cotton-tipped swabs, penlight, stethoscope, sphygmomanometer (with cuff sized to fit the child's arm)
- Supplies for seizure precautions (padding for sharp corners and bed, no tongue blades or any other device to fit in mouth) and suction equipment, if needed
- Enteral feeding supplies, if ordered
- Orthopedic appliances or assistive devices to reduce spasticity, facilitate bodily alignment, and increase mobility

Safety requirements
- Standard precautions for infection control and waste and sharps disposal

- System to assist compliance with complex medication regimen, including nutrition therapy
- Activity restrictions
- Emergency plan and access to functional phone and list of emergency phone numbers
- Fire evacuation plan, functional smoke detectors, and access to functional fire extinguisher
- Signs and symptoms requiring notification of physician
- Night-light
- Identification and correction of environmental hazards and patient-specific concerns (for example, floors cleared of small objects, loose rugs secured, sharp corners of furniture or appliances cushioned, electrical cords removed from walkways, and unused electrical outlets covered)
- Correct application and use of orthopedic appliances, if used
- Seizure precautions, if child has seizures
- Child safety precautions with an easy-to-remember key such as A through E:

All children sit in back seats.

Buckle only one child in each safety belt.

Car seat or booster seat should be used for each small child.

Distractions should be handled by first pulling to the side of the road.

Emergency phone numbers and information should be kept in the car.

Major diagnostic codes
- Cerebral palsy, athetoid/unspecified/spastic hemiplegic/quadriplegic 333.7/343.9/343.1/343.2

Defense of homebound status

- Difficulty ambulating requiring assistance due to impaired gait and frequent falls
- Inability to climb stairs due to spasticity, hemiplegia, or involuntary movement
- Confinement to wheelchair, requiring assistance of two persons to transfer

Selected nursing diagnoses and patient outcomes

Risk for injury related to inability to control movements and impaired mobility

The patient or caregiver will:
- identify factors that increase the risk of injury   (N, HCA, OT, PT)
- relate an intent to use safety measures to prevent injury (for example, remove throw rugs or anchor them)
(N, OT, PT)
- remain free from injury throughout care period   (N, HCA, OT, PT)
- demonstrate correct application and use of assistive devices as appropriate
(N, OT, PT)
- exhibit improved mobility within functional limitations.
(N, OT, PT)

Knowledge deficit related to management of therapeutic regimen secondary to insufficient knowledge of (specify: disease process, pharmacologic regimen, activity program, community resources, orthopedic appliances, or nutritional needs)

The patient or caregiver will:

- verbalize an understanding of (specify)   (N, D, OT, PT)
- display less anxiety about fear of the unknown, fear of loss, or misconceptions   (N, OT, PT, SW)
- describe causes and factors contributing to symptoms and the regimen for symptom control   (N, OT, PT)
- use measures to enhance health behaviors and prevent complications
(N, D, OT, PT, SP)
- demonstrate adequate skills necessary to care for the child.
(N, D, OT, PT)

Altered growth and development related to impaired ability to achieve developmental tasks

The patient or caregiver will:
- demonstrate progression in behaviors in personal, social, language, cognition, or motor activities appropriate to age-group (specify behaviors)
(N, OT, PT, SP, SW)
- exhibit achievement of appropriate developmental milestones within limits of functional ability.
(N, OT, PT, SP, SW)

Altered family processes related to adjustment requirements for situation (specify: for example, time, emotional, and physical energy, financial, or physical care)

The patient or caregiver will:
- verbalize feelings openly
(N, HCA, OT, PT, SP, SW)
- participate in care of family member with special health care needs
(N, HCA, OT, PT, SP, SW)
- facilitate return of family member with special health care needs from sick role to well role
(N, HCA, OT, PT, SP, SW)

- maintain a functional system of mutual support for each family member
(N, HCA, OT, PT, SP, SW)
- seek appropriate external resources when needed. (N, SW)

Risk for altered parenting related to (specify: abuse, rejection, or overprotection secondary to inadequate resources or coping mechanisms)

The patient or caregiver will:

- share feelings regarding parenting
(N, HCA, OT, PT, SP, SW)
- identify factors that interfere with effective parenting (N, SW)
- describe appropriate disciplinary measures (N, SW)
- identify resources available for assistance with parenting. (N, SW)

Skilled nursing services

Care measures

- Perform an initial skilled assessment of all body systems with emphasis on neurologic, integumentary, and musculoskeletal systems; assess growth and development.
- Assess level of care provided by patient and caregiver, including observations of attention to safety precautions and administration of medications and treatments.
- Assess effectiveness of treatment regimen, including monitoring blood levels of analeptics and other medications.
- Perform baseline and follow-up developmental screenings and consult with other disciplines.
- Evaluate seizure activity, including frequency, type, onset, and care measures employed.

- Assess swallowing ability and institute aspiration precautions.
- Assess skin integrity and status of any wounds present, including size, color, drainage, and extent of healing; perform wound care, if indicated.
- Assess mobility status and risk of injury, including safety needs; use of orthopedic, assistive, or adaptive devices; and exercise program.
- Provide for grief responses and provide hope and guidance for parents in forming a relationship with their child.

Patient and family teaching

- Teach about disease process.
- Explain medication regimen, including drug actions, adverse effects, precautions, interactions, and methods of administration.
- Discuss seizure and safety precautions, including aspiration precautions such as placing food far back in mouth to facilitate swallowing.
- Review skin care, especially involving areas in contact with orthopedic braces, splints, and assistive or adaptive devices.
- Provide anticipatory guidance for family regarding growth and development, transition to adulthood, sexual development, and needs throughout life cycle.
- Discuss exercise program, which should include activities such as sucking lollipops to develop muscle control to minimize drooling.
- Demonstrate application and use of orthopedic, assistive, or adaptive devices.

Interdisciplinary actions

Physical therapist
- Development of home exercise program
- Ambulation, gait, and transfer training
- Fitting and use of orthopedic appliance or assistive devices
- Physical measures (such as moving and turning child carefully to reduce muscle spasms) to treat symptoms

Occupational therapist
- Assistive devices (such as splints, adaptive eating utensils, and a low toilet seat with arms) for activities of daily living
- Exercise program
- Play or riding therapy to promote balance and improved proprioception

Speech pathologist
- Speech evaluation and training
- Swallowing training
- Hearing evaluation

Dietitian
- Nutritional status evaluation
- Nutritional support program and development of individual meal plans

Social worker
- Referral for community resources
- Counseling and stress management, including discussion of the importance of not forming an overly protective environment
- Assistance with financial, emotional, and social needs

Home care aide
- Assistance with personal care and hygiene
- Assistance with ADLs

Discharge plan
- Safe, independent management of child with cerebral palsy with follow-up services of physician, school nurse (if attending school), and therapists
- Referral for continued outpatient physical and occupational therapy
- Referral to local community cerebral palsy organization for follow-up and continued assistance

Documentation requirements
- Assessment data for all systems, including weight, vital signs, skin integrity, nutritional status, Denver II Developmental Screening test or other developmental screening test results, and medication blood levels
- Activity level of child, including type of play and changes in mobility status, language and speech, swallowing, and functional ability
- Seizure activity, if any, measures used to control seizure activity
- Response to medication therapy, including adverse reactions
- Use, type, and care of all durable medical equipment
- Use of and ability to apply orthopedic or assistive and adaptive devices
- Patient's and family's adjustment to and ability to cope with illness
- Resources available for support
- Caregiver teaching and demonstrated responses to teaching
- Communication with physician and other members of the health care team
- Patient and caregiver participation in care

• Patient and caregiver progress toward educational goals, including feelings of being overwhelmed and the need for repeated instructions
• Complications (evidence or lack thereof)
• Patient's and caregiver's independence with care and therapy regimen
• Safety, aspiration, and seizure precautions implemented
• Signs and symptoms to be reported

Reimbursement reminders

• Care of children with cerebral palsy is covered under the Individuals with Disabilities Education Act and the Katie Beckett Act. Guidelines and funding are administered in many states by Medicaid. Children who aren't eligible for other medical assistance programs because their parents' income or assets are too high may be eligible for medical assistance through the Katie Beckett Act.
• Record any barriers to learning, such as physical deformities; visual impairment; cultural, language, and literacy barriers; and lack of or overburdened support person.

Insurance hints

• Report complete assessment data from each visit, including changes in condition since last visit, such as seizures, injury, or skin breakdown.
• Describe the response of the child and family to care at each visit, including follow-through with instructions and the child's ability to attend school.
• Include a report on the child's and family's use and care of equipment at each visit, including settings and frequency of use.

• Describe gains in knowledge such as skills and concepts mastered in medication administration, seizure precautions, nutritional therapy, and use of orthopedic devices.
• Present specific data on homebound status, such as improved ambulation with assistive device, continued inability to ambulate because of spasticity, number of persons needed to assist patient out of chair, continued limitation in ambulation distance, or development of any injury related to disease process.

Cystic fibrosis

Cystic fibrosis, an inherited genetic abnormality affecting the organs that produce mucus, leads to the destruction of the lungs, pancreas, liver, and intestines. The mucus produced by these organs becomes salty, thick, and tenacious — destroying rather than protecting the organs.

Cystic fibrosis is the number one genetic killer of children and young adults in the world today. The average life expectancy for a person with the disease is about 30 years; females usually die at a younger age than males. Cystic fibrosis primarily affects whites; about 5% of the white American population is asymptomatic, with a single mutant version of genes. Approximately 1 in 2,500 children of European descent carries 2 defective gene copies and has the disease. The United States has a total of 30,000 persons with cystic fibrosis; approximately 1,000 new cases are diagnosed each year. Home health care of children with cystic fibrosis focuses on thinning and removing mucus from respiratory passages, treating chronic infections, providing enzyme and nutritional supplements, and providing support to the child and family. Gene therapy is currently in clinical trials and may radically change treatment in the next few years.

Previsit checklist

Physician orders and preparation
- Genetic testing to detect the presence of cystic fibrosis transmembrane conductance regulator (known as CFTR) in deoxyribonucleic acid
- Inclusion in clinical trial for gene replacement therapy, if warranted
- Gene replacement therapy including dosage, route (usually intranasal, via bronchoscopy or inhaled nebulizer), frequency (one dose is ineffective), and preparation of child for therapy
- Laboratory studies, such as sputum culture, arterial blood gases, or serum electrolyte levels
- Frequency and duration of chest physiotherapy to loosen and remove mucus, including chest percussion, vibration, postural drainage, and suctioning (if needed)
- Peak flow monitoring, including target ranges and warning levels
- Medications, including oral or inhaled glucocorticosteroids, inhaled bronchodilators, oxygen, oral or inhaled cromolyn, and inhaled dornase alpha
- Antibiotic therapy for chronic or recurrent infections
- Nutritional support, including pancreatic enzyme supplements, multiple vitamins (including vitamin E), vitamin K for infants, and nutritional supplements (oral, parenteral, or enteral)
- Replacement fluids and chloride; total parenteral nutrition, if needed
- Method of delivery for all ordered medications and treatments, including settings, routes, frequency, and dosage
- Activity orders and restrictions
- Dietitian evaluation for nutritional status, nutritional support program, and replacement
- Respiratory therapy evaluation for chest physiotherapy and endurance training
- Respiratory therapist evaluation for adequacy of aeration and functional breathing ability
- Home care aide assistance with activities of daily living (ADLs) and hygiene
- Social worker evaluation for community resources and assistance with long-term care needs

Equipment and supplies
- Supplies for standard precautions and proper waste and sharps disposal
- Delivery devices for use with medications and treatments, such as a nebulizer; air compressor; suction catheter; suction machine; peak flow meter; pulse oximeter; vibrator; chest percussor; oxygen delivery equipment, such as a tank, flowmeter, and tubing; I.V. administration supplies, including fluids, replacement electrolytes and, preferably, needleless system via a central access device
- Safety devices, such as OXYGEN IN USE and NO SMOKING signs; securing devices for oxygen tanks; notification of fire and police departments and utility companies that oxygen is in use in the home
- Nutritional support equipment and supplies (parenteral or enteral), such as formulas and a feeding pump

- Assessment equipment, stethoscope, thermometer, and sphygmomanometer (with cuff sized to fit the child's arm)

Safety requirements

- Standard precautions for infection control, waste and sharps disposal
- System to assist adherence to complex medication regimen, including nutrition therapy
- Emergency plan and access to functional phone and list of emergency phone numbers
- Fire evacuation plan, functional smoke detectors, and access to functional fire extinguisher
- Night-light
- Oxygen precautions, safe handling and placement of home oxygen equipment, and notification of local fire and police departments of oxygen use in the home
- Information on medications, including dosage, adverse effects, interactions, and safe storage
- Activity restrictions
- Signs and symptoms requiring notification of physician
- Child safety precautions, including keeping matches and lighters out of child's reach, plugging only one heat-producing appliance in each outlet, never running electric cords under rugs or close to drapes, and repairing or discarding frayed electrical cords

Major diagnostic codes

- Bronchitis, chronic without/with exacerbation 491.20/491.21
- Constipation 564.0
- Cystic fibrosis without/with mention of meconium ileus 277.0/277.01
- Failure to thrive 783.4
- Ileus/intussusception 560.1/560.0

Defense of homebound status

- Unable to ambulate farther than 10′ (3 m) due to respiratory distress
- Invasive medical equipment requiring confinement to bed during use
- Restricted to first floor of home secondary to extreme fatigue and shortness of breath
- Restricted to home for infection control and prevention of infection from exposure to others
- Restricted to home secondary to required treatment (specify, such as total parenteral nutrition or antibiotic therapy)

Selected nursing diagnoses and patient outcomes

Ineffective airway clearance related to increased mucopurulent secretions
The patient or caregiver will:
- demonstrate effective coughing and increased air exchange in lungs
(N, RT)
- use appropriate positioning techniques to promote drainage of secretions
(N, RT)
- demonstrate ability to perform chest physiotherapy and suction secretions from airway as needed   (N, RT)
- verbalize measures to humidify atmosphere.
(N)

Altered nutrition: Less than body requirements related to the need for increased calories and protein secondary to impaired intestinal absorption, loss of fat, and fat-soluble vitamins in stools
The patient or caregiver will:

- exhibit a gain in weight and decrease in fatty stools (N)
- describe nutritional effects of cystic fibrosis (N, D)
- adhere to medication therapy regimen for pancreatic enzyme replacement (N)
- demonstrate ability to provide nutrition, orally, enterally, or parenterally, as appropriate. (N, D)

Knowledge deficit related to management of therapeutic regimen secondary to insufficient knowledge of (specify: disease process, pharmacologic regimen, activity program, community resources, or orthopedic appliances)

The patient or caregiver will:
- report a decrease in anxiety about fear of the unknown, fear of loss, or misconceptions (N, SW)
- describe cystic fibrosis, causes and factors contributing to symptoms, and the regimen for symptom control (N)
- demonstrate adherence to medication regimen (N)
- identify possible complications and associated contributing factors (N)
- institute health behaviors needed or desired for prevention of complications. (N, D, RT)
- demonstrate understanding of rationale and procedure for treatments (N, PT, RT)

Activity intolerance related to impaired respiratory function and nutritional status

The patient or caregiver will:
- demonstrate energy conservation measures (N, RT)
- use oxygen therapy as necessary and ordered to enhance functional ability (N)

- participate in ADLs and personal care with assistance (N, HCA)
- exhibit ability to gradually increase ambulation distance throughout plan of care (N, PT)
- participate in a home exercise program. (N, HCA, PT)

Altered growth and development related to impaired ability to achieve developmental tasks

The patient or caregiver will:
- demonstrate an increase in behaviors in personal, social, language, cognition, or motor activities appropriate to age-group (specify behaviors) (N, SW)
- achieve appropriate developmental milestones for age. (N, PT, SW)

Altered family processes related to adjustment requirements for situation (specify: time, emotional and physical energy, financial, and physical care)

The patient or caregiver will:
- verbalize feelings openly (N, SW)
- actively participate in care (N, HCA, PT, RT)
- facilitate return of family member with special health care needs from sick role to well role (N, PT, RT, SW)
- maintain functional system of mutual support for each member (N, SW)
- seek appropriate external resources when needed. (N, SW)

Skilled nursing services

Care measures
- Perform an initial skilled assessment of all body systems, with emphasis on respiratory, GI, and immune systems.

• Assess level of care provided by patient and caregiver, such as observation of and attention to all safety precautions as well as, administration of medications and treatments.

• Assess effectiveness of treatment regimen, including nutritional and hydration status, oxygen saturation levels, peak flow readings, and breath sounds.

• Assess vital signs, weights, sputum production, and complaints of shortness of breath and dyspnea at each visit.

• Monitor oxygen therapy use, including rate, frequency, and duration of use.

• Institute nutritional support therapy as ordered.

• Evaluate consistency of stools on each visit.

• Obtain laboratory tests such as sputum culture as indicated.

• Provide for grief responses; provide hope and guidance to parents in forming relationship with their child.

Patient and family teaching

• Teach about medications, including actions, adverse effects, precautions, interactions, and methods of administration.

• Explain mucus plug removal after use of bronchodilators to avoid fatal rebound bronchospasm.

• Emphasize importance of nutritional support, hydration, and chest physiotherapy.

• Provide anticipatory guidance to family regarding patient's growth and development, disability process, and needs throughout life cycle.

• Discuss genetic counseling, including availability of or participation in clinical trials for genetic replacement therapy for cystic fibrosis.

• Explain self-care measures to use during a minor illness such as a common cold.

• Review infection control measures such as frequent hand washing.

• Identify signs and symptoms to report to physician.

Interdisciplinary actions

Physical therapist
• Endurance training
• Home exercise program

Respiratory therapist
• Chest physiotherapy
• Airway clearance vest (such as ThAIRapy Vest) recommendations

Dietitian
• Nutritional status evaluation and development of menu plans incorporating food preferences

Social worker
• Referral to community resources
• Crisis intervention
• Counseling and assistance with long-term needs
• Advocacy regarding air quality issues

Home care aide
• Assistance with personal care and hygiene
• Assistance with ADLs

Discharge plan

• Independent, safe management of child with cystic fibrosis in the home, with follow-up services of physician and school nurse (if attending school)

- Referral for episodic follow-up by dietitian for nutritional changes related to disease process and growth and development of child and social services for crisis intervention
- Referral to community agencies for support
- Patient and caregiver understanding and control of disease process; knowledge of preventative measures and signs and symptoms of recurrence

Documentation requirements

- Vital signs, signs and symptoms of infection, and breath sounds
- Nutritional assessment data, including weight and skin turgor, characteristics of stools
- Activity level of child, including type of play and limitations
- Patient's response to care
- Results of laboratory studies, including sputum cultures and arterial blood gases, if ordered
- Activity restrictions and adherence to endurance training
- Complications (evidence or lack thereof)
- Patient's and caregiver's independence with care and therapy regimen
- Response to medication and nutritional supplements, including adverse reactions, if any
- Durable medical equipment (DME) used, at what settings, and care of equipment
- Status, use, and care of any access devices
- Caregiver teaching and demonstrated responses to teaching
- Patient and caregiver instruction

- Medication therapy, including drug, dosage, frequency, adverse effects, and signs and symptoms to report
- Activity restrictions and energy conservation measures
- Nutritional therapy, chest physiotherapy and oxygen use and suctioning as appropriate
- Safety measures, including oxygen safety measures
- Signs and symptoms to be reported
- Changes in plan of care, including changes in medication dosages based on sputum or blood studies as well as patient and caregiver understanding of changes
- Patient's activity tolerance
- Patient's compliance with instructions and therapy regimen

Reimbursement reminders

- Care of children with cystic fibrosis is covered under the Individuals with Disabilities Education Act and the Katie Beckett Act. Guidelines and funding are administered in many states by Medicaid. The Katie Beckett Act allows many children to qualify for medical assistance even if their parents' income or assets would otherwise make them ineligible for medical assistance. Coverage includes skilled nursing in the home and school, dietitian and social work services, and DME rentals. Use of needleless infusion systems, while more expensive, is an appropriate safeguard against sharps injuries in the community.
- Describe stool and sputum characteristics objectively, including color and consistency.
- Identify positive and negative changes in child's activity level, including changes specifically related to

treatment measures such as use of bronchodilators or chest physiotherapy.

• Provide evidence of the need for nutritional support, such as weight, skin turgor, and intake (via dietary history or recall).

Insurance hints

• Review complete assessment data each visit, including changes in condition since last visit, such as an increase or change sputum color, decrease in fatty stools, improved activity tolerance, or trends in weight.

• Note response of child and family to care each visit, including ability to follow through with instructions and comply with treatment regimen.

• Record presence, use, and care of equipment each visit, including settings and rates, specifically the frequency and duration of use and the need for oxygen and nutritional support.

• Note all teaching of child and family and response to teaching each visit; include problems encountered, such as caregiver's feelings of being overwhelmed, difficulty planning times for chest physiotherapy, child's lack of adherence to medication regimen.

• List all communication with physician and other disciplines, including plans for physical therapist, dietitian, and social worker.

• Identify environmental situations that may affect child's susceptibility to respiratory distress episodes. For example, document exposure to environmental tobacco smoke, high pollen counts, code red and orange days (high heat and humidity), toxic spraying in child's environment, such as for insect control, exposure to others in households with infection.

Down syndrome

Down syndrome results from one of several trisomy genetic disorders caused by the addition of a third gene to the usual pair. It's characterized by slow physical development and a flat skull and facial features and is always accompanied by moderate to severe mental retardation, autism, or attention deficit with hyperactivity. Down syndrome is also sometimes associated with heart defects and vision or hearing impairment.

Home care of the child with Down syndrome focuses on supporting growth and development, cardiovascular and respiratory function, and nutrition. It also is focused on health care maintenance, prevention of debilitation, and promotion of independence.

Previsit checklist

Physician orders and preparation

• Seizure control and prevention; seizure precautions, including suction, if needed

• Thyroid or pituitary hormone replacement medications as needed

• Medications such as digoxin to reduce workload of heart if defects present

• Laboratory testing as indicated for serum levels of analeptics, hormone replacements, and other medications

• Physical therapy evaluation for home exercise program, pulmonary exercises, and environmental safety

• Occupational therapy evaluation for assistive devices and activities of daily living (ADL) training

- Audiologic evaluation to assess hearing
- Speech and language therapist evaluation for language function
- Home care aide assistance with personal care and ADLs
- Social worker for community referrals, support, and counseling
- Dietitian consultation for assessment of nutritional status

Equipment and supplies

- Supplies for standard precautions and proper sharps disposal
- Supplies for Denver II Developmental Screening test or other developmental assessment test, as appropriate (some agencies supply standardized kits; otherwise, bring supplies as specified in test)
- Physical assessment and neurologic testing equipment, including cotton wisps, cotton-tipped swabs, penlight, stethoscope, sphygmomanometer (with cuff sized to fit the child's arm)
- Supplies for seizure precautions (padding for sharp corners and bed, no tongue blades or any other device to fit in mouth) and suction equipment, if needed
- Orthopedic appliances or assistive devices to facilitate body alignment, and increase mobility
- Oxygen administration during sleep; continuous positive airway pressure or other positive pressure delivery device as needed

Safety requirements

- Standard precautions for infection control and sharps disposal
- Identification and correction of environmental hazards and patient-specific concerns (for example, floors cleared of small objects, loose rugs secured, sharp corners of furniture or appliances cushioned, electrical cords removed from walkways, and unused electrical outlets covered)
- Oxygen precautions, safe handling and placement of home oxygen equipment, and notification of local fire and police departments of oxygen use in the home
- Emergency plan and access to functional phone and list of emergency phone numbers
- Fire evacuation plan, functional smoke detectors, and access to functional fire extinguisher
- Night-light
- Signs and symptoms requiring notification of physician
- Correct use of orthopedic and assistive devices, with frequent skin checks under orthopedic appliances, if used
- Seizure precautions, if child has seizures
- General safety precautions: child facing away from faucet when in the tub, not allowing water to remain in tubs or buckets (drowning can occur in 2″ of water), furniture positioned far from windows so child can't lean against the window or screen and fall out.

Major diagnostic codes

- Down syndrome 758.0
- Mild mental retardation 317

Defense of homebound status

- Poor endurance and inability to ambulate farther than 10′ (3 m) due to cardiovascular and respiratory difficulties

• Unable to be left alone secondary to severity of developmental deficits

Selected nursing diagnoses and patient outcomes

Ineffective breathing pattern related to decreased expansion secondary to decreased muscle tone, inadequate mucus drainage, and mouth breathing

The patient or caregiver will:
• perform hourly deep-breathing (sigh) exercises and cough sessions as needed   (N, HCA, PT)
• demonstrate maximum pulmonary function   (N)
• relate importance of daily pulmonary exercises   (N, HCA, PT)
• exhibit respiratory rate and depth and breath sounds within acceptable parameters.   (N, PT)

Knowledge deficit related to management of the therapeutic regimen secondary to insufficient knowledge of (specify: disease process, pharmacologic regimen, activity program, or community resources)

The patient or caregiver will:
• report a decrease in anxiety about fear of the unknown, fear of loss, or misconceptions   (N, SW)
• describe syndrome, causes and factors contributing to symptoms, and the regimen for symptom control   (N)
• demonstrate effective health behaviors needed or desired for prevention of complications.   (N)

Altered growth and development related to an impaired ability to achieve developmental tasks

The patient or caregiver will:

• demonstrate an increase in behaviors in personal, social, language, cognition, or motor activities appropriate to age-group   (N, OT, PT)
• demonstrate adequate skills necessary to care for child.   (N, OT, PT)

Altered family processes related to adjustment requirements for situation (specify: for example, time, emotional and physical energy, financial, and physical care)

The patient or caregiver will:
• verbalize feelings openly
                    (N, HCA, OT, PT, SC, SP, SW)
• participate in care of family member with special health care needs
                    (N, HCA, OT, PT, SP, SW)
• facilitate return of family member with special health care needs from sick role to well role
                    (N, HCA, OT, PT, SP, SW)
• maintain functional system of mutual support for each member
                             (N, SC, SW)
• seek appropriate external resources when needed.   (N, SC, SW)

Skilled nursing services

Care measures

• Perform an initial skilled assessment of all body systems, including neurologic (vision and hearing), cardiovascular, endocrine, integumentary, and musculoskeletal systems; assess growth and development.
• Assess level of care provided by patient and caregiver; observe attention to all safety precautions, and administration of medications and treatments.
• Assess effectiveness of treatment regimen: obtain blood levels of analeptics and other medications, perform

baseline and follow-up developmental screenings, and evaluate mobility and cognitive status.
- Evaluate seizure activity, including frequency, type, onset, and care measures.
- Assess mobility status and risk of injury, including safety needs; use of orthopedic, assistive, or adaptive devices; and adherence to exercise program.

Patient and family teaching
- Review disease process.
- Teach about medications, including actions, adverse effects, precautions, interactions, and methods of administration.
- Discuss seizure and safety precautions, including aspiration precautions.
- Describe skin care, especially involving areas in contact with orthopedic braces or splints, and assistive or adaptive devices.
- Provide anticipatory guidance to family regarding patient's growth and development, life skills, transition to adulthood, employment issues, and patient's needs throughout life cycle.
- Emphasize importance of exercise.
- Demonstrate application and use of orthopedic, assistive, or adaptive devices.

Interdisciplinary actions

Physical therapist
- Development of home exercise program
- Ambulation, gait, and transfer training
- Fitting and use of orthopedic appliance or assistive devices

Occupational therapist
- ADL training
- Play therapy or riding therapy to promote balance and improved proprioception

Speech pathologist
- Speech training
- Communication methods if hearing is affected

Social worker
- Referral for community resources
- Counseling and stress management
- Assistance with financial, emotional, and social needs

Home care aide
- Assistance with personal care and hygiene
- Assistance with ADLs

Discharge plan
- Safe, independent management of child with Down syndrome in the home with follow-up services by physician and school nurse (if attending school)
- Referral to community services for crisis intervention, counseling, and support
- Referral for continued outpatient physical and occupational therapy

Documentation requirements
- Weight, vital signs, and signs or symptoms of infection or cardiac or respiratory involvement
- Nutritional assessment data, including weight and height
- Activity level of child, including type of play and changes in mobility status,

language and speech, and functional ability

• Seizure activity, if any, and control of seizure activity

• Response to medication, including adverse reactions

• Use, type, and care of all durable medical equipment (DME)

• Use and ability to apply orthopedic or assistive and adaptive devices

• Patient's and family's adjustment to and ability to cope with illness

• Resources available for support

• Caregiver teaching and demonstrated responses to teaching

• Communication with physician and other disciplines

• Patient and caregiver participation in care

• Patient's and caregiver's independence with care and therapy regimen

• Complications (evidence or lack thereof)

• Safety and seizure precautions

• Communication methods

• Danger signs and symptoms to be reported

Reimbursement reminders

• Care of children with Down syndrome is covered under the Individuals with Disabilities Education Act and the Katie Beckett Act. Guidelines and funding are administered in many states by Medicaid. The Katie Beckett Act extends medical assistance coverage to some children whose parents' income or assets are too high. This includes skilled nursing and skilled therapies in the home and school, and dietitian and social worker services as well as DME rentals.

• Record any barriers to learning such as physical deformities, visual impairments, and the lack of availability or overwhelming of support person.

Insurance hints

• Report complete assessment data each visit, including changes in condition since last visit, such as seizures, injury, and skin breakdown.

• Describe response of child and family to care each visit, including follow through with instructions.

• Describe gains in knowledge, such as skills and concepts mastered in medication administration, seizure precautions, and use of orthopedic or assistive devices.

• Objectively report child's developmental level and optimal level of functioning.

• Document goals and achievements aimed at preventing institutionalization of patient.

Failure to thrive

Failure to thrive or lack of expected physiologic development was once believed to be a form of child abuse or neglect that resulted from a caregiver's refusal to provide food to an infant or child. Failure to thrive is now recognized as an early warning sign of a number of diseases or syndromes and is also associated with the use of inappropriate growth charts for a child's ethnic group or medical condition. Home health care of children with failure to thrive focuses on nutritional support, developmental screening, and support of the family.

Previsit checklist

Physician orders and preparation
- Dietitian evaluation for nutritional program, supplementation, dietary guidelines, and calorie requirement and allotment
- Speech therapist evaluation of swallowing or sucking
- Occupational therapist evaluation for feeding skills and play therapy as required
- Social worker evaluation for community resources, counseling, and crisis intervention
- Laboratory testing such as serum protein levels
- Baseline weight and vital sign parameters for contacting the physician
- Nutritional supplement or replacement, including type, formula, and route of administration
- Fluid requirements, including I.V. therapy, if indicated

Equipment and supplies
- Supplies for standard precautions and proper sharps disposal
- Supplies for Denver II Developmental Screening test or other developmental assessment test as appropriate (some agencies supply standardized kits; otherwise, bring supplies as specified in the test)
- Physical assessment and neurologic testing equipment, including cotton wisps, cotton-tipped swabs, penlight, stethoscope, and sphygmomanometer (with cuff sized to fit the child's arm)
- Suction equipment as needed
- Growth charts appropriate for ethnic group and disease or disability of child; if unknown, standard growth charts. Usually, differences by ethnic

group are not great; however, significantly different. Growth charts exist for children with the following disorders: cerebral palsy, Down syndrome, myelomingocele, and syndromes such as Aader Willis Marfan, Noonam, Turner, fragile X; or sickle cell disease. Growth charts also exist for infants born prematurely.
- Equipment for measuring growth: tape measure in inches and centimeters, scale, and skin calipers
- Phlebotomy equipment
- Nutritional therapy supplies, such as feeding tube, formula, and feeding pump

Safety requirements
- Standard precautions for infection control and sharps disposal
- Identification and correction of environmental hazards and patient-specific concerns (for example, floors cleared of small objects, loose rugs secured, sharp corners of furniture or appliances cushioned, electrical cords removed from walkways, and unused electrical outlets covered)
- Emergency plan and access to functional phone and list of emergency phone numbers
- Fire evacuation plan, functional smoke detectors, and access to functional fire extinguisher
- Night-light
- Signs and symptoms requiring notification of physician
- Seizure precautions, if child has seizures
- Child safety precautions: not allowing child to play in cabinets (permitting such behavior establishes tight spaces with doors as a safe place to be) and teaching toddlers to go up and

down stairs on their behinds (sitting is a safer way to navigate the stairs than standing.)

Major diagnostic codes
- Feeding difficulties and mismanagement 783.3
- Lack of expected normal physiological development 783.4
- Pica 307.52
- Psychogenic rumination disorder 307.53

Defense of homebound status
- Poor endurance related to lack of expected growth and development and impaired nutritional status
- Invasive treatment requiring restriction to home

Selected nursing diagnoses and patient outcomes

Knowledge deficit related to altered nutritional status secondary to the disease process

The patient or caregiver will:
- demonstrate and verbalize purpose of nutritional supplements, such as medium-chain triglyceride oil or mixed polysaccharides, in quantities ordered (N, D)
- record food and fluid intake and count diapers every 24 hours (N)
- schedule rest periods for child if excessive cardiovascular or respiratory effort has increased child's nutritional requirements (N)

- prepare child for laboratory and other testing to determine cause of nutritional deficit: for example, if child is suspected of having celiac disease, blood testing will precede colon biopsy (N)
- report usual family dietary pattern and relevant cultural nutritional practices (N, D)
- demonstrate appropriate feeding measures to improve child's nutritional intake (N, D, OT, SP)
- feed child appropriately and safely by GI access device if sucking or swallowing are impaired (N)
- perform swallowing exercise program (N, SP)
- demonstrate use of assistive devices for self-feeding, if upper body weakness or spasticity are present (N, OT)
- count stools and note odor and if fat or mucus are present, especially if malabsorption is suspected (N)
- assist child in therapy as ordered if the child has psychiatric disease, such as pica or rumination (N)
- verbalize understanding of "catching up" processes and the extra metabolic demands of syndromes, such as bronchopulmonary dysplasia, if child was born at low birth weight. (N, D)

Altered nutrition: Less than body requirements related to inadequate intake, secondary to lack of emotional and sensory stimulation or lack of knowledge of caregiver

The patient or caregiver will:
- verbalize child's need for adequate nutrition (N, D)
- demonstrate appropriate feeding techniques (N, D, OT, SP)

- display age-appropriate intake (N, D)
- demonstrate age-appropriate growth and development (N)
- demonstrate adherence to treatment plan including medications. (N, MD)

Skilled nursing services

Care measures
- Perform an initial skilled assessment of all body systems with emphasis on GI, cardiovascular, respiratory, neurologic, and endocrine systems; and assess growth and development.
- Assess level of care provided by patient and caregiver, including ability to complete feeding routines, administer nutritional support therapy, use assistive self-feeding devices, and adhere to medications and treatments.
- Observe interaction with child, including eye contact (be sure to take cultural variances into account).
- Assess effectiveness of treatment regimen, including nutrition and hydration status
- Obtain laboratory tests as ordered, such as medication blood levels.
- Perform baseline and follow-up developmental screenings.
- Monitor weight for trends and measure child's height and head circumference at each visit.
- Institute nutritional support therapy, as ordered. Assess caregiver's ability to provide therapy and child's response to it.
- Evaluate consistency of stools on each visit.

Patient and family teaching
- Teach about medications, including actions, adverse effects, precautions, interactions, and methods of administration.
- Discuss nutritional support, feeding techniques, sucking and swallowing exercises (such as using a straw or lollipop to improve feeding ability), and hydration.
- Provide anticipatory guidance to family regarding patient's growth and development, underlying disease process, and possible needs throughout life cycle.
- Discuss interaction techniques with child.
- Review guidelines in preparation for diagnostic tests to determine underlying cause.

Interdisciplinary actions

Occupational therapist
- Feeding skills
- Play therapy

Speech pathologist
- Sucking and swallowing evaluation and studies
- Exercise program for sucking or swallowing

Dietitian
- Dietary need evaluation
- Calorie allotment
- Meal planning
- Nutritional supplements and therapy

Social worker
- Referral to community resources
- Crisis intervention
- Counseling for child abuse or neglect if warranted

Discharge plan

- Independent safe management of child in the home with follow-up services by physician, and school nurse (if attending school)
- Referral for continued outpatient speech or occupational therapy for swallowing and sucking exercises
- Referral for periodic evaluation and episodic follow-up by dietitian for nutritional changes related to disease process and growth and development of child
- Referral to community agencies for support and crisis intervention

Documentation requirements

- Vital signs
- Nutritional assessment data, including summary of intake and output; weight, height (length), and head circumference; and skin turgor
- Trends in growth rate according to appropriate growth chart
- Activity level of child, including type of play
- Interaction between child and caregiver during feeding and child's response
- Response to medication and nutritional supplements, including adverse reactions, if any
- Ability to swallow or suck and any changes related to therapy
- Results of laboratory tests
- Caregiver teaching and demonstrated responses to teaching, including danger signs and symptoms to report and nutritional support therapy

- Feeding routines and use of assistive devices
- Communication with physician and other members of health care team
- Objective data pertaining to suspected abuse. This information must be reported to the proper authorities because failure to do so constitutes a crime. Document what was reported and to whom.

Reimbursement reminders

- Care of children with failure to thrive may be covered as part of health care for an underlying disease (medical or psychiatric condition).
- Care of child may be covered as part of care administered by child's local protective services agency, if disorder is a consequence of parental neglect or abuse.
- Ensure careful reporting of assessment data, which is key in determining cause.
- Use appropriate growth charts for child's ethnic group and disease or disability, which is essential to accurate assessment, and cite growth chart used each visit; make sure age of child is corrected for prematurity, if necessary, to ensure that growth parameters are plotted accurately.

Insurance hints

- Describe complete assessment data each visit, including changes in condition, specifically weight trends, laboratory results, feeding ability, and child-caregiver interaction, since last visit.

- Elaborate on current plan for determining possible underlying disorder.
- Report response of child and family to care each visit, including ability to follow through with instructions and comply with treatment regimen, noting changes in ability to cope.
- Substantiate need for equipment at each visit, including use, frequency, settings, and rates.
- Record all teaching of child and family and response to teaching each visit, such as swallowing or sucking exercise program and feeding techniques.

Heavy metal toxicity

All heavy metals can cause illness, ranging from subtle subclinical effects on learning and behavior and blood forming processes to death from toxicity. Heavy metals include lead, cadmium, mercury, arsenic, beryllium, chromium, manganese, antimony, copper, iron, and nickel. Very small amounts of manganese, copper, chromium, zinc, and iron are needed for adequate nutrition; these are most safely eaten as constituents of foods (preferably free from pesticides, herbicides, and toxic fertilizers).

Home health care of children experiencing heavy metal toxicity focuses on providing nutritional support, administering medications as needed, and developmental screening. It may include collaborating with public and environmental health officials to identify the source of the toxicity and obtaining samples for testing.

Previsit checklist

Physician orders and preparation
- Diagnostic testing
- Chelating medication (depends on heavy metal present; dosage depends on age and size of child and other medications taken by child)
- Dietitian for evaluation and meal planning, including nutritional support during chelation therapy
- Social worker for crisis intervention, and advocacy regarding heavy metal agents and other environmental toxins
- Home care aide assistance with personal care and activities of daily living
- Toxic substance abatement in home (may require verification by local health department or environmental health inspector)

Equipment and supplies
- Supplies for standard precautions and proper sharps disposal
- Supplies for Denver II Developmental Screening test or other developmental assessment test (some agencies supply standardized kits; otherwise, bring supplies as specified in the test)
- Physical assessment and neurologic testing equipment, including cotton wisps, cotton-tipped swabs, penlight, stethoscope, and sphygmomanometer (with cuff sized to fit the child's arm)
- Supplies for laboratory specimen collection, including collection of samples from blood, urine, and soil (substance-specific collection kits may be

necessary)

• Supplies for seizure precautions, including suction equipment, if needed

Safety requirements

• Standard precautions for infection control and sharps disposal
• Emergency plan and access to functional phone and list of emergency phone numbers
• Fire evacuation plan, functional smoke detectors, and access to functional fire extinguisher
• Night-light
• Identification and correction of environmental hazards and patient-specific concerns (for example, floors cleared of small objects, loose rugs secured, sharp corners of furniture or appliances cushioned, electrical cords removed from walkways, and unused electrical outlets covered)
• Signs and symptoms requiring notification of physician
• Seizure precautions, if child has seizures
• Installation of home water purifier if heavy metal agent is thought to be waterborne and use of only purified water in caring for child (distilled water if water purifier can't be installed), including for cooking, preparing beverages, brushing teeth, and any water contact with mucous membranes (*Note:* Boiled tap water shouldn't be used because boiling may concentrate toxins or heavy metals in water supply.)
• Installation of home air filtration system if agent is thought to be airborne
• Child safety precautions: hot water heater thermostat set to 120° F (48.9° C), safety adapters for electrical outlets installed, toy labels checked for age-appropriateness

Major diagnostic codes

• Disorder of written expression 315.2
• Lead poisoning 984.9
• Learning disorder not otherwise specified 315.7
• Mathematics disorder 315.1
• Mild mental retardation 317
• Reading disorder 315.00
• Toxic effect of:
  – antimony and its compounds 985.4
  – arsenic and its compounds 985.1
  – beryllium and its compounds 985.3
  – brass fumes, iron compounds, copper salts, nickel compounds 985.8
  – cadmium and its compounds 985.5
  – chromium and its compounds 985.6
  – lead (including from all sources except medicinal substances)/inorganic/organic 984.0/984.1
  – manganese and its compounds 985.2
  – mercury and its compounds (Minamata disease) 985.0
  – unspecified metal 985.9

Defense of homebound status

• Unable to engage in usual activities due to fatigue or dyspnea
• Confined to bed secondary to toxic effects of heavy metal, such as gait disturbance, nausea and vomiting
• Unsafe to be left alone due to central nervous system effects such as confusion

Selected nursing diagnoses and patient outcomes

Ineffective community coping related to environmental sources of heavy metal toxicity, such as contaminated air, water, dust, and environmental surfaces

The patient or caregiver will:
- access information to improve coping (N, SW)
- use communication channels to access assistance (N, SW)
- determine and remove or abate point sources of environmental contamination. (N, SW)

Altered protection related to neurologic, cardiovascular, or genitourinary effects of heavy metal toxicity

The patient or caregiver will:
- identify factors that can be controlled by patient or caregiver (N)
- make decisions regarding child's care, treatment, and future whenever possible (N)
- exhibit a return to optimal level of system function as metal is removed from body. (N)

Altered growth and development related to neurologic effects of heavy metal toxicity

The patient or caregiver will:
- demonstrate a progression in behaviors in personal, social, language, cognition, or motor activities, appropriate to age-group (N, SW)
- participate in age-appropriate activities to achieve developmental milestones. (N, HCA, SW)

Activity intolerance related to insufficient oxygen, secondary to diminished red blood cell count

The patient or caregiver will:
- identify factors that reduce activity tolerance (N)
- demonstrate progress to highest level of social function, mobility, and cognition possible (N, SW)
- exhibit a decrease in hypoxic signs and increased activity. (N)

Knowledge deficit related to management of therapeutic regimen secondary to insufficient knowledge of causes, prevention, and signs and symptoms of complications

The patient or caregiver will:
- relate less anxiety about fear of the unknown, fear of loss, and misconceptions (N, SW)
- describe heavy metal toxicity, causes and factors contributing to symptoms, and the regimen for symptom control (N)
- demonstrate appropriate health behaviors needed or desired for prevention of complications. (N)

Skilled nursing services

Care measures
- Perform an initial skilled assessment of all body systems with a focus on the neurologic, cardiovascular (including hematopoietic), and genitourinary systems.
- Assess level of care provided by patient and caregiver, including attention to all safety precautions, administration of medications and treatments, awareness of effects of heavy metal agent on patient and family.

- Assess effectiveness of treatment regimen; obtain or arrange for laboratory tests of heavy metal levels, complete blood counts, serum chemistries and urinalysis for evaluation of kidney function.
- Evaluate for expected rebound of serum heavy metal levels as treatment continues — this is a sign of effectiveness indicating the heavy metal is being extracted from tissues. Maintain ongoing assessments for medication–heavy metal interactions and for adverse effects of medications.
- Observe for signs and symptoms of treatment-related nutritional deficits; continue or adjust meal plans to promote a healthy diet and evaluate its effectiveness in mediating symptoms.
- Evaluate effectiveness of heavy metal removal or abatement related to child's symptoms.
- Evaluate seizure activity, including frequency, type, onset, care measures and outcome.
- Discontinue medication for attention deficit disorder or hyperactivity under supervision and skilled nursing surveillance while testing and chelation treatment occur if necessary, resume therapy after completing course of treatment for heavy metal toxicity.

Patient and family teaching

- Explain health effects of heavy metal in child's environment.
- Review symptoms of heavy metal toxicity, which are often mistaken for attention deficit disorder and hyperactivity.
- Discuss possible sources of heavy metal agents (now often associated with air, water, soil; hobby-related activities; remodeling; environmental sur-

faces and contamination at parent's workplace).
- In conjunction with physician's orders and dietitian's recommendations, emphasize the importance of diet high in dietary sources of vitamins A and C, zinc, copper, and iron, such as brightly colored fruits and vegetables, citrus, cabbage, potatoes, legumes, and seeds to prevent treatment-related anemia and protect against adverse effects of chelation medications.
- Explain need to remove heavy metals from the child's environment completely, permanently, and as quickly as possible, using a licensed contractor trained in safe abatement practices.
- Discuss use of noncontaminated water — purified or distilled. (Boiled water isn't always recommended because boiling may concentrate the toxin).
- Explore potential need for air purification system in the home and alternative measures if not a viable option.

Interdisciplinary actions

Dietitian
- Dietary evaluation
- Meal planning, including nutritional support during chelation therapy

Social worker
- Crisis intervention and counseling
- Advocacy regarding heavy metal agents and other environmental toxins
- Assistance with financial issues or relocation needs during abatement procedures

Discharge plan

- Independent, safe management of child with heavy metal toxicity in the home (or temporary shelter if home evacuation is required during abatement of heavy metal agent) with physician, school nurse (if attending school), and local environmental health services follow ups for chelation administration
- Complete heavy metal agent removal without recurrence
- Return to optimal level of functioning with minimal or no residual effects from heavy metal poisoning
- Referral for episodic follow-up by a dietitian for nutritional changes related to disease process or growth and development of child
- Referral for social services for crisis intervention and activism regarding source of heavy metal agent on outpatient basis

Documentation requirements

- Weight, vital signs, and signs or symptoms related to toxicity
- Nutritional assessment data, including the response to nutritional supplements and dietary changes during and after chelation therapy
- Activity level of child, including type of play and objectively describing any attention deficit or hyperactivity in child
- Response to medication, including adverse reactions, if any
- Measures instituted for removal of heavy metal agent from child and environment
- Caregiver teaching and demonstrated responses to teaching

- Disease process, including complications (evidence or lack thereof)
- Patient's and caregiver's independence with care and therapy regimen, including chelation therapy
- Safety and seizure precautions
- Signs and symptoms to be reported

Reimbursement reminders

- Care of children with heavy metal toxicity is covered under the Individuals with Disabilities Education Act and the Katie Beckett Act. Guidelines and funding are administered in many states by Medicaid. The Katie Beckett Act provides medical assistance to some children whose parents' income or assets are too high to normally qualify them for medical assistance. Coverage includes skilled nursing in the home and school and dietitian and social worker services as well as durable medical equipment rentals.
- Record any barriers to learning, such as physical deformities, visual impairments, and a lack of availability or overwhelming of support person.
- In rental housing, the landlord may be responsible for all costs related to abatement and possibly to chelation or other treatment. Rental housing codes vary from state to state.

Insurance hints

- Report complete assessment data each visit, including changes in condition since last visit (such as seizures) and results of laboratory studies.
- Describe response of child and family to care each visit, including follow through with instructions.
- Identify gains in knowledge, such as skills and concepts mastered in chelation therapy administration, seizure

precautions, and required nutritional therapy.

● Present specific data on homebound status, such as changes in ability to ambulate or reversal of toxic effects on body systems with improved functional ability.

Incontinence care

Control of bowel and bladder function in children is a developmental task that depends on the innervation of perineal, urinary tract, and intestinal structures, including the sphincter muscles. Some children, such as those with developmental disabilities, never develop control; others develop control but later lose it. Some children become incontinent due to surgery, such as abdominal-perineal pull-through or creation of augmented bladders or stomas for elimination. Other children experience incontinence in conjunction with mental illness or emotional trauma or as a result of poisoning. Home care of the child with incontinence focuses on measures to deal with the problem, maintain skin integrity, and promote effective parenting. All children should be evaluated for a bowel or bladder regimen that will afford them the opportunity to become continent.

Previsit checklist

Physician orders and preparation
● Diagnostic testing to determine causes of incontinence and evaluate effectiveness of treatment

● Medications and nutritional measures to regulate bowel or bladder function

● Social worker evaluation for stress management and referrals for community support

● Home care aide to assist with personal care, skin care, and activities of daily living

Equipment and supplies
● Supplies for standard precautions and proper sharps disposal

● Denver II Developmental Screening test (some agencies supply standardized kits; otherwise, bring supplies as specified in test)

● Physical assessment and neurologic testing equipment, including cotton wisps, cotton-tipped swabs, penlight, stethoscope, and sphygmomanometer (with cuff sized to fit the child's arm)

● Supplies for laboratory specimen collection

● Diapers or disposable underpants sized to fit infant or child

● Supplies for bowel program or urinary catheterization as appropriate

Safety requirements
● Standard precautions for infection control and sharps disposal

● Emergency plan and access to functional phone and list of emergency phone numbers

● Fire evacuation plan, functional smoke detectors, and access to functional fire extinguisher

● Night-light

● Identification and correction of environmental hazards and patient-specific concerns (for example, floors cleared of small objects)

- Signs and symptoms requiring physician notification
- Child safety precautions: keeping plastic bags and packaging completely out of reach; favoring Mylar balloons over latex ones to reduce the risk of choking

Major diagnostic codes
- Anal sphincter incontinence 787.6
- Urinary incontinence 788.30
  – Overflow incontinence 788.39
  – Stress (female) incontinence 625.6
  – Stress (male) incontinence 788.32
  – Urge incontinence 788.31
  – Urge and stress incontinence 788.33

Defense of homebound status
- Unable to leave home due to inability to control bowel or bladder function
- Bedridden or confined to wheelchair

Selected nursing diagnoses and patient outcomes

Bowel incontinence related to (specify)
  The patient or caregiver will:
- report evacuation of a soft, formed stool daily, every other day, or every third day   (N, HCA)
- demonstrate measures to control bowel elimination   (N)
- participate in bowel training program.   (N)

Urinary incontinence related to (specify underlying cause)
  The patient or caregiver will:

- remain dry during the sleep cycle (if maturational enuresis)   (N, HCA)
- exhibit residual volume of less than 1⅔ oz (50 ml)   (N)
- verbalize nature and cause of enuresis (if maturational enuresis)   (N)
- assist in eliminating or reducing incontinent episodes (if functional enuresis)   (N)
- remove or minimize environmental barriers from home   (N, SW)
- describe causative factors for incontinence   (N)
- assist child to use triggering mechanisms to initiate reflex voiding or catheterize child every 4 to 6 hours, using clean technique (if reflex or total incontinence)   (N, HCA)
- report child's ability to stay dry with assistive measures (if reflex or total incontinence).   (N)

Risk for altered parenting related to embarrassment, shame, or frustration to bowel or bladder incontinence of child
  The patient or caregiver will:
- verbalize feelings about child's condition and its effect on parenting   (N, SW)
- identify factors that interfere with effective parenting   (N, SW)
- describe appropriate disciplinary measures   (N, SW)
- identify resources available to assist with parenting.   (N, SW)

Skilled nursing services

Care measures
- Perform an initial skilled assessment of all body systems with emphasis on GI, genitourinary, neurologic, and musculoskeletal systems.

- Obtain specimens for laboratory testing, such as blood for chemistries, urine for analysis and culture, and stool for analysis, culture, and parasite detection.
- Inspect skin, especially around perineal area.
- Assess level of care provided by patient and caregiver, including attention to skin care, safety precautions, administration of medications, bowel or bladder programs, and interaction with child.
- Assess effectiveness of treatment regimen, including episodes of control over bowel and bladder elimination or increased episodes of incontinence.
- Obtain specimens for diagnostic tests and note results, including radiographic or sonographic examinations.
- Perform baseline and follow-up developmental screenings
- Carefully note caregiver reports regarding child's elimination patterns and caregiver and child interaction.

Patient and family teaching
- Review incontinence type, cause, and methods of control.
- Discuss bowel or bladder program, including procedures for enema, catheterization, and skin care.
- Teach about medications, including actions, adverse effects, precautions, interactions, and methods of administration.
- Describe nutritional supplements to aid in stimulating peristalsis and softening stool.
- Provide anticipatory guidance to the family regarding patient's growth and development as well as long-term needs throughout life cycle.
- Teach coping mechanisms to grief responses.

- Teach parenting techniques and interventions to help form positive relationship with child who has special needs.
- Demonstrate use of clean technique in care of equipment and catheterization, if required.

Interdisciplinary actions

Home care aide
- Assistance with personal care and hygiene
- Assistance with ADLs

Social worker
- Referral to community resources
- Counseling and stress management
- Assistance with financial, emotional, and social needs

Discharge plan
- Independent safe management of child with incontinence in the home with physician and school nurse (if attending school) follow-up services
- Referral to community agencies for support
- Return to optimal level of bowel or urinary function within limits of child's underlying disease process

Documentation requirements
- Assessment data for all systems, including weight and vital signs, signs and symptoms of infection, and type of incontinence and frequency of episodes
- Activity level of child, including type of play
- Response to medication, including adverse reactions, if any

- Ability of caregiver to carry out measures to control incontinence, including use of and care of equipment
- Caregiver teaching and demonstrated responses to teaching, including bowel program or catheterization
- Specific measures used for controlling incontinence and maintaining skin integrity
- Improvement or continuation of incontinence despite interventions
- Complications (evidence or lack thereof)
- Patient's and caregiver's independence with care and therapy regimen
- Signs and symptoms to be reported
- Coping strategies for effective parenting

Reimbursement reminders
- Care of children with incontinence may be covered under insurance for underlying condition.
- Ensure that the range of covered needs to be evaluated is part of the initial assessment.
- Diapers and disposable underpants aren't typically covered by insurance; catheterization supplies usually are reimbursed, although quantities may be limited.

Insurance hints
- Report complete assessment data each visit, including changes in condition since last visit, such as control of incontinence, effectiveness of program, and skin integrity.
- Describe the response of child and family to care each visit, including questions asked and answers given.
- Report on the use and care of equipment at each visit, including care and reuse of supplies as needed.

- Describe all teaching of child and family and response to teaching each visit, especially related to measures to control bowel and bladder elimination.

Postoperative care

Because of changes in insurance coverage and in an attempt to prevent perioperative infection and emotional distress, more and more children go home within 23 hours of surgery, many within 1 hour of surgery. Postoperative care of children at home focuses on careful assessment of the wound and invasive devices, cardiovascular and respiratory support, fluid and nutrition support, and pain control.

Previsit checklist

Physician orders and preparation
- Care of wound or invasive devices
- Nutritional support, including enteral feeding
- Medication orders, such as for pain, including route, dosage, and frequency
- Infusion orders, including type, route, duration, and rate
- Laboratory tests, such as complete blood counts, electrolyte levels, and wound cultures

Equipment and supplies
- Physical assessment equipment, including penlight, pediatric stethoscope, and sphygmomanometer (with cuff sized to fit the child's arm)
- Wound care supplies
- Phlebotomy supplies
- Camera, film, and consent form for photographing wound

- Developmental assessment tool such as the Denver Developmental Screening test
- Infusion therapy supplies
- Scale

Safety requirements

- Standard precautions for infection control and sharps disposal
- Night-light, working smoke detectors on all floors of home, and fire escape plan
- Identification and correction of environmental hazards and patient-specific concerns (for example, floors cleared of small objects, loose rugs secured, sharp corners of furniture or appliances cushioned, electrical cords removed from walkways, and unused electrical outlets covered
- Danger signs and symptoms and what they mean
- Emergency plan and access to functional phone and list of emergency phone numbers, including physician, home health or nursing agency, durable medical equipment provider, emergency medical services, fire department, police, and utility providers
- Notification of power company and local fire and police departments that oxygen and medically necessary electrical equipment are in use in the home. For extended illnesses, notify the telephone company that a sick person is in residence.

Major diagnostic codes

- Appendectomy 47.09
- Appendicitis 540.1
- Attention to artificial opening of urinary tract V55.6

- Attention to surgical dressing and sutures V58.3
- Bone marrow transplant, surgical 41.00
- Constipation 564.0
- Dehydration, postoperative 998.0
- Diabetes mellitus, type 1, with complications 250.91
- Hernia repair, inguinal 53.00
- Hernia repair, umbilical 53.49
- Infection of implanted device 996.69
- Insertion of totally implantable venous access device 86.07
- Otherwise healthy infant or child receiving care V20.1
- Spinal cord injury, traumatic, unspecified 952.9
- Wound dehiscence 998.3
- Wound infection   998.5

Defense of homebound status

- Altered level of consciousness or pain requiring medical management, secondary to effects of surgery

Selected nursing diagnoses and patient outcomes

Risk for infection related to surgical invasion of bodily defenses
  The caregiver will:
- wash hands thoroughly before and after caring for child's surgical site or invasive device   (N)
- demonstrate clean or sterile technique in caring for child's surgical site or invasive device   (N)
- monitor child for signs and symptoms of infection including lethargy, increase in temperature, redness at surgical site or site of invasive device, purulent or foul-smelling drainage, in-

creased pain, feeding difficulties, and vomiting (N, HCA)
• Report signs and symptoms of infection to nurse and physician. (N, HCA)

Breathing pattern, ineffective related to inability to maintain adequate rate and depth of respirations secondary to postanesthesia state, postoperative immobility, and pain
The caregiver will:
• assist child with repositioning frequently, at least every hour (N, HCA)
• encourage child to perform deep breathing and controlled cough or sigh exercises or will hold child while rocking to elicit deep breaths (N, HCA)
• gradually increase child's activity to usual level (N, HCA)
• provide medication for pain. (N)

Pain related to physical, biological, or chemical agents (specify, such as presence of incision, invasive device, and flatus)
The caregiver will:
• provide medication for pain (N)
• perform treatments such as wound care or care of invasive device in firm, gentle manner to avoid increased pain (N)
• note child-specific signs of pain (N, HCA)
• provide comfort by holding or rocking child. (N, HCA)

Nutrition alteration: Less than body requirements related to increased protein and vitamin requirements for wound healing and decreased intake secondary to pain, nausea, vomiting and diet restrictions
The caregiver will:

• gradually increase child's food intake as ordered by physician and as child tolerates (N, MD)
• describe causes for child to be at risk for altered nutrition (N)
• describe rationale and procedure for gradual dietary increases toward normal pattern. (N)

Management of therapeutic regimen, ineffective, family, related to insufficient knowledge of home care, incisional care or care of invasive device, signs and symptoms of complications, activity restriction, and follow-up care
The caregiver will:
• relate less anxiety about fear of the unknown, fear of loss, or misconceptions. (N)
• describe postoperative healing process, causes and factors contributing to symptoms, and the regimen for symptom control. (N)
• relate an intent to practice health behaviors needed or desired for prevention of complications. (N)

Skilled nursing services

Care measures
• Assess vital signs, bleeding, and drainage.
• Perform a skilled assessment of integumentary, cardiovascular, neurologic, respiratory, and immune systems as well as specific system corrected or treated by surgical procedure.
• Assess level of care by caregiver: Observe attention to all safety precautions, administration of medications and treatments, and interaction with child.
• Assess effectiveness of treatment regimen, including wound healing, in-

tegrity of invasive device, child's vital signs and dietary intake, and activity level.

● Assess wound site for proper healing and absence of infection, and photograph as ordered and per agency protocol.

Patient and family teaching

● Teach family and caregivers about all medications, including actions, adverse effects, precautions, methods of administration, and all interactions with over-the-counter drugs, foods, and other prescribed drugs.

● Reinforce preoperative teaching on type and purpose of surgical procedure and any specific needs.

Interdisciplinary actions

Home care aide

● Bathing and personal care
● Assistance with ambulation
● Meal preparation

Discharge plan

● Caregiver will safely manage care of postoperative child in the home, with follow-up care scheduled with physician.

Documentation requirements

● Assessment data for all systems, including vital signs, signs or symptoms of infection, and wound

● Activity level of child, including type of play

● Response to medication, including adverse reactions and pain level rated

3 or less on a 0-to-10 scale at least 80% of the time.

● All durable medical equipment used, settings of equipment, appropriate care of equipment, caregiver verbalization of who to contact in case of equipment failure during and after regular business hours

● Status, use, and care of any access devices

● All patient and caregiver teaching and demonstrated responses to teaching

● All communication with physician and other team members

● Any change to the plan of care

Reimbursement reminders

● Postoperative care of children may be covered by insurance for child's underlying condition, so verify coverage details during initial assessment.

● Identify positive and negative changes in child's activity level, including changes specifically related to treatment measures such as analgesia and deep-breathing exercises.

● Provide evidence of need for nutritional support, such as weight, skin turgor, and intake (via dietary history or recall).

Insurance hints

● Review complete assessment data each visit, including changes in condition since last visit, such as decrease in wound size or pain level, increase in activity level, and developmental changes.

● Note response of child and family to care each visit, including ability to follow through with instructions and comply with treatment regimen.

- Report presence, use, and care of equipment each visit, including settings and rates, ensuring they comply with physician's orders.
- Note all teaching of child and family and response to teaching each visit; include problems encountered, such as caregiver's feelings of being overwhelmed, difficulty planning times for infusion therapy, and adverse reactions to medication.

Sickle cell anemia

Sickle cell anemia encompasses a group of inherited red blood cell disorders, characterized by chronic hemolytic anemia; high susceptibility to infections; and damage to the spleen, liver, and kidneys. Intermittent microvascular occlusion by elongated red blood cells (caused by abnormal hemoglobins S, A, and Q), results in both acute and chronic pain. Home health care of the child with sickle cell anemia focuses on hydration (including presurgical blood transfusion to dilute the concentration of abnormal red blood cells), pain management by use of oxygen, medications to reverse sickling and treat pain, and prevention of crisis episodes by avoiding such risk factors as infection, high temperatures, and high atmospheric pressure.

Previsit checklist

Physician orders and preparation
- Medications for pain and to reverse sickling
- I.V. fluid therapy and preoperative blood transfusions to dilute concentration of abnormal red blood cells

- Oxygen therapy, including rate and delivery devices
- Nutritional support, including folic acid and iron supplements to sustain body's manufacture of red blood cells
- Inclusion in clinical trials for stem cell transplantation; if there is a healthy sibling donor, bone marrow transplantation preparation
- Social worker evaluation for referral to community support agencies, financial assistance, and psychosocial assessment
- Home care aide assistance with personal hygiene and activities of daily living (ADLs)

Equipment and supplies
- Supplies for standard precautions and proper sharps disposal
- Equipment for I.V. infusion (preferably needleless infusion system), access tubings, infusion pump, dressings, and heparin or normal saline solution for flushes
- Oxygen and delivery devices as needed
- Physical assessment and neurologic testing equipment, including cotton wisps, cotton-tipped swabs, penlight, stethoscope, and sphygmomanometer (with cuff sized to fit the child's arm)
- Blood drawing equipment

Safety requirements
- Standard precautions for infection control and sharps disposal
- Emergency plan and access to functional phone and list of emergency phone numbers
- Fire evacuation plan, functional smoke detectors, and access to functional fire extinguisher

- Power outage plan (many local power companies need to know if a patient in the home requires electrical power for life-support equipment)
- Oxygen precautions, safe handling and placement of home oxygen equipment, and notification of local fire and police departments of oxygen use in the home
- Signs and symptoms requiring notification of physician
- Child safety precautions, such as ensuring that all caregivers have completed emergency room forms and information, including an authorization to treat form, emergency contacts, pediatrician's name and phone number, allergic reactions, and current medication list

Major diagnostic codes
- Dehydration 276.5
- Sickle cell anemia without/with crisis 282.61/282.62
- Sickle cell trait 282.5

Defense of homebound status
- Unable to ambulate farther than 10′ (3 m) due to profound fatigue secondary to pain and lack of oxygen to tissues
- Bedridden or confined to chair secondary to severe pain and weakness

Selected nursing diagnoses and patient outcomes

Altered peripheral tissue perfusion related to viscous blood and occlusion of microcirculation

The patient or caregiver will:

- identify factors that improve peripheral circulation such as adequate hydration (N)
- identify necessary lifestyle changes, such as avoidance of very hot or high atmospheric pressure situations (N)
- identify medical regimen, diet, medications, and activities that promote vasodilation (N, MD)
- describe signs and symptoms that require contacting physician or health care professional. (N)

Pain related to viscous blood and tissue hypoxia

The patient or caregiver will:
- identify the source of the pain (N)
- identify activities that increase and decrease pain (N)
- report relief after a satisfactory relief measure, such as medication or rest of affected area. (N, HCA)

Knowledge deficit related to management of therapeutic regimen secondary to insufficient knowledge of hazards, signs and symptoms of complications, fluid requirements, and heredity factors

The patient or caregiver will:
- relate less anxiety about fear of the unknown, fear of loss, or misconceptions (N, SW)
- describe sickling process, causes and factors contributing to symptoms, and the regimen for symptom control (N)
- institute health behaviors needed or desired for prevention of complications (N)
- verbalize feelings related to genetically transmitted disease and effects on future children (N, SW)
- demonstrate measures to adequately manage the disorder. (N, SW)

Skilled nursing services

Care measures

• Perform an initial skilled assessment of all body systems including neurologic, cardiovascular, respiratory, GI, genitourinary, and musculoskeletal systems.

• Assess level of care provided by caregiver, including attention to all safety precautions and administration of medications and treatments.

• Assess effectiveness of treatment regimen.

• Evaluate pain level and effectiveness of medication, oxygen, and rest.

• Assess child's vital signs, especially temperature, for changes.

• Investigate any complaints, being especially alert for signs and symptoms of sickle cell crises (pale lips, lethargy, difficulty awakening, severe pain, fever of 104° F (40° C) or low grade fever lasting 2 or more days, and upper abdominal pain).

• Assess activity level and its effect on pain and the patient's condition.

• Initiate fluid replacement and I.V. infusions as indicated; monitor skin turgor, hydration, nutritional status, and weight.

• Obtain or arrange for laboratory studies and report results to physician.

Patient and family teaching

• Emphasize importance of routine well-child care and keeping immunization status up-to-date.

• Teach about medications, including actions, adverse effects, precautions, interactions, and methods of administration.

• Review signs and symptoms of sickle cell anemia.

• Describe measures to prevent red blood cell sickling.

• Discuss infection control and prevention measures, including long-term antibiotic therapy, careful hand washing before and after care of child, and influenza vaccine annually and pneumococcal vaccine.

• Review signs and symptoms of infection, including lethargy, increase in temperature, skin discoloration, purulent or foul-smelling drainage, increased pain, feeding difficulties, and vomiting.

• Discuss both pharmacologic and nonpharmacologic measures to alleviate pain.

• Explain nutritional requirements and needs, including appropriate food and fluid choices, such as foods with folic acid and plenty of water or juice.

• Emphasize need to verbalize feelings related to disorder.

Interdisciplinary actions

Social worker

• Coordination with school nurse

• Referral to community agencies

• Assistance with finances

• Psychosocial assessment and intervention

Home care aide

• Assistance with personal care and hygiene

• Assistance with ADLs

Discharge plan

• Independent, safe management of the child with sickle cell anemia in the home with physician, school nurse (if attending school), and skilled nursing (for infusion therapy) follow-up services

- Return to pre-exacerbation level of function
- Referral to community support groups

Documentation requirements

- Assessment data for all systems, including weight and vital signs, signs or symptoms of infection or sickling crisis
- Nutritional assessment data, including weight, intake and output, fluid needs, and I.V. therapy
- Activity level of child, including type of play and any association with pain
- Response to medication and nutritional supplements, including adverse reactions
- Use of durable medical equipment, including settings and frequency
- Status of I.V. insertion sites
- Caregiver teaching and demonstrated responses to teaching, including ability to follow through with pain relief measures, prevent infection and crises, and maintain optimal level of functioning

Reimbursement reminders

- Care of children with sickle cell anemia is covered under the Individuals with Disabilities Education Act and the Katie Beckett Act, administered in many states by Medicaid. The Katie Beckett Act provides medical assistance for some children whose parents' income or assets are otherwise too high for medical assistance. Coverage includes skilled nursing in the home and school, dietitian and social worker services, and durable medical equipment rentals.
- Use of needleless infusion system, while more expensive, is an appropriate safeguard against sharps injuries in the community.

Insurance hints

- Report complete assessment data each visit, including changes in condition since last visit, such as increased or decreased pain, fever, and signs of infection.
- Describe the response of child and family to care each visit, including follow through with instructions and ability to control symptoms and prevent crises.
- Include a report on the child's and family's use and care of equipment, such as oxygen and I.V. therapy, at each visit, including settings and frequency of use.
- Describe gains in knowledge, such as skills and concepts mastered in medication administration, nutritional therapy, and use of equipment and pain relief measures.
- Present specific data on homebound status, such as improved ambulation or continued inability to ambulate because of pain or profound fatigue.
- Relate communication with physician, including report of laboratory test results.

Spina bifida

Spina bifida results from incomplete closure of the covering and spinal support structure of the spinal cord before birth. It varies in severity according to the degree of incompleteness of spinal cord closure and the site of incomplete closure. Disabilities range from quadriplegia to weakness of the lower extremities. Spina bifida is also associated with hydrocephalus and with Arnold-Chiari syndrome, characterized by cyst formation within the spinal cord and requiring ongoing drainage. Children with spina bifida often have or are at risk for developing latex allergies.

Home health care of children with spina bifida focuses on neurologic and musculoskeletal support, with respiratory support as needed.

Previsit checklist

Physician orders and preparation

- Medications, including respiratory support drugs and anticonvulsants
- Activity orders and restrictions
- Braces or orthopedic appliances
- Shunt site care if hydrocephalus present
- Peak flow meter, suctioning, and respiratory support measures such as oxygen
- Laboratory tests and testing for blood drug levels
- Physical therapy evaluation for home exercise program, transfer and gait training, muscle strengthening, and assistive devices
- Occupational therapy evaluation for play and adaptations with activities of daily living (ADLs)
- Seizure precautions
- Social worker evaluation for counseling and referral to support groups

Equipment and supplies

- Supplies for standard precautions and proper sharps disposal
- Physical assessment and neurologic testing equipment, including cotton wisps, cotton-tipped swabs, penlight, stethoscope, and sphygmomanometer (with cuff sized to fit the child's arm)
- Blood drawing equipment
- Supplies for seizure precautions and suctioning if needed
- Delivery devices for use with medications and treatments, including oxygen therapy
- Fragrance-free soaps, lotions, cleaning supplies, and latex-free gloves
- Assistive devices, such as braces or orthopedic appliances

Safety requirements

- Standard precautions for infection control and sharps disposal
- Multiple chemical sensitivity precautions, including not wearing perfume or cologne, being aware of and avoiding child's allergens, using vinyl gloves rather than latex gloves (this should be a routine practice for the patient with spina bifida), using fragrance-free cleaning products, and avoiding strong household cleaners
- Emergency plan and access to functional phone and list of emergency phone numbers
- Oxygen precautions, safe handling and placement of home oxygen equipment, and notification of local fire and police departments of oxygen use in the home
- Instructions on signs and symptoms of medical emergency and actions to take
- Seizure precautions if needed
- Child safety precautions: install cabinet and drawer latches, toilet-lid locks, security gates, tub-spout guard, doorknob covers, and stove knob guards (or remove the knobs when stove isn't in use); and use a bath mat

Major diagnostic codes
- Spina bifida 741.9
- Spina bifida occulta 756.17
- Spina bifida with hydrocephalus 741.0

Defense of homebound status
- Unable to ambulate farther than 10′ (3 m) without assistance
- Bedridden or confined to wheelchair secondary to profound weakness or quadriplegia

Selected nursing diagnoses and patient outcomes

Knowledge deficit related to management of therapeutic regimen secondary to insufficient knowledge of (specify: disease process, pharmacologic regimen, activity program, community resources, or orthopedic appliances)

The patient or caregiver will:
- relate less anxiety about fear of the unknown, fear of loss, or misconceptions (N, SW)
- describe disabling process, causes and factors contributing to symptoms, and the regimen for symptom control (N, PT)
- identify health behaviors needed or desired for prevention of complications (N, OT, PT)
- demonstrate measures to optimize functional ability. (N, OT, PT)

Altered growth and development related to impaired ability to achieve developmental tasks

The patient or caregiver will:

- demonstrate progress in behaviors in personal, social, language, cognition, or motor activities appropriate to age group (specify the behaviors) (N, OT, PT)
- demonstrate achievement of developmental milestones within limitations of disease (N, PT, SP)
- participate in activity-related treatment program. (N, HCA, OT, PT)

Altered family processes related to adjustment requirements for situation (for example, time, emotional and physical energy, financial, and physical care)

The patient or caregiver will:
- verbalize feelings about situation (N, HCA, SW)
- participate in care as much as possible (N, HCA, OT, PT)
- facilitate the return of the family member with special care needs from sick role to well role (N, HCA, PT, SW)
- maintain functional system of mutual support for each family member (N, SW)
- seek appropriate external resources when needed (N, SW)
- identify factors that interfere with effective parenting and family function (N, SW)
- describe appropriate disciplinary measures. (N, SW)

Skilled nursing services

Care measures
- Perform an initial skilled assessment of all body systems with emphasis on neurologic, integumentary, and musculoskeletal systems; and assess growth and development.

- Assess level of care provided by patient and caregiver, including attention to all safety precautions, administration of medications and treatments, exercise program, and respiratory support as needed.
- Assess effectiveness of treatment regimen; obtain or arrange for laboratory studies, and perform baseline and follow-up developmental screenings.
- Evaluate degree of respiratory and musculoskeletal impairment and institute treatment measures to enhance functioning.
- Assess mobility status and risk of injury, including safety needs; use of orthopedic, assistive, or adaptive devices; and exercise program.
- Inspect shunt site, as appropriate, for signs and symptoms of functioning and infection; assess signs and symptoms of increasing intracranial pressure related to shunt and subsequent recurrence of hydrocephalus.
- Provide for grief responses and provide hope and guidance to parents in forming relationship with their child.

Patient and family teaching
- Teach about medications, including actions, adverse effects, precautions, interactions, and methods of administration.
- Provide anticipatory guidance of family regarding patient's growth and development, disability process, and needs throughout life cycle.
- Emphasize importance of forming a relationship with child.
- Describe skin care, especially involving areas with use of orthopedic braces and assistive or adaptive devices and shunt site.
- Discuss exercise program.

- Demonstrate application and use of orthopedic, assistive, or adaptive devices.

Interdisciplinary actions

Physical therapist
- Orthopedic appliance or assistive device fitting and use
- Exercise program
- Physical measures to treat symptoms
- Transfer and gait training

Occupational therapist
- Assistive devices for facilitating ADLs, including fitting and use
- Play therapy

Respiratory therapist
- Chest physiotherapy
- Pulmonary evaluation

Social worker
- Referral for community resources
- Counseling and stress management
- Assistance with financial, emotional, respite, and social needs

Speech pathologist
- Audiologic evaluation

Home care aide
- Assistance with personal care and hygiene
- Assistance with ADLs

Discharge plan
- Independent safe management of child with spina bifida in the home, with follow-up services by physician, school nurse (if attending school), and skilled therapist

- Achievement of optimal level of functioning within limits of disease
- Referral to community agencies for support and assistance
- Referral for continued physical and occupational therapy on an outpatient basis

Documentation requirements

- Assessment data for all systems, including weight and vital signs, shunt site, and level of consciousness
- Activity level of child, including type of play and functional ability, use of or need for assistive devices
- Response to medication, including adverse reactions, if any
- All durable medical equipment used, including settings and frequency of use
- Use and ability to apply orthopedic or assistive and adaptive devices and perform shunt site care as appropriate
- Patient's and family's adjustment to illness and ability to cope with it
- Resources available for support and respite care
- Caregiver teaching and demonstrated responses to teaching
- Communication with physician and other disciplines, including report of laboratory test results
- Patient and caregiver progress toward educational goals, including feelings of being overwhelmed, and need for repeated instructions
- Patient and caregiver instructions
- Complications (evidence or lack thereof)
- Patient's and caregiver's independence with care and therapy regimen
- Safety precautions, including proper installation of a car safety seat

- Skin care measures, including care of shunt site
- Signs and symptoms to be reported

Reimbursement reminders

- Care of children with spina bifida is covered under the Individuals with Disabilities Education Act and the Katie Beckett Act. Guidelines and funding are administered in many states by Medicaid. The Katie Beckett Act provides medical assistance for some children whose parents' income or assets are otherwise too high for medical assistance. Coverage includes skilled nursing and skilled therapies in the home and school as well as durable medical equipment rentals.
- Barriers to learning, such as physical deformities, visual impairments, and a lack of availability or overwhelming of support person should be recorded.

Insurance hints

- Report complete assessment data each visit, including changes in condition since last visit, such as injury, skin breakdown, and signs of increased intracranial pressure.
- Describe the response of child and family to care each visit, including follow through with instructions.
- Include a report on the child's and family's use and care of equipment each visit, including settings and frequency of use.
- Describe gains in knowledge, such as skills and concepts mastered in medication administration and use of orthopedic devices.
- Present specific data on homebound status, such as improved ambulation with assistive device, continued in-

ability to ambulate because of weakness, number of persons needed to assist patient out of chair, continued limitation in ambulation distance, or development of any injury related to disease process.

Spinal muscular atrophy

Spinal muscular atrophy (SMA) is a disease of the anterior horn cells, located in the spinal cord. It affects the voluntary muscles for such activities as crawling, walking, head and neck control, and swallowing. SMA mainly affects muscle groups proximal to the trunk, with leg weakness usually greater than arm weakness. Fasciculations (abnormal twitching) of muscles such as the tongue may be present. Senses and feelings are normal, as is intellectual activity. In fact, it's often observed that patients with SMA are unusually bright and sociable. There are three levels of severity of SMA:

• Type I acute (severe) is also called Werdnig-Hoffmann Disease. Diagnosis is usually made between ages 3 and 6 months; there may be a lack of fetal movement in the final trimester of pregnancy. The child with type I SMA is never able to lift his head or accomplish normal physical milestones. Swallowing and feeding as well as managing secretions may be difficult. Intercostal and accessory muscle weakness requires diaphragmatic breathing; and the chest appears concave.

• Type II (intermediate) is usually diagnosed between ages 15 months and 2 years. Children with type II SMA may sit unsupported but must be assisted to sitting position. They may progress to standing by use of a bracing, parapodium, or standing frame. Feeding and swallowing problems are rare; when present, a feeding tube may become necessary. Finger or tongue fasciculations may be present. Diaphragmatic breathing is present in children with type II SMA.

• Type III (mild), also called Kugelberg-Welander syndrome or juvenile spinal muscular atrophy is usually diagnosed between age 18 months and adolescence. The child can sit alone and walk but may show difficulty with walking and getting up from a seated or bent-over position. Tongue fasciculations are rare, but fasciculations in outstretched fingers are common.

SMA is nonprogressive or very slowly progressive. Diagnosis is made by spinal motor neuron probes, which detect the absence of gene sequences in 90% to 94% of patients with SMA, and is confirmed by needle muscle biopsy, done under local anesthetic to avoid compromise of already weakened respiratory function. Home health care of children with SMA focuses on respiratory, nutritional, and developmental support.

Previsit checklist

Physician orders and preparation

• Chest physical therapy and suctioning techniques
• Nutritional support, such as nasogastric or gastrostomy tube feedings
• Port-a-Lung (negative pressure ventilation) or biphasic positive airway pressure respiratory support (biPap); use of intermittent positive pressure

breathing (IPPB) and incentive spirometer respiratory support

- Aquatic therapy, physical, and mental stimulation
- Respiratory assistive devices, including oxygen rate if needed
- Medications, including dosage, route, and frequency
- Nutritional supplements, including type, volume, rate, route, and access device, if any
- Assistive devices for standing and sitting
- Physical therapy evaluation, therapeutic exercise programs, fit and application of assistive devices, and chest physiotherapy
- Occupational therapy evaluation for adaptations in activities of daily living (ADLs) and play therapy
- Social work evaluation for referrals and assistance with long-term care needs
- Home care aide assistance with personal care and ADLs

Equipment and supplies

- Supplies for standard precautions and proper sharps disposal
- Physical assessment and neurologic testing equipment, including cotton wisps, cotton-tipped swabs, penlight, stethoscope, and sphygmomanometer (with cuff sized to fit the child's arm)
- Delivery devices for use with medications and treatments, such as nebulizers, air compressor, suction catheters, suction machine, peak flow meter, ventilatory support, and oxygen
- Assistive devices, orthopedic braces, adaptive devices as indicated
- Enteral feeding supplies

Safety requirements

- Standard precautions for infection control and sharps disposal
- Emergency plan and access to functional phone and list of emergency phone numbers
- Fire evacuation plan, functional smoke detectors, and access to functional fire extinguisher
- Power outage plan (many local power companies need to know if a patient in the home requires electrical power for life-support equipment)
- Oxygen precautions, safe handling and placement of home oxygen equipment, and notification of local fire and police departments of oxygen use in the home
- Identification and correction of environmental hazards and patient-specific concerns (for example, floors cleared of small objects and loose rugs secured)
- Signs and symptoms requiring notification of physician
- Constant observation of child when exercising in water to prevent aspiration of water or secretions; make sure water temperature is 90° to 100° F (32.2° to 37.7° C) and that water doesn't reach child's head or neck
- Correct application and frequent checks of skin under orthopedic devices, if used
- Child safety precautions: colorful decals affixed to glass doors to make them visible; wall hooks to hold long cords out of child's reach

Major diagnostic codes

- Spinal muscular atrophy 335.10

Defense of homebound status

- Unable to ambulate farther than 10′ (3 m) without assistance
- Confined to wheelchair
- Assistance of two persons required for transfer from bed to chair

Selected nursing diagnoses and patient outcomes

Knowledge deficit related to management of therapeutic regimen secondary to insufficient knowledge of (specify: for example, disease process, pharmacologic regimen, activity program, community resources, or orthopedic appliances)

The patient or caregiver will:
- relate less anxiety about fear of the unknown, fear of loss, or misconceptions (N, SW)
- describe disabling process, causes and factors contributing to symptoms, and the regimen for symptom control (N, OT, PT, RT, SW)
- demonstrate appropriate health behaviors needed or desired for prevention of complications (N, OT, PT, RT)
- demonstrate adequate skills necessary to care for child. (N, OT, PT, RT)

Altered growth and development related to impaired ability to achieve developmental tasks secondary to muscle atrophy

The patient or caregiver will:
- demonstrate progression in behaviors in personal, social, language, cognition, or motor activities appropriate to age-group (N, OT, PT)

- exhibit achievement of appropriate developmental milestones within limits of functional ability (N, OT, PT, SP, SW)
- identify methods to foster achievement of milestones. (N, OT, PT, SW)

Altered family processes related to adjustment requirements for situation (for example, time, emotion and physical energy, financial, and physical care)

The patient or caregiver will:
- verbalize feelings openly (N, HCA, OT, PT, SP, SW)
- participate in care of family member with special care needs (N, HCA, OT, PT, SP, SW)
- maintain functional system of mutual support for each member (N, HCA, OT, PT, SP, SW)
- seek appropriate external resources when needed. (N, SW)

Risk for altered parenting related to (specify: such as abuse, rejection, overprotection secondary to inadequate resources or coping mechanisms)

The patient or caregiver will:
- share feelings regarding parenting (N, HCA, OT, PT, RT, SP, SW)
- identify factors that interfere with effective parenting (N, SW)
- describe appropriate disciplinary measures (N, SW)
- identify resources available for assistance with parenting. (N, SW)

Risk for injury related to impaired voluntary muscle activity

The patient or caregiver will:
- remain free from injury (N, HCA, OT, PT, RT)

• integrate the use of adaptive and assistive devices appropriately and correctly   (N, HCA, OT, PT, RT)
• demonstrate use of respiratory support devices when indicated. (N, RT)

Skilled nursing services

Care measures
• Perform an initial skilled assessment of all body systems with emphasis on neurologic, integumentary, respiratory and musculoskeletal systems; also assess growth and development.
• Assess level of care provided by patient and caregiver, including attention to all safety precautions, administration of medications, respiratory support measures, nutritional support, and exercise program.
• Assess effectiveness of treatment regimen; obtain or arrange for laboratory tests as indicated and perform baseline and follow-up developmental screenings.
• Evaluate respiratory status including need for IPPB, biPap, or negative pressure ventilation.
• Inspect skin, especially those areas under orthopedic and assistive devices.
• Assess mobility status and risk of injury, including safety needs as well as use of orthopedic, assistive, or adaptive devices and exercise program.
• Provide for grief responses and provide hope and guidance in forming relationship with their child who happens to have special needs.

Patient and family teaching
• Teach about disease process.
• Explain medication regimen, including actions, adverse effects, pre-cautions, interactions, and methods of administration.
• Discuss fall and safety precautions.
• Demonstrate skin care, especially involving areas with use of orthopedic braces or splints and assistive or adaptive devices.
• Review such skills as respiratory support, and enteral tube feedings.
• Provide anticipatory guidance of family regarding growth and development, disability process, and needs throughout life cycle.
• Review dangerous signs and symptoms.

Interdisciplinary actions

Physical therapist
• Orthopedic appliance or assistive device fitting and use
• Home exercise program
• Transfer, gait, and ambulation training as appropriate
• Use of physical measures to treat symptoms

Occupational therapist
• Assistive devices for ADLs
• Exercise program
• Play therapy

Respiratory therapist
• Chest physiotherapy
• Pulmonary evaluation
• Education of family members in use of respiratory equipment

Social worker
• Referral for community resources
• Counseling and stress management
• Assistance with long-term financial, emotional, and social needs

Home care aide
- Assistance with personal care and hygiene
- Assistance with ADLs

Discharge plan
- Independent, safe management of child with SMA in the home with follow-up services by physician and school nurse (if attending school)
- Episodic follow-up by skilled services for nutritional changes related to disease process and growth and development of child
- Referral for outpatient crisis intervention
- Referral for continued physical therapy and occupational therapy on an outpatient basis
- Achievement of optimal level of functioning within limitations of disease

Documentation requirements
- Assessment data for all systems, including weight, vital signs, skin integrity, nutritional status, Denver II Developmental Screening test or other screening test results, and laboratory test results
- Activity level of child, including type of play and changes in mobility status, language and speech, and functional ability
- Response to medication, respiratory therapy, and enteral nutrition therapy, including adverse reactions
- Use, type, and care of all durable medical equipment, such as IPPB, bi-Pap, ventilator, oxygen, and feeding pump
- Use and ability to apply orthopedic and assistive or adaptive devices

- Patient's and family's adjustment to illness and ability to cope with it
- Resources available for support
- Caregiver teaching and demonstrated responses to teaching
- Communication with physician and other disciplines, including laboratory results and changes in patient's condition
- Patient and caregiver participation in care
- Patient and caregiver progress toward educational goals, including feelings of being overwhelmed, and need for repeated instructions
- Patient and caregiver instructions
- Complications (evidence or lack thereof)
- Patient's and caregiver's independence with care and therapy regimen
- Safety precautions
- Signs and symptoms to be reported

Reimbursement reminders
- Care of children with SMA is covered under the Individuals with Disabilities Education Act and the Katie Beckett Act. Guidelines and funding are administered in many states by Medicaid. The Katie Beckett Act provides medical assistance for some children whose parents' income or assets are otherwise too high for medical assistance. Coverage includes skilled nursing and skilled therapies in the home and school as well as durable medical equipment rentals.
- Respiratory, rather than physical, therapy may be used to initiate respiratory care measures, depending on the requirements of the insurance.

Insurance hints

● Report complete assessment data each visit, including changes in condition since last visit such as weight loss, injury, or skin breakdown.

● Describe the response of child and family to care each visit, including follow through with instructions.

● Include a report on the child's and family's use and care of equipment such as oxygen, feeding pump, and biPap each visit, including settings and frequency of use.

● Describe gains in knowledge such as skills and concepts mastered in medication administration, nutritional therapy, and use of orthopedic devices.

● Present specific data on homebound status, such as improved ambulation with assistive device, continued inability to ambulate because of profound weakness, number of persons needed to assist patient out of chair, continued limitation in ambulation distance, or development of any injury related to disease process.

10 Psychiatric disorders and treatments

Anxiety

Anxiety disorders encompass a complex of symptoms and behaviors that range from mild concern to out-of-control panic. More than 14% of the general population is believed to have experienced severe anxiety sometime in their lives, and anxiety disorders are some of the most common psychiatric illnesses in the elderly and in individuals with chronic medical problems.

Anxious feelings are the emotional response to stressful or threatening situations. Mild to moderate anxiety can give us heightened alertness and help us focus on a problem, blocking out nonessential information in the search for an appropriate response. Severe anxiety causes such extreme focus on the problem that the individual may not be able to think clearly. If the feelings escalate to panic, they can result in loss of control, distortion of perceptions, and a sense of impending doom. Prolonged or severe anxiety symptoms may indicate a disabling anxiety disorder. Physical signs of stress, such as shortness of breath, heart palpitations, diaphoresis, dizziness, nausea, and flushes or chills, can impair an individual's ability to carry out normal daily activities. Over time, these stress responses can elevate blood pressure or alter fat and protein metabolism. Anxiety disorders can interfere with healing and recovery during a medical illness.

Like depression, anxiety may or may not be the primary diagnosis for a home care patient, but it often accompanies other diagnoses. When anxiety symptoms are present, they should be reported and addressed in the plan of care. Common anxiety disorders include generalized anxiety, panic disorder, obsessive-compulsive disorder, phobias, and posttraumatic stress disorder. Treatment of most anxiety disorders is usually successful with behavioral therapy and, sometimes, with medications.

Previsit checklist

Physician orders and preparation
* Medications such as anxiolytics
* Behavior therapy and stress reduction techniques

- Suicide precautions
- Laboratory testing, if indicated
- Social worker evaluation for crisis intervention, counseling, and referral to community agencies
- Review current (nonpsychotropic) medications to rule out anxiety as an adverse drug effect

Equipment and supplies
- Supplies for standard precautions and proper sharps disposal

Safety requirements
- Standard precautions for infection control and sharps disposal
- System to assist compliance with complex medication regimen, including supervision
- Depression and suicide precautions
- Emergency contact person and crisis intervention phone numbers
- Emergency plan and access to functional phone and list of emergency phone numbers
- Fire evacuation plan, functional smoke detectors, and access to functional fire extinguisher
- Night-light

Major diagnostic codes
- Agoraphobia with/without panic attacks 300.21/300.22
- Anxiety depression 300.4
- Anxiety state, unspecified 300.00
- Generalized anxiety disorder 300.02
- Hysteria 300.1
- Obsessive-compulsive disorder 300.3
- Organic anxiety syndrome 293.84
- Other phobias 300.29
- Panic disorder 300.01
- Phobia, unspecified 300.20
- Phobic disorders 300.2

- Social phobia 300.23

Defense of homebound status
- Inability to leave home because of severe anxiety, panic attacks, or phobias
- Agoraphobia interfering with ability to leave home

Selected nursing diagnoses and patient outcomes

Knowledge deficit related to management of anxiety disorder (for example, medications, management of anxiety level, safety measures, and suicide precautions)

The patient or caregiver will:
- state correct dose and time for each medication prescribed as well as adverse effects and precautions for each and demonstrate adherence to medication regimen (N)
- state signs and symptoms of adverse effects related to medications that require reporting to physician (N)
- demonstrate or verbalize knowledge of measures to lower anxiety level (N, SW)
- verbalize knowledge of resources and assistance, such as counseling, local support groups, spiritual or pastoral support, and crisis intervention hotlines that are available to the patient and caregiver (N, SW)
- demonstrate or verbalize knowledge of and compliance with keeping psychotherapeutic appointments (N, SW)
- demonstrate or verbalize knowledge of and adherence to home safety practices and suicide precautions. (N, SW, OT)

Ineffective individual coping related to inability to manage stressors

The patient or caregiver will:

• demonstrate or verbalize understanding of methods to control and manage anxiety　　　　(N, SW, OT)
• demonstrate or verbalize progressive relaxation techniques (N, SW, OT)
• verbalize knowledge of stimulants that create anxiety and should be avoided　　　　　　(N, SW, OT)
• participate in treatment programs.
　　　　　　　　　　　　(N, SW)

Impaired social interaction related to severity of anxiety and inability to leave home

The patient or caregiver will:

• demonstrate calmer speech patterns and decreased anxious verbalization
　　　　　　　　　　　　(N, SW)
• demonstrate increased involvement in care and activities　　(N, SW, OT)
• experience a decrease in the number of or have no panic attacks (N, SW)
• verbalize feelings and accept reassurances of others　　　　　(N)
• communicate needs to others
　　　　　　　　　　　　(N, SW)
• demonstrate ability to leave home with or without caregiver (N, SW, OT)
• demonstrate adequate socialization by increased or improved communication with family and caregivers (N, SW)
• express appropriate interests in activities and in others.　　(N, SW)

Skilled nursing services

Care measures
• Perform an initial skilled assessment of all body systems; assess family and environmental factors.

• Assess nonverbal and verbal indications of anxiety and stress.
• Evaluate physical symptoms of stress response, both short-term and long-term.
• Assess patient's knowledge and understanding of anxiety, medications, and resources.
• Assess for psychosomatic symptoms, such as problems with sleeping, eating, and elimination.
• Evaluate medication therapy regimen, including compliance with and adherence to treatment.
• Investigate patient's participation in stress reduction and behavior therapy techniques.

Patient and family teaching
• Teach about medication management and compliance.
• Teach skills for coping, forming relationships, self-care, mental well-being, and independence.
• Explain constructive verbalizing of and listening to feelings.
• Discuss home safety concerns and issues, including suicide precautions and managing situational crises.
• Stress importance of therapy and medical follow-up and compliance.
• Detail available resources.
• Identify feelings and triggering events or stresses.
• Review signs and symptoms of anxiety and ways to alleviate them; discuss ways to maintain a therapeutic environment.
• Emphasize need for social contact and involvement with others.

Interdisciplinary actions

Social worker

- Assessment of the social and emotional factors related to the patient's illness
- Referral to community resources and support groups
- Psychotherapy by licensed clinical social worker
- Crisis intervention
- Brief counseling (two or three visits) for patient's family or caregiver when needed to resolve direct impediments to patient's recovery

Occupational therapist

- Assessment of rehabilitation needs and development of home activity plan
- Therapeutic activities designed to increase cognitive abilities and functional participation in activities of daily living
- Plan to maximize home safety

Discharge plan

- Independent, safe management of patient with anxiety at home with appropriate follow-up
- Compliance with therapy program
- Referral to community agencies for support and crisis interventions
- Demonstration of decreased anxiety, improved coping skills, and increased social interaction

Documentation requirements

- History, including usual patterns of coping, previous episodes of anxiety, and family history (psychiatric)
- Signs and symptoms of anxiety

- Review of adverse effects of all medications taken by patient
- Medication regimen and effectiveness as well as medication changes and subsequent effects
- Patient and caregiver progress toward educational goals
- Patient's progress or lack of progress in symptoms of anxiety, social interaction, and ability to provide self-care
- Patient's response to interventions, including an objective description of interventions and subsequent responses
- Triggers or significant stressors associated with anxiety and family dysfunctions that affect the patient
- Patient's statements about subjective feelings
- Patient and caregiver participation in care
- Assessment of patient's suicide potential
- Psychiatric nursing interventions in response to anxious thought patterns expressed by patient and patient's response to them
- Specific knowledge deficits and evidence of progress as seen in medication management, self-care, social interaction, and verbalized concepts
- Patient and caregiver instructions
- Relaxation techniques, measures to control crises, and coping strategies

Reimbursement reminders

- The patient must have an Axis I Diagnosis (clinical disorder) for the *DSM-IV,* which must match the diagnosis that the ordering physician is treating or for which the patient was hospitalized; the diagnosis must be fully documented in the record.
- Home care orders for psychiatric nursing don't require the signature of

the patient's psychiatrist; the primary care or attending physician's signature is acceptable.

• Home care nurses caring for patients with a psychiatric condition must be qualified by experience, education, or certification to provide specialized psychiatric nursing; evidence of the nurse's qualifications should be maintained in the nurse's personnel file for examination as needed by regulatory bodies and third-party payers. Some Medicare intermediaries insist on reviewing and approving a nurse's credentials for providing psychiatric evaluation and therapy in home care *before* the nurse can render psychiatric services.

Insurance hints

• Establish reasonable goals that can realistically be achieved. Decreasing or shortening inpatient care may be an achievable and reimbursable goal.

• Present objective data about homebound status, including the severity of the patient's anxiety and how it interferes with ability to leave home.

• Describe additional underlying conditions that may impact patient's homebound status.

• Provide objective assessment findings and changes, identify specific signs and symptoms experienced and their frequency, and include any reports of an increase or decrease in frequency.

• Detail specific findings about medication effects and changes.

• Report specifics about patient education progress, including ability to demonstrate relaxation techniques and effectiveness.

• Present objective assessment of patient's progress or lack of progress toward symptom control, self-care, and stated feelings.

Bipolar disorder

Bipolar disorder, also known as manic-depressive disorder, is a chronic and disabling affective disease characterized by episodes of serious mania and depression. The patient typically experiences mood swings that range from sadness and hopelessness to extremely high activity and irritability, and then back again. Between the episodes of mood swings, the patient usually displays a normal mood. The severity and duration of the affective episodes varies. Sometimes mania is the main problem, with infrequent depression, and sometimes the patient is primarily depressed with only an occasional manic episode. The disorder is a lifelong affliction that typically begins in adolescence or early adulthood, and affects at least 2 million Americans.

Bipolar disorder is an extremely disruptive disease — for the patient and for the patient's family members, friends, and employers. The illness causes serious behavior problems, such as excessive spending sprees or abusive binges involving sex, drugs, or alcohol. The consequences of many of these behaviors are long lasting and may include divorce, job loss, financial ruin, and suicide. Many people with bipolar disorder don't recognize the severity of their illness and may not feel they need help. Home care nurses usually see patients with this condition after they have been hospitalized for an acute episode and are on medications that may still need some dosage adjustments. Because the disease causes family disruptions and often runs in families, the home care nurse may find herself dealing with a dysfunctional family situation. Patient and caregiver education is the primary goal of home care.

Previsit checklist

Physician orders and preparation
- Medications, including mood stabilizers
- Laboratory testing (for example, blood levels for drug monitoring)
- Psychiatric therapy and treatment program
- Suicide precautions
- Social worker evaluation for crisis intervention, community referrals, and assistance with measures to ensure compliance

Equipment and supplies
- Supplies for standard precautions and proper sharps disposal

Safety requirements
- Standard precautions for infection control and sharps disposal
- Emergency plan and access to functional phone and list of emergency phone numbers
- Fire evacuation plan, functional smoke detectors, and access to functional fire extinguisher
- Night-light
- System to assist compliance with complex medication regimen, including supervision
- Depression and suicide precautions
- Emergency contact person and crisis intervention phone numbers
- Phlebotomy supplies

Major diagnostic codes
- Atypical depressive disorder 296.82
- Bipolar affective disorder
  - depressed, unspecified 296.50
  - manic, unspecified 296.40
  - mixed, unspecified 296.60
  - unspecified 296.7
- Major depressive disorder, recurrent episode, unspecified/single episode, unspecified 296.30/296.20
- Manic disorder, recurrent episode, unspecified 296.10

Defense of homebound status
- Inability to leave home because of extreme lethargy from depression
- Behavior that poses risk to self or others
- Unsafe outside the home because of impaired judgment and potential for harm
- Inability to leave home because of extreme irritability
- Acute mania with aberrant and antisocial behavior
- Supervision required because of impaired judgment

Selected nursing diagnoses and patient outcomes

Knowledge deficit related to management of bipolar disorder (for example, medications, coping skills, safety issues, and suicide precautions)

The patient or caregiver will:
- verbalize the correct dose and time for each medication prescribed and demonstrate adherence to medication regimen   (N)

- state signs and symptoms of bipolar disorder and understanding of chronic lifetime nature of the disorder (N)
- relate possible adverse effects of medications that require notification of physician (N)
- verbalize knowledge of resources and assistance, such as counseling, local support groups, spiritual or pastoral support, and crisis intervention hotlines that are available (N, SW)
- demonstrate and verbalize knowledge of and compliance with keeping psychotherapeutic appointments (N, SW)
- demonstrate and verbalize knowledge of and adherence to home safety practices and suicide precautions. (N, SW, OT)

Altered thought processes related to psychiatric disorder and wide-ranging mood swings

The patient or caregiver will:
- exhibit decreased symptoms of mania or depression (N, SW)
- demonstrate measures to continue working toward optimal reality orientation within disease limitations (N, SW, OT)
- demonstrate ability to orient and assist patient with realistic thought processes as needed (N, SW, OT)
- verbalize and demonstrate an ability to maintain a supportive environment (N, SW, OT)
- participate in treatment programs. (N, SW)

Risk for injury to self or others related to altered thought processes and problems with reality orientation

The patient or caregiver will:
- verbalize signs and symptoms of suicidal or hostile intentions (N, SW)

- demonstrate understanding of need for patient to have supervision (N, SW)
- demonstrate ability to create a safe environment for patient. (N, SW, OT)

Noncompliance related to life-long illness requiring complex treatment regimen

The patient or caregiver will:
- verbalize understanding of necessity for compliance with treatment (N)
- state importance of taking medications as ordered even when patient doesn't feel they're necessary (N)
- demonstrate planning for renewal or reorder of medications to ensure continuity of treatment (N, SW)
- state the importance of periodic serological testing for therapeutic levels of medication. (N)

Skilled nursing services

Care measures
- Take a thorough medical and psychiatric history and list all medications patient is taking, along with pertinent potential adverse effects.
- Perform an initial skilled assessment of all body systems; assess family and environmental factors.
- Assess nonverbal and verbal indications of a depression or mania.
- Evaluate behaviors indicative of patient's mood.
- Assess patient's knowledge and understanding of disease, medications, and resources.
- Assess interactions with significant others and coping skills.
- Perform a skilled assessment of suicide potential.

• Institute suicide precautions, including having the patient sign a contract that he won't injure himself.

• Assess level of orientation and reorient patient to reality as necessary; define acceptable behaviors.

• Obtain or arrange for laboratory studies as indicated.

Patient and family teaching

• Describe medication management and compliance.

• Discuss coping and relationship skills.

• Review symptom recognition and response.

• Identify home safety concerns and issues; detail suicide precautions.

• Discuss need for readily available access to therapist's or clinic's telephone number.

• Explain importance of therapy, medical follow-up, and compliance.

• Emphasize maintenance of lifestyle with a balance of rest and activity and balanced nutrition.

Interdisciplinary actions

Social worker

• Referral to community resources and support groups

• Counseling and crisis intervention

• Counseling (two or three visits) to assist family members in coping with behaviors of the bipolar patient or to resolve impediments to the patient's recovery

• Assistance with finances to aid in medication compliance

• Education regarding disease cycles, management, and suicide precautions

Occupational therapist

• Rehabilitation needs and development of a home activity plan

• Therapeutic activities designed to increase cognitive abilities and functional participation in activities of daily living

• Development of a plan to maximize home safety

Discharge plan

• Independent, safe management of patient with bipolar disorder in the home with physician and community follow-up services

• Compliance with medication and treatment therapy, including any serologic testing necessary to ensure therapeutic medication levels

• Referral to community resources for assistance and support

• Demonstration of appropriate behaviors with control of mood swings

Documentation requirements

• Signs and symptoms of depression and mania

• Medication therapy regimen and effects of medication regimen

• Patient and caregiver progress toward educational goals, such as understanding of need for medication, suicide precautions, and effects of mood swings

• Patient's progress or lack of progress in behavior, social interaction, feelings, and ability to provide self-care

• Patient's response to interventions, including psychiatric therapy

• Triggers or significant stressors associated with mood swings and family dysfunctions that affect patient

- Patient's statements about subjective feelings
- Patient and caregiver participation in care
- Assessment of patient's suicide potential
- Laboratory test results, including blood drug levels and changes to dosage or plan of care after speaking with physician
- Patient and caregiver instructions
- Medication therapy, including signs and symptoms of adverse effects and toxicity
- Signs and symptoms of mood swings
- Suicide and home safety precautions
- Coping strategies and measures to control crisis
- Dangerous signs and symptoms

Reimbursement reminders

- The patient must have an Axis I Diagnosis (clinical disorder) for the *DSM-IV,* which must match the diagnosis that the ordering physician is treating or for which the patient was hospitalized; the diagnosis must be fully documented in the record.
- Home care orders for psychiatric nursing don't require signature of patient's psychiatrist; the attending or primary care physician's signature is acceptable.
- Home care nurses caring for patients with a psychiatric condition must be qualified by experience, education, or certification to provide specialized psychiatric nursing; evidence of nurse's qualifications should be maintained in personnel files for examination as needed by regulatory bodies and third-party payers. Some Medicare intermediaries insist on reviewing and approving a nurse's credentials for providing psychiatric evaluation and therapy in home care before nurse can render psychiatric services.

- Patient may need separate services by both a psychiatric nurse and a social worker, so be careful to avoid duplication of services in areas such as patient counseling.
- Record destructive thought patterns expressed by patient and patient's response to psychiatric nursing interventions.
- Document specific knowledge deficits that show evidence of progress as seen in medication management, self-care, social interaction, and verbalized concepts.

Insurance hints

- Establish reasonable goals that can realistically be achieved. Decreasing or shortening inpatient care may be an achievable and reimbursable goal.
- Present objective data about homebound status specifically addressing the effect of the patient's mood swings on ability to go outside the home.
- Describe objective assessment findings and changes, emphasizing potential findings associated with suicide ideation.
- Relate specific findings about medication effects and changes; report actual laboratory results of blood drug levels.
- Discuss specific details about patient education progress; include direct patient and caregiver statements related to understanding of disease process, coping, therapy, and medications.
- Present objective assessment of patient's progress or lack of progress toward improved affect, self-care, and stated feelings.

Dementia

Dementia is an organic mental disorder that causes memory impairment; loss of other intellectual abilities, such as abstract thinking, judgment, and language; and, sometimes, personality changes. An estimated 4 to 5 million Americans, including 15% of those over age 65, have cognitive failure in some form and degree, with dementia the most common syndrome. Dementia may be caused by disease, such as Parkinson's and Huntington's disease, thyroid disease, infection, meningitis, syphilis, or acquired immunodeficiency syndrome; such disorders as stroke, brain tumor, or hydrocephalus; or other conditions such as drug reactions, nutritional deficiencies, head injuries, or alcoholism.

Alzheimer's disease is the most common form of dementia, followed by multi-infarct dementia. Most dementias begin slowly and develop gradually over many months or years, and are considered chronic and irreversible. Some disorders that produce dementia are reversible and may require prompt treatment to prevent brain damage. It's important to determine the underlying cause of dementia symptoms before deciding on a course of treatment and care.

The risk of dementia increases dramatically with advancing age; the number of people with Alzheimer's disease is projected to increase to 14 million by the year 2050 if no cure or prevention is found. New medications may halt or slow the progression of Alzheimer's, but some of them have significant adverse effects and require diligent monitoring.

Many older home care patients suffer from some form of dementia, even if it isn't the principle reason for home care visits. The home care plan of care for any patient that exhibits even mild dementia should address the special concerns that arise from this condition. Home care nurses will be concerned with teaching caregivers about safety, following the medical regimen, and preserving as much cognitive, social, physical, and psychological function as possible.

Previsit checklist

Physician orders and preparation
- Medications and review of current medication regimen for any adverse effects that may present as dementia
- Specific orders related to other disease conditions and assurance that those conditions are being treated appropriately and adequately
- Laboratory studies, such as liver function tests and blood drug levels
- Occupational therapy evaluation for home exercise program, home safety, and endurance training
- Home care aide assistance with personal care and activities of daily living (ADLs)
- Social worker evaluation for assistance with long-term needs and referrals for community support and counseling for caregivers

Equipment and supplies
- Supplies for standard precautions and proper sharps disposal

Safety requirements

- Standard precautions for infection control and sharps disposal
- System to assist compliance with complex medication regimen, including supervision
- Emergency plan and access to functional phone and list of emergency phone numbers
- Fire evacuation plan, functional smoke detectors, and access to functional fire extinguisher
- Identification and correction of environmental hazards and patient-specific concerns (for example, floors cleared of small objects and other fall hazards, and installation of bathroom grab rails)
- Patient identification bracelet or tag and wandering precautions
- Emergency contact person and crisis intervention phone numbers
- Supervised smoking
- Assistance with ambulation including devices
- Supervised care of ADLs

Major diagnostic codes

- Presenile dementia with delirum/delusional features/depressive features 290.11/290.12/290.13
- Arteriosclerotic dementia with delirium/delusional features/depressive features 290.41/290.42/290.43
- Senile dementia with delirium/delusional features/depressive features 290.3/290.20/290.21

Defense of homebound status

- Unable to leave home unattended and remain safe due to (specify)

- 24-hour supervision necessary for safety of self (wandering) and others
- Patient not oriented to time, place, or person
- Risk to self or others secondary to behavior
- Unable to ambulate without assistance of additional person, secondary to unsteady gait and confusion

Selected nursing diagnoses and patient outcomes

Knowledge deficit related to disease and management of care (specify: medications, ADLs, safety issues, or caregiver support)

The patient or caregiver will:
- state correct dose and time for each medication prescribed and demonstrate adherence to medication regimen   (N)
- verbalize adverse effects related to medications that require notification of physician   (N)
- verbalize understanding of necessity for laboratory tests (such as liver function studies and drug levels) ordered by the physician as evidenced by demonstrating compliance with the test schedule   (N)
- demonstrate and verbalize knowledge of patient's daily hygiene, skin care, nutritional, fluid, and elimination needs   (N)
- verbalize and demonstrate ability to recognize signs and symptoms of illness or infection that patient may be unable to communicate   (N)
- demonstrate and verbalize understanding of communication techniques (distraction and reorientation, for example) useful in dealing with an individual with dementia   (N, SW)

- verbalize knowledge of resources and assistance, such as local support groups and information resources, available to caregiver and patient   (N, SW)
- demonstrate and verbalize knowledge of and adherence to home safety practices.   (N, OT)

Altered thought processes related to underlying disease process

The patient or caregiver will:

- exhibit preservation of existing cognitive function, evidenced by patient's intellectual abilities stabilizing without additional noticeable decline   (N, SW, OT)
- demonstrate continued working toward optimal cognitive functioning within disease limitations (N, SW, OT)
- evidence ability to orient and assist patient with realistic thought processes as needed   (N, SW, OT)
- verbalize and demonstrate ability to maintain a supportive environment and avoid actions that will disturb the patient   (N, SW, OT)
- verbalize and demonstrate understanding of patient's optimal environment, how to enhance communication, and how to promote activity and task accomplishment.   (N, SW, OT)

Self-care deficit related to cognitive difficulties and memory impairments

The patient or caregiver will:

- demonstrate increased involvement in care and daily activities   (N, HCA, OT)
- communicate needs to others   (N, HCA, OT)
- cooperate in hygiene and mealtime activities   (N, HCA, OT)
- maintain self-care within disease limitations, with or without assistance or assistive devices, as indicated by patient's condition and as evidenced by appropriate personal hygiene and fluid and nutritional intake   (N, OT)
- participate in a home exercise program to increase strength and endurance   (N, HCA, PT, OT)
- demonstrate ability to assist appropriately in ADLs as needed or supervise self-care activities while encouraging patient's independence   (N, OT)
- demonstrate ability to keep patient adequately groomed, hydrated, and nourished.   (N, OT)

Risk for violence directed at others related to cognitive impairments and increased level of frustration

The patient or caregiver will:

- exhibit an absence of hostility in affect and conduct, evidenced by a lack of agitation, frustration, and combative behavior   (N, OT)
- institute measures to prevent violence based on identified causes of agitation and combative behavior   (N, OT)
- demonstrate understanding of patient's need to retain as much control over environment and activities as possible   (N, OT)
- demonstrate or verbalize ways to eliminate or minimize stimuli and situations that cause agitation or frustration to the patient.   (N, OT)

Risk for injury related to wandering and impaired judgment

The patient or caregiver will:

- identify hazards to patient in home   (N, OT)
- institute measures to maintain the patient's safety   (N, OT)

• obtain a patient identification tag or bracelet for notification in case of wandering.   (N, SW)

Skilled nursing services

Care measures
• Take a thorough medical and psychiatric history and list all medications patient is taking, along with pertinent potential adverse effects.
• Perform an initial skilled assessment of all body systems, family dynamics, and caregiver's ability and willingness to provide care.
• Explore memory deficits; orientation to time, place, and person; and general cognitive abilities.
• Assess medication therapy and evaluate for effectiveness and possible adverse effects.
• Assess patient's behavior, verbal and nonverbal.
• Investigate sleeping, eating, and elimination patterns.
• Institute wandering and home safety precautions.
• Assess patient's level of orientation and reorient to person, place, and time as necessary.
• Obtain or arrange for laboratory tests as ordered.

Patient and family teaching
• Teach about disease process, progression, and ongoing care.
• Review orientation-based stimulation, such as clocks, calendars, crossword puzzles, and clear verbal interactions.
• Describe approach to and treatment of patient during times of inappropriate or difficult behavior.

• Discuss stimuli and environmental stress reduction measures, such as reducing noise and excessive lighting.
• Emphasize need for adequate hydration, nutrition, and consistent daily routine.
• Identify home safety concerns and review fall precautions.
• Describe personal hygiene and preventive skin care.
• Review medications, including purposes, dosages, and possible adverse effects.
• Teach about medical regimen, including physician follow-up and laboratory testing.
• Discuss available resources and community support groups.

Interdisciplinary actions

Social worker
• Referrals to community resources and support groups
• Crisis intervention counseling
• Supportive counseling to assist family members in coping with needs of the patient with dementia
• Planning for future and options for long-term care, including possible need for long-term institutional placement

Occupational therapist
• Assessing rehabilitation needs and develop home activity plan
• Teaching therapeutic activities designed to increase cognitive abilities and functional participation in ADLs
• Developing plan to maximize home safety

Home care aide
(Infrequently reimbursed or covered only on a short-term basis)

- Assistance with personal care and hygiene
- Assistance with ADLs, including feeding and adequate nutrition intake
- Respite care for caregivers

Discharge plan

- Independent, safe management of patient with dementia in home with physician follow-up services and community support
- Safe management of the medication regimen at home
- Referral to community agencies for support
- Referral of patient to respite care as indicated
- Successful coping strategies for patient's special needs and daily care
- Referral to long-term care facility because of symptom severity and caregiver exhaustion

Documentation requirements

- Signs and symptoms of cognitive impairment
- Medication regimen, including effectiveness
- Patient and caregiver progress toward educational goals, such as use of wandering and home safety precautions and understanding of disease progression
- Patient progress or lack of progress in managing levels of agitation and ability to participate in self-care
- Patient response to interventions, including episodes of wandering or agitation
- Triggers or significant stressors associated with agitation and family dysfunctions that affect patient

- Caregiver's participation in patient care, including problems that suggest need for respite care
- Patient and caregiver instructions
- Signs and symptoms of disease progression
- Dangerous signs and symptoms
- Wandering and home safety precautions
- Measures to maintain and promote patient independence

Reimbursement reminders

- Medicare and most other third-party payers will only pay for a brief period of care when the patient is first diagnosed, although the needs of patients with dementia are ongoing and progressive.
- Home care aide services for the care of a patient with dementia may or may not be reimbursed. However, if reimbursed, these services are usually only permitted on a short-term basis.
- Thorough documentation of the teaching that the caregiver receives in how to care for the patient is essential.
- If assessment reveals that patient can't be safely cared for at home, these findings must be reported. Focus is then on discharge planning and helping family, caregiver, and patient make the transition to institutional care. If patient or family refuse institutional care, the home care nurse must document that home care can't adequately meet the patient's needs and conduct a discharge planning conference to set a discharge date.

Insurance hints

- Present objective data about homebound status, specifically patient's cognitive level. Also include any functional limitations that impact the patient's status such as other underlying disease conditions.

• Describe objective assessment findings and changes, emphasizing potential findings associated with behavior, agitation, and wandering.

• Relate specific findings about medication effects and changes; report actual laboratory results if indicated.

• Discuss specific details about patient education progress; include direct patient and caregiver statements related to understanding disease process, coping, therapy, and medications.

• Present objective assessment of patient's progress or lack of progress toward improved behavior, cognition, and self-care.

• Present objective assessment of caregiver's ability to care for patient and of caregiver's progress toward care goals including any safety issues that may impact the ability of the patient to remain at home.

Depression

Characterized by feelings of sadness, pessimism, and poor self-esteem, depression is the most common geriatric psychiatric disorder, and is the principal mental disorder that nurses will encounter in home care. Almost five million older Americans suffer from clinically significant depression. While it may or may not be the primary diagnosis in a patient receiving home care, it frequently occurs as a secondary condition that requires attention in the plan of care.

A disabling affective disorder, depression is typically demonstrated by a disturbed or despondent mood, flattened affect, and impaired social interaction. Depression may be caused by an event, such as sickness or the loss of a loved one. It may also have a genetic or biochemical cause, or be the result of a variety of family, environmental, or societal influences. Depression is more common in women than in men and is seen frequently in the homebound or chronically ill patient due to isolation, illness, and decreased social responsibilities. Depression should be considered life-threatening, because severely depressed elderly are more likely to commit suicide than individuals in any other age group. Medication regimens can be remarkably effective over time, but must be managed carefully, particularly in the elderly. Medication effectiveness must be monitored frequently until a stable therapeutic response is achieved. In addition, lifestyle changes and improved thinking patterns are often necessary to achieve long-term control of depression.

Home care nurses will strive to monitor medication effectiveness and achieve changes in thought patterns, behavioral responses, and daily routines, primarily through patient teaching. Caregivers and patients need to be taught about medications, positive coping skills, maintaining a safe environment, and achieving feelings of well-being.

Previsit checklist

Physician orders and preparation

• Medication therapy regimen, including antidepressants

- Laboratory studies, including blood drug levels
- Behavior and psychological therapy
- Physical therapy evaluation for home exercise program and endurance training and home safety evaluation
- Social worker evaluation for referral to community services, crisis intervention and counseling, and coping strategies
- Home care aide assistance with personal care and activities of daily living (ADLs)

Equipment and supplies
- Supplies for standard precautions and proper sharps disposal

Safety requirements
- Standard precautions for infection control and sharps disposal
- Phlebotomy equipment
- System to assist compliance with complex medication regimen, including supervision
- Emergency plan and access to functional phone and list of emergency phone numbers
- Fire evacuation plan, functional smoke detectors, and access to functional fire extinguisher
- Night-light
- Emergency contact person and crisis intervention phone numbers

Major diagnostic codes
- Arteriosclerotic dementia with depressive features 290.43
- Atypical depressive disorder 296.82
- Depression, postpartum 648.4
- Depressive disorder 311
- Depressive type psychosis 298.0

- Major depressive disorder, single episode/recurrent 296.2/296.3
- Neurotic depression 300.4
- Organic affective syndrome 293.83
- Senile dementia with depressive features 290.21

Defense of homebound status
- Inability to leave home because of extreme lethargy resulting from depressive disorder
- Constant supervision required because of potential to harm self

Selected nursing diagnoses and patient outcomes

Knowledge deficit related to management of depressive disorder (specify: medications, coping skills, safety issues, or suicide precautions)

The patient or caregiver will:
- state correct dose and time for each medication prescribed and adverse effects and precautions for each; as well as demonstrate adherence to medication regimen (N)
- identify signs and symptoms of adverse effects related to medications that require notification of physician (N)
- demonstrate and verbalize knowledge of depressive illness and measures to decrease depression (N, SW)
- verbalize knowledge of resources and assistance, such as counseling, local support groups, spiritual or pastoral support, and crisis intervention hotlines, that are available to patient and caregivers (N, SW)

• demonstrate and verbalize knowledge of and compliance with keeping psychotherapeutic appointments
(N, SW)
• demonstrate or verbalize knowledge of and adherence to home safety practices and suicide precautions.
(N, OT, SW)

Ineffective individual coping related to feelings of sadness, pessimism, and poor self-esteem
The patient or caregiver will:
• demonstrate or verbalize lifestyle changes that relieve depression
(N, SW, OT)
• demonstrate or verbalize understanding of relationship between depressive feelings and causative events or sensations
(N, SW)
• identify reasons for depressive feelings
(N, SW)
• participate in treatment programs.
(N, OT ,SW)

Self-esteem disturbance related to depressive symptoms and underlying factors responsible for depression
The patient or caregiver will:
• demonstrate brighter mood and affect
(N, SW, OT)
• verbalize feelings and accept reassurances of others
(N, SW, OT)
• communicate needs to others
(N, SW)
• show improved appearance and interest in self-care
(N, SW, OT)
• participate in home exercise program to enhance participation in activities.
(N, OT)

Impaired social interaction related to feelings of isolation and illness
The patient or caregiver will:

• demonstrate ability to leave home with or without caregiver (N, SW, OT)
• show improved eye contact and behavior around others
(N, SW)
• demonstrate adequate socialization by increased or improved communication with the family and caregivers
(N, SW)
• express appropriate interests in activities, in personal appearance, and in others.
(N, SW, OT)

Hopelessness related to social isolation, despondency, and illness
The patient or caregiver will:
• demonstrate decreased negative verbalization
(N, SW)
• verbalize at least one positive thought each day
(N, SW)
• contract to refrain from harming self
(N, SW)
• discuss feelings of anger, frustration, and fear openly
(N, SW)
• demonstrate use of positive coping skills.
(N, SW, OT)

Skilled nursing services

Care measures
• Take a thorough medical and psychiatric history; list all medications patient is taking, along with pertinent potential adverse effects.
• Perform an initial skilled assessment of all body systems; assess family and environmental factors indicative of isolation, stress, or limited social contact.
• Assess nonverbal and verbal indications of depression, including poor eye contact, flat affect, slow or monotone speech, and slumped posture.
• Evaluate defense mechanisms, self-preoccupation, and feelings of loneli-

ness, rejection, hostility, and poor self-esteem.

- Assess patient's knowledge and understanding of depression, medications, and resources.
- Perform skilled assessment of psychosomatic symptoms, such as problems with sleeping, eating, or elimination.
- Institute suicide precautions and perform skilled assessment.
- Monitor medication compliance and effectiveness of suicide potential at each visit.
- Obtain or arrange for laboratory studies as ordered.

Patient and family teaching

- Teach medication management and compliance.
- Describe measures to identify and manage depressive feelings and triggering stresses.
- Teach coping and relationship skills.
- Emphasize need to verbalize and listen to feelings in constructive ways.
- Review signs and symptoms of depression.
- Identify home safety concerns and issues; discuss suicide precautions.
- Emphasize importance of therapy, medical follow-up, and compliance, including serological testing for medication levels.
- Identify available resources.

Interdisciplinary actions

Social worker

- Referral to community resources and support groups
- Counseling and crisis intervention
- Brief counseling (two or three visits) to assist family members in coping

with needs of the depressed patient or to resolve impediments to patient's recovery

- Assistance with finances to aid in medication compliance
- Education regarding the disease, management of it, and suicide precautions

Occupational therapist

- Assessment of rehabilitation needs and development of home activity plan
- Instruction in therapeutic activities designed to increase cognitive abilities and functional participation in ADLs
- Development of plan to maximize home safety

Discharge plan

- Safe, independent management of the patient with depression in home with physician and community follow-up services
- Patient and caregiver management of medication regimen at home
- Compliance with medication and treatment therapy
- Referral to community resources for assistance and support
- Referral for continued psychotherapy as indicated on outpatient basis
- Demonstration of appropriate behaviors with control of depressive symptoms

Documentation requirements

- Signs and symptoms of depression
- Effects of medication regimen, including signs and symptoms of adverse effects and toxicity
- Patient and caregiver progress toward educational goals, such as un-

derstanding of the need for medication, suicide precautions, and effects of depressive symptoms
• Patient progress or lack of progress in affect, behavior, social interaction, feelings, and ability to provide self-care
• Patient response to interventions, including psychiatric therapy
• Triggers or significant stressors associated with depression and family dysfunctions that affect patient
• Patient's statements about subjective feelings
• Patient and caregiver participation in care, including evidence of increasing participation in all activities and observations of improved grooming and hygiene
• Assessment of patient's suicide potential, including actions taken and their outcomes
• Patient and caregiver instructions
• Suicide and home safety precautions
• Coping strategies and measures to control crisis
• Dangerous signs and symptoms

Reimbursement reminders

• The patient must have an Axis I Diagnosis for the *DSM-IV,* which must match the diagnosis that the ordering physician is treating or for which the patient was hospitalized; the diagnosis must be fully documented in the record.
• Home care orders for psychiatric nursing don't require the signature of the patient's psychiatrist; the attending or primary care physician's signature is acceptable.
• Home care nurses caring for patients with a psychiatric condition must be qualified by experience, education, or certification to provide specialized psychiatric nursing; evidence of the nurse's qualifications should be maintained in the nurse's personnel file for examination as needed by regulatory bodies and third-party payers. Some Medicare intermediaries insist on reviewing and approving a nurse's credentials for providing psychiatric evaluation and therapy in home care before the nurse can render psychiatric services.
• The patient may need separate services by both a psychiatric nurse and a social worker, so be careful to avoid duplication of services in areas such as patient counseling.
• Record destructive thought patterns expressed by the patient and the patient's response to psychiatric nursing interventions.
• Document specific knowledge deficits that show evidence of progress as seen in medication management, self-care, affect, social interaction, and verbalized concepts.

Insurance hints

• Establish reasonable goals that can realistically be achieved; decreasing or shortening inpatient care may be an achievable and reimbursable goal.
• Present objective data about homebound status specifically addressing the effect of the patient's depression, including complaints of lethargy or fatigue or inability to go outside the home.
• Describe objective assessment findings and changes, actions taken, and patient outcomes; emphasize potential findings associated with suicide ideation.
• Relate specific findings about medication effects and changes; report actual laboratory results of blood drug levels.

• Discuss specific details about patient education progress; include direct patient and caregiver statements related to understanding disease process, coping, therapy, and medications.

• Present objective assessment of patient's progress or lack of progress toward improved affect, self-care, and stated feelings.

Paranoid disorder

Paranoia or paranoid thinking can be a prominent feature in dementia, personality disorders, affective disorders, schizophrenia, and manic-depressive psychoses. It's a syndrome in which a person thinks that other people are plotting against, harassing, or somehow trying to harm him. The patient commonly suffers from the systematic delusion that everything that happens is about the patient, or is self-referent. The most trivial incidents will be interpreted irrationally by the patient, such as seeing the home care nurse talking privately to a family member and assuming that the nurse and family member are criticizing or plotting against the patient.

Paranoia varies in the degree of its severity, ranging from abnormal suspicion in an otherwise normal and functional individual to an unshakable highly elaborate delusional system involving massive conspiracies directed against the patient. Paranoid disorders can cause serious problems in a patient's relationships with others; in other respects, the individual may have normal or near-normal intellectual function and personality. Severe paranoia is believed by some experts to be a variety of schizophrenia. Delusions of persecution and delusions of grandeur are two of the more common manifestations of paranoid syndromes. The patient is usually completely convinced of the truth of these delusional convictions, as indicated by an eagerness to accept anything, no matter how flimsy the evidence, to support the belief, and a total unwillingness to hear anything that contradicts it.

Paranoid disorders are normally treated with antipsychotic drugs on a long-term basis. The home care nurse is responsible for monitoring the medications and their effectiveness, teaching the patient and caregiver about the medications and adverse effects, and helping the patient and caregiver with reality orientation and relationship issues.

Previsit checklist

Physician orders and preparation

• Medication therapy, including antipsychotics

• Laboratory testing, such as blood levels for drug monitoring

• Psychiatric therapy and treatment program

• Suicide precautions

• Social worker evaluation for crisis intervention, community referrals, and assistance with measures to ensure compliance

Equipment and supplies

• Supplies for standard precautions and proper sharps disposal

Safety requirements

• Standard precautions for infection control and sharps disposal

- Emergency plan and access to functional phone and list of emergency phone numbers
- Fire evacuation plan, functional smoke detectors, and access to functional fire extinguisher
- Night-light
- System to assist compliance with complex medication regimen, including supervision
- Suicide precautions
- Emergency contact person and crisis intervention phone numbers
- Phlebotomy equipment

Major diagnostic codes

- Chronic paranoid psychosis 297.1
- Organic delusional syndrome 293.8
- Other specific paranoid states 297.8
- Paranoia 297.1
- Paranoid state induced by drugs/simple 292.11/297.0
- Paraphrenia 297.2
- Shared paranoid disorder 297.3
- Unspecified paranoid state 297.9

Defense of homebound status

- Refusal to leave home due to paranoid delusions
- Severe paranoia that causes fear of contact with others
- Unsafe in public due to extreme paranoia with hostile behavior
- Inability to leave home because of fearful behavior resulting from paranoid disorder
- Behavior that poses risk to self or others
- Supervision necessary due to impaired judgment

Selected nursing diagnoses and patient outcomes

Knowledge deficit related to management of paranoid disorder (specify: medications, coping skills, safety, or suicide precautions)

The patient or caregiver will:

- state correct dose and time for each medication prescribed and demonstrate adherence to medication regimen (N)
- verbalize signs and symptoms of adverse effects related to medications that require notification of physician (N)
- demonstrate or verbalize knowledge of paranoid disorder (N, SW)
- verbalize knowledge of resources and assistance, such as counseling, local support groups, spiritual or pastoral support, and crisis intervention hotlines, that are available to the patient and caregivers (N, SW)
- demonstrate or verbalize knowledge of and compliance with keeping psychotherapeutic appointments (N, SW)
- demonstrate or verbalize knowledge of and adherence to home safety practices and suicide precautions. (N, SW)

Altered thought processes related to paranoid thinking and delusions

The patient or caregiver will:

- exhibit decreased symptoms of paranoid thinking and delusions (N, SW)
- demonstrate continued working toward optimal reality orientation within disease limitations (N, SW)
- evidence ability to orient and assist patient with realistic thought processes as needed (N, SW)

• verbalize or demonstrate ability to maintain a supportive environment and avoid actions that will disturb the patient (N, SW)

• verbalize or demonstrate understanding of patient's optimal environment, how to enhance communication, and how to promote appropriate interpretations of events. (N, SW)

Risk for violence directed at self or others related to delusions and suspicions
The patient or caregiver will:

• exhibit an absence of hostility in affect and conduct, evidenced by a lack of agitation, frustration, and combative behavior (N, SW)

• participate in treatment programs (N, SW)

• demonstrate understanding and acceptance of need for supervision (N, SW)

• institute measures to prevent violence based on identified causes of agitation and combative behavior (N, SW)

• demonstrate ability to provide a calm, reassuring, supportive, supervised environment (N, SW)

• verbalize signs and symptoms of suicidal or hostile intentions. (N, SW)

Impaired social interaction related to delusions of persecution and grandeur
The patient or caregiver will:

• demonstrate ability to leave home with or without caregiver (N, SW)

• demonstrate adequate socialization by increased or improved communication with family and caregivers (N, SW)

• express appropriate responses to personal interactions with others (N, SW)

• exhibit an absence of hostility in affect and conduct. (N, SW)

Skilled nursing services

Care measures

• Take a thorough medical and psychiatric history; list all medications patient is taking, along with pertinent potential adverse effects.

• Perform an initial skilled assessment of all body systems; assess family and environmental factors affecting patient.

• Assess patient's self-referent thinking and other symptoms of paranoia, including threats to personal safety and others.

• Assess nonverbal and verbal indications of paranoid thinking.

• Evaluate patient's knowledge and understanding of paranoid disorder, medications, and resources.

• Assess interactions with significant others and coping skills.

• Perform a skilled assessment of suicide potential.

• Institute suicide precautions and safety measures.

• Assess level of orientation and reorient to reality as necessary; define acceptable behaviors.

• Obtain or arrange for laboratory studies as indicated.

Patient and family teaching

• Teach medication management and adherence with medical regimen.

• Review dangerous signs and symptoms, including those of antipsychotic medications and signs indicating danger to self or others.

• Identify home safety concerns and issues; discuss suicide precautions.

• Emphasize importance of therapy, medical follow-up, and compliance.

• Review symptoms that should be reported to physician.

- Discuss methods for coping with paranoid behavior and orienting patient to reality.

Interdisciplinary actions

Social worker
- Referral to community resources and support groups
- Counseling and crisis intervention
- Brief counseling (two or three visits) to assist family members in coping with needs of the patient with paranoia or to resolve impediments to patient's recovery
- Assistance with finances to aid in medication adherence with regimen
- Education regarding disease, management, and suicide precautions

Discharge plan
- Independent, safe management of patient with paranoid disorder in the home with physician and community follow-up services
- Adherence to medication and treatment therapy
- Referral to community resources for assistance and support
- Referral for continued psychotherapy as indicated on outpatient basis
- Demonstration of appropriate behaviors with control of paranoia

Documentation requirements
- Signs and symptoms of paranoia and delusions
- Effects of medication regimen
- Patient and caregiver progress toward educational goals, such as understanding of need for medication,

suicide precautions, and effects of antipsychotic medications
- Patient progress or lack of progress in reality orientation, social interaction, feelings, and delusional convictions
- Patient response to interventions, including crisis intervention, psychiatric therapy, and antipsychotic medications
- Triggers or significant stressors associated with paranoid thoughts and family dysfunctions that affect patient
- Patient's statements about feelings
- Patient and caregiver participation in care
- Assessment of the patient's suicide potential
- Laboratory test results, including blood drug levels with report to physician
- Patient and caregiver instructions
- Medication therapy, including signs and symptoms of adverse effects and toxicity
- Suicide and home safety precautions
- Coping strategies and measures to control crisis
- Dangerous signs and symptoms

Reimbursement reminders
- The patient must have an Axis I Diagnosis (clinical disorder) for the *DSM-IV*, which must match the diagnosis that the ordering physician is treating or for which the patient was hospitalized; the diagnosis must be fully documented in the record.
- Home care orders for psychiatric nursing don't require the signature of the patient's psychiatrist; any physician's signature is acceptable.
- Home care nurses caring for patients with a psychiatric condition must be

qualified by experience, education, or certification to provide specialized psychiatric nursing; evidence of the nurse's qualifications should be maintained in the nurse's personnel files for examination as needed by regulatory bodies and third-party payers. Some Medicare intermediaries must review and approve a nurse's credentials for providing psychiatric evaluation and therapy in home care before the nurse can render psychiatric services.

● Document psychiatric nursing interventions into destructive thought patterns expressed by patient and the patient's responses, including documentation reflecting communication with the physician.

● The patient may need separate services by both a psychiatric nurse and a social worker, so be careful to avoid duplication of services in areas such as patient counseling.

● Specific knowledge deficits and evidence of progress as seen in medication management, self-care, affect, social interaction, reality orientation, and absence of delusions are crucial for reimbursement of care.

Insurance hints

● Establish reasonable goals that can be realistically achieved; decreasing or shortening inpatient care may be an achievable and reimbursable goal.

● Present objective data about homebound status, specifically addressing the effect of the patient's behavior, including delusions, and risks to self and others on ability to go outside the home.

● Describe objective assessment findings and changes, emphasizing potential findings associated with suicide.

● Relate specific findings about medication effects and changes; report actual laboratory results of blood drug levels ideation and evidence of adverse effects of antipsychotic medications.

● Discuss specific details about patient education progress; include direct patient and caregiver statements related to understanding disease process, coping, therapy, and medications.

● Present objective assessment of patient's progress or lack of progress toward improved reality orientation, relationship skills, and presence or absence of delusional convictions.

Substance abuse

Overuse or abuse of such substances as alcohol, tobacco, and other drugs will eventually affect every part of the body and every aspect of the patient's life. Substance abuse is an expensive disorder, and pervasive in American society. Much of the health care bill in the United States is for tobacco-, alcohol-, and other drug-related expenses. Substance abuse is linked to homicides, suicides, accidents, and many diseases of all ages.

Addiction to alcohol and other drugs is no longer considered by experts to be a moral or character problem, but a chronic, and possibly inherited, illness that causes complicated and possibly irreversible changes in the brain. While using or abusing drugs is a behavior that an individual can choose to control, actual addiction is a disease of the brain that requires aggressive treatment and major lifestyle changes. Using alcohol, tobacco, or other drugs in this addicted state is a compulsive behavior that the abuser may feel powerless to change. Often, only through intense education can most patients learn to change. Home care focuses on helping the patient's family and friends learn not to blame the patient for having a substance abuse disorder. Through education in lifestyle changes, the home care nurse will help the patient stay with a plan of treatment that will achieve long-term success.

Previsit checklist

Physician orders and preparation
- Medications
- Substance abuse therapy
- Suicide precautions
- Social worker evaluation for crisis intervention, community referrals, and assistance with measures to ensure compliance
- Laboratory studies as indicated

Equipment and supplies
- Supplies for standard precautions and proper sharps disposal

Safety requirements
- Standard precautions for infection control and sharps disposal
- System to assist compliance with complex medication regimen, including supervision
- Emergency plan and access to functional phone and list of emergency phone numbers
- Fire evacuation plan, functional smoke detectors, and access to functional fire extinguisher
- Night-light
- Suicide precautions
- Emergency contact person and crisis intervention phone numbers
- Phlebotomy equipment

Major diagnostic codes
- Alcohol withdrawal delirium 291.0
- Drug-induced hallucinosis 292.12
- Drug-induced organic delusional syndrome 292.11
- Drug withdrawal syndrome 292.0
- Other specified drug-induced mental disorders 292.8
- Pathological drug intoxication 292.2
- Unspecific drug-induced mental disorder 292.9

Defense of homebound status
- Unsafe for patient to leave home unsupervised due to addictive use of (specify substance)
- Inappropriate behavior that renders patient unsafe outside the home due to substance abuse
- 24-hour supervision necessary due to drug- or alcohol- induced psychosis
- Acutely ill and unable to leave home due to alcohol or drug withdrawal
- Unsteady, requiring assistance to ambulate due to alcohol- or drug-related illness
- Paranoid or hallucinatory condition induced by substance abuse interfering with patient's safety outside the home
- Behavior risk to self or others
- Impaired judgment making patient unsafe without supervision

Selected nursing diagnoses and patient outcomes

Knowledge deficit related to management of substance abuse (specify: medications, lifestyle changes, safety, or effects of substance abuse)

The patient or caregiver will:

- state correct dose and time for each medication prescribed as well as adverse effects and precautions for each and demonstrate adherence to medication regimen   (N)
- identify adverse effects related to medications that require reporting to physician   (N)
- demonstrate or verbalize knowledge of substance abuse and its effects on the body and mind   (N, SW)
- verbalize knowledge of resources and assistance, such as counseling, local support groups, spiritual or pastoral support, and crisis intervention hotlines, that are available to the patient and caregiver   (N, SW)
- demonstrate or verbalize knowledge of and compliance with keeping psychotherapeutic appointments (N, SW)
- demonstrate or verbalize knowledge of and adherence to home safety practices   (N, SW)
- demonstrate or verbalize knowledge of necessary lifestyle changes. (N, SW)

Ineffective individual coping related to dependence and abuse of substance

The patient or caregiver will:

- demonstrate or verbalize lifestyle changes necessary for dealing with substance abuse such as attending a support group   (N, SW)
- demonstrate or verbalize understanding of relationship between substance abuse and its effects on patient's current situation   (N, SW)
- participate in treatment programs.   (N, SW)

Altered thought process related to effects of substance abuse on body systems

The patient or caregiver will:

- demonstrate or verbalize adequate thought processes, evidenced by orientation to reality and to environment   (N)
- demonstrate or verbalize appropriate thought processes as evidenced by awareness that alcohol or drugs have caused alteration in thought.   (N)

Skilled nursing services

Care measures

- Perform an initial skilled assessment of all body systems, family dynamics, and support systems.
- Assess evidence of memory deficits and other cognitive impairment resulting from substance abuse.
- Evaluate patterns of daily living and patient's willingness or ability to change destructive patterns in current lifestyle.
- Assess patient's knowledge and understanding of disease, medications, and resources.
- Evaluate psychosomatic symptoms, such as problems with sleeping, eating, or elimination.
- Assess interactions with significant others and coping skills.
- Perform a skilled assessment of suicide potential.
- Institute suicide precautions.

Patient and family teaching

- Identify feelings and events or stressors that trigger substance use.
- Review coping skills and alternative ways of coping.
- Discuss verbalization of feelings.
- Describe addictive behavior.
- Emphasize need for social contact and involvement with others.
- Explain medication management and compliance.

- Review relationship skills.
- Discuss home safety concerns and issues.
- Emphasize importance of therapy, medical follow-up, and compliance.
- Discuss community resources.

Interdisciplinary actions

Social worker
- Referral to community resources and support groups
- Counseling and crisis intervention
- Referral to substance abuse group such as Alcoholics Anonymous
- Brief counseling (two or three visits) to assist family members in coping with needs of the substance abuser or to resolve impediments to patient's recovery
- Education regarding disease cycles, management, and suicide precautions

Discharge plan
- Independent, safe management of patient with substance abuse disorder in the home, with physician and community follow-up services
- Compliance with medication and treatment therapy
- Referral to community resources for assistance and support
- Referral for continued psychotherapy as indicated on outpatient basis
- Demonstration of appropriate behaviors with control of substance abuse
- Initiation and continuation of participation in community substance abuse–related program

Documentation requirements
- Signs and symptoms of substance abuse or withdrawal from substance
- Medication therapy if ordered and effects of medication regimen
- Patient and caregiver progress toward educational goals, such as understanding of need for treatment program, suicide precautions, effects of substance abuse on self and others
- Patient progress or lack of progress in abuse of substances, affect, social interaction, feelings, and ability to provide self-care
- Patient response to interventions, including abstinence from substance use
- Triggers or significant stressors associated with substance abuse and family dysfunctions affecting the patient
- Patient's statements about subjective feelings
- Patient and caregiver participation in care
- Assessment of patient's suicide potential
- Laboratory test results
- Patient and caregiver instructions
- Suicide and home safety precautions
- Coping strategies and measures to control crisis
- Dangerous signs and symptoms

Reimbursement reminders
- The patient must have an Axis I Diagnosis (clinical disorder) for the *DSM-IV*, which must match the diagnosis that the ordering physician is treating or for which the patient was hospitalized; the diagnosis must be fully documented in the record.

● Home care orders for psychiatric nursing don't require the signature of the patient's psychiatrist; any physician's signature is acceptable.

● Home care nurses caring for patients with a psychiatric condition must be qualified by experience, education, or certification to provide specialized psychiatric nursing; evidence of the nurse's qualifications should be maintained in the nurse's personnel files for examination as needed by regulatory bodies and third-party payers. Some Medicare intermediaries must review and approve a nurse's credentials for providing psychiatric evaluation and therapy in home care before the nurse can render psychiatric services.

● The patient may need separate services by both a psychiatric nurse and a social worker, so be careful to avoid duplication of services in areas such as patient counseling.

● Home care aide services for the care of a patient with a psychiatric disorder may not be covered. Several state-specific reimbursement programs for home care aide services may be available; however, these programs vary greatly. It's always best to check with the agency and insurance company.

● Record psychiatric nursing interventions into destructive thought patterns expressed by the patient, and the patient's response, as evidence to substantiate the need for home care.

● Document specific knowledge deficits and evidence of progress as seen by management of substance abuse and medication or therapy regimen.

Insurance hints

● Establish reasonable goals that can be realistically achieved; decreasing or shortening inpatient care may be an achievable and reimbursable goal.

● Present objective data about homebound status specifically addressing the effect of the patient's substance abuse on ability to go outside the home and be safe.

● Describe objective assessment findings and changes, emphasizing potential findings associated with suicide ideation and evidence of withdrawal.

● Discuss specific details about patient education progress; include direct patient and caregiver statements related to understanding disease process, coping, therapy, and treatment programs.

● Present objective assessment of patient's progress or lack of progress toward control of addictive behavior and substance abuse; report episodes of substance abuse or recurrent substance abuse behavior after initiation of therapy.

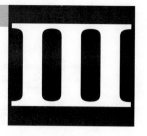

PART

III

Clinical
pathways
in
home care

Using clinical pathways in home care

Clinical pathways are widely used as a documentation tool in home care, long-term care, and acute care settings. Pathways emerged in health care in the 1980s, a time when hospitals had to initiate a system that linked reimbursement with diagnosis-related groups. Hospitals implemented clinical pathways for high-volume diagnoses or high-acuity admissions, finding that the pathways helped reduce the patient's length of stay, decrease costs, and improve outcomes of care. In the early 1990s, other areas of health care, including hospices and home health care agencies, also began using clinical pathways.

Definition

Also known as critical paths, care maps, or care guidelines, clinical pathways are one of the major tools used to manage patient outcomes. They have been described as road maps that outline the entire course of care that should be provided to the patient. As such, they remind the user (nurses as well as other members of the health care team) to address certain issues during treatment and work toward meeting established goals.

Clinical pathways can be developed for a specific diagnosis (such as heart failure) or a surgical procedure (such as coronary artery bypass grafting). They help make a complicated case much easier to manage because they lay out the assessment, care plan, and evaluation of the patient's progress. As an added benefit, they provide patients with a clear plan about the care they will receive and the time frame in which their outcomes will be achieved.

Primary benefits of pathways

Each completed pathway tells a story about the patient's progress toward meeting established goals. For various reasons, a specified expected outcome may not be achieved. This is called a *variance*. By analyzing the data on the variances that occur, a clearer picture of the services provided in relation to the patient outcomes can be obtained. This helps identify trends that need to be studied. For example, is there something that an agency can do to improve patient outcomes? Is there something the nurse or therapist can do? Clinical pathways can provide data to justify procedural changes or expenditures.

Case management and coordination

The case manager in home care is usually the nurse. Clinical pathways allow the case manager to have a simple tool to organize the daunting tasks required. They serve as both a plan of care and a documentation system coordinated by a single professional (usually the case manager). This person is responsible for:

• ensuring that nothing is missed in the treatment or education of the patient and the family

• coordinating care so that planned events occur as expected without gaps or overlaps in services.

Time management

With the sheer volume of documentation required on admission, due in part to the Outcome Assessment Information Set (OASIS) B form and the documentation necessary to ensure compliance with state, federal, and other agencies, it's crucial to have a tool to help organize data for improved time management. The home health care provider has a lot to accomplish in a limited amount of time. The clinical pathway simplifies this process. The home care nurse need only complete the appropriate pathway related to the patient's primary diagnosis, and much of the work is already done. This greatly reduces the amount of time the nurse previously used in documenting visit patterns, expected outcomes, guidelines for patient teaching, and treatment. This one tool can accomplish all

of that and needs only to be personalized for the individual patient by the nurse.

Standardization of care

Clinical pathways can also decrease variations in treatment. They define specific visit patterns and outcomes to be achieved on each visit. Because the pathways are the same for all patients, the nurse can be sure that everyone is receiving the same high standard of care on each visit. Many cues help the nurse complete the specific goals for each visit. Any deviation from these goals is documented as a variance. The goals or outcomes are then moved to the next visit for completion.

The nurse becomes familiar with the outcomes for each visit because they're standardized. Also, another nurse that is required to visit the patient when the primary nurse or case manager isn't available for visits can pick up exactly where the case manager left off.

Quality care

Everyone wins when the patient receives high-quality care. Increased patient satisfaction can improve future business volume by referrals and possible future admissions of the patient, who will be more likely to choose the same agency for care. Pathways also assist in coordinating services and measuring outcomes, allowing the home health care team to evaluate the care the patient receives. The home health care provider can tell at a glance if the patient has received the expected treatments and reached the desired outcomes. This makes the job of both the performance improvement team and surveyors much easier.

Skilled services provided on each visit are clearly indicated. The chart tells the story of the patient's progress toward meeting goals and the reasons why certain outcomes were not met.

Often, when a standardized plan like the pathway isn't used, it's much more difficult to extract the necessary data from a chart. With clinical pathways, each visit is organized with specific steps and procedures to be followed, making it easy for anyone to identify what occurred on any given visit.

When pathways are initiated, members of the health care team and the patient, family, or legal guardian review them. In this way, a patient still participates in the planning of his care. He is aware of the outcomes that are expected to occur as a result of the interventions of the home health care team, and he has a clear view of when outcomes will be achieved.

Clinical pathways are kept in the patient's chart and are initialed and dated by home health care team members as treatments are provided. In home care, this is done on a per-visit basis. Deviations from the pathway are recorded as variances. Codes are assigned to these variances and the data is aggregated. This aggregate pathway data is then used by the quality improvement team to evaluate and identify potential opportunities for improvement. This evaluation also allows the team to determine if a patient is meeting the expected outcomes. When these variances are tracked, it helps the team to determine if there is a need to improve or modify patient services or care in some way. As a result, clinical pathways are continuously being evaluated. As new information becomes available, the quality improvement team can change the pathways to better meet the needs of their patients.

Other benefits

Clinical pathways also serve other purposes. When the Joint Commission on Accreditation of Healthcare Organizations set standards requiring coordination of care, agencies needed a system to evaluate multidisciplinary care. With clinical pathways, disciplines work together to achieve better patient outcomes and costs are reduced.

When the health care team works together to follow the pathway, care is provided in a logical sequence that progresses toward desired outcomes at regular intervals. Use of pathways also enhances patient satisfaction. This may be due to the patient's increased knowledge of what to expect from home care.

Finally, clinical pathways aid in cost containment because they:
- streamline documentation, thereby increasing staff efficiency
- decrease fragmented care
- limit delays in delivery of care
- reduce hospital re-admissions.

Developing specific clinical pathways

Each home health care agency must review its patient population and determine which procedures and disorders would benefit from the use of clinical pathways. The most common factor is high-volume or high-cost services. For example, agencies specializing in infusion therapy might choose pathways on I.V. hydration, and those with a rehabilitation facility would probably have pathways for postoperative joint replacement.

Who develops clinical pathways?

Usually, a multidisciplinary team from the home health agency works to develop each pathway. This team should include all representatives of the health care team. The pathway should include:

• clinical practice guidelines on which the pathway is based

• ancillary and support activities that make the practice guideline a reality

• intermediate and end-state outcomes that the patient is to achieve.

Guidelines for development

When developing a clinical pathway, the team should:

• obtain internal leadership input

• involve all participants

• discuss supplier costs and quality outcomes

• question the status quo

• develop a consensus for change

• consider all opportunities

• identify information sources

• identify high-cost or high-volume procedures

• gather specific information about the procedures

• compare the data to identify the best practices

• standardize supplies and procedures

• define expected patient outcomes

• implement the pathway

• monitor variances and measure outcomes

• evaluate the pathway using variance reports.

Evaluating clinical pathways

It's important for a home health care agency to evaluate the pathways it's currently using. The most common way to do this is through variance reports.

Any failure to meet an expected outcome for a visit is documented on the variance report. The cause may be attributed to the patient, the provider, or the system:

• A *patient variance* is any factor associated with the patient that prevented the outcome from occurring (such as inability to ambulate because of dizziness).

• A *provider variance* is any deviation from the plan of care because of the home care provider. For example, if she didn't show up for the visit or forgot to bring essential equipment.

• A *system variance* is attributed to the home health care agency or to external influences (for example, a home care provider missing a visit because of a scheduling problem or denial of care by a third-party payer).

Some agencies have very detailed variance reports broken down into categories that are much more specific than those stated here. The variances should be specific to the outcomes that are expected. When variances from an outcome occur, the pathway should be reviewed to determine whether there is a need to change it.

The quality improvement team will look for trends or patterns of variation, and specific revisions may be made to the pathway to improve patient outcomes. Continuous evaluation is vitally important to ensure that the tools chosen to refine documentation remain up-to-date with current regulations and care guidelines and enhance the care the patient receives.

The sample clinical pathways that follow reflect the beginning of an evolutionary process. As data are compiled and research is analyzed, some of the specifics listed here will undoubtedly change.

Acute myelogenous leukemia

PLAN OF CARE	HOME CARE Visit 1
Diagnostic tests	• Complete blood count • Electrolyte levels • Blood chemistries
Medications	• Administer chemotherapeutic agents as ordered. • Evaluate the effects and adverse effects of prescription and over-the-counter medications.
Procedures	• Perform an in-depth physical assessment as a baseline. • Evaluate vascular access device (VAD) site and patient compliance with home maintenance of VAD. • Check vital signs (VS).
Diet	• Encourage diet as tolerated to maintain enough calories for metabolic needs.
Activity	• Evaluate the level of fatigue and impact on activity.
Elimination	• Evaluate for constipation or diarrhea as adverse effects of chemotherapy.
Hygiene	• Inspect oral and perineal areas to determine the patient's ability to maintain hygiene.
Patient teaching	• Discuss medication and VAD care as needed. • Reinforce the schedule of follow-up visits and therapy. • Teach home chemotherapy precautions and home safety needs.
Discharge planning	Social services: • Perform a comprehensive needs assessment related to financial, occupational, social, psychological, and spiritual needs.

Visit 2	Visit 3
• Same as previous visit	• Same as previous visit
• Repeat care given at previous visit.	• Repeat care given at previous visit.
• Evaluate for signs and symptoms of infection, neutropenia, anemia, and thrombocytopenia. • Assess VAD site and site care. • Check VS. • Weigh patient and compare to baseline.	• Repeat care given at previous visit.
• Determine amount and calories consumed in 24-hour diet recall. • Adjust plan of care based on findings.	• Encourage a diet high in protein, vitamins, minerals, and fluids.
• Encourage progressive activity.	• Repeat care given at previous visit.
• Repeat care given at previous visit.	• Repeat care given at previous visit.
• Inspect oral and perineal areas to determine the patient's ability to maintain hygiene. • Consider contacting home care aide services.	• Repeat care given at previous visit.
• Discuss psychosocial concerns (for example, fear of recurrence, changes in family roles, survivorship issues, reproductive concerns, and sexuality issues) with the patient and family.	• Repeat care given at previous visit.
Social services: • Refer to vocational counseling. • Refer to occupational therapy. • Refer to psychological counseling. • Refer to community support agencies and groups.	Social services: • Repeat care given at previous visit.

Alzheimer's type dementia

PLAN OF CARE	HOME CARE Visit 1
Diagnostic tests	• Any indicated
Medications	• Give tacrine (Cognex). • Give antipsychotic (low dose). • Assess for effectiveness and adverse effects of medications. • Assess for proper administration (when administered, with or without food, and so forth).
Procedures	• Check vital signs. • Assess home for safety factors. • Assess mental status. • Assess structure in environment. • Assess effect of reality orientation. • Assess effect of reminiscence therapy.
Diet	• Assess nutritional status, especially intake. • Assess for chewing or swallowing problems.
Activity	• Assess for sleep activity. • Monitor living area for safety. • Establish exercise program (consult with physician or physical therapist).
Elimination	• Assess skin integrity. • Assess bowel movement pattern.
Hygiene	• Assess for problems related to urinary incontinence. • Assess hygiene.
Patient teaching	• Teach the caregiver to recognize signs and symptoms of the progressive stages of dementia and to prioritize care. • Teach the caregiver how to manage emotions (recognize feelings and deal with them through support groups or a counselor). • Teach caregiver to build a collaborative partnership with health care provider to help deal with the personal, social, and financial problems the caregiver will encounter.
Discharge planning	• Reinforce the benefits of support groups for the patient and caregiver. • Help make contacts with community support services. • Plan a family meeting to obtain help from patient's other family members, if feasible. • Facilitate identification of needs, and plan a schedule for intervention from family members.

Visit 2	Visit 3
• Any indicated	• Any indicated
• Assess for compliance with the medication regimen. • Assess for effectiveness and adverse effects of medications.	• Repeat care given at previous visit.
• Repeat care given at previous visit.	• Repeat care given at previous visit.
• Repeat care given at previous visit. • Refer to dietary counseling if needed.	• Repeat care given at previous visit.
• Repeat care given at previous visit.	• Repeat care given at previous visit.
• Repeat care given at previous visit.	• Repeat care given at previous visit.
• Repeat care given at previous visit.	• Repeat care given at previous visit.
• Assess learning since the last visit. • Teach the caregiver how to control and prevent crisis. • Teach the caregiver how to overcome denial through expressing emotions and joining support groups. • Teach the caregiver how to balance needs (caregiver's as well as patient's) with resources. • Teach problem-solving techniques to the caregiver.	• Assess learning since the last visit. • Assess for further teaching needs of caregiver. • Reinforce all teaching with caregiver.
• Reinforce previous visit.	• Help caregiver evaluate possible options for the patient's final days. • If possible, include the patient in the decision-making process.

Asthma

PLAN OF CARE	HOME CARE Visit 1
Diagnostic tests	• Complete blood count • Serum electrolyte levels • Theophylline level
Medications	• Evaluate the effectiveness and adverse effects of medications. • Evaluate compliance with the drug regimen.
Procedures	• Refer to respiratory therapy (RT), if indicated. • Observe patient performing postural drainage and deep breathing (DB) exercises. • Assess proper use of oxygen and other respiratory equipment (if ordered). • Assess vital signs, breath sounds, sputum production (amount and color), use of accessory muscles for breathing, and presence of cyanosis.
Diet	• Assess nutritional intake. • Assess medication interactions with food. • Encourage to force fluids, 2 to 3 L/day.
Activity	• Assess sleep pattern. • Assess response to activity.
Elimination	• Assess urine output.
Hygiene	• Evaluate the home environment for allergens. • Encourage oral hygiene before and after medications.
Patient teaching	• Discuss signs and symptoms to report to the physician and when to seek medical care. • Reinforce postural drainage and DB exercises. • Discuss medication (name, dosage, purpose, time and route of administration, adverse effects, and food interactions). • Teach safe use of RT equipment necessary for drug administration. • Explain the need to control allergens and cigarette smoke in the environment. • Teach the patient to avoid being outdoors on high-humidity days and to check the air quality index (if poor, stay inside). • Teach relaxation measures (imagery and DB exercises) to decrease anxiety to stimuli.
Discharge planning	• Assess home support and resource needs (for example, economic means to purchase medication and equipment). • Refer to appropriate agency or social services as indicated.

Visit 2	Visit 3
• Arterial blood gases and pulmonary function tests (referral to physician if indicated)	• Same as previous visit
• Evaluate compliance with the drug regimen. • Assess for effectiveness and adverse effects of drug therapy.	• Repeat care given at previous visit.
• Repeat care given at previous visit. • Refer to RT (if indicated).	• Repeat care given at previous visit.
• Reinforce previous visit. • Refer to dietary counseling if indicated.	• Repeat care given at previous visit.
• Reinforce previous visit.	• Repeat care given at previous visit.
• Reinforce previous visit.	• Repeat care given at previous visit.
• Reinforce previous visit.	• Repeat care given at previous visit.
• Define factors that trigger asthma attacks. • Discuss lifestyle modifications and environmental control measures, smoking cessation, and the need for regular follow-up care.	• Reinforce and evaluate teaching sessions from previous home visits.
• Assess home support and resource needs. • Refer to RT and a counselor, if indicated.	• Assess home support and resource needs.

Breast cancer

PLAN OF CARE	HOME CARE Visit 1
Diagnostic tests	• Complete blood count • Electrolyte levels
Medications	• Evaluate preoperative medications. • Evaluate the need for and frequency of pain medications. • Determine adverse reactions to medications.
Procedures	• Inspect the surgical wound and surgical dressing. • Inspect the suture line. • Inspect the drain sites.
Diet	• Encourage a high-protein diet as tolerated. • Evaluate for nausea or anorexia.
Activity	Physical therapist (PT): • Evaluate the need for postmastectomy exercise and ways to decrease lymphedema, if present.
Elimination	• Assess drainage from the surgical drain.
Hygiene	• Assist hygiene needs. • Assess caregiver abilities.
Patient teaching	• Discuss concerns related to sexuality, resumption of sexual intercourse, and other psychosocial needs. • Discuss prosthesis and reconstruction. • Discuss maintenance of a safe home environment.
Discharge planning	• Reinforce the schedule of follow-up visits with surgeon. • Discuss schedules for radiation therapy and chemotherapy as needed.

Visit 2	Visit 3
None	None
• Determine the effectiveness of and adverse reactions to medications.	• Repeat care given at previous visit.
• Inspect the surgical wound for infection, flap necrosis, and seroma formation.	• Repeat care given at previous visit.
• Encourage diet as tolerated.	• Repeat care given at previous visit.
• Progress postmastectomy exercises as prescribed by PT. • Monitor lymphedema levels.	• Repeat care given at previous visit.
• Assess for constipation.	• Repeat care given at previous visit.
• Repeat care given at previous visit.	• Repeat care given at previous visit.
• Provide information related to planned adjuvant therapies, such as chemotherapy, radiation therapy, and tamoxifen therapy.	• Teach about new symptoms since last visit that should be reported, such as new back pain, weakness, shortness of breath, confusion, and constipation (may indicate metastasis).
• Encourage participation in community support programs, such as I Can Cope, Look Good Feel Better, and Reach to Recovery. • Discuss potential referrals for lymphedema management if needed in future.	• After 6 weeks and with physician's approval, begin aerobics, water exercise, and overall fitness program.

Cerebrovascular accident

PLAN OF CARE	HOME CARE Visit 1
Diagnostic tests	• Oxygen saturation • Prothrombin time (PT)
Medications	• Assess compliance with and effectiveness of drug therapy. • Assess for adverse effects of drugs.
Procedures	• Check vital signs and perform a neurologic assessment. • Assess lung and heart sounds. • Assess for signs and symptoms (S/S) of cerebrovascular accident (CVA): bleeding, headache, edema, increased or new blurred vision, weakness, immobility, and slurred speech. • Assess for S/S of seizure activity.
Diet	• Assess nutritional and fluid intake. • Teach the patient to eat small, frequent, and supplemental feedings, if indicated. • Teach the patient to avoid foods that may cause choking, such as mashed potatoes, large pieces of meat, and soft breads.
Activity	• Assess mobility and the ability to perform activities of daily living. • Assess safe and appropriate use of assistive devices. • Consult a physical therapist if needed. • Encourage the patient to plan rest periods daily. • Encourage range-of-motion exercises for extremities and regular daily exercise.
Elimination	• Assess urinary and bowel elimination. • Reinforce bladder training program.
Hygiene	• Assess skin integrity. • Assess the oral cavity. • Encourage frequent oral hygiene.

Visit 2	Visit 3
• PT	• PT
• Repeat care given at previous visit.	• Repeat care given at previous visit.
• Repeat care given at previous visit.	• Repeat care given at previous visit.
• Repeat care given at previous visit.	• Repeat care given at previous visit.
• Assess compliance with rest periods. • Repeat care given at previous visit.	• Repeat care given at previous visit.
• Repeat care given at previous visit.	• Repeat care given at previous visit.
• Repeat care given at previous visit.	• Repeat care given at previous visit.

(continued)

Cerebrovascular accident *(continued)*

PLAN OF CARE	HOME CARE Visit 1
Patient teaching	• Teach S/S of CVA. • Teach S/S to report to the physician. • Teach safety precautions related to anticoagulant therapy. • Teach the patient and family ways of adapting the home for accessibility. • Reinforce physical therapy training related to use of wheelchair, crutches, or walker. • Teach the family or caregiver proper body mechanics and how to protect the caregiver's back when assisting the patient. • Teach safety measures to prevent falls. • Encourage speech exercises daily. • Teach the family to engage in communication with patient as much as possible. • Teach the family to develop competency in the following (if needed): home ventilation, suctioning, positioning techniques, parenteral or enteral home nutrition, and tracheostomy care.
Discharge planning	• Assess the availability of pertinent phone numbers (pharmacy, durable medical equipment, occupational therapy, physical therapy, speech pathology, and social services). • Assess resource and support needs. • Consult a psychological counselor if needed. • Discuss the importance of follow-up care. • Assess the need for modifications in the home environment, and refer to social services, if needed.

Visit 2	Visit 3
• Reinforce previous teaching. • Teach definitions and S/S of CVA. • Teach risk factors (high blood pressure, blood clot in neck vessels or brain, high cholesterol, athero-sclerosis, excessive stress in presence of other risk factors, and tobacco use in presence of other risk factors). • Teach the importance of follow-up care. • Teach the need to consult an occupational thera-pist, a physical therapist, a speech pathologist (SP), social services, and a psychological counselor as needed. • Evaluate understanding of teaching.	• Reinforce previous teaching. • Evaluate understanding of teach-ing.
• Assess resources and support needs. • Evaluate patient and family understanding of follow-up care. • Evaluate patient and family seeking appropriate support groups. • Consult a psychological counselor if needed. • Discuss the importance of follow up care. • Assess the need for modifications in the home environment and refer to social services, if needed.	• Repeat care given at previous vis-it. • Plan for more visits if necessary. • Encourage continued visits from occupational therapist, physical therapist, SP, social services, and psychological counselor, if needed.

Chronic renal failure

PLAN OF CARE	HOME CARE Visit 1
Diagnostic tests	• Blood urea nitrogen • Complete blood count • Serum electrolyte levels • Urine and serum creatinine • Osmolarity • Urinalysis • Electrocardiogram
Medications	• Assess the effectiveness of medications. • Assess compliance with the drug regimen.
Procedures	• Check vital signs. • Assess breath and heart sounds. • Evaluate mental status. • Observe coping and family processes.
Diet	• Assess nutritional intake. • Evaluate compliance with dietary restrictions (protein, potassium, and sodium). • Assess the presence of nausea, vomiting, and anorexia (conditions that cause the loss of needed nutrients). • Refer to a dietitian, if indicated. • Weigh the patient.
Activity	• Assess sleep pattern. • Assess ability to perform activities of daily living. • Instruct patient to turn, cough, and deep breathe q 2 hr if immobile.
Elimination	• Assess intake and output (I&O). • Assess for presence of edema. • Encourage exercise and sufficient dietary bulk.
Hygiene	• Assess the dialysis site. • Assess skin integrity. • Encourage oral hygiene before and after meals.

Visit 2	Visit 3
• Same as previous visit if indicated	• Same as previous visit if indicated
• Repeat care given at previous visit. • Assess for effectiveness and adverse effects of drug therapy.	• Repeat care given at previous visit.
• Repeat care given at previous visit.	• Repeat care given at previous visit.
• Reinforce care given at previous visit. • Weigh the patient.	• Repeat care given at previous visit.
• Reinforce care given at previous visit.	• Reinforce care given at previous visit.
• Reinforce care given at previous visit.	• Reinforce care given at previous visit.
• Reinforce care given at previous visit.	• Reinforce care given at previous visit.

(continued)

Chronic renal failure *(continued)*

PLAN OF CARE	HOME CARE Visit 1
Patient teaching	• Discuss signs and symptoms (S/S) to report to the physician. • Teach the importance of avoiding persons who have respiratory infections. • Teach the importance of good hand-washing techniques for patient and others in close contact with the patient. • Teach how to measure blood pressure (BP), and instruct to check BP daily at same time; keep daily record and report changes to the physician. • Advise the patient to avoid over-the-counter drugs without a physician's approval. • Encourage daily rest periods. • Discuss medications (name, dosage, purpose, time and route of administration, and adverse effects). • Teach I&O procedure, and instruct to report changes in output to the physician. • Instruct the patient to weigh himself daily wearing the same clothing, at same time, and using the same scale. • Instruct the patient to avoid laxatives and antacids that contain magnesium. • Advise the use of stool softeners to avoid straining during bowel movements.
Discharge planning	• Assess home and support resource needs. • Refer to a psychological counselor if indicated.

Visit 2	Visit 3
• Teach the definition of and factors that cause chronic renal failure.	• Reinforce and evaluate teaching sessions from previous home visits.
• Teach S/S of edema, hyperkalemia, hyperphosphatemia, hypermagnesemia, and hypocalcemia.	• Observe the patient and family performing dialysis access device or catheter care, BP, and I&O procedures.
• Teach the purpose of dialysis.	• Assess the home environment for hygienic measures.
• Teach care of the dialysis access device or catheter.	
• Discuss measures that decrease the risk of injury and infection of the dialysis access device or catheter.	
• Instruct to report S/S of redness, pain, swelling or drainage from the dialysis access device or catheter to the physician.	
• Teach S/S of urinary tract infection (dysuria, foul-smelling urine, and fever), and instruct the patient to report them to the physician.	
• Teach S/S or pericarditis (pericardial friction rub and chest pain).	
• Tell the patient not to measure BP or allow venipuncture in the arm that has the dialysis access device in place.	
• Assess home and support resource needs.	• Refer to an appropriate agency or social services as indicated.

Chronic obstructive pulmonary disease

PLAN OF CARE	HOME CARE Visit 1
Diagnostic tests	• Complete blood count • Serum electrolyte levels
Medications	• Evaluate the effectiveness and adverse effects of medications. • Evaluate compliance with the drug regimen. • Explain the need to avoid over-the-counter medication without a physician's approval.
Procedures	• Assess vital signs, breath and heart sounds, and the thorax. • Observe the patient performing pursed-lip, abdominal, and deep breathing (DB) exercise techniques. • Assess proper and safe use of oxygen (O_2) and other respiratory equipment. • Assess proper sitting techniques. • Refer to a respiratory therapist, if indicated.
Diet	• Have patient force fluids to 2 to 3 L/day if tolerated. • Assess weight. • Assess nutritional intake. • Encourage high-protein, low-carbohydrate foods. • Assess sodium intake if steroid dependent. • Refer to a dietitian, if indicated.
Activity	• Assess exercise tolerance. • Assess O_2 needs. • Assess the ability to perform activities of daily living.
Elimination	• Assess presence of edema. • Instruct to keep a daily weight log.
Hygiene	• Assess the home environment for factors likely to cause a recurrence (adequate heating and cooling, absence of persons with infections, fresh air, and lack of dust and other irritants). • Encourage frequent oral hygiene. • Assess skin integrity.

Visit 2	Visit 3
• Arterial blood gases and chest X-ray (refer to physician if indicated)	• Same as previous visit
• Evaluate compliance with the drug regimen. • Assess for effectiveness and adverse effects of drug therapy.	• Repeat care given at previous visit.
• Review lab work with the patient and family. • Repeat care given at previous visit.	• Repeat care given at previous visit.
• Reinforce care given at previous visit. • Explain the importance of diet maintenance. • Refer to a dietitian if indicated.	• Reinforce care given at previous visit.
• Repeat care given at previous visit.	• Repeat care given at previous visit.
• Assess the presence of edema. • Evaluate the daily weight log.	• Reinforce care given at previous visit.
• Reinforce care given at previous visit.	• Reinforce care given at previous visit.

(continued)

Chronic obstructive pulmonary disease *(continued)*

PLAN OF CARE	HOME CARE Visit 1
Patient teaching	• Discuss signs and symptoms to report to the physician. • Reinforce pursed-lip, abdominal breathing, and DB exercise techniques. • Explain the need to slow down the disease process. • Teach to continue O_2 use during meals. • Instruct to eat a balanced diet in frequent and small portions. • Teach O_2 safety and use. • Discuss medication (name, dosage, purpose, time and route of administration, and adverse effects).
Discharge planning	• Assess home support and resource needs (for example, economic means to purchase medications and equipment). • Refer to appropriate agency or social services as indicated.

Visit 2	Visit 3
• Discuss the definition and causes of chronic obstructive pulmonary disease, lifestyle modifications, and risk factor reduction (for example, smoking cessation). • Refer to physical therapist, occupational therapist, and psychosocial counselor, if indicated and explain the need for regular follow-up care.	• Reinforce and evaluate teaching sessions from previous home visits.
• Assess home support and resource needs.	• Assess home support and resource needs.

Colostomy

PLAN OF CARE	HOME CARE Visit 1
Diagnostic tests	• Complete blood count • Blood chemistries • Electrolyte levels • Blood urea nitrogen • Chest X-ray
Medications	• Evaluate adherence to drug regimen; effectiveness and adverse effects of prescribed antibiotics, analgesics, and antiemetics. • Determine over-the-counter (OTC) medication use. • Observe for undissolved medications in ostomy pouch.
Procedures	• Determine specific ostomy type and location (for example, single barrel versus double barrel; and transverse, ascending, or descending). • Evaluate the patient's ability to manage ostomy care. • Inspect the surgical wounds and dressings. • Take baseline vital signs (VS).
Diet	• Take baseline weight. • Determine calorie intake. • Evaluate 24-hour diet recall for appropriate calorie, vitamin, mineral, protein, and residue intake.
Activity	• Determine the level of activity since discharge. • Determine the patient's tolerance for activity. • Perform a home safety evaluation.
Elimination	• Assess the quality, amount, and odor of colostomy effluent. • Inspect the urine amount, concentration, and color.
Hygiene	• Inspect oral, perineal, and general body hygiene. • Consider home care aide services.
Patient teaching	• Reinforce prior teaching. • Reteach concepts as necessary. • Request return demonstration on peristomal skin preparation and care, pouch emptying, pouch application, and ostomy irrigation.
Discharge planning	• Evaluate the amount and quality of home care supplies, such as skin barrier and pouches.

Visit 2	Visit 3
None	• Electrolyte levels
• Observe for adverse effects of prescription and OTC drugs, particularly diarrhea or constipation. • Inspect ostomy pouch for undissolved medications.	• Repeat care given at previous visit.
• Inspect peristomal skin for signs of yeast infection, bacterial infection, and excoriation. • Evaluate the color and size of the stoma. • Evaluate the healing of surgical wounds. • Check VS.	• Repeat care given at previous visit.
• Weigh the patient. • Determine if body weight has been maintained or if loss or gain has occurred. • Evaluate daily dietary consumption.	• Repeat care given at previous visit.
• Determine the level of activity since discharge. • Determine the patient's tolerance for activity.	• Repeat care given at previous visit.
• Recommend dietary and fluid adjustments based on colostomy and urine outputs.	• Repeat care given at previous visit.
• Inspect oral, perineal, and general body hygiene.	• Repeat care given at previous visit.
• Reinforce prior teaching. • Reteach concepts as necessary. • Request return demonstration on peristomal skin preparation and care, pouch emptying, pouch application, and ostomy irrigation. • If radiation or chemotherapy is to follow, begin teaching specific to these therapies.	• Repeat care given at previous visit.
• Determine compliance with follow-up visits to such health care providers as a surgeon, medical oncologist, and radiation oncologist.	• Provide the patient and family with written information on how to contact local support agencies, such as the American Cancer Society and Ostomy Society.

Coronary artery bypass surgery

PLAN OF CARE	HOME CARE Visit 1
Diagnostic tests	• Complete blood count • Serum electrolyte levels • Blood urea nitrogen • Creatinine level
Medications	• Assess compliance with the drug regimen. • Evaluate the schedule of self-medication. • Assess over-the-counter medication use.
Procedures	• Evaluate the sternal wound, graft sites, and previous chest tube sites for infection and stage of healing. • Assess vital signs (VS) and peripheral pulses.
Diet	• Give diet instructions for a cardiac-prudent diet: low-fat, low-sodium, and low-cholesterol. • Consult with a dietitian as needed. • Weigh the patient.
Activity	• Physical therapy evaluation. • Progressive cardiac rehabilitation, electrocardiogram-monitored exercise (also called Phase 2).
Elimination	• Evaluate for nocturia and frequency of urination.
Hygiene	• Evaluate the need for home care aide services.
Patient teaching	• Discuss early identification of medical problems, especially during exercise.
Discharge planning	• Investigate participation in community cardiac-related support groups and educational programs.

Visit 2	Visit 3
None	• Serum potassium, if on a diuretic
• Evaluate cardiovascular and respiratory systems for adverse effects of drug therapy, including shortness of breath, edema, and rapid weight gain.	• Recommend to physician increases or decreases in medication dosages as indicated by the patient's physical status.
• Review the results of previous tests with the patient and family. • Check VS. • Evaluate surgical wound sites. • Palpate peripheral pulses.	• Check VS. • Review weight and heart rate logs. • Palpate peripheral pulses.
• Reinstruct on foods high in potassium and low in cholesterol, saturated fat, and sodium. • Weigh the patient.	• Provide additional instructions on dietary choices and modifications within the prescribed nutrient range. • Weigh the patient.
• Review the heart rate log. • Determine the level of compliance with prescribed exercise. • Evaluate the effects of the exercise regimen.	• Focus on increasing exercise capacity in such activities as walking, jogging, and weight training.
• Evaluate for constipation or straining during defecation.	• Reassess the need for a diuretic, stool softener, or laxative.
• Assess as needed.	• Assess as needed.
• Discuss risk reduction behaviors, such as smoking decrease or cessation.	• Discuss psychosocial needs of the patient and family to minimize episodes of anxiety and depression. • Discuss the ability to resume sexual activities with physician approval.
• Refer to occupational therapy as needed to assist in return to occupational and leisure activities.	• Provide the patient and family with community support necessary for continuing lifestyle changes.

Diabetes mellitus

PLAN OF CARE	HOME CARE Visit 1
Diagnostic tests	• Review home glucose monitor use with patient as necessary.
Medications	• Observe the patient's self-administration of insulin, oral hypoglycemic agent, or both.
Procedures	• Assess vital signs (VS). • Inspect skin and mucous membranes. • Palpate pedal pulses. • Perform neurologic assessment.
Diet	• Evaluate compliance with a reduced-calorie, reduced-fat, increased-fiber diet as recommended by the American Diabetes Association. • Evaluate alcohol intake. • Weigh the patient.
Activity	• Evaluate compliance with the prescribed activity plan. • Determine the appropriateness of the shoes the patient uses for exercise. • Assess home safety.
Elimination	• Assess for constipation, frequent urination, and nocturia.
Hygiene	• Assess the need for home care aide services.
Patient teaching	• Request a demonstration of self-monitoring of blood glucose. • Reteach components as needed. • Establish daily schedule for glucose testing. • Teach appropriate needle disposal and storage of insulin.
Discharge planning	• Evaluate the appropriateness, the quantity, and correct storage of the patient's diabetic supplies. • Evaluate the patient's financial ability to purchase medical supplies and nutritionally appropriate food. • Establish a patient checklist and diabetes care record.

Visit 2	Visit 3
• Same as previous visit	• Same as previous visit
• Repeat care given at previous visit.	• Ask the patient about episodes of hypoglycemia or hyperglycemia. • Ask about the relationship of food intake to blood glucose fluctuations.
• Assess VS. • Inspect skin and mucous membranes. • Palpate pedal pulses.	• Repeat care given at previous visit.
• Review food and meal selections for previous week with patient and family. • Provide written instructions as necessary to reinforce previous dietary teaching or to add new concepts. • Weigh the patient.	• Repeat care given at previous visit.
• Review the activity log, if available. • Inspect the lower extremities; if patient is bedbound, inspect back.	• Repeat care given at previous visit.
• Repeat care given at previous visit.	• Repeat care given at previous visit.
• Assist as needed.	• Repeat care given at previous visit.
• Arrange for a dietitian to teach the patient advanced dietary management, such as reading and interpreting food labels, adjusting nutrients as needed, and eating away from home.	• Discuss methods to prevent complications from diabetes. • Review blood glucose control up to this point.
• Provide videotapes, audiotapes, and other education materials as necessary for home use. • Provide information about local diabetic support groups, screenings, and educational programs for the public. • Assess the need for ongoing maintenance and custodial care; initiate referrals as needed.	• Help the patient schedule routine medical check-ups and follow-up appointments for foot care, eye care, and dental care.

Heart failure

PLAN OF CARE	HOME CARE Visit 1
Diagnostic tests	• Blood urea nitrogen • Creatinine, digoxin, and potassium levels
Medications	• Assess compliance with the drug regimen. • Assess for effectiveness and adverse effects of drug therapy.
Procedures	• Perform a comprehensive assessment to establish a baseline.
Diet	• Assess compliance with a dietary restrictions. • Restrict sodium (Na) and fluids as necessary. • If the patient is on diuretic therapy, instruct on dietary sources of potassium.
Activity	• Assess exercise tolerance. • Restrict activities, if necessary. • Refer to a physical or occupational therapist for energy conservation appraisal, if needed.
Elimination	• Assess intake and output (I&O) patterns. • Assess for nocturia, urinary frequency, and constipation.
Hygiene	• Provide assistance as needed. • Evaluate for need of home care aide services.
Patient teaching	• Provide the patient and family with written educational materials from such sources as the American Heart Association. • Teach lifestyle modifications and risk factor reduction, such as smoking cessation. • Reinforce the permanence of the therapeutic regimen.
Discharge planning	• Assess home support and resource needs, such as transportation needs for follow-up visits to health care providers, long-term durable medical equipment needs, and home care aide needs. • Make sure the patient has an accurate scale for taking daily weight.

Visit 2	Visit 3
• Same as previous visit	• Same as previous visit
• Assess compliance with the drug regimen. • Assess for the effectiveness and adverse effects of drug therapy. • Reinforce permanence of the drug regimen.	• Repeat care given at previous visit.
• Review the results of previous tests with the patient and family. • Reassess vital signs, lungs, and the cardiovascular and peripheral vascular systems. • Reassess mental status. • Reevaluate for the presence of edema. • Evaluate the weight log. • Evaluate the carotid pulse log.	• Repeat care given at previous visit.
• Assess compliance with a therapeutic diet.	• Repeat care given at previous visit.
• Assess exercise tolerance and tolerance of activities of daily living, including sexual activity.	• Repeat care given at previous visit.
• Assess I&O patterns.	• Repeat care given at previous visit.
• Assist as needed.	• Repeat care given at previous visit.
• Teach the importance of regular follow-up visits with health care providers, effects of increased Na and fluid intake, and exercise and activity restrictions as necessary. • Teach patient about hidden sources of Na (such as antacids). • Teach food and drug interactions.	• Reinforce and evaluate teaching sessions from previous home visits.
• Assess home support and resource needs.	• Repeat care given at previous visit.

Hypertension

PLAN OF CARE	HOME CARE Visit 1
Diagnostic tests	• Serum electrolyte and creatinine levels • Blood urea nitrogen
Medications	• Validate antihypertensive medication type, dosage, and sequencing, including diuretics, adrenergic inhibitors, angiotensin-converting enzyme inhibitors, and calcium antagonists. • Assess for medication interactions with other drugs and with foods.
Procedures	• Measure blood pressure (BP) carefully: take initially in both arms and subsequently in the arm with the higher reading; measure BP in sitting, supine, and standing positions. • Weigh the patient
Diet	• Review the prescribed diet. • Establish dietary goals with the patient and family for weight loss as necessary. • Make sure a scale is available, if needed.
Activity	• Establish goals and parameters for incrementally increasing activity levels. • Focus on achieving long-term adherence to increased activity levels.
Elimination	• Evaluate for nocturia, hematuria, frequent urination, urine retention, and constipation.
Hygiene	• Evaluate the need for home care aide services.
Patient teaching	• Communicate BP reading to the patient, and explain its significance as necessary. • Reinforce the need for lifelong antihypertensive therapy. • Review understanding of medication dosage and sequencing. • Reinforce relaxation and stress-management techniques.
Discharge planning	• Evaluate the patient's financial resources necessary for compliance with antihypertensive therapy. • Consult social services if financial resources appear inadequate to ensure long-term compliance with therapy.

Visit 2	Visit 3
• Serum electrolyte levels	• Serum electrolyte levels
• Evaluate for expected effects of BP medications. • Make recommendations to physician for alterations in type and dose of medications, if needed. • Evaluate medications for adverse effects.	• Evaluate for adverse effects of BP medications (such as, depression, weakness, dry mouth, impotence, sedation, orthostatic hypertension). • Address interactions.
• Measure BP carefully. • Assess for edema of lower extremities. • Weigh the patient. • Determine adherence to medication regimen.	• Measure BP and note variances and trends from previous visits. • Assess for edema. • Weigh the patient.
• Take 24-hour recall of food intake. • Review food choices that are appropriate or inappropriate as necessary.	• Look for "hidden" sources of sodium and fat (such as canned foods, processed foods, and antacids). • Review "dining out" habits; stress the need to avoid "fast foods."
• Review the patient's participation in the exercise regimen since last visit. • Revise activity goals if indicated.	• Encourage participation in aerobic exercises, such as walking, after evaluation by the physician.
• Evaluate urinary and bowel patterns.	• Evaluate urinary and bowel patterns.
• Assess as needed.	• Assess as needed.
• Instruct the patient not to miss doses of medications, "double up" on doses, "borrow" BP medications from others, or abruptly discontinue medications. • Discuss how to manage orthostatic hypertension: change positions slowly, do leg exercises, lie or sit down when dizzy.	• Teach the patient that most adverse reactions to BP medication will diminish over time. • Begin teaching the patient or family member how to take BP measurements if willing, capable, and reliable.
• Begin to evaluate the patient's and family's potential for long-term compliance with all aspects of therapy. • Refer to smoking cessation courses as needed.	• Evaluate long-term lifestyle modification and medication compliance. • Ensure that the patient and family have written instructions on therapy and that they're following them.

Ileostomy

PLAN OF CARE	HOME CARE Visit 1
Diagnostic tests	• Complete blood count • Blood urea nitrogen, creatinine, and electrolyte levels • Urinalysis and urine osmolarity
Medications	• Caution the patient not to use over-the-counter (OTC) or prescription laxatives. • Evaluate compliance with and adverse effects of prescribed antibiotics, analgesics, and antiemetics. • Observe for undissolved medications in ostomy pouch (especially enteric-coated medicines)
Procedures	• Evaluate the patient's ability to perform care of the ostomy. • Inspect and evaluate perianal and abdominal wounds, staples, dressing, tubes, and drains as appropriate. • Take baseline vital signs.
Diet	• Evaluate hydration status by assessing mucous membranes and skin turgor. • Obtain 24-hour diet recall from the patient. • Evaluate for evidence of food blockage of stoma. • Evaluate for nausea and vomiting (N/V). • Weigh the patient.
Activity	• Perform a home safety assessment. • Determine the patient's level and tolerance of activity since discharge.
Elimination	• Determine quality, consistency, and amount of ileostomy effluent in 24 hours (should be approximately 800 to 1,000 ml/24 hr). • Determine color, concentration, and urine output.
Hygiene	• Evaluate peristomal and perirectal skin areas for signs of redness, excoriation, and denuding.
Patient teaching	• Use correct terminology for wounds, equipment, and supplies. • Ask for return demonstrations on care of the ostomy as appropriate.
Discharge planning	• Evaluate amount, quality, and appropriateness of home care supplies. • Replenish supplies as needed.

Visit 2	Visit 3
• Urine osmolarity	• Electrolyte levels • Urine osmolarity
• Observe for adverse affects of prescription and OTC drugs, particularly diarrhea or constipation. • If still on antibiotics, observe peristomal skin for signs of fungal or yeast superinfection.	• Observe for adverse effects of prescription and OTC drugs. • If on antibiotics, observe peristomal skin for superinfection. • Inspect ostomy pouch for partially dissolved medications.
• Inspect stoma for signs of pallor, discoloration, bleeding, strangulation, hernia, or retraction. • Inspect peristomal skin for signs of yeast infection, bacterial infection, or contact with fecal drainage. • Evaluate healing of all surgical wound sites.	• Repeat care given at previous visit.
• Evaluate hydration status. • Evaluate for evidence of food blockage of stoma. • Evaluate for N/V. • Weigh the patient; from patient weight record determine if body weight loss or gain has occurred. • Evaluate daily food and fluid consumption. • Identify "problem foods" for the patient.	• Repeat care given at previous visit.
• Increase activity level as appropriate. • Determine the need for assistive equipment. • Repeat care given at previous visit.	• Repeat care given at previous visit.
• Recommend dietary fluid adjustments based on ostomy and urine outputs.	• Repeat care given at previous visit.
• Consider home care aide assistance with hygiene as needed.	• Repeat care given at previous visit.
• Use correct terminology. • Ask for return demonstrations on care of the ostomy; reteach concepts as needed.	• Repeat care given at previous visit.
• Determine compliance with follow-up visits to a health care provider.	• Provide written information and telephone numbers of local support groups and organizations.

Lower extremity amputation

PLAN OF CARE	HOME CARE Visit 1
Diagnostic tests	• Serum electrolyte levels • Complete blood count • Prothrombin and activated partial thromboplastin time • International normalized ratio
Medications	• Assess use of analgesics and antispasmodics. • Monitor insulin (if diabetic).
Procedures	• Check vital signs and perform a physical assessment. • Assess the stump incision site, patient's ability to perform incision care, safety needs in home environment, pain management, and presence of contractures. • Assist with and reiterate postoperative conditioning exercises: sit-ups, trunk flexion, and hopping in place. • Massage the stump toward the suture line as ordered. • Reapply compression wrap on postsurgical cast. • Assist with prosthesis management.
Diet	• Assess nutritional intake. • Encourage high-protein foods.
Activity	• Assess patient performance of walker and crutch ambulation, muscle strengthening exercises, and transfer techniques.
Elimination	• Assess urine output and bowel movements.
Hygiene	• Assess cleanliness of the stump and wrap. • Teach the patient and family proper hand-washing techniques.
Patient teaching	• Assess the patient's comprehension of in-hospital teaching and ability to learn. • Teach environmental safety, nonpharmacologic pain relief measures, incision care, use of mirror to view all aspects of stump, application of compression ace bandage wraps, and signs and symptoms to report to the physician. • Instruct to follow in-home physical therapy exercise program. • Reinforce correct use of walkers and crutches. • Reinforce prosthesis application teaching.
Discharge planning	• Assess need for crutches, walker. • Consult social services, physical therapist, or psychological counselor if needed. • Assess access to phone communication with durable medical equipment company. • Assess availability of transportation for needed appointments.

Visit 2	Visit 3
• Any indicated	• Any indicated
• Repeat care given at previous visit.	• Repeat care given at previous visit.
• Repeat care given at previous visit.	• Repeat care given at previous visit.
• Repeat care given at previous visit.	• Repeat care given at previous visit.
• Repeat care given at previous visit.	• Repeat care given at previous visit.
• Repeat care given at previous visit.	• Repeat care given at previous visit.
• Assess cleanliness of stump and wrap and patient's ability to perform stump care.	• Assess cleanliness of the stump and wrap.
• Reinforce previous teaching. • Observe patient and family performing incision care, compression bandage wrap, muscle strengthening exercises, walker ambulation, and prosthetic application.	• Reinforce previous teaching.
• Explain the importance of follow-up care. • Assist with arrangements for follow-up visits. • Promote expression by the patient and family about impact of surgery. • Consult with a psychological counselor, if needed.	• Reinforce previous visits. • Promote expression by the patient and family about the impact of surgery. • Consult psychological counselor if needed.

Lung cancer

PLAN OF CARE	HOME CARE Visit 1
Diagnostic tests	• Pulse oximetry • Complete blood count • Electrolyte levels • Blood chemistries
Medications	• Evaluate compliance with usage of prescription and over-the-counter medications (such as bronchodilators and aspirin). • Evaluate the effects of pain medications. • Assess for adverse reactions to medications.
Procedures	• Evaluate breath sounds carefully and compare to baseline data. • Evaluate for hoarseness. • Weigh the patient. • Examine oxygen (O_2) delivery system and services. • Assess for right-sided heart failure; note signs and symptoms such as peripheral edema, weight gain, edema of dependent body parts, and jugular vein distention and unrelieved pain.
Diet	• Evaluate for dysphagia. • Evaluate whether calorie consumption is adequate for metabolic needs.
Activity	Physical therapist (PT) and occupational therapist (OT): • Evaluate the need for assistive devices, such as canes, walkers, wheelchairs, and mobile O_2 devices.
Elimination	• Assess for constipation.
Hygiene	• Evaluate the need for home care aide services.
Patient teaching	• Teach about smoking cessation, adequate food and fluid intake, and need for follow-up appointments. • Teach about operating and trouble-shooting home devices.
Discharge planning	• Refer to OT, PT, and pulmonary rehabilitation as needed. • Evaluate the knowledge and use of community support services. • Provide information about living wills and assist patient as needed.

Visit 2	Visit 3
• Pulse oximetry	• Same as previous visit
• Repeat care given at previous visit.	• Repeat care given at previous visit.
• Evaluate pain, breath sounds, hoarseness, and O_2 delivery system. • Weigh the patient.	• Repeat care given at previous visit.
• Repeat care given at previous visit.	• Repeat care given at previous visit.
PT and OT: • Teach patient and family use of prescribed assistive devices.	PT and OT: • Repeat care given at previous visit.
• Repeat care given at previous visit.	• Repeat care given at previous visit.
• Encourage the use of a bedside commode or shower bench as needed.	• Repeat care given at previous visit.
• Discuss specifics related to chemotherapy and radiation therapy prescribed for the patient as adjuvant therapy.	• Teach the patient and family signs and symptoms to report that could indicate progression of the disease. • Reinforce teaching related to chemotherapy and radiation therapy.
• Refer to community programs, such as I Can Cope and CanSurmount. • Refer to vocational counseling as appropriate.	• Refer to community hospice program if indicated.

Major depression

PLAN OF CARE	HOME CARE Visit 1
Diagnostic tests	• Any indicated
Medications	• Give antidepressants as prescribed. • Assess the patient's knowledge of antidepressants (name, dosage, schedule, adverse effects, and contraindications). • Assess the effectiveness of antidepressants. • Assess compliance with antidepressant regimen. • Administer stool softeners or laxatives as indicated.
Procedures	• Perform psychosocial assessment. • Perform suicide assessment. • Provide one-on-one intervention as needed. • Ask the patient to identify strengths and accomplishments. • Ask the patient to identify goals to work on for the next visit. • Teach the patient about support groups for depression. • Teach the patient about cognitive distortion log and have the patient do a log as an assignment.
Diet	• Assess nutritional intake; refer to a dietitian if indicated. • Give low tyramine diet if taking a monoamine oxidase inhibitor.
Activity	• Assess sleep pattern. • Assess activity level.
Elimination	• Encourage fluids, 2 to 3 L/day.
Hygiene	• Encourage hygiene activities, such as dressing and haircuts.
Patient teaching	• Teach strategies for prevention of relapse (recognizing symptoms of depression when they first occur: change in mood, such as becoming more depressed; decrease in energy; isolating self; not participating in activities; tired; sleep disturbances; appetite changes; and suicidal thoughts.) • Teach not to stop taking antidepressants unless told by physician. • Teach how to set up structured daily schedule. • If symptoms occur, teach the patient to see his physician quickly. • Review medication instructions and evaluate patient understanding.
Discharge planning	• Emphasize the importance of ongoing outpatient care. • Emphasize the importance of support group participation. • Emphasize the importance of following the antidepressant regimen.

Visit 2	Visit 3
• Any indicated	• Any indicated
• Repeat care given at previous visit	• Repeat care given at previous visit.
• Repeat care given at previous visit. • Ask the patient to evaluates the goals from the previous visit. • Discuss the patient cognitive distortion log. Role-play situations from log using assertiveness techniques. • Have the patient continue thought distortion log. • Monitor and increase social interactions. • Evaluate teaching from previous visit.	• Repeat care given at previous visit.
• Repeat care given at previous visit.	• Repeat care given at previous visit.
• Repeat care given at previous visit. • Assess for spontaneity.	• Repeat care given at previous visit.
• Reinforce previous visit.	• Reinforce previous visit.
• Reinforce previous visit.	• Reinforce previous visit.
• Evaluate understanding of previous teaching.	• Evaluate patient understanding of previous teaching.
• Reinforce previous visit.	• Reinforce previous visit.

Myocardial infarction

PLAN OF CARE	HOME CARE Visit 1
Diagnostic tests	• Serum electrolyte levels • Blood urea nitrogen • Creatinine level • Activated partial thromboplastin time • Digoxin level
Medications	• Assess medication compliance, including aspirin, stool softener, beta-adrenergic blocker, digoxin, diuretic, and analgesic as indicated.
Procedures	• Perform comprehensive assessment to establish home care baseline data set.
Diet	• Assess compliance with a diet low in calories, sodium, and fat. • Weigh the patient. • Consult a dietitian as needed.
Activity	Physical therapist and occupational therapist: • Continue planned cardiac physical rehabilitation at home.
Elimination	• Assess intake and output patterns. • Assess for nocturia and constipation.
Hygiene	• Evaluate the need for home care aide services.
Patient teaching	• Assess the level of understanding of and compliance with previous cardiac teaching. • Assess ability to verbalize personal risk factors.
Discharge planning	• Assess the home environment for stressors. • Determine the need for home medical equipment, such as a bedside commode, and shower bench.

Visit 2	Visit 3
None	None
• Assess for compliance with the medication regimen. • Assist with modification in medications and dosage as needed. • Assess the adverse effects of medications.	• Assess medication compliance. • Assess for adverse effects of medications. • Reinforce the permanence of the medication regimen.
• Review results of previous laboratory work with patient and family. • Reassess vital signs (VS) and the cardiovascular, respiratory, and peripheral vascular systems. • Evaluate for denial, anger, depression, fear, and despondency.	• Assist with scheduling of outpatient stress testing, cardiac catheterization as needed. • Reassess VS and VS log if available. • Reassess the cardiac and respiratory systems.
• Assess dietary compliance. • Weight the patient. • Evaluate food choices and meal composition.	• Weigh the patient and monitor for downward trend as indicated. • Reteach components as needed.
• Discuss activity limitations and planned rest periods. • Demonstrate home exercises.	• Reinforce consultation with physician before resuming sexual activity, driving, work, and traveling.
• Assess for edema in the lower extremities.	• Assess for edema. • Evaluate the consistency of stool.
• Progressive independence in self-care activities as tolerated.	• Repeat care given at previous visit.
• Evaluate the use of alcohol and tobacco products in the home setting. • Stress the need for permanent lifestyle changes.	• Reinforce teaching of symptoms that require immediate medical attention.
• Determine the need for assistance with transportation to attend outpatient cardiac rehabilitation and for follow-up visits to health care providers.	• Provide the patient with information about local cardiac support groups, organizations, and services.

Pain

PLAN OF CARE	HOME CARE Visit 1
Diagnostic tests	• Determine blood levels of adjuvant medications, such as carbamazepine, as indicated.
Medications	• Assess the effectiveness of the prescribed pharmacologic pain regimen using 0-to-10 pain scale.
Procedures	• Check vital signs (VS). • Evaluate sleep and rest cycle.
Diet	• Adjust patient's nutrient and calorie intake as prescribed. • Weigh the patient.
Activity	Home physical therapist consultation: • Assess the need for transcutaneous electrical nerve stimulation therapy, dermal stimulation, and heat and cold therapy.
Elimination	• Evaluate the pattern and consistency of bowel movements.
Hygiene	• Assess the need for home care aide services.
Patient teaching	• Teach the patient and family what type of pain the patient should expect and how long pain is likely to last, emphasizing that pain is an individual experience.
Discharge planning	• Evaluate the need for home medical equipment, such as canes, walker, and a bedside commode.

Visit 2	Visit 3
None	None
• Evaluate for evidence of overdosing or underdosing of pain medications. • Assess pain using 0-to-10 pain scale.	• Assess for adverse effects of pain regimen, such as oversedation, constipation, itching, respiratory depression, and nausea. • Assess pain using 0-to-10 pain scale.
• Check VS. • Evaluate sleep and rest cycle. • Assess for tolerance to pain medication.	• Check VS. • Evaluate sleep and rest cycle.
• Ensure adequate fluid intake to prevent constipation • Weigh the patient	• Weigh the patient.
• Progress with physical rehabilitation as pain allows.	• Repeat care given at previous visit.
• Repeat care given at previous visit.	• Repeat care given at previous visit.
• Assist as needed.	• Assist as needed.
• Teach how to use and store opioids safely. • Teach effects of opioids on driving and operating equipment.	• If increasing doses of opioids are needed to tolerate pain, reinforce teaching related to the concept of tolerance.
• Refer the patient to local acute or chronic pain support groups.	• Ensure that patient and family understand the importance of participating in outside activities to lessen preoccupation with pain and to provide distraction.

Panic disorder without agoraphobia

PLAN OF CARE	HOME CARE Visit 1
Diagnostic tests	• Any indicated
Medications	• Assess the effectiveness of antianxiety drugs. • Assess the effectiveness of antidepressants. • Identify target symptoms.
Procedures	• Perform a psychosocial assessment. • Perform a suicide assessment. • Have the patient perform progressive muscle relaxation. • Evaluate the patient's goals for anxiety reduction. • Evaluate the anxiety or stress reduction log. • Have the patient practice breathing exercises. • Monitor outpatient therapy.
Diet	• Assess nutritional status.
Activity	• Have the patient perform activities as tolerated. • Assess the patient's sleep pattern. • Discuss exercise and start a daily plan with patient (for example, walking or aerobics).
Elimination	• Assess for any problems.
Hygiene	• Assess for any problems.
Patient teaching	• Discuss disease process of panic disorder. • Review medications: antianxiety agents and antidepressants. • Discuss progressive muscle relaxation. • Review anxiety or stress log. • Teach about support groups.
Discharge planning	• Emphasize the importance of ongoing care. • Emphasize the importance of support group. • Emphasize the importance of compliance with the medication regimen.

Visit 2	Visit 3
• Any indicated	• Any indicated
• Assess the effectiveness of antianxiety drugs. • Assess the effectiveness of antidepressants. • Assess compliance with the medication regimen. • Evaluate patient knowledge of medications from previous session.	• Repeat care given at previous visit.
• Perform a psychosocial assessment. • Perform a suicide assessment. • Have the patient perform a self-evaluation of relaxation goals. • Discuss and evaluate anxiety and the stress reduction log (cognitive restructuring). • Have patient perform role playing. • Review patient's goals for anxiety reduction. • Monitor outpatient therapy.	• Perform psychosocial assessment. • Perform suicide assessment. • Have patient perform self-evaluation: relaxation, goals, assertive behaviors, thought stopping. • Discuss and evaluate anxiety or stress reduction log (cognitive restructuring). • Have patient perform role playing. • Review patient's goals for anxiety reduction. • Monitor outpatient therapy.
• Encourage diet as tolerated.	• Repeat care given at previous visit.
• Assess the benefits of the exercise program. • Continue with exercise program.	• Repeat care given at previous visit.
• Repeat care given at previous visit.	• Repeat care given at previous visit.
• Repeat care given at previous visit.	• Repeat care given at previous visit.
• Evaluate learning from previous session. • Review thought stopping. • Discuss assertiveness.	• Evaluate learning from previous session. • Review problem-solving techniques and time management.
• Reinforce previous visit. • Emphasize assertiveness.	• Reinforce previous visit. • Emphasize time management and problem solving.

Parkinson's disease

PLAN OF CARE	HOME CARE Visit 1
Diagnostic tests	• Blood urea nitrogen • Hematocrit • Hemoglobin
Medications	• Assess compliance with medication therapy. • Monitor the effectiveness and adverse effects of medications.
Procedures	• Check vital signs and breath sounds. • Evaluate level of consciousness, orientation, neurologic status, and home safety.
Diet	• Assess nutritional and fluid intake. • Weigh the patient. • Observe ability to swallow.
Activity	• Monitor disabilities related to activities of daily living (ADLs). • Assess compliance with physical therapy (PT), occupational therapy (OT), and speech therapy (ST) programs. • Evaluate patient performance of stretching and range-of-motion (ROM) exercises and ambulation.
Elimination	• Assess urinary and bowel elimination patterns, and evaluate urinary control.
Hygiene	• Evaluate degree of self-care. • Encourage frequent oral hygiene.
Patient teaching	• Teach about medications: names, dosage, purpose, route, time, and adverse effects. • Teach the definition and causes of Parkinson's disease. • Discuss signs and symptoms of Parkinson's disease (tremors, rigid movement, unstable posture) and late-stage Parkinson's disease (expressionless face, drooling, infrequent blinking, rapid rolling movement of fingers, tremors at rest, soft and expressionless voice). • Teach home safety. • Evaluate patient and caregiver understanding of instruction.
Discharge planning	• Assess accessibility to pertinent phone numbers for durable equipment, pharmacy, PT, OT, ST, and physician. • Assess resource and support needs. • Refer to social services or psychological counselor if indicated. • Discuss the importance of follow-up care.

Visit 2	Visit 3
• Same as previous visit	• Same as previous visit
• Repeat care given at previous visit.	• Repeat care given at previous visit.
• Repeat care given at previous visit.	• Repeat care given at previous visit.
• Repeat care given at previous visit.	• Repeat care given at previous visit.
• Repeat care given at previous visit.	• Repeat care given at previous visit.
• Repeat care given at previous visit.	• Repeat care given at previous visit.
• Repeat care given at previous visit.	• Repeat care given at previous visit.
• Reinforce previous teaching. • Instruct in proper feeding. • Reinforce PT, OT, and ST teaching about stretching, strengthening, ROM exercises; speech pattern exercises; daily routine skills and safety with ADLs; and proper use of adequate equipment. • Evaluate understanding of teaching.	• Reinforce previous teaching. • Evaluate patient understanding of teaching.
• Repeat care given at previous visit.	• Repeat care given at previous visit.

Pneumonia

PLAN OF CARE	HOME CARE Visit 1
Diagnostic tests	• Complete blood count and white blood cell count • Serum electrolyte levels
Medications	• Evaluate the effectiveness of medications. • Assess adverse effects of medication. • Evaluate compliance with the drug regimen.
Procedures	• Observe the patient performing deep-breathing (DB) exercises and postural drainage. • Assess vital signs (VS), breath sounds, and the thorax. • Assess proper use of vaporizer or humidifier and oxygen (O_2).
Diet	• Weigh the patient. • Have the patient force fluids to 3 L/day unless contraindicated. • Assess nutritional intake (avoid high-calorie diet if overweight).
Activity	• Assess exercise tolerance. • Explain the importance of 2 to 3 rest periods per day. • Evaluate O_2 needs.
Elimination	• Assess the presence of fever, diaphoresis, night sweats, and persistent cough.
Hygiene	• Evaluate the home environment for factors likely to cause a recurrence (adequate heat and cooling, absence of persons with infections, and fresh air).
Patient teaching	• Explain the need to prevent recurrence (convalesce gradually, keep warm, avoid chills and persons with infections, receive vaccinations for influenza and pneumonia as recommended by physician). • Discuss symptoms to report to physician (elevated temperature, chills, night sweats, diaphoresis, dyspnea, and persistent cough). • Discuss medication (name, dosage, purpose, time and route of administration, and adverse effects). • Explain methods of avoiding transmission of the disease. • Teach O_2 use and safety and inhaler use, if necessary.
Discharge planning	• Assess home support and resource needs (for example, economic means to purchase medication and equipment). • Refer to appropriate agency or social services as indicated.

Visit 2	Visit 3
• Chest X-ray (referral, if indicated)	• Same as previous visit
• Evaluate compliance with drug regimen. • Assess for positive and adverse effects of drug therapy. • Explain the need to avoid over-the-counter drugs without physician approval.	• Repeat care given at previous visit.
• Review results of laboratory work with the patient and family. • Reassess VS, thorax, and breath sounds. • Reassess proper and safe use of equipment and O_2. • Reassess DB exercises.	• Reassess VS, thorax, and breath sounds. • Reassess proper equipment use. • Encourage to continue DB exercises q.i.d. for 6 to 8 weeks.
• Weigh the patient. • Explain the importance of diet maintenance and fluid intake.	• Reinforce previous visit. • Take 24-hour recall of food intake.
• Repeat care given at previous visit.	• Reinforce previous visit.
• Repeat care given at previous visit.	• Repeat care given at previous visit.
• Repeat care given at previous visit.	• Repeat care given at previous visit.
• Discuss lifestyle modification and risk factor reduction (for example, smoking decrease or cessation and the need for regular follow-up care).	• Reinforce and evaluate teaching sessions from previous home visits.
• Assess home support and resource needs.	• Repeat care given at previous visit.

Pressure ulcer (stage IV)

PLAN OF CARE	HOME CARE Visit 1
Diagnostic tests	• Review of recent hospital laboratory data • Complete blood count • Electrolyte levels • Fasting blood glucose level
Medications	• Administer a high-potency multivitamin and mineral supplement daily. • Administer a systemic antibiotic for wound infection. • Treat with topical antibiotic ointment (triple antibiotic or silver sulfadiazine) in clean, nonhealing, exudative pressure ulcers (PUs) after 2 to 3 weeks of appropriate care. • Don't use topical antibiotics or antiseptics in clean wounds. • Use systemic antibiotic therapy in patients with bacteremia, sepsis, advancing cellulitis, or osteomyelitis. • Administer analgesics if nonpharmacologic treatments aren't sufficient.
Procedures	• Assess the wound and patient for signs and symptoms (S/S) of wound infection. • Perform complete admission history and physical assessment to establish baseline data. • Complete initial wound assessment, and document location, size, color, edges, exudate, sinus tract, tunneling, undermining, necrotic tissue, periwound skin color, temperature, edema, maceration, induration, and pain. • Mutually establish treatment goals with the patient or caregiver. • Determine the need to debride necrotic tissue using autolytic, enzymatic, or sharp debridement. *PU care:* • Clean PU and surrounding skin with normal saline solution (NSS); pat skin dry. • Irrigate wound, undermining, and tunnels with NSS using 35-ml syringe with 19G angiocath. • Loosely fill dead space, undermining, and tunnels with saline- or gel-moistened gauze. • Manage exudate with absorbent dressing (moist gauze, calcium alginate, foam, hydrocolloid, paste or granules, copolymer starch). • Apply secondary cover dressing. • Depending on type of dressing, change dressing daily to three times per day as needed to prevent strike-through, leakage, and skin maceration. • Monitor dressing near the anus for rolled edges. • Avoid massaging over bony prominences.

Visit 2	Visit 3
None	• If the wound appears infected, obtain wound fluid for a Gram stain or obtain a wound culture.
• Repeat care given at previous visit. • Assess wound for decreased S/S of infection and medicate as appropriate.	• Repeat care given at previous visit.
• Review the results of laboratory work with the patient or caregiver. • Continue ongoing assessment for wound infection. • Perform comprehensive PU assessment, including ongoing assessment for complications and monitoring for worsening of PU. • Perform focused physical assessment, including vital signs and mental status. • Measure PU size weekly. • Review treatment goals, and document progress in meeting goals. *PU care:* • Repeat care given at previous visit. • Debride necrotic tissue as needed using autolytic, enzymatic, or sharp debridement.	• Repeat care given at previous visit. • When patient is on systemic antibiotics, monitor for S/S of secondary infection, such as diarrhea, nausea, and rash. • Revise the treatment plan and goals as needed; document progress in meeting goals. • Debride necrotic tissue as needed using autolytic, enzymatic, or sharp debridement. *PU care:* • Repeat care given at previous visit. • Using valid PU assessment tool (for example, Bates-Jensen Pressure Sore Assessment Tool), assess wound for healing: size (length, width, depth); periwound skin color, intactness, edema, maceration, induration, and wound edges (open or closed); character and amount of exudate; formation of granulation tissue; reepithelialization; necrotic tissue, slough; and evidence of

(continued)

Pressure ulcer (stage IV) *(continued)*

PLAN OF CARE	HOME CARE Visit 1
Procedures *(continued)*	*Infected PU care:* • Teach the patient or caregiver the purpose of infected wound care. • Obtain an order for systemic antibiotics and noncytotoxic topical antiseptics. • Avoid occlusive dressing if PU is infected. • Using aseptic technique, clean wound and surrounding skin with NSS; pat skin dry. • Irrigate wound, undermining, and tunnels with gauze moistened with noncytotoxic concentration of topical antiseptic. • Cover with nonocclusive secondary dressing to manage exudate (calcium alginate, foam, gauze). • Change dressing daily to three times per day as needed to prevent strike-through, leakage, and skin maceration. (Teach the family to change second dressing.) • Consider using a dressing that can be left in place for several days as recommended by the Agency for Health Care Policy and Research. • Manage PU pain by covering wound, repositioning, analgesics, or nonpharmacologic intervention (imagery, relaxation techniques, music therapy). • Instruct caregiver or patient to keep pain log using pain scale and to record pain intensity and effect of dressing, turning, and medication.
Diet	• Assess current diet, fluid intake, appetite, and ability to feed self. • Encourage diet high in protein and calories unless contraindicated. • Endure adequate fluids to approximately 2.5 L/day unless contraindicated. • Assess skin turgor and mucous membranes. • Take baseline weight.
Activity	• Assess activity level: ability to ambulate and assist moving self in bed or chair. • Assess for contractures, joint mobility, and pain. • Evaluate home environment for safety; teach measures to prevent falls. • Evaluate the need for assistive devices. • Encourage the patient to perform an exercise regimen: stretching, isometric, or light weight-training exercises.

Visit 2	Visit 3
Infected PU care:	sinus tract, tunneling, or undermining.
• Reinforce teaching.	*Infected PU care:*
• Continue with the wound care regimen.	• Assess PU odor, exudate, and wound bed for response to systemic and local therapy.
• Evaluate the wound for decreasing S/S of infection.	• Revise antibiotic therapy based on wound culture if necessary.
• Assess the effectiveness of the pain management regimen.	• Reevaluate the effectiveness of pain management; adjust the plan as necessary.
• Repeat care given at previous visit.	• Repeat care given at previous visit.
• Initiate food and fluid intake record.	• Assess adequacy of intake.
• Weigh the patient.	• Initiate dietary consult if necessary.
	• Assess nutritional status every 3 months.
	• Report significant unexpected weight gain or loss (change of 3 lb/wk) to the physician.
• Confirm assessments and initiate physical therapy (PT) consult as needed.	• Reinforce PU prevention instructions.
• Assess patient or caregiver compliance.	• Initiate PT consult if needed.
	• Assess patient or caregiver compliance.

(continued)

Pressure ulcer (stage IV) *(continued)*

PLAN OF CARE	HOME CARE Visit 1
Elimination	• Assess elimination pattern, laxative use, and incontinence. • Initiate instruction on skin care following voiding or bowel movement (BM). • Keep skin clean and dry. • Apply moisture barrier after each voiding or BM. • Assess and treat incontinence. • Assess the need for a male external catheter, a fecal pouch, antidiarrheal medication, or disimpaction. • Use reusable (not disposable) underpads. • Establish voiding schedule. • Measure intake and output (I&O).
Hygiene	• Assess self-care ability, cleanliness, grooming needs, and body odor. • Teach caregiver or patient bathing schedule and routine. • Keep skin clean with mild soap and lukewarm water; rinse well and pat dry. • Avoid hot water and excessive friction. • Apply humectants, emollients, or moisturizers to dry skin. • Apply cornstarch or power between skin folds; wash skin folds twice per day.
Patient teaching	• Orient to home health care agency and services. • Involve caregiver or patient in ongoing care planning and meeting treatment goals. • Initiate PU teaching: stage, risk factors, prevention, prevention of infection, PU care to promote healing, and conditions necessary for healing (nutrients, fluid, pressure relief, uninfected wound, correct dressing changed as often as necessary). • Provide written PU information. *Managing tissue loads:* • Provide written instructions to: – avoid positioning on PU and donut ring devices – use positioning device to raise PU off surface (head or heel) – post written repositioning schedule – avoid positioning immobile patients on trochanters and ischial tuberosities – prevent direct contact between bony prominences (knees or ankles) with a pillow or blanket. • Don't raise the head of the bed to greater than 30 degrees unless contraindicated by medical condition or tube feeding. • Limit lateral position to less than 30 degrees. • Reposition bed-bound patients at least every 2 hr; chair-bound patients, hourly.

Visit 2	Visit 3
• Continue instruction to patient or caregiver on skin care after voiding or BM. • Measure I&O	• Evaluate caregiver, patient, or home care aide implementation of skin protection after voiding or BM. • Measure I&O.
• Assess skin for dryness, cleanliness, intactness, rash, and itching.	• Repeat care given at previous visit.
• Teach the importance of regular follow-up visits with health care providers. • Continue teaching, assessing comprehension, follow-though, and compliance. *Managing tissue loads:* • Assess caregiver and patient understanding of moisture, pressure, friction, and shear in PU etiology. • Assess the caregiver's or patient's ability to reduce and distribute tissue loading.	• Answer patient's, caregiver's, or family's questions. • Continue teaching caregiver and patient PU care and prevention. • Document patient's or caregiver's understanding and performance.

(continued)

Pressure ulcer (stage IV) *(continued)*

PLAN OF CARE	HOME CARE Visit 1
Patient teaching *(continued)*	• Teach chair-bound patients to shift weight every 15 minutes. • Have patient perform range-of-motion exercises (ROM) exercises every 4 hr while awake. • Support patient's feet with foot board. • Lift the patient; avoid pulling or sliding. • Manage moisture or perspiration and humidity. *Support surfaces:* • Work with the caregiver, patient, or payer for reimbursement of medically necessary equipment. • Teach the need for pressure-reducing support surface based on the patient's condition and risk for developing PUs: – comfort only or no risk: sheepskin, convoluted high-density foam – medium risk: air-filled static or alternating-pressure overlay or pads – high risk: low air-loss bed, dynamic floatation mattress – ultra high risk: air-fluidized bead bed. • Provide pressure-reducing cushion for chair-bound patient. • Initiate teaching to prevent further PUs or worsening of current PU. • Instruct patient who can walk about the importance of ambulating in home at least three times per day. • Teach caregiver or home care aide: – to reposition or encourage repositioning in bed or chair. – to have the patient perform complete ROM exercises three to four times per day (for patient who gets up in chair with assistance) – to change patient position hourly (for patient in chair) – to perform ROM exercises every 4 hr while patient is awake (for patient who is immobile or requires bed rest) – to position patient in alignment, with body weight evenly distributed. • Teach patient to shift weight every 15 minutes when up in chair. • Cover chair with sheet or blanket. • Teach patient to turn, cough, and deep breathe q 2 hr.
Discharge planning	• Assess resources: availability and skill of caregiver, patient understanding, and equipment needs. • Arrange for home care aide visits. • Discuss home care aide service with the patient or caregiver.

Visit 2	Visit 3
Support surfaces: • Assess comprehension and compliance.	*Support surfaces:* • Initiate support surface intervention. • Evaluate PU preventive measures.
• Assess caregiver's need for rest and sleep, and ability to provide care. • Evaluate home care aide care.	• Determine progress toward meeting goals of care.

Pulmonary tuberculosis (TB)

PLAN OF CARE	HOME CARE Visit 1
Diagnostic tests	• Complete blood count • Purified protein derivative testing of family and contacts
Medications	• Evaluate for adverse effects of drug therapy. • Evaluate compliance with drug regimen and develop an action plan as needed to increase adherence to the medication regimen. • Explain the need to avoid over-the-counter medication without physician approval.
Procedures	• Check vital signs. • Assess breath sounds and signs of difficulty breathing. • Assess presence of diaphoresis and night sweats. • Observe the patient's deep breathing exercises and postural drainage. • Assess maintenance of respiratory isolation. • Assess proper and safe use of any respiratory therapy equipment.
Diet	• Have patient force fluids to 2 to 3 L/day if tolerated. • Assess weight and nutritional intake. • Encourage a high-protein, high-carbohydrate diet. • Refer to dietary consult if indicated.
Activity	• Assess response to activity. • Explain the importance of frequent rest periods.
Elimination	• Evaluate fluid intake. • Instruct to keep daily weight and fluid intake log.
Hygiene	• Assess home for sanitary equipment necessary for good hygiene: disposable waste bags and covered trash containers. • Assess home for sleeping conditions, crowding, persons with upper respiratory infections (URIs), children, elderly, and others susceptible to infection.
Patient teaching	• Discuss signs and symptoms to report to the physician • Discuss medication (name, dosage, purpose, and adverse effects). • Instruct patient to avoid crowds and persons with URIs • Teach respiratory isolation techniques. • Explain the importance of hygiene measures and hand washing.
Discharge planning	• Assess home support and resource needs (for example, economic means to purchase medications and supplies and to maintain isolation in home until acceptable medication levels are attained). • Refer to appropriate agency or social services as indicated.

Visit 2	Visit 3
• Arterial blood gases (referral to physician if indicated) • Chest X-ray (referral to physician if indicated)	• Same as previous visit
• Repeat care given at previous visit.	• Repeat care given at previous visit.
• Repeat care given at previous visit.	• Repeat care given at previous visit.
• Review laboratory work with the patient and family. • Reinforce previous visit. • Explain the importance of diet maintenance.	• Reinforce previous visit.
• Reinforce previous visit.	• Reinforce previous visit.
• Evaluate daily weight and fluid intake log.	• Evaluate daily weight and fluid intake log.
• Repeat care given at previous visit.	• Repeat care given at previous visit.
• Discuss causes and treatment of TB. • Reinforce previous teaching. • Evaluate the maintenance of respiratory isolation. • Explain the importance of regular follow-up care.	• Reinforce and evaluate teaching sessions from previous home visits.
• Assess home support and resource needs.	• Repeat care given at previous visit.

Sepsis

PLAN OF CARE	HOME CARE Visit 1
Diagnostic tests	• Complete blood count • Electrolyte levels • Blood urea nitrogen • Creatinine level
Medications	• Administer I.V. anti-infective as prescribed or assess compliance with oral anti-infectives.
Procedures	• Perform comprehensive assessments to establish baseline.
Diet	• Assess compliance with diet high in protein, carbohydrates, and calories. • Weigh the patient.
Activity	• Evaluate tolerance for exercise and activities of daily living.
Elimination	• Assess for urinary tract infection.
Hygiene	• Evaluate the need for home care aide services.
Patient teaching	• Teach about anti-infective therapy (take as prescribed, follow dosage schedule, and don't skip doses).
Discharge planning	• Assess home support and resource needs (financial ability to purchase anti-infectives; and medical equipment needs).

Visit 2	Visit 3
None	None
• Repeat care given at previous visit.	• Repeat care given at previous visit.
• Review results of laboratory work with the patient, family, and physician. • Assess vital signs, particularly temperature. • Evaluate any wounds for signs of infection. • Evaluate the I.V. site if present. • Assess for cough and sputum characteristics.	• Repeat care given at previous visit. • Reassess vital signs, lungs, and cardiovascular systems. • Assess mental status.
• Assess for anorexia, nausea, and vomiting. • Determine weight change. • Assess compliance with diet.	• Repeat care given at previous visit.
• Repeat care given at previous visit.	• Repeat care given at previous visit.
• Repeat care given at previous visit.	• Repeat care given at previous visit.
• Assist as needed.	• Repeat care given at previous visit.
• Provide teaching specific to the patient's risk for sepsis. • Discuss the importance of complying with the diet, exercise, and medication regimen.	• Reinforce and evaluate teaching sessions from previous home visits.
• Assess home support and resource needs.	• Reinforce the importance of keeping follow-up appointments.

Total knee replacement

PLAN OF CARE	HOME CARE Visit 1
Diagnostic tests	• Prothrombin time (PT) • International normalized ratio (INR)
Medications	• Assess effectiveness and adverse effects of analgesics for pain relief and anticoagulants to prevent blood clots. • Assess compliance with the therapeutic regimen.
Procedures	• Check vital signs and physical assessment. • Assess the incision site for drainage and the condition of the surrounding tissue. • Assess incision care. • Assess safety needs in home environment. • Assess the affected leg for color, motion, edema, and sensation.
Diet	• Assess food and fluid intake.
Activity	• Assess mobility status. • Assess patient walking at least 70′ (21 m) with assistive device. • Assess patient's performance of muscle strengthening exercises. • Assess transfer and ambulation techniques.
Elimination	• Assess elimination patterns and need for laxatives.
Hygiene	• Assess the ability to perform activities of daily living.
Patient teaching	• Evaluate comprehension of in-hospital teaching. • Teach appropriate transfer and ambulation safety precautions. • Teach incision care. • Teach the importance of progressive ambulation. • Instruct to follow in-home physical therapy program. • Instruct to progressively increase exercise activities. • Teach safe technique for immobilizer application (if ordered). • Teach how to rewrap the elastic bandage. • Teach safe use of ice packs to knee every 20 to 30 minutes for swelling, pain, or stiffness. • Teach signs and symptoms (S/S) to report to the physician. • Teach home safety measures. • Teach nonpharmacologic pain relief measures and medication instruction.
Discharge planning	• Consult with a physical therapist, if needed. • Assess access to phone communication with durable medical equipment company. • Assess availability of appropriate assistive devices. • Consult with social services if needed.

Visit 2	Visit 3
• PT • INR • Complete blood count	• PT • INR
• Repeat care given at previous visit.	• Repeat care given at previous visit.
• Repeat care given at previous visit.	• Repeat care given at previous visit.
• Repeat care given at previous visit.	• Repeat care given at previous visit.
• Repeat care given at previous visit.	• Repeat care given at previous visit.
• Repeat care given at previous visit.	• Repeat care given at previous visit.
• Repeat care given at previous visit.	• Repeat care given at previous visit.
• Reinforce previous teaching. • Observe patient and family performing incision care. • Observe patient using safety measures in transfer and ambulation. • Observe patient and family compliance with home safety measures. • Observe patient and family performing application of immobilizer (if ordered), elastic bandage rewrap, and ice pack. • Reevaluate safety in the home.	• Reinforce previous teaching.
• Explain the importance of follow-up care. • Assist with arrangements for follow-up visits.	• Assess patient's and family's understanding of importance of follow-up care.

Urinary incontinence

PLAN OF CARE	HOME CARE Visit 1
Diagnostic tests	• Urinalysis • Catheterization for residual urine if indicated
Medications	• Assess the effectiveness and adverse effects of medication. • Assess compliance with drug therapy.
Procedures	• Check vital signs. • Observe the patient performing catheter care.
Diet	• Assess compliance with weight reduction diet. • Refer to nutrition consult if indicated. • Assess fluid intake.
Activity	• Assess exercise program (Kegel exercises). • Assess patient's performance on activities of daily living. • Assess bladder training program.
Elimination	• Assess intake and output. • Assess catheter patency and leakage.
Hygiene	• Assess skin integrity. • Assess catheter site. • Assess control of urine odor.
Patient teaching	• Teach signs and symptoms (S/S) of skin impairment, early action to take, and when to report to physician. • Reinforce establishment and maintenance of voiding program. • Encourage performance of exercise program (Kegel exercises) daily if appropriate. • Review techniques to control urine odor. • Teach catheter care if appropriate (site cleaning, checking for patency, self-catheterization, storage and cleaning of equipment, catheter removal). • Discuss medications (name, dosage, purpose, time and route of administration, and adverse effects).
Discharge planning	• Assess home support and resource needs (for example, economic status to purchase medication and equipment). • Refer to appropriate agency or social services as indicated.

Visit 2	Visit 3
• Urine culture and sensitivity if indicated	• Same as previous visit
• Assess for effectiveness and adverse effects of drug therapy.	• Repeat care given at previous visit.
• Repeat care given at previous visit.	• Repeat care given at previous visit.
• Repeat care given at previous visit.	• Repeat care given at previous visit.
• Repeat care given at previous visit.	• Repeat care given at previous visit.
• Repeat care given at previous visit.	• Repeat care given at previous visit.
• Repeat care given at previous visit.	• Repeat care given at previous visit.
• Teach about incontinence, especially the patient's specific type; urine retention; S/S of bladder distention; catheter function; and problem solving. • Reinforce the need to evaluate episodes of incontinence for precipitating factors and to make changes in schedules and training as necessary. • Instruct the patient to report continued incontinence.	• Reinforce and evaluate previous teaching sessions. • Stress the need for regular follow-up care.
• Repeat care given at previous visit.	• Repeat care given at previous visit.

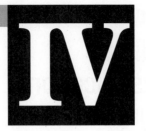

PART

IV

Appendices

APPENDIX A

Fifth-digit subclassification of diagnoses

To ensure appropriately detailed documentation for quality assurance and billing purposes, use the fifth-digit subclassifications listed below for the appropriate categories. More detailed information about ICD-9-CM and ICD-10-CM is available on the World Health Organization Web site at *www.who.int.*

Abdominal and pelvic symptoms

For use with categories 789.0, 789.3, 789.4, and 789.6:
0 Unspecified site
1 Right upper quadrant
2 Left upper quadrant
3 Right lower quadrant
4 Left lower quadrant
5 Periumbilic
6 Epigastric
7 Generalized
9 Other specified site (includes multiple sites)

Abuse, substance (including alcoholism)

For use with categories 303, 305.0, and 305.2 through 305.9:
0 Unspecified
1 Continuous
2 Episodic
3 In remission

Affective psychoses

For use with categories 296.0 through 296.6:
0 Unspecified
1 Mild
2 Moderate
3 Severe, without mention of psychotic behavior
4 Severe, specified as with psychotic behavior
5 In partial or unspecified remission
6 In full remission

Asthma

For use with category 493:
0 Without mention of status asthmaticus
1 With status asthmaticus (therapy doesn't reduce symptoms)

Burns

For use with category 948 to denote percentage of body surface with third-degree burns:
0 Less than 10 percent or unspecified
1 10 to 19 percent
2 20 to 29 percent
3 30 to 39 percent
4 40 to 49 percent
5 50 to 59 percent
6 60 to 69 percent
7 70 to 79 percent
8 80 to 89 percent
9 90 percent or more of body surface

Diabetes mellitus

For use with category 250:
0 Type 2 or unspecified (non-insulin-dependent or adult onset), controlled
1 Type 1 (insulin-dependent or juvenile onset), controlled
2 Type 2 (non-insulin-dependent or adult onset), uncontrolled
3 Type 1 (insulin-dependent or juvenile onset), uncontrolled

Epilepsy

For use with categories 345.0, 345.1, and 345.4 through 345.9:
0 Without mention of intractable epilepsy
1 With intractable epilepsy (resistant to medication)

Fracture of vertebral column without spinal cord injury

For use with categories 805.0 and 805.1 to specify affected cervical vertebrae:
0 Unspecified level
1 First
2 Second
3 Third
4 Fourth
5 Fifth
6 Sixth
7 Seventh
8 Multiple

Gastritis and duodenitis

For use with category 535:
0 Without mention of hemorrhage
1 With hemorrhage

Hemiplegia and hemiparesis

For use with categories 342.0 through 342.9:
0 Affecting unspecified side
1 Affecting dominant side
2 Affecting nondominant side

Hepatitis B

For use with categories 070.2 and 070.3:
0 Acute or unspecified, without mention of hepatitis D
1 Acute or unspecified, with hepatitis D
2 Chronic, without mention of hepatitis D
3 Chronic, with hepatitis D

Hypertensive heart and renal disease

For use with category 404:
0 Without mention of heart or renal failure
1 With heart failure
2 With renal failure
3 With heart and renal failure

Hypertensive renal disease

For use with category 403:
0 Without mention of renal failure
1 With renal failure

Intracranial injury

For use with categories 851 through 854:
0 Specified state of consciousness
1 With no loss of consciousness (LOC)
2 With brief (less than 1 hour) LOC
3 With moderate (1 to 24 hours) LOC
4 With prolonged (more than 24 hours) LOC and return to preexisting level of consciousness
5 With prolonged (more than 24 hours) LOC and without return to preexisting level of consciousness
6 With LOC of unspecified duration
9 With concussion, unspecified

Malignant neoplasm of lymphatic and hematopoietic tissue

For use with categories 200 through 202:
0 Unspecified site, extranodal and solid organ sites
1 Lymph nodes of head, face, and neck
2 Intrathoracic lymph nodes
3 Intra-abdominal lymph nodes
4 Lymph nodes of axilla and upper-limb
5 Lymph nodes of inguinal region and lower limb
6 Intrapelvic lymph nodes
7 Spleen
8 Lymph nodes of multiple sites

Multiple myeloma and immunoproliferative neoplasms

For use with categories 203 through 208:
0 Without mention of remission
1 Remission (symptoms reduced in degree or intensity)

Musculoskeletal system and connective tissue diseases

For use with categories 711, 712, 715, 716, 718, 719, and 730:
0 Site unspecified
1 Shoulder region
2 Upper arm
3 Forearm
4 Hand
5 Pelvic region and thigh
6 Lower leg
7 Ankle and foot
8 Other specified sites (such as head, neck, and trunk)
9 Multiple sites

Myocardial infarction, acute

For use with category 410:
0 Episode of care unspecified
1 Initial episode of care (first episode of care for a newly diagnosed myocardial infarction [MI])
2 Treatment for an MI that has received initial treatment but is still less than 8 weeks old

Perinatal conditions

For use with categories 764 through 765 (to denote birthweight):
0 Unspecified weight
1 Less than 500 g (1.1 lbs)
2 500 to 749 g (1.11 to 1.67 lbs)
3 750 to 999 g (1.68 to 2.23 lbs)
4 1,000 to 1,249 g (2.24 to 2.78 lbs)
5 1,250 to 1,499 g (2.79 to 3.34 lbs)
6 1,500 to 1,749 g (3.35 to 3.9 lbs)
7 1,750 to 1,999 g (3.91 to 4.5 lbs)
8 2,000 to 2,499 g (4.51 to 5.59 lbs)
9 2,500 g or more (5.6 lbs)

Precerebral artery occlusion and stenosis

For use with category 433:
0 Without mention of cerebral infarction
1 With cerebral infarction

Pregnancy, labor, and delivery

For use with categories 640 to 648, 651 to 659, and 670 to 676:
0 Unspecified as to episode of care or not applicable
1 Delivered, with or without mention of antepartum condition
2 Delivered, with mention of post-partum complication
3 Antepartum condition or complication
4 Postpartum condition or complication

Schizophrenic disorders

For use with category 295:
0 Unspecified
1 Subchronic
2 Chronic
3 Subchronic with acute exacerbation
4 Chronic with acute exacerbation
5 In remission

Spina bifida

For use with category 741:
0 Unspecified region
1 Cervical region
2 Dorsal (thoracic) region
3 Lumbar region

Tuberculosis

For use with categories 010 to 018:
0 Unspecified
1 Bacteriological or histological examination not done
2 Bacteriological or histological examination unknown (at present)
3 Tubercle bacilli found (in sputum) by microscopy
4 Tubercle bacilli found by bacterial culture
5 Tuberculosis confirmed histologically
6 Tuberculosis confirmed by other methods (inoculation of animals)

Ulcer, gastric, duodenal, peptic, or gastrojejunal

For use with category 531 to 534:
0 Without mention of obstruction
1 With obstruction

Hospice care

Hospice refers to a concept of care, a team approach with a core philosophy of allowing patients the ability to choose how they will spend their final months with as much freedom from pain as possible. It's a special system of care for a terminally ill patient whose life expectancy is 6 months or less.

Hospice isn't about dying. Rather, it's about enhancing the quality of a person's life with an emphasis on the dignity and strength of the patient and his family. Hospice team members give care when a cure is no longer possible; that is, the patient is no longer receiving treatment toward a cure. One major goal of hospice is to help patients and their families find a sense of peace.

Hospice and care delivery

The hospice concept is a system of medical, emotional, and spiritual care. This care is directed largely by the patient and his loved ones in conjunction with a physician and the hospice team, which includes physicians, nurses, social workers, home care aides, spiritual counselors, volunteers, and occupational, physical, and speech therapists. Medical treatment focuses on the patient's physical comfort and mental alertness. Although all hospices have one or more physicians on their team, a patient's personal physician is encouraged to continue caring for the patient in addition to the hospice team.

Patients and their caregivers have access to hospice team members on an on-call basis 24 hours per day, 7 days per week.

General requirements for a hospice agency

Requirements for hospice agencies vary depending on state and local laws and mandates. The list below presents general requirements based on federal standards for operation. For a more detailed and complete list, refer to the operation standards from state and local licensing agencies and the Code of Federal Regulations. In general, a hospice agency must:

• be a public agency or private organization primarily engaged in providing care to terminally ill individuals (life expectancy of 6 months or less if the illness runs its normal course)

• have a medical director who is employed by the agency and who is a doctor of medicine or osteopathy

• provide nursing services, physician services, drugs, and biologicals routinely on a 24-hour basis

• provide for all other covered services on a 24-hour basis to the extent necessary to meet the needs of the patient and reasonably achieve management and palliation of the terminal illness and other related conditions

• provide bereavement counseling

- provide all services in a manner consistent with accepted standards of practice, including documentation requirements (federal, state, and local laws and mandates)
- establish a written plan of care that must be reviewed and updated at specified intervals
- designate an interdisciplinary group or groups composed of individuals who provide or supervise care (should at least include a doctor of medicine or osteopathy, registered nurse, social worker, pastoral or other counselor, and home care aide)
- provide ongoing training for employees and volunteers
- use and maintain a volunteer staff to provide administrative or direct patient care in an amount that equals at least five percent of patient care hours of all paid hospice employees and contact staff
- make reasonable efforts to arrange for visits of clergy or members of other religious organizations if requested by the patient and advise the patient of availability of this service
- be licensed if state or local law provides for licensing of hospices
- keep clinical records in accordance with federal, state, and local standards of operation
- provide nursing care and services under the supervision of a registered nurse (for exceptions to this, see Code of Federal Regulations, Title 42, Chapter IV, part 418.83)
- provide medical social services by a qualified social worker and under the direction of a physician
- make counseling services available to the patient and family members, including bereavement, dietary, spiritual, and any other counseling needs necessary to meet identified problems
- provide physical, occupational, and speech therapy as needed
- make homemaker and home care aide services available and frequent enough to meet the needs of the patient
- provide medical supplies and appliances, including drugs and biologicals, for palliation and management of the terminal illness (this will vary depending on the reimbursement agency)
- arrange for or provide inpatient care for pain control, symptom management, and respite services.

Payment for hospice

Medicare, Medicaid, and the Civilian Health and Medical Programs for the Uniformed Services all have special hospice benefits. Most other private insurance companies and health plans also have some form of hospice coverage. Because these plans vary, written confirmation of coverage should be obtained before starting service. Hospice care and services aren't limited to a home environment. They can be provided in other settings, such as hospitals, long-term care facilities, and hospice residential facilities.

Accreditation

Most home health care agencies now have a hospice program that operates as part of their services, a benefit that allows a smooth transition from regular home health care into hospice care. Thus, patients and families don't have to make the adjustment to a new agency.

An increase in hospice agencies has resulted in many insurance companies looking for some measurement of quality and certification on a national level. Regulations for hospice agencies vary greatly from state to state and region to region. Currently, only the Joint Commission on Accreditation of Healthcare Organizations and the Social Security Administration (Medicare) have national accrediting standards for hospice agencies. More and more independent insurance companies are relying on these standards as conditions for participation and reimbursement for services. Other agencies, such as the National Hospice Organization, represent the interests of American hospices in Congress and the general public but aren't regulatory or accrediting agencies. Membership in these national agencies is recommended as a resource for networking, education, information, and support.

Hospice team requirements

Hospice team education and training requirements vary according to state and local mandates. Federal law, which must be followed if serving Medicare patients (see Code of Federal Regulations, Title 42, Part 418, Sections 418.50 to 418.72), states that all hospice team members must have valid licenses in their field of practice (if a license is required to practice). Additionally, the medical director must be a hospice employee who is a doctor of medicine or osteopathy, and orientation and training must be consistent with acceptable standards of hospice practice.

A hospice must provide an ongoing program for training its employees. Although volunteer training requirements vary from state to state and region to region, in most cases a minimum of 22 hours of training is required.

Hospice nursing certification

Registered nurses may seek certification as hospice nurses from the National Board for Certification of Hospice and Palliative Nurses (NBCHPN). This certification is a written examination offered in most states twice per year (March and September). To sit for certification, a registered nurse must be currently licensed in the United States or the equivalent in Canada. The NBCHPN recommends that a candidate have at least 2 years of experience in hospice and palliative nursing because the examination content is based on the competencies normally achieved through 2 years of practice in end-of-life care.

Patient requirements for admission

For a patient to be eligible for hospice services, a physician must give written certification that the patient's life expectancy is 6 months or less if the illness runs its normal course. When certification has been made, the patient (or his representative) must sign a statement that contains the following:
• name of the hospice service that will provide care
• patient's or representative's acknowledgment that he has been given a full understanding of the palliative rather than curative nature of hospice care, especially as it relates to the individual's terminal illness
• acknowledgment of the extent of insurance reimbursement and any co-pays or financial responsibilities
• effective date of service.

State and local mandates may require additions to or expansions of these statements. This information can be obtained from state and local licensing agencies.

Revocation of hospice care

A patient or his representative may revoke the election of hospice care at any time. For this to occur, a statement must be filed with the servicing hospice that includes the following:
• name of patient or representative and the servicing hospice
• date the revocation is to be effective (the patient or representative may not designate an effective date earlier than the date the revocation is made)
• statement acknowledging that the patient or representative comprehends that all hospice care will end on the revocation date (a patient can be reinstated into hospice care at any time if he meets initial hospice criteria)
• patient's or representative's signature.

Change to another agency

A patient or representative may elect to change hospice agencies. Some reimbursement agencies have set limits on how often this may occur in a certification period. For example, Medicare states that this may occur once in each election period. To change hospice agencies, the patient or representative must file a signed statement with the hospice from which care has been received and the newly designated hospice. The statement should include the following information:
• name of the hospice from which the patient has received care and the name

of the hospice from which he plans to receive care
• date the change is to be effective.

Common concerns and guidelines

Hospice patients, caregivers, and family members all have special needs that should be addressed by the hospice nurse or other team members. A thorough assessment of the care environment and patient-family relationships is necessary. The patient and his family may require counseling services as well as the services of community agencies for financial assistance, respite, and group support. An assessment of the patient's cultural and spiritual beliefs about death, dying, and burial should also be made. A nurse isn't expected to know all the different cultural and religious practices she may encounter but she should be aware of practices and traditions to which a patient or his family may adhere. She should use the resources of local clergy and cultural centers to meet these diverse needs.

Throughout a patient's hospice care, various situations commonly develop that may require advanced planning or prompt intervention. It seems that these concerns commonly occur *after* typical agency operating hours. However, because the hospice team is available 24 hours per day, 7 days per week, awareness of these situations and use of specific guidelines helps to promote the patient's well-being.

After-hours medication needs

After hours medication need should be addressed *before* such a situation arises. To prepare, the following guidelines are helpful:

- Work with a hospice pharmaceutical provider. More and more hospice agencies are working with national pharmaceutical providers that focus solely on meeting the needs of terminally ill patients, providing not only medication but up-to-date information on palliative care and medication use guidelines. They commonly assist a hospice agency in acquiring standing orders that cover in-home starter or emergency kits. They can also make local pharmacy connections for after-hours emergency medications. These agencies normally charge a per-day, per-patient rate that is lower than individual medication costs.

- Obtain standing orders and an in-home starter or emergency kit . The kit provides for after-hours increases in medication and changes in the plan of care, such as adding an antianxiety drug for restlessness or an antiemetic for nausea or vomiting. The kit can reduce the number of unnecessary visits and after-hours physician calls.

- If possible, arrange with a local pharmacy for after-hours emergency service for hospice medications, or check with the local physician or hospital pharmacy about obtaining medications during the middle of the night and on holidays. These actions are often very appropriate for patients living in rural areas, but arrangements need to be made in advance and in writing to save confusion and frustration.

Inadequate pain relief

To address inadequate pain relief for hospice patients, the following guidelines are helpful:

- Obtain a standing order for analgesia that includes parameters for increasing pain medication or phoning an on-call provider for an order.
- Assess for other causes of pain such as anxiety. (Teaming antianxiety drugs with analgesics is often more effective than using analgesics alone.)
- Obtain standing orders and an in-home starter or emergency kit or the phone number of a 24-hour pharmacy.
- Obtain an order and document any increase or change in medication, the patient's reaction to medication, and when pain will be reassessed. Reassessment should occur within the "peak action" time of the medication (taking into consideration the patient's age and condition). Also, document any other support methods used by the patient or caregiver, such as distraction, visualization, and change of position.

Nausea and vomiting

To address nausea and vomiting, the following guidelines are helpful:

- Assess for the cause of nausea, such as constipation or bowel obstruction, medication adverse effects, anxiety, and the disease process.
- If constipation is present, use a standing order or obtain a new order for restoring bowel function from the on-call provider.
- If vomiting is the problem, use a standing order or obtain a new order for an antiemetic from the on-call provider.
- Obtain standing orders and an in-home starter or emergency kit or the phone number of a 24-hour pharmacy.
- Document the order, assessment findings, support methods (such as an enema) used to assist with alleviating nau-

sea or vomiting, the patient's reaction to the medication, and when reassessment will occur. Reassessment should occur within the "peak action" time of the medication (taking into consideration the patient's age and condition).

Death of the patient

Patient and family preparations

To address the patient's pending death, the following guidelines are helpful:

• Assess the patient's condition and how close he appears to death during the visit.

• Determine what the patient and family know and comprehend regarding hospice service and palliative care.

• Assess what the patient and family want and expect.

• Find out what interventions are already being used and what support services are in place.

• Assess the patient's cultural and religious beliefs and traditions and whether arrangements have been made to accommodate them.

• Determine whether the patient and family are making plans or whether they're still in denial.

• Encourage the patient and family to preplan the funeral and put plans in writing.

• If possible, determine the person who will be designated to make the telephone call to the funeral home and home care agency.

• Assess how family members and the patient communicate with each other and the professional staff; assist in this communication when needed.

• Suggest that the patient write letters or make a video for family members and help him, if necessary.

• Evaluate which ethical, financial, and social decisions the patient and family have to make.

• Inform the family and patient about the community resources that are available to them.

• Allow family members and the patient time to verbalize concerns, fears, and grief.

• Teach the family and caregivers about pain control, comfort measures, diet, medications, hydration, palliative care, skin care, the indwelling urinary catheter, oxygen, suction, and I.V. therapy.

• Document all identified issues and instructions as well as patient, caregiver, and family responses. Document all referrals and any conferences with supportive services.

What the family should do

To address what the family should do to prepare for the patient's death, the following guidelines are helpful:

• Post written instructions in the home next to the phone. (They should be simple and bulleted, in bold lettering.)

• Review with the family and the caregiver what to do when the patient dies.

• Describe everyone's role, including the steps to be performed by the nurse right after death.

• Make sure the caregiver and family members know what to expect and what will occur at the moment of death.

• Document instructions given and the family's comprehension of and reaction to them. Be specific, documenting individual family members' responses.

When the patient dies

To address what should happen when the patient dies, the following guidelines are helpful:

• Follow the agency protocol, which is based on federal, state, and local laws and mandates.

• Advise the designated family member to call the funeral home and hospice agency to inform them of the patient's death.

Do-not-resuscitate order

To address a do-not-resuscitate (DNR) order, the following guidelines are helpful:

• The physician and the patient or his representative sign a DNR order, usually at the time of admission into hospice care. A copy of the order must be kept in the patient's home as well as in the agency's medical records. The physician should also keep a copy.

• Inform the family that if they take a hospice patient to the emergency room or call an ambulance, the DNR may not be honored. Paramedics and other emergency responders working outside the hospital generally have a duty to provide cardiopulmonary and other forms of resuscitation when needed.

Over half of the states now have "prehospital" DNR programs so that a physician's DNR order can be honored outside of the hospital setting. The state's Emergency Medical Services department or state medical associations usually administer these programs. The programs vary from state to state, but some common features include:

• standardized documents that responders can recognize quickly, which may be posted prominently in the home (responders know to look for them)

• DNR bracelets or medallions that communicate to the responder the DNR status (responders are trained to look for these)

• physician involvement (a physician generally must sign DNR orders before responders will honor them)

• nonwithholding of comfort treatment (responders are still required to alleviate pain)

• documentation (for any questions or discussions with family members, the patient, or the physician regarding DNR orders, a copy must be kept in the medical record).

Bereavement follow-up and care

Bereavement follow-up and care typically continue for 1 year after the patient dies. These services extend to the patient's family and significant caregiver. To address this concern, the following guidelines are helpful:

• Make the initial bereavement visit at the time of the patient's death.

• If possible, attend the patient's funeral or memorial service, which comes under the scope of bereavement care (This action is recommended but not required.)

• Offer the services of support groups, counseling services, and other community resources to the bereaved.

• Follow up with phone calls according to the agency's policy.

• Document each contact or visit with the bereaved and their responses, referrals or conferences with support services, and the bereaved's progress through the grief process.

When the patient is a child

When the hospice patient is a child, the hospice nurse must address special concerns beyond the standard ones.

Safety of patient and siblings

To address the safety of the patient and his siblings, the following guidelines are helpful:

- Keep all medications in a locked cupboard.
- Teach standard precautions for prevention and spread of infection to the patient, siblings, and parents.
- Don't assume that the parents will teach younger children about precautions as a matter of routine. For example, teach younger children to wash hands thoroughly and cover the mouth when coughing and sneezing.
- Document all teaching and responses as well as safety measures instituted.

Sibling confusion about death

To address feelings of confusion the patient's sibling may have about death, the following guidelines are helpful:

- Provide counseling for siblings.
- Enlist the aid of school guidance counselors as appropriate.
- Encourage all hospice team members, including social workers, volunteers, and clergy, to interact with siblings during home visits to assess for confusion, determine their needs, and provide support.
- Encourage parents to include siblings in the treatment plan; inclusion during the dying process often makes it easier for siblings to be included in the grief process and assists with holding together the family structure.
- Document identified concerns and interventions used to assist with or alleviate these concerns as well as the responses to interventions.

Sibling's loss of parental contact

To address the sibling's loss of parental contact, the following guidelines are helpful:

- Encourage parents to take turns with care of the patient and care of siblings. Commonly, one parent becomes the primary patient caregiver and siblings begin to crave attention from that parent. (The reverse may also be true.)
- Provide volunteer or extended family support to care for the patient on a regularly scheduled basis, thus allowing time for the parent to interact with the siblings. In single-parent homes, the parent is often so involved with caring for the dying child that siblings are often unintentionally overlooked.
- Encourage parents to use this time to play, read to, and shop with siblings.
- Document identified concerns and interventions used to assist with or alleviate concern and responses to interventions.

Bereavement follow-up

To address bereavement follow-up, the following guidelines are helpful:

- Arrange for a referral for individual grief counseling.
- Refer the family to support groups for siblings and parents.
- Contact school counselors, teachers, and the principal for in-school assistance with grief and possible assistance with class work.
- Encourage parents to allow siblings time to talk with them about their deceased brother or sister.
- Urge the parents to include siblings in funeral preparations and service (as much as is age-appropriate).
- Remember that children have the same need to grieve as adults do.
- Document identified concerns and referrals to and conferences with schools and support services. Also, document family responses to referrals and suggested interventions.

Resources for professionals, patients, and caregivers

General Web sites for health care professionals and patients

* *www.healthfinder.gov* — From the U.S. government, this large searchable database has links to Web sites, support groups, government agencies, and not-for-profit organizations that provide health care information for patients.

* *http://healthweb.org* — From a group of librarians and information professionals at academic medical centers in the Midwest, this site offers a searchable database of evaluated Web sites for patients and health care professionals.

* *www.medmatrix.org/reg/login. asp* — This site includes journal articles, abstracts, reviews, conference highlights, and links to other major sources for health care professionals.

* *www.mwsearch.com* — Medical World Search searches thousands of selected medical sites for you.

* *www.wellweb.com* — Wellness Web, The Patient's Network is designed for patients. This site includes conventional as well as complementary medicine, nutrition, and fitness information.

Organizations

* *www.aafp.com* — American Academy of Family Physicians, includes "Family Medicine Online," offering handouts and other resources to patients and health care professionals as well as links to other sites

* *www.jcaho.org* — Joint Commission on Accreditation of Healthcare Organizations (JCAHO)

* *www.healthcareforums.com* — Worldwide Healthcare Forum for healthcare professionals worldwide; in English as well as Spanish, French, and German

Government agencies

* Specialized Information Services and U.S. Government Resources (online listing of government bureaus with links to their sites), *http://sis.nlm.nih. gov/tehwwg.htm*

* Department of Health and Human Services (DHHS), *www.dhhs.gov*

* Administration on Aging, *www.aoa.dhhs.gov*

- Agency for Health Care Policy and Research and National Guideline Clearinghouse, *www.ahcpr.gov. Note:* name has been changed to the Agency for Healthcare Research and Quality (AHRQ, pronounced "arc"). AHRQ also has additional functions. TDD (888) 586-6340 (hearing impaired only)
- Centers for Disease Control and Prevention, *www.cdc.gov.* Also check under entries for diseases, injuries and disabilities, health risks, and prevention guidelines.
- Food and Drug Administration, *www.fda.gov*
- Health Care Financing Administration (HCFA), *www.hcfa.gov*
- National Center for Complementary and Alternative Therapy, *http://nccam.nih.gov*

- National Board for Certification of Hospice and Palliative Nurses: *hpna.org/NBCHN/nbchpn_main.htm*
- Hospice Patients Alliance: *www.hospicepatients.org*
- Death, What You Can Expect: *www.emanon.net/~kcabell*
- Death, Dying, and Grief: *www.betterknown.com* (click on life events, then death and dying)

Links to Spanish language sites
- CancerNet: *cancernet.nci.nih.gov/sp_menu.htm*
- Healthfinder: *www.healthfinder.com* (click on espanol)
- Vaccination schedule for adults: *www.immunize.org*

Home health care
- American Federation of Home Health Agencies (AFHHA): *www.his.com/~afhha/usa.html*
- Home Care Association of America (HCAA): *www.hcaa-homecare.com*
- Home Health Care Nurse Web Page: *http://junior.apk.net/~nurse*
- National Association for Home Care (NAHC): *www.nahc.org*

Hospice
- National Hospice Organization Standards and Accreditation Committee Medical Guidelines Task Force: To find hospice in patient's area, call (800) 658-8888.
- National Hospice Organization, *www.nho.org:* (800) 658-8898
- *Code of Federal Regulations,* Title 42, Volume 2, Parts 400 to 429: *www.hospicepatients.org/law.html*

Condition-specific sites

AIDS/HIV/STDs
- Centers for Disease Control and Prevention, Division of HIV and AIDS Prevention: *www.cdc.gov/nchstp/hiv_aids/dhap.htm*
- National Prevention Information Network (formerly the National AIDS Clearinghouse): *http://www.cdcnpin.org*
- HIV and AIDS Treatment Information Service: *sis.nlm.nih.gov/aids/aidstrea.html, www.hivatis.org,* (800) TRIALS-A, (800) 448-0440 (Spanish available) TTY (888) 430-3739

- JAMA Women's Health Sexually Transmitted Disease Information Center: *www.ama-assn.org/special/std/std.htm*
- National AIDS Hotline: (800) 342-AIDS; Spanish (800) 344-SIDA; TTY (800) 243-7889
- Office of AIDS Research (OAR): *http://sis.nlm.nih.gov/aids/oar.html*

Allergies and asthma

- Allergy and Asthma Network Mothers of Asthmatics: *www.aanma.org*
- Allergy, Asthma, and Immunology Online: *www.allergy.mcg.edu*
- American Academy of Allergy, Asthma, and Immunology: *www.aaaai.org*
- Allergy and Asthma Disease Management Center: *www.aaaai.org/aadmc*
- Global Initiative for Asthma: A Pocket Guide for Physicians and Nurses: *www.ginasthma.com/PRACTICAL/PRACTICAL.HTML*
- JAMA's Asthma Information Center: *www.ama-assn.org/special/asthma*
- National Institute of Allergy and Infectious Diseases: *www.niaid.nih.gov*

Aging

- Agency on Aging: *www.aoa.dhhs.gov*
- American Society on Aging (ASA): *www.asaging.org*
- National Institute on Aging: *www.nih.gov/nia*, (800) 222-2225; TTY (800) 222-4225

Alzheimer's disease

- AHCPR's Clinical Guidelines and Patient and Family Guide: *www.ahcpr.gov/clinic/alzcons.htm*
- AHCPR's Recognition and Assessment Guideline: *www.ahcpr.gov/clinic/alzover.htm*
- Alzheimer Europe: *www.alzheimer-europe.org*
- Alzheimer's Association: *www.alz.org*
- Alzheimer's Disease Education and Referral (ADEAR): *www.alzheimers.org*
- AlzWell Caregiver Page: *www.alzwell.com*
- Rush Alzheimer's Disease Center: *www.rush.edu/Departments/Alzheimers*

Arthritis

- American Autoimmune Related Diseases Association, Inc. (AARDA): *www.aarda.org*
- American College of Rheumatology: *www.rheumatology.org*
- Arthritis Foundation: *www.arthritis.org*
- National Institute of Arthritis and Musculoskeletal and Skin Diseases: *www.nih.gov/niams*

Attention deficit (hyperactivity) disorder

- ADD links: *www.cadvision.com/pchoate/links.htm*
- Children and Adults with Attention-Deficit Disorder: *www.chadd.org*
- Internet Resources for Special Children (IRSC): *www.irsc.org*
- National Attention Deficit Disorder Association: *www.add.org*
- University of Virginia/ Office of Special Education: Attention Deficit Disorder links: *http://teis.virginia.edu:0080/go/cise/ose/categories*

Cancer

- American Cancer Society: *www.cancer.org*, (800) ACS-2345
- CancerNet (National Cancer Institute): *http://cancernet.nci.nih.gov*

• CancerLit Topic Searches (National Cancer Institute): *http://cnetdb. nci.nih.gov/cancerlit.shtml*
• Cancer News on the Net: *www.cancernews.com*
• National Center for Chronic Disease Prevention and Health Promotion: *www.cdc.gov/nccdphp/cancer.htm*
• National Comprehensive Cancer Network: *www.nccn.org*
• Y-Me, National Organization for Breast Cancer Information and Support: *www.y-me.org,* (800) 221-2141
• Cancer Care, Inc. and the National Cancer Care Foundation: *www.cancercareinc.org,* (800) 813-HOPE
• Susan G. Komen Breast Cancer Foundation: (800) 462-9273
• National Breast Cancer Awareness Month: *www.nbcam.org*
• National Cancer Institute, International Cancer Information Center: (800) 4-CANCER or (800) 422-6237
• Cancer Trials, National Cancer Institute: *http://cancertrials.nci.nih.gov.*

Cardiac
• American Heart Association, *www.americanheart.org,* (800) 242-8721
• National Stroke Association, (800) STROKES
• Mayo Health Oasis Heart Resource Center, *www.mayohealth.org*
• National Heart, Lung, and Blood Institute, *www.nhlbi.nih.gov*

Diabetes
• American Association of Diabetes Educators, *www.aadenet.org,* (800) 338-3633

• American Diabetes Association: *www.diabetes.org,* (800) 232-3472 (membership information); *(www.diabetes.org/diabetesforecast* offers full text articles from the journal *Diabetes Care,* which publishes annual *Buyer's Guide to Diabetes Supplies* — (800) 232-6733 [to order publications])
• Diabetes self-care equipment for the visually impaired: Palco Labs: (800) 346-4488, *www.palcolabs.com;* Lighthouse: (800) 829-0500
• Joslin Diabetes Center: *www.joslin.harvard.edu/wlist.html*
• National Diabetes Information Clearinghouse: *www.niddk.nih.gov*
• National Institute of Diabetes and Digestive and Kidney Disorders: *www.niddk.nih.gov*

Disabilities
• University of Virginia, General Resources About Disabilities: *http://curry.edschool.virginia.edu/go/cise/ose/resources/general.html*
• University of Virginia, Assistive Technology Resources: *http://curry.edschool.virginia.edu/go/cise/ose/resources/asst_tech.html*

Elder abuse
• National Center on Elder Abuse (NCEA): *www.gwjapan.com/NCEA* (case-sensitive Web address)
• National Victim Center: *www.nvc.org*
• U.S. Administration on Aging, Elder Abuse Sites: *www.aoa.dhhs.gov/aoa/webres/abuse.htm*

Gastrointestinal disorders
• American Liver Foundation: (800) GO LIVER (465-4837)

- National Digestive Diseases and Education and Information Clearinghouse: *www.niddk.nih.gov,* (301) 654-3810
- National Kidney Foundation: *www.kidney.org,* (800) 622-9010

Musculoskeletal disorders

- National Osteoporosis Foundation: *www.nof.org*
- National Association of Physically Handicapped, Inc.: *www.naph.net*
- Amputee Coalition of America: (888) AMP-KNOW; (888) 267-5669
- National Institutes of Health, Osteoporosis and Bone Related National Resource Center: (800) 624-BONE
- Arthritis Answers: *www.arthritis.org,* (800) 283-7800
- American College of Foot and Ankle Surgeons: (888) 843-3338
- Amputee Support Online: *http://vandyke.digiweb.com, www.amputee-online.com* (provides information, magazines, discussion groups, addresses of support groups, and other items of interest to amputees)

Neurology

- National Institute of Neurological Disorders and Stroke (NINDS): *www.ninds.nih.gov*
- National Institute on Deafness and Other Communication Disorders (NIDCD): *www.nih.gov/nidcd*
- Association of Late-Deafened Adults, Inc., 10310 Main St., #274, Fairfax, VA 22030; TTY (404) 289-1596; Fax (404) 284-6862
- National Federation of the Blind: *www.nfb.org,* 1800 Johnson St., Baltimore, MD 21230; (410) 659-9314
- National Association of the Deaf: NADinfo@nad.org

- The EAR Foundation/The Meniere's Network *www.earfoundation.org,* 1817 Patterson St., Nashville, Tennessee 37203; (800) 545-HEAR, TDD (615) 329-7807, FAX (615) 329-7935
- The American Academy of Otolaryngology: 1 Prince St., Alexandria, VA 22314; (703) 836-4444
- American Brain Tumor Association: (800) 866-2282
- The ALS Association National Office: *www.alsa.org;* information and referral service (800) 782-4747, all others (818) 880-9007

Pediatrics

- National Institute of Child Health and Human Development (NICHD): *www.nichd.nih.gov*
- National Pediatric AIDS Network (NPAN): *www.npan.org*
- Children with Diabetes: *www.childrenwithdiabetes.com*
- United Cerebral Palsy: *www.ucpnatl@ucpa.org,* (800) 872-5827
- Cystic Fibrosis Mutation Data Base: *www.genet.sickkids.on.ca/cftr*
- CFUSA-Cystic Fibrosis USA: *www.cfusa.org*
- Cystic Fibrosis Foundation: *www.cff.org,* (800) FIGHT-CF; (800) 344-4823
- Parents of Down Syndrome, Inc.: (301) 984-5792
- Down Syndrome: *www.healthlinkusa.com/down Mdrome.htm*
- Down's Heart Group: *www.downs-heart.downsnet.org*
- Sickle Cell Information Center: *www.emory.edu* (enter "sickle cell" in the search box), (404) 616-3572
- Sickle Cell Association: *www.goHamptonRoads.com*

- Spina Bifida Association of America: *www.sbaa.org,* (800) 621-3141
- Families of S.M.A. (Spinal Muscular Atrophy): *www.fsma.org,* (800) 886-1762
- Growth and Prematurity Web site: *www.comeunity.com* (click on Prematurity)
- Growth Charts for Children with Down Syndrome Web site: *www.growthcharts.com*
- Adoption from Vietnam Growth Charts (Chinese) for boys and girls: *www.csd.net/~merlin*

Psychiatric disorders

- National Alliance for the Mentally Ill: *www.nami.org,* (800) 950-NAMI (6264)
- National Mental Health Association: *www.nmha.org,* (800) 969-6642
- Suicide Awareness and Voices of Education: *www.save.org*
- Mental Health Net: *http://mentalhelp.net*
- The Center for Mental Health Services: *www.mentalhealth.org,* (800) 789-CMHS (2647)
- American Psychological Association: *www.apa.org,* (800) 374-3120
- National Depressive and Manic Depressive Association: *www.ndmda.org,* (800) 826-3632

Respiratory disorders

- Allergy and Asthma Network, Mothers of Asthmatics: *www.aanma.org,* (800) 878-4403
- Allergy, Asthma, and Immunology Online: *www.allergy.mcg.edu*
- American Academy of Allergy, Asthma, and Immunology: *www.aaaai.org,* (800) 822-2762

- American Association for Respiratory Care: *www.aarc.org*
- American Heart Association: (800) 242-8721 (smoking cessation information)
- American Lung Association: *www.lungusa.org,* (800) LUNG-USA (local affiliates answer)
- Joint Commission of Allergy, Asthma, and Immunology: *www.jcaai.org*
- National Asthma Education and Prevention Program: *www.nhlbi.nih.gov/nhlbi/othcomp/opec/naepp/naeppage.htm*
- National Emphysema Foundation: *www.xmission.com/~gastown/herpmed/respi.htm*
- National Heart, Lung, and Blood Institute Information Center: *www.nhlbi.nih.gov,* (301) 592-8573 (information center, answered by a person)

Skin disorders

- National Pressure Ulcer Advisory Panel (NPUAP) (information on the PUSH tool and monitoring ulcers): *www.npaup.org*
- Wound, Ostomy, and Continence Nurses Society: *www.wocn.org,* (888) 224-WOCN
- Wound Care Information Network, by Dr. Allen Freedline, information for patients and professions, including support groups: *www.medicaledu.com*
- Wound Care Institute; newsletter, free products for financial hardships: *www.woundcare.org,* (305) 919-9192
- *Advances in Wound Care,* journal for healthcare providers: *www.springnet.com* (click on wound care), (800) 950-0879

Substance abuse

- Alcoholics Anonymous:
www.alcoholics-anonymous.org
(Spanish and French options)
- National Institute on Alcohol Abuse and Alcoholism:
www.niaaa.nih.gov, (301) 443-3860
- National Council on Alcoholism and Drug Dependence:
(800) NCA-CALL (622-2255)
- Narcotics Anonymous:
www.wsoinc.com
- S.M.A.R.T. Recovery:
www.smartrecovery.org
- The QuitNet: *www.quitnet.org*
- Al-Anon and Alateen:
www.al-anon.alateen.org,
(888) 4AL-ANON (425-2666)
- Substance abuse and mental health services administration:
www.samhsa.gov
- Office on Smoking and Health Centers for Disease Control and Prevention: *www.cdc.gov/tobacco*

Women's health

- American Heart Association:
http://women.americanheart.org
- American Medical Women's Association: *www.amwa-doc.org*
- American College of Cardiology:
www.acc.org
- HeartPoint: *www.heartpoint.com*
- Heart Information Network:
www.heartinfo.org
- Journal of the American Medical Association's Women's Health Information Center: *www.ama-assn.org/womh*
- Johns Hopkins Intelihealth: *www.intelihealth.com/specials/htMain.htm*
(search for "women heart disease")
- National Women's Health Resource Center: *www.healthywomen.org* (click

on search, click health center, under "all topics" click heart disease)
- Office on Women's Health and U.S. Public Health Service:
www.4women.gov/owh
- Womens' Heart Initiative (WHI):
www.nhlbi.nih.gov/whi

Durable medical equipment coverage

Durable medical equipment (DME) is equipment that withstands repeated use, serves a medical purpose (such that the patient wouldn't use it in the absence of injury or illness), and is appropriate for use in the patient's home. DME is partially reimbursed based on a set amount listed in a fee schedule, but reimbursement is much more complex than that. Criteria and limits for coverage of DME are very specific. And, of course, the paperwork must be in order.

Patients and family members must be notified that Medicare part B covers 80% of DME costs as listed on the fee schedule, and the patient (or supplemental insurance) is responsible for the other 20%. The difference between "medically necessary" and luxury or deluxe items must be detailed for the patient, as these items or features won't be covered by insurance. For example, even if a patient could benefit from an emergency response system (such as wearing an emergency button around the neck) and the physician is willing to write a prescription for it, it's considered a luxury and won't be reimbursed.

The home care nurse must explain to the third-party payer why the DME is needed and respond to any questions if the DME doesn't easily fit the criteria for coverage. For example, a con-

tinuous passive motion (CPM) machine isn't normally covered for an operation involving the femur but if it involved the distal portion of the femur and the surgeon is worried about joint involvement, the case manager may give DME authorization if informed of these pertinent facts.

A Certificate of Medical Necessity (CMN) must be signed by the patient's physician. The CMN is filled out by the DME supplier and sent to the physician to certify that the patient needs the specified DME. A CMN is valid for up to 12 months, at which time another CMN may be submitted.

To ensure reimbursement, the nurse must use the correct form (Health Care Financing Administration Form 1500 for Medicare; other payers generally require specific forms that can be obtained from authorized DME suppliers) and to contact the appropriate supplier. In addition, specific criteria must be met for the charge to be allowed. For instance, CPM devices are covered as DME for patients who have received total knee replacements, but use of the device must begin within 2 days after surgery and coverage is limited to the first 3 weeks after surgery. For general guidelines on which DME supplies are covered and official rationales for denial or coverage, consult the following table.

EQUIPMENT	COVERAGE STATUS
Air cleaners	Denied — environmental control equipment; not primarily medical in nature
Air conditioners	Denied — environmental control equipment; not primarily medical in nature
Ambulation aids: walker, quad cane, and crutches	Covered if the patient's condition impairs ambulation
Bathtub lifts	Denied — convenience item; not primarily medical in nature
Bathtub seats	Denied — comfort or convenience item; hygienic equipment; not primarily medical in nature
Bed baths (home type)	Denied — hygienic equipment; not primarily medical in nature
Bedboards	Denied — not primarily medical in nature
Bed pans	Covered if the patient is bedridden
Blood glucose monitor	Covered if the patient meets certain conditions
Canes	Covered if the patient's condition impairs ambulation
Catheters	Denied — nonreusable disposable supply
Commodes	Covered if the patient is confined to bed or room (payment may also be made if a patient's medical condition confines him to a floor of the home and there is no bathroom located on that floor)
Communicator	Denied — convenience item; not primarily medical in nature
Continuous passive motion device	Covered for patients who have received total knee replacements (To qualify for coverage, use of the device must commence within 2 days after surgery. In addition, coverage is limited to the 3-week period after surgery during which the device is used in the patient's home. There is insufficient evidence to justify coverage of these devices for longer periods of time or for other applications.)
Continuous positive airway pressure (CPAP) device	Covered under Medicare when used in adult patients with moderate or severe obstructive sleep apnea for whom surgery is a likely alternative to CPAP
Dehumidifiers (room or central heating system type)	Denied — environmental control equipment; not primarily medical in nature

(continued)

EQUIPMENT	COVERAGE STATUS
Elevators	Denied — convenience item; not primarily medical in nature
Exercise equipment	Denied — not primarily medical in nature
Face masks (oxygen)	Covered if oxygen is covered
Grab bars	Denied — self-help device; not primarily medical in nature
Heat and massage foam cushion pad	Denied — not primarily medical in nature; personal comfort item
Heating pads or heat lamps	May be covered if medical condition is one for which the application of heat via a heating pad is therapeutically effective
Hospital beds	Covered if physician prescription and documentation establish the medical necessity for a hospital bed due to one of the following reasons: positioning of the body required in a way not feasible in an ordinary bed or patient requiring special attachments that can't be fixed and used on an ordinary bed
Humidifiers (room or central heating system types)	Denied — environmental control equipment; not medical in nature
Infusion pumps	Some coverage for enteral or parenteral infusion
Injectors (hypodermic jet devices for injection of insulin)	Denied — noncovered self-administered drug supply
Intermittent positive-pressure breathing machines or fluidic breathing assister	Covered if the patient's ability to breathe is severely impaired
Lamb's wool pads	Covered if patient has, or is highly susceptible to, decubitus ulcers and patient's physician has specified that he will be supervising its use in connection with his course of treatment
Massage devices	Denied — personal comfort items; not primarily medical in nature
Mattress	Covered only where hospital bed is medically necessary (separate charge for replacement mattress shouldn't be allowed where hospital bed with mattress is rented)
Muscle stimulators	Covered for certain conditions
Nebulizers	Covered if the patient's ability to breathe is severely impaired

EQUIPMENT	COVERAGE STATUS
Oxygen	Covered for patients with significant hypoxemia who meet the medical documentation, laboratory evidence, and health conditions specified (also includes special coverage criteria for portable oxygen systems)
Oxygen humidifiers and tents	Covered if prescribed for use in connection with medically necessary durable medical equipment for purposes of moisturizing oxygen
Oxygen regulators (medical) and flow-meter	Covered if the patient's ability to breathe is severely impaired
Pacemaker monitor: self-contained or digital	Covered when prescribed by a physician for a patient with a cardiac pacemaker
Patient lifts	Covered if contractor's medical staff determines the patient's condition is such that periodic movement is necessary to effect improvement or to arrest or retard deterioration in condition
Percussors	Covered for mobilizing respiratory tract secretions in patients with chronic obstructive lung disease, chronic bronchitis, or emphysema (when the patient or operator of powered percussor has received appropriate training by a physician or therapist or no one is available to administer manual therapy)
Portable oxygen systems	• Regulated (adjustable): Covered under certain conditions • Emergency, first-aid, or not adjustable; oxygen is essentially not therapeutic in nature and will be denied payment
Postural drainage boards	Covered if patient has a chronic pulmonary condition
Preset portable oxygen units	Denied — emergency, first-aid, or precautionary equipment; essentially not therapeutic in nature
Raised toilet seats	Denied — convenience item; hygienic equipment; not primarily medical in nature
Rolling chairs	• Limited to rollabout chairs with casters of at least 5″ (12.7 cm) in diameter, specifically designed to meet the needs of ill, injured, or otherwise impaired individuals • Denied for the wide range of chairs with smaller casters as are found in general use — not primarily medical in nature (coverage is based on medical need and is determined and prescribed by the patient's physician [in lieu of a wheelchair])

(continued)

EQUIPMENT	COVERAGE STATUS
Safety roller	Possibly appropriately covered for some patients who are obese, have severe neurological disorders, or are restricted to the use of one hand, making it impossible to use a wheeled walker that doesn't have the sophisticated braking system found on safety rollers (This item is routinely reviewed and, if an alternative or modification is available, the allowable charge is reduced to that amount.)
Seat lift	Covered if evidence shows that the item is included in the physician's course of treatment, is likely to effect improvement or arrest or retard deterioration in the patient's condition, and severity of the condition is such that the alternative would be chair or bed confinement (added cost for a recliner feature not covered)
Sitz bath	Covered for an infection or injury of the perineal area but must be prescribed by the patient's physician as part of the home care treatment
Spare tanks of oxygen	Denied — convenience or precautionary supply
Speech teaching machine	Denied — education equipment; not primarily medical in nature
Standing table	Denied — convenience item; not primarily medical in nature
Suction machine	Covered if the contractor's medical staff determines that the machine specified in the claim is medically required and appropriate for home use without supervision
Support hose	Denied — nonreusable
Telephone alert systems	Denied — emergency communications systems; don't serve a diagnostic or therapeutic purpose
Telephone arms	Denied — convenience item; not medical in nature
Toilet seats	Denied — not medical equipment
Traction equipment	Covered if the patient has an orthopedic impairment that requires traction equipment that prevents ambulation during the period of use (devices used during ambulation, such as a cervical traction collar, are covered under the brace provision)
Trapeze bars	Covered if the patient is bedridden and requires a trapeze bar to sit up because of respiratory condition, to change body position for other medical reasons, or to get in and out of bed
Treadmill exerciser	Denied — exercise equipment; not primarily medical in nature

EQUIPMENT	COVERAGE STATUS
Ultraviolet cabinet	Covered for selected patients with generalized intractable psoriasis but only allowed if other no alternative (such as outpatient department of a hospital) is available
Urinals (autoclavable)	Covered if patient is bedridden
Vaporizers	Covered if patient has a respiratory illness
Ventilators	Covered for treatment of neuromuscular diseases, thoracic restrictive diseases, and chronic respiratory failure consequent to chronic obstructive pulmonary disease (includes both positive and negative pressure types)
Wheelchairs	Covered if the patient's condition is such that without the use of a wheelchair he would otherwise be bedridden or confined to a chair. (an individual may qualify for a wheelchair and still be considered bedridden)
Wheelchairs (power operated and those with other special features)	Covered if the patient's condition is such that a wheelchair is medically necessary and the patient is unable to operate the wheelchair manually (payment for special features is limited to those that are medically required because of the patient's condition; a power-operated vehicle that may appropriately be used as a wheelchair can be covered)
Whirlpool bath equipment	Covered if the patient is homebound and has a condition for which the whirlpool bath can be expected to provide substantial therapeutic benefit justifying its cost (where the patient isn't homebound but has such a condition, payment is restricted to the cost of providing the services elsewhere [such as the outpatient department of a participating hospital] if that alternative is less costly)
Whirlpool pumps	Denied
White cane	Denied

Gordon's functional health patterns

Gordon has described a functional health pattern system to help identify and formulate nursing diagnoses. Based on general categories, this system allows for easy organization of basic nursing information obtained during your initial assessment. Flexible and adaptable, these functional health patterns can be used for patients in various states of health and illness, in any age-group, and in any clinical specialty. Presented below is a brief outline of Gordon's functional health patterns.

Learning to incorporate Gordon's concepts into your assessment format may require time and practice; however, the rewards of understanding the patient and identifying specific areas where you can intervene are well worth the effort. When using the following health pattern categories, obtain the nursing history from the patient's perspective through a series of specific questions designed to elicit information in an organized manner.

1. Health perception and health management pattern
- General health
- Health practices
- Concerns about illness
- Responsibility for health restoration and maintenance

2. Nutritional and metabolic pattern
- Daily food and fluid intake
- Weight loss or gain
- Appetite
- Dietary restrictions
- Healing potential of skin wounds or lesions
- General body status or condition

3. Elimination pattern
- Bowel elimination pattern or problem
- Urinary elimination pattern or problem
- Perspiration pattern or problem

4. Activity and exercise pattern
- Energy level
- Exercise pattern
- Perceived ability for (use the functional level code*):

Bathing _____
Bed mobility _____
Cooking _____
Dressing _____
Feeding _____
General mobility _____
Grooming _____
Home maintenance _____
Shopping _____
Toileting _____

5. Sleep and rest pattern
- Sleep problems
- Rested or not rested after sleep
- Use of sleep aids

6. Cognitive and perceptual pattern
- Sensory status: visual, auditory, olfactory, tactile, gustatory
- Memory
- Intelligence
- Pain or discomfort

7. Self-perception and self-concept pattern
- Feelings about self
- Body image
- Self-esteem
- Emotional state

8. Role and relationship pattern
- Living arrangement
- Family or significant others
- Communication
- Role and responsibilities in family
- Socialization
- Finances

9. Sexuality and reproductive pattern
- Sexual relations
- Sexual satisfaction or dissatisfaction
- Contraceptive use and problems
- Reproductive and menstrual history

10. Coping and stress-tolerance pattern
- Stressors
- Coping mechanisms
- Major life changes
- Problem management

11. Value and belief pattern
- Satisfaction with life
- Spirituality and religious beliefs
- Religious practices
- Conflicts

12. Other
- Concerns not already discussed

* Functional level code
0 = Completely independent
1 = Requires use of equipment or device
2 = Requires help, supervision, or teaching from another person
3 = Requires help from another person and equipment or device
4 = Dependent; doesn't participate in activity

English-Spanish medical translations

If you can greet your patient in his native language, you'll make him feel more at ease. Here are some phrases you can use to converse with your Spanish-speaking patients and learn some basic information about their health.

Greetings

Hello.	¡Hola!
Good morning.	Buenos días.
Good afternoon.	Buenas tardes.
Good evening.	Buenas noches.
Come in please.	Pase Ud. por favor.
My name is _____.	Me llamo _____.
Who is the patient?	¿Quién es el (la) paciente?
What is your name?	¿Cómo se llama Ud.?
It's nice to meet you.	Mucho gusto en conocerle.
How are you?	¿Cómo está Ud.?
Goodbye.	Hasta luego or adiós

Basic phrases

Please	Por favor
Thank you	Gracias
Yes	Sí
No	No
Maybe	Quizás or tal vez
Sometimes	A veces
Never	Nunca
Always	Siempre
Date	Fecha
Signature	Firma
How are you feeling?	¿Cómo se siente Ud.?
What time is it?	¿Qué hora es?
What day is it?	¿Qué día es hoy?
What is the date?	¿A qué fecha estamos?
Where are you?	¿Dónde está Ud.?
How old are you?	¿Cuántos años tiene Ud.?

Did you come alone?	¿Vino Ud. solo(a)?
Who brought you?	¿Quién lo (la) trajo?
Where were you born?	¿Dónde nació Ud.?
Where do you live?	¿Dónde vive Ud.?
What is your address?	¿Cuál es su dirección?

Family

Do you live alone?	¿Vive Ud. solo(a)?
Who lives with you?	¿Quién vive con Ud.?
– Parents?	– ¿Sus padres?
– Spouse?	– ¿Su esposo(a)?
– Children?	– ¿Sus hijos?
Son?	¿Su hijo?
Daughter?	¿Su hija?
Grandchildren?	¿Sus nietos?
– Mother?	– ¿Su madre?
– Father?	– ¿Su padre?
– Uncle?	– ¿Su tío?
– Aunt?	– ¿Su tía?
– Grandfather?	– ¿Su abuelo?
– Grandmother?	– ¿Su abuela?
– Cousin?	– ¿Su primo(a)?
– Friend?	– ¿Su amigo(a)?
– Other relative?	– ¿Otro pariente?
Are you:	¿Es Ud.:
– single?	– soltero(a)?
– married?	– casado(a)?
– divorced?	– divorciado(a)?
– widowed?	– viudo(a)?
– separated?	– ¿(Está Ud.) separado(a)?
Do you have any children?	¿Tiene Ud. hijos?
– How many?	– ¿Cuántos?

School and work

Did you go to school?	¿Asistió Ud. a la escuela?
– How many grades did you complete?	– ¿Cuántos años completó Ud.?
– Did you go to college?	– ¿Hizo Ud. estudios universitarios?
Do you work outside the home?	¿Trabaja Ud. fuera de casa?
– What type of work do you do?	– ¿Qué tipo de trabajo hace?
Accountant?	¿Contador(a)?
Architect?	¿Arquitecto(a)?
Banker?	¿Banquero(a)?

Bus driver?	¿Conductor(a) de autobuses?
Businessperson?	¿Persona de negocios?
Computer operator?	¿Operador(a) de computadoras?
Designer?	¿Diseñador(a)?
Doctor?	¿Doctor(a)?
Engineer?	¿Ingeniero(a)?
Factory worker?	¿Obrero(a) en una fábrica?
Farmer?	¿Campesino(a)?
Lawyer?	¿Abogado(a)?
Mechanic?	¿Mecánico(a)?
Salesperson?	¿Vendedor(a)? or ¿Dependiente?
Secretary?	¿Secretario(a)?
Student?	¿Estudiante?
Taxi driver?	¿Chofer de taxi?
Teacher?	¿Maestro(a)?
Truck driver?	¿Camionero(a)?
Waiter?	¿Camarero?
Waitress?	¿Camarera?
Where do you work?	¿Dónde trabaja Ud.?

Hobbies

Do you have any hobbies?	¿Tiene Ud. pasatiempos favoritos?
– Movies?	– ¿Cine?
– Music?	– ¿Música?
– Painting?	– ¿Arte?
– Photography?	– ¿Fotografía?
– Reading?	– ¿Leer?
– Sewing?	– ¿Coser?
– Sports?	– ¿Deportes?
Baseball?	¿Béisbol?
Basketball?	¿Baloncesto?
Football?	¿Fútbol americano?
Golf?	¿Golf?
Hockey?	¿Hockey?
Running?	¿Correr?
Soccer?	¿Fútbol?
Tennis?	¿Tenis?
– Theater?	– ¿Teatro?

Days

Monday	lunes
Tuesday	martes
Wednesday	miércoles
Thursday	jueves

Friday	viernes
Saturday	sábado
Sunday	domingo

Months

January	enero
February	febrero
March	marzo
April	abril
May	mayo
June	junio
July	julio
August	agosto
September	septiembre
October	octubre
November	noviembre
December	diciembre

Seasons

Spring	La primavera
Summer	El verano
Fall	El otoño
Winter	El invierno

Cardinal numbers

1	Uno
2	Dos
3	Tres
4	Cuatro
5	Cinco
6	Seis
7	Siete
8	Ocho
9	Nueve
10	Diez
11	Once
12	Doce
13	Trece
14	Catorce
15	Quince
16	Diez y seis *or* dieciséis
17	Diez y siete *or* diecisiete
18	Diez y ocho *or* dieciocho
19	Diez y nueve *or* diecinueve
20	Veinte

30	Treinta
40	Cuarenta
50	Cincuenta
60	Sesenta
70	Setenta
80	Ochenta
90	Noventa
100	Cien
1,000	Mil
10,000	Diez mil
100,000	Cien mil
100,000,000	Cien millones

Ordinal numbers

First	Primero(a)
Second	Segundo(a)
Third	Tercero(a)
Fourth	Cuarto(a)
Fifth	Quinto(a)
Sixth	Sexto(a)
Seventh	Séptimo(a)
Eighth	Octavo(a)
Ninth	Noveno(a)
Tenth	Décimo, diez (in dates)
Eleventh	Once
Twelfth	Doce
Thirteenth	Trece

Time

Second	Segundo
Minute	Minuto
Fifteen minutes	Quince minutos
Thirty minutes	Treinta minutos
Hour	Hora
In the morning	Por la mañana
At noon	Al mediodía
In the afternoon	Por la tarde
In the evening	Por la noche
At midnight	A medianoche

Meals

Breakfast	El desayuno
Lunch	El almuerzo
Midafternoon snack	Bocadillo a media tarde
Dinner	La cena

Bedtime snack	Bocadillo a la hora de acostarse

Colors

Black	Negro
Blue	Azul
Brown	Café
Gray	Gris
Green	Verde
Orange	Anaranjado *or* color naranja
Pink	Rosa *or* rosado
Purple	Morado *or* vio leta
Red	Rojo
White	Blanco
Yellow	Amarillo

Opposites

Alive/dead	Vivo/muerto
Better/worse	Mejor/peor
Central/peripheral	Central/periférico
Dark/light	Oscuro/claro
Fat/thin	Gordo/delgado
Flat/raised	Plano/en relieve
Healthy/sick	Saludable/enfermo
Heavy/light	Pesado/ligero
High/low	Alto/bajo
Hot/cold	Caliente/frío
Large/small	Grande/pequeño
Long (length)/short (length)	Larga (longitud)/corta (longitud)
Loud/soft	Fuerte/suave
Many/few	Muchos/pocos
Open/closed	Abierto/cerrado
Painful/painless	Doloroso/indoloro
Regular/irregular	Regular/irregular
Smooth/rough	Liso/áspero
Soft/hard	Blando/duro
Sweet/sour	Dulce/agrio
Symmetric/asymmetric	Simétrico/asimétrico
Tall/short	Alto/bajo
Thick/thin	Grueso/fino
Weak/strong	Débil/fuerte
Wet/dry	Mojado/seco

Weights and measures

Centimeter	Centímetro
Circumference	Circunferencia

Cubic centimeter	Centímetro cúbico
Deciliter	Decilitro
Depth	Profundidad
Gram	Gramo
Height	Altura
Kilogram	Kilo
Length	Longitud
Liter	Litro
Meter	Metro
Microgram	Microgramo
Milligram	Miligramo
Milliliter	Mililitro
Millimeter	Milímetro
Tablespoon	Cucharada
Teaspoon	Cucharadita
Volume	Volumen
Weight	Peso
Width	Ancho *or* anchura

Everyday items

Blanket	Manta *or* frazada
Brush	Cepillo
Comb	Peine
Deodorant	Desodorante
Lotion	Loción
Mouthwash	Enjuague para la boca
Pillow	Almohada
Pillowcase	Funda de almohada
Razor	Navaja de afeitar
Sanitary napkin	Toalla sanitaria
Shampoo	Champú
Shaving cream	Crema de afeitar
Sheet	Sábana
Soap	Jabón
Tampon	Tampón
Toothbrush	Cepillo de dientes
Toothpaste	Pasta de dientes
Towel	Toalla
Washcloth	Paño para lavarse la cara *or* el cuerpo
Water	Agua

Doctors

Doctor	Doctor(a)
Anesthesiologist	Anestesista
Cardiologist	Cardiólogo

Dermatologist	Dermatólogo
Endocrinologist	Endocrinólogo
Gastroenterologist	Gastroenterólogo
Gynecologist	Ginecólogo
Hematologist	Hematólogo
Internist	Internista
Nephrologist	Nefrólogo
Neurologist	Neurólogo
Nutritionist	Especialista en nutrición
Obstetrician	Obstetra
Oncologist	Oncólogo
Ophthalmologist	Oftalmólogo
Orthopedist	Ortopedista
Otolaryngologist	Otolaringólogo
Pediatrician	Pediatra
Pneumonologist	Neumonólogo
Psychiatrist	Psiquiatra
Psychologist	Psicólogo
Radiologist	Radiólogo
Surgeon	Cirujano

Nurses and other health care personnel

Practical nurse	Technica
Registered nurse	Enfermero(a) calificado(a)
Nurse's aid	Asistente de enfermero(a)
Volunteer	Voluntario(a)
Physical therapist	Terapeuta físico *or* terapista
Occupational therapist	Terapeuta ocupacional or terapista
Nurse practitioner	Enfermera(o) practicante
Janitor	Empleado(a) de limpieza *or* conserji
Electrician	Electricista
Medical technician	Técnico de medicina
Medical assistant	Ayudante de medicina
Medical transcriptionist	Persona que transcribe documentos médicos
Admissions clerk	Empleado de ingresos
Laboratory technician	Ayudante de laboratorio
Intravenous nurse	Enfermera(o) especialista en procedimientos intravenosos
Dentist	Dentista
Dental hygienist	Higienista dental
Social worker	Trabajador(a) social
Respiratory therapist	Terapeuta respiratorio(a) or terapista
X-ray technician	Técnico de radiografía

■ Selected references

Allen, A. "Breath of Life," *The Washington Post Magazine,* October 1999.

Bateman, S. "Using a Team Approach: Diabetics and Wound Care Management in the Home," *Rehab Management,* Aug/Sep 1999.

Boaden, A. "Know How. Coming to Terms with Stoma Surgery," *Community Nurse* 5(8):48-9, September 1999.

Carpenito, L.J., ed. *Nursing Diagnosis: Application to Clinical Practice,* 8th ed. Philadelphia: Lippincott Williams & Wilkins, 2000.

Davis, K.M., and Mathew, E. "Pharmacologic Management of Depression in the Elderly," *Nurse Practitioner* 23(6):16-18, 26, 28, passim, June 1998.

Dollemore, D. "Enzyme May Protect Against Brain Disorders," National Institute of Health News Release, (2000, June 7): *www.nih. gov/nia/news/pr/2000/06-07.htm,* [2000, July 6].

Duggal, H.S., et al. "Gasoline Inhalation Dependence and Bipolar Disorder," *Australian and New Zealand Journal of Psychiatry* 34(3):531-2, June 2000.

Funnell, M.M., et al., eds. *A Core Curriculum for Diabetes Education,* 3rd ed. Chicago: American Association of Diabetes Educators, 1998.

Halpin-Landry, J.E., and Goldsmith, S. "Feet First: Diabetes Care," *AJN* 99(2):26-33, February 1999.

Huang, C.C., et al. "Measurement of the Urinary Lactate: Creatinine Ratio for the Early Identification of Newborn Infants at Risk for Hypoxic-Ischemic Encephalopathy," *New England Journal of Medicine* 341(5):328-35, July 1999.

Krasner, D. "Diabetic Ulcers of the Lower Extremity: A Review of Comprehensive Management," *Ostomy/ Wound Management* 44(4): 56-58, 60-62, 64, passim, April 1998.

Marrelli, T.M. *Handbook of Home Health Standards and Documentation Guidelines for Reimbursement,* 3rd ed. St. Louis: Mosby–Year Book, 1998.

Smeltzer, S.C., and Bare, B.G. *Brunner and Suddarth's Textbook of Medical-Surgical Nursing,* 9th ed. Philadelphia: Lippincott Williams & Wilkins, 2000.

Tanaka, P.K. *ICD-9-CM Easy Coder.* Montgomery: Unicor Medical, 1998.

"Tobacco Use Among Middle and High School Students — United States, 1999, *Morbidity and Mortality Weekly Report* 49(03):49-53, January 2000.

Underwood, Anne. "The Perils of Pasta," *Newsweek,* October 1999.

Wilson, R.L. "Optimizing Nutrition for Patients with Cancer," *Clinical Journal of Oncology Nursing* 4(1):23-8, January-February 2000.

■ Index

C

Cancer
  breast, 578-579
  causes of, 157
  diagnostic codes for, 158
  discharge planning for, 160
  documentation requirements for, 160-161
  homebound status of patients with, 158
  interdisciplinary actions for, 160
  lung, 606-607
  nursing diagnosis and outcomes in, 159
  nursing services for, 159-160
  previsit checklist for, 157-158
  reimbursement tips for, 161
  safety requirements for patients with, 158
Cancer care
  children's response to, 489
  diagnostic codes for, 490
  discharge planning for, 492
  documentation requirements for, 492
  homebound status of patients receiving, 490
  interdisciplinary actions for, 492
  nursing diagnosis and outcomes in, 490-491
  nursing services for, 491-492
  previsit checklist for, 489-490
  reimbursement tips for, 493
  safety requirements for patients receiving, 490
Cardiomyopathy
  causes of, 164
  diagnostic codes for, 164
  discharge planning for, 165
  documentation requirements for, 166
  homebound status of patients with, 164
  interdisciplinary actions for, 165
  nursing diagnosis and outcomes in, 165
  nursing services for, 165
  previsit checklist for, 164
  reimbursement tips for, 166
  safety requirements for patients with, 164
Cardiovascular disorders
  diagnostic codes for, 162
  discharge planning for, 163
  documentation requirements for, 163
  homebound status of patients with, 162
  interdisciplinary actions for, 163
  nursing diagnosis and outcomes in, 162-163
  nursing services for, 163
  previsit checklist for, 161
  reimbursement tips for, 163-164
  safety requirements for patients with, 161-162
Caregivers
  incompetent, 51-52
  noncompliance by, 51
Care maps. *See* Clinical pathways.
Case management, clinical pathways and, 569
Case Management Society of America, 19
Case manager, role in home care, 19-20

Cast care
  diagnostic codes for, 167
  discharge planning for, 169
  documentation requirements for, 169
  homebound status of patients receiving, 167
  interdisciplinary actions for, 168
  nursing diagnosis and outcomes in, 167-168
  nursing services for, 168
  previsit checklist for, 166
  reimbursement tips for, 169
  safety requirements for patients receiving, 166-167
Cellulitis
  causes of, 169
  diagnostic codes for, 170
  discharge planning for, 172
  documentation requirements for, 172
  homebound status of patients with, 170-171
  interdisciplinary actions for, 172
  nursing diagnosis and outcomes in, 171
  nursing services for, 171-172
  previsit checklist for, 170
  reimbursement tips for, 172-173
  safety requirements for patients with, 170
Centers for Disease Control and Prevention, 10, 73
Cerebral palsy
  causes of, 493
  diagnostic codes for, 494
  discharge planning for, 497
  documentation requirements for, 497-498
  homebound status of patients with, 495
  interdisciplinary actions for, 497
  nursing diagnosis and outcomes in, 495-496
  nursing services for, 496
  previsit checklist for, 493-494
  reimbursement tips for, 498
  safety requirements for patients with, 494
Cerebrovascular accident
  causes of, 173
  clinical pathway for, 580-583
  diagnostic codes for, 174
  discharge planning for, 178
  documentation requirements for, 178
  homebound status of patients with, 174
  interdisciplinary actions for, 177-178
  nursing diagnosis and outcomes in, 174-177
  nursing services for, 177
  previsit checklist for, 173
  reimbursement tips for, 178-179
  safety requirements for patients with, 173-174
Certification
  quality care issues and, 31
  requirements for home care agencies, 10-12
Certified nurse administrator, 18
Certified nurse administrator, advanced, 18
Cesarean section postcare
  diagnostic codes for, 450
  discharge planning for, 452-453